KU-623-653

Infection, Resistance, and Immunity

Second Edition

Books are to be returned on or before
the last date below.

LIVERPOOL
J MOORES UNIVERSITY
AVRIL ROBARTS LRC
TITHEBARN

7-DAY

LIVERPOOL JMU LIBRARY

3 1111 01027 3116

LIVERPOOL
J MOORES UNIVERSITY
AVRIL ROBARTS LRC
TITHEBARN STREET
LIVERPOOL L2 2ER
TEL. 0151 231 4022

Infection, Resistance, and Immunity

Second Edition

Julius P. Kreier

Professor Emeritus of Microbiology
The Ohio State University

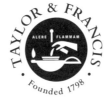

USA	Publishing Office:	TAYLOR & FRANCIS
		29 West 35th Street
		New York, NY 10001
		Tel: (212) 216-7800
		Fax: (212) 564-7854
	Distribution Center:	TAYLOR & FRANCIS
		7625 Empire Drive
		Florence, KY 41042
		Tel: 1-800-624-7064
		Fax: 1-800-248-4724
UK		TAYLOR & FRANCIS
		27 Church Road
		Hove
		E. Sussex, BN3 2FA
		Tel: +44 (0) 1273 207411
		Fax: +44 (0) 1273 205612

INFECTION, RESISTANCE, AND IMMUNITY, Second Edition

Copyright © 2002 Taylor & Francis. All rights reserved. Printed in the United States of America. Except as permitted under the United States Copyright Act of 1976, no part of this publication may be reproduced or distributed in any form or by any means, or stored in a database or retrieval system, without prior written permission of the publisher.

1 2 3 4 5 6 7 8 9 0

Printed by Sheridan Books, Ann Arbor, MI, 2002.

A CIP catalog record for this book is available from the British Library.
   The paper in this publication meets the requirements of the ANSI Standard Z39.48-1984 (Permanence of Paper).

Library of Congress Cataloging-in-Publication Data
CIP information available from publishers.

ISBN 90-5702-595-7

Contents

PREFACE   xiii
CONTRIBUTORS   xv

Chapter 1 – Introduction to Infection, Resistance, and Immunity   1
Samuel J. Black

Introduction   1
The Immune System   1
Host and Pathogen Interactions   7
Public Health Measures   9
Summary   10
Suggestions for Further Reading   10
Questions   11

Chapter 2 – Host-Parasite Relationships   13
Julius P. Kreier

Introduction   13
Types of Host-Parasite Relationships   15
The Normal Microbial Populations On and In Multicellular Organisms   18
Microbial Populations Normally Associated with Humans   19
Koch's Postulates and Their Limitations   22
Summary   24
Suggestions for Further Reading   25
Questions   25

Chapter 3 – Constitutive Host Resistance   27
Cynthia Baldwin

Introduction   27
The External Defense Systems   27
The Internal Defense Systems   30
Summary   41

Suggestions for Further Reading   41
Questions   42

Chapter 4 – The Inflammatory Response: A Bridge Between the
    Constitutive and Inducible Systems   45
Samuel J. Black

Introduction   45
Overview   45
Local Inflammatory Events   46
Systemic Consequences of the Inflammatory Reaction   55
Summary   56
Suggestions for Further Reading   57
Questions   58

Chapter 5 – The Inducible System: History of Development of
    Immunology as a Component of Host-Parasite Interactions   61
Ralph A. Sorensen

Introduction   61
Immunization   61
The Nature of Inducible Immunity   62
Theories to Explain Inducible Immunity   64
Self-Recognition in Immunology   69
The Structure and Behavior of Antibodies   74
Monoclonal Antibodies   75
The Genetics of the Immune Response   77
Hormonal Substances Induced in Immunity   78
Summary   81
Suggestions for Further Reading   82
Questions   82

Chapter 6 – The Inducible System: Antigens   85
Ralph A. Sorensen

Introduction   85
Characteristics of Antigens   86
The Hapten-Carrier Concept   89
Sites on Antigens Recognized by Antibodies   91
Mapping Epitopes and Antigen-Binding Sites   94
The Strength of Antigen Binding   95
Cross-Reactivity of Antigens   97
The Genotype of the Responding Animal   99
Superantigens   99
Routes of Antigen Administration   100
Adjuvants   101
Summary   101
Suggestions for Further Reading   102
Questions   103

Chapter 7 – The Inducible Defense System: Antibody Molecules and Antigen-Antibody Reactions 105
Diane Wallace Taylor

Introduction   105
Nature of Antibodies   106
Structure of Antibodies   107
The B-Cell Receptor (BCR)   113
Antibody Diversity   114
Changes in the Affinity and Class of Antibodies During the Course of the Immune Response   116
Functions of Immunoglobulin Classes   118
Detection of Antibodies: Basic Principles and Concepts Behind Serological Assays   119
Summary   127
Suggestions for Further Reading   128
Questions   129

Chapter 8 – The Inducible Defense System: The Induction and Development of the Inducible Defense   131
Michael A. Hickey and Diane Wallace Taylor

Introduction   131
Cells of the Inducible Immune System   131
The Immune System   136
Development of the Immune System   138
Activation of the Immune System by Antigen   145
Summary   153
Suggestions for Further Reading   154
Questions   155

Chapter 9 – Specific Host Resistance: The Effector Mechanisms   157
Ralph A. Sorensen

Introduction   157
Antibody-Mediated Effector Mechanisms   158
Complement-Mediated Effector Mechanisms   162
Cell-Mediated Effector Mechanisms   168
Summary   178
Suggestions for Further Reading   178
Questions   179

Chapter 10 – Immunologically Mediated Diseases and Allergic Reactions   181
Kim A. Campbell and Caroline C. Whitacre

Introduction   181
Autoimmune Diseases   181
The Hypersensitivities   184

Summary   197
Suggestions for Further Reading   198
Questions   198

**Chapter 11 – The Host Response to Grafts and Transplantation
    Immunology   201**
Armead H. Johnson

The Phenomenon of Rejection   201
Types of Grafts   202
Forms of Graft Rejection   202
Histocompatibility Antigens   205
Immunologic Mechanisms of Allograft Rejection   208
T Cell AlloRecognition Pathways   209
T Lymphocyte Activation   211
Cytokines   212
Cytokine Promoter Region Polymorphism   213
Mixed Lymphocyte Cultures   213
Generation and Detection of Cytotoxic T Lymphocytes   213
Clinical Strategies for Avoidance of Graft Rejection   215
Special Considerations: Retransplants   218
Special Considerations: Transplantation of Specific Tissues   219
Summary   219
Suggestions for Further Reading   220
Questions   221

Chapter 12 – The Immunological System and Neoplasia   223
K.A. Schat

Introduction   223
Experimental Tumor Immunology   224
Escape of Tumor Cells from Immune Responses   229
Immunity to Virus-Induced Neoplasia   231
Hepatocellular Carcinoma   238
Conclusions from Immunization Studies against Viral-Induced
    Neoplasia   241
Immunological Approaches for the Control of Tumors   241
Prospects for Immunological Control of Neoplasia   242
Summary   242
Suggestions for Further Reading   242
Questions   243

Chapter 13 – Comparative Immunology   247
Ian Tizard

Introduction   247
Immunity in Invertebrates   247
Immunity in Fish   251
Immunity in Amphibians   254

Immunity in Reptiles   256
Immunity in Birds (and Dinosaurs)   258
Immunity in Mammals   260
Summary   262
Suggestions for Further Reading   263
Questions   263

Chapter 14 – Pathogenicity and Virulence   265
Lola Winter

Introduction   265
Factors Mediating Adherence to Host Cells   266
Invasion of Host Cells   269
Prevention of Phagocytosis   270
Survival within the Phagocyte   274
Siderophores and Iron Acquisition   277
Toxins   277
R Factors and Pathogenicity Islands   280
Summary   280
Suggestions for Further Reading   281
Questions   281

Chapter 15 – Bacteria   283
Patrick R. Dugan

Introduction   283
Ubiquity and Size of Microorganisms   284
Shape and Grouping Among Prokaryotes   285
Synopsis of Nutrition, Metabolism, and Growth   286
Prokaryotic Cell Structure   288
Taxonomy and Phylogenetic Relationships   296
Some Medically Important Bacteria and the Diseases They Cause   298
Mechanisms of Immunity and Resistance to Bacterial Infection   312
Summary   314
Suggestions for Further Reading   317
Questions   317

Chapter 16 – The Viruses   319
Michael D. Lairmore

Introduction   319
Morphology and Structure of Viruses   319
Classification and Replication Strategies of Viruses   320
Viral Pathogenesis   325
Anti-Viral Strategies of the Host Cell and Immune System   327
Anti-Viral Drugs   329
Diagnosis of Viral Infections   329
Immunization against Viral Infections   331
Selected Diseases Resulting from Acute Viral Infections   333

Selected Diseases Resulting from Viral Infections that
    Resolve or Persist   337
Selected Diseases Associated with Persistent Viral Infections   341
Summary   346
Suggestions for Further Reading   347
Questions   347

Chapter 17 – The Parasitic Protozoa and Helminth Worms   349
F.E.G. Cox

Outline   349
Introduction   349
Parasitic Protozoa   351
Parasitic Nematodes   361
Parasitic Trematodes (Flukes)   366
Cestodes (Tapeworms)   368
Summary   372
Suggestions for Further Reading   373
Questions   374

Chapter 18 – The Fungi   379
Lola Winter

Introduction   379
Classification of Mycotic Diseases   379
Laboratory Diagnosis   388
Therapy   389
Summary   389
Suggestions for Further Reading   389
Questions   390

Chapter 19 – Immunization   393
Michael F. Para, Susan L. Koletar, and Carter L. Diggs

Introduction   393
General Principles   394
Host Response to Vaccination   398
Complications Resulting from Vaccination   400
Vaccine Development and Production   401
Challenges in Vaccinology   408
Summary   409
Suggestions for Further Reading   409
Questions   409

Chapter 20 – Immunological Tests for Diagnosis of Disease and
    Identification of Molecules   413
Frank Petersen

Introduction   413

Immunological Tests   413
Monoclonal Antibody Production   431
Summary   431
Suggestions for Further Reading   433
Questions   433

**Chapter 21 – Epidemiology, Disease Transmission, Prevention,
    and Control   435**
Gabriel A. Schmunis

Introduction   435
Terminology   436
Epidemiological Investigation   437
Epidemiological Surveillance   440
Infectious Diseases   441
Infectious Organisms   444
Emerging and Reemerging Diseases   445
The Host   446
The Environment   448
Transmission Mechanisms   450
Prevention and Control   453
Summary   456
Suggestions for Further Reading   457
Questions   457

INDEX   459

Preface

This book is designed to introduce the student to the field of host-parasite interaction. The text was developed through teaching an undergraduate course in introductory immunology and pathogenic microbiology at The Ohio State University. In this course we provide the student a holistic view of the interaction of parasites with their hosts, including host defensive measures and the parasites' countermeasures.

In most immunology courses, the student receives considerable instruction on the mechanisms of the inducible immune response and somewhat less on the constitutive resistance mechanisms, but little effort is made to treat host-parasite interaction as an entity.

After completing an immunology course, the student may take courses in infectious diseases and study pathogenic mechanisms; then, the student may piece together the relationship between immunology and infection and disease. In this text we aid the student in grasping the role of immunity in the broader relationship between the parasite and the host.

There are many excellent, comprehensive texts on immunology that are suitable for advanced courses in immunology. These texts are very up-to-date and present all available information on immunology. The books are frequently a pleasure for a professor to read. In them, he finds much new and exciting information on the subject. For the beginning student, they contain too much information and too much detail. They are often so massive, they discourage the student.

The various chapters of this book have been written by various authors, following the editor's guidelines, and have been edited to a standard format and appropriate content. Some chapters in this second edition have been revised and updated by the original authors; but for other chapters, different authors have undertaken the task of revision. In the years between the first and second editions, the editor lost contact with many of the original authors and had to select new authors. In some cases, new chapters were added as well as new authors.

The editor acknowledges the contributions of the original authors and thanks them for their efforts. The new authors' treatment of chapters carried over from the first edition have ranged from composition of a completely new text to various degrees of modification of the existing text. The revision was dictated by the development of knowledge in the subjects covered by each chapter, as determined by the new author's judgment.

The editor thanks Edna Chandler for turning out a clean manuscript in a standard form from the variety of computer formats and my extensive handwritten editing. My thanks also go to Sue Ridge and Sally Cheney of Gordon and Breach Editorial Services, Inc.

In conclusion, I wish to emphasize that this text is designed to be a beginning text, not a reference book. It contains the amount of material a student can be expected to assimilate in a one-semester course. I hope it will provide the beginning student in biology, premedical, preveterinary, and allied medical fields with an introduction to the host parasite relationship which, perhaps will lead him to the study of host parasite interaction.

Contributors

Cynthia Baldwin
Department of Veterinary and Animal
  Sciences
University of Massachusetts

Samuel J. Black
Department of Veterinary and Animal
  Sciences
University of Massachusetts

Kim A. Campbell
Department of Medical Microbiology and
  Immunology
College of Medicine
The Ohio State University

F.E.G. Cox
Department of Infectious and Tropical
  Diseases
London School of Hygiene and Tropical
  Medicine
University of London

Carter L. Diggs
Malaria Vaccine Development Program
United States Agency for International
  Development

Patrick R. Dugan
Professor Emeritus, Department of
  Microbiology
College of Biological Sciences
The Ohio State University

Michael A. Hickey
Department of Biology
Georgetown University

Armead H. Johnson
Department of Pediatrics
Division of Immunogenetics
Georgetown University Medical Center

Julius P. Kreier
Professor Emeritus, Department of
  Microbiology
College of Biological Sciences
The Ohio State University

Michael D. Lairmore
Department of Veterinary Biosciences
College of Veterinary Medicine
The Ohio State University

Frank Petersen
Department of Food Sciences
Cook College
Rutgers University

K.A. Schat
Department of Microbiology and
  Immunology
College of Veterinary Medicine
Cornell University

Gabriel A. Schmunis
Communicable Diseases Program
Pan-American Health Organization
Regional Office of the World Health
  Organization

Ralph A. Sorensen
Department of Biology
Gettysburg College

Diane Wallace Taylor
Department of Biology
Georgetown University

Ian Tizard
Department of Veterinary Pathobiology
The Texas Veterinary Medical Center

Lola Winter
Department of Microbiology and
  Immunology
College of Veterinary Medicine
Cornell University

Caroline C. Whitacre
Department of Medical Microbiology and
  Immunology
College of Medicine
The Ohio State University

INTRODUCTION
THE IMMUNE SYSTEM
Constitutive Immunity
Adaptive or Inducible
    Immunity
Vaccination
Passive Immunity
HOST AND PATHOGEN
    INTERACTIONS
Immune Evasion Strate-
    gies of Pathogens
Host Selection By Disease
PUBLIC HEALTH
    MEASURES
Personal Health Measures
Impact of Public and Per-
    sonal Health Measures on
    Pathogens
SUMMARY
SUGGESTIONS FOR
    FURTHER READING
QUESTIONS
ANSWERS

CHAPTER 1

Introduction to Infection, Resistance, and Immunity

Samuel J. Black

INTRODUCTION

This chapter is designed to provide an overview of the material that is covered in the rest of the text. We hope that it helps the student to grasp the field as a whole by tying together and integrating the material handled in the various chapters that follow. The student may find that rereading this chapter at various times as the course progresses will aid in obtaining a grasp of how the components of infection, resistance, and immunity work together to maintain our health.

THE IMMUNE SYSTEM

All life-forms on planet Earth are constructed from the same materials, and assembled in basically the same way. All compete for the same resources and each is rich in directly utilizable processed materials. Each life-form provides an opportunity for creative exploitation by others, i.e., can enhance reproductive fitness of other life forms by being food or shelter, or by making it easier to obtain food or shelter. In short, life-forms on this planet did not, and do not, get on by ignoring each other.

Although assembled from the same units, each speck of life flaunts its individuality through the array of molecules on its surface and announces its presence by a unique perfume of metabolites and other secretory products. From the very beginning, mutation and selection equipped life-forms with receptors to pick up cues from other life-forms, and with biochemical pathways that linked cue to response, be the response gene activation or movement to engulf and kill prey or release of secretions to capture scarce resources or to attract mates or to repel predators.

By the time metazoa arose through evolution, neighboring organisms were already equipped to perceive and prey on them, whilst the metazoa most likely had a

Table 1.1. The nature of lymphoid organs and of immune responses of vertebrates of various classes.

| Vertebrate Class | Lymphoid organs | Functional activity | |
		Graft rejection	Antibody formation
Jawless fishes, e.g., hagfish	No thymus equivalent present	+/-	+
Cartilaginous fishes, e.g., sharks	Thymus equivalent present	+	+
	Spleen present		
Bony fishes	Thymus equivalent present	+	+
	Spleen present		
	Lymphoid cell aggregates present		
Amphibians			
Newts/Salamanders	Thymus-like organ present	+	+
	Spleen present		
Frogs/Toads	Thymus-like organ present	+	+
	Spleen present		
	Lymph nodes present		
Reptiles			
Alligators/Crocodiles	Spleen present	?	?
	Thymus not described		
Lizards/Turtles/Snakes	Bursa-like organ present	+	+
	Thymus equivalent present		
	Lymph nodes present		
Birds	Bursa with a defined inner structure present	+	+
	Thymus and spleen present		
	Lymph nodes present		
Mammals	No bursa (bone marrow is the probable bursal equivalent)	+	+
	Thymus, spleen, lymph nodes, and lymphatic duct system all present		

variety of counterdefenses to frustrate this process. These primitive immune systems continued to develop during evolution under the selective pressure of pathogens. At present, numerous types of immune systems exist. They differ in fairly substantial ways between phyla and in more subtle ways between species (Table 1.1). The systems are least complex in invertebrates, which lack adaptive immune components, and most complex in mammals, which are the focus of this text. See chapter 13 (Comparative Immunology) for further discussion of this subject.

The immune system plays an essential role in ensuring our survival. We are exposed to viruses, bacteria, fungi, and parasites that can use our bodies both as niche and nutrient source. The level of exposure is regulated by public and personal health practices, but excellent public and personal health programs alone do not prevent disease. Even in our hygiene-conscious society, most individuals occasionally incubate infections. Individuals with defective immune systems, e.g., patients who have certain genetic defects, or are maintained on immunosuppressive therapy to prevent graft rejection, or who are infected with, for example, the immune system-destructive acquired immunodeficiency syndrome (AIDS) virus, can develop life-threatening disease often with organisms usually considered to be of little or no pathogenicity.

The immune system is our primary defense against disease. It is composed of interacting molecules, cells, and organs that can discriminate environmental agents (nonself) from one's own tissues (self) and prevent or limit the extent to which the body is colonized by nonself. It is important to be aware that there are many components making up the immune system, each with its own set of functions. Some aspects and functions of the immune systems are outlined in Figure 1.1 and are listed below:

Constitutive Immunity: (1) Barrier Immunity—Prevents the initial invasion of the body by other organisms. (2) The Inflammatory Response—Rapidly responds to pathogens that bypass barrier immunity and creates conditions that limit their replication at the site of invasion.

Adaptive Immunity—Mounts, over a period of several days, immune responses that eliminate invading organisms and their products in a highly specific manner.

Passive Immunity—Protects the fetus and newborn from infection during the development of its immune system.

Constitutive Immunity
Barrier Immunity
In this type of immunity, just as with martial arts, all parts of the body are used in defense and as weapons against the foe, here, disease-causing organisms. The surfaces that come into intimate contact with the environment both present a physical barrier to environmental pathogens and are endowed with antimicrobial activities. The skin of the frog and the silkworm contains short hydrophobic peptides, called cecropins, that lyse fragile protozoan parasites. Mammal skin is dotted with hair follicles and associated sebaceous glands that secrete antimicrobial lactic and fatty acids. Antimicrobial agents in sweat, tears, and saliva limit growth of microorganisms in these secretions. Pathogens that are inhaled are often trapped in mucin at mucosal surfaces, expelled back into the mouth, swallowed, and exposed to damaging treatment with acid, bile, and enzymes of the digestive tract. Sneezing, coughing, vomiting, diarrhea, and urination all play a role in removal of infectious agents from the body. Products of adaptive immune responses also participate in the maintenance of barrier immunity, e.g., pathogen-reactive antibodies of the IgA class, are secreted at mucosal surfaces and help to reduce infection by binding to structures on microbes that facilitate invasion.

The Inflammatory Response
Mere physical and mechanical barriers are often an inadequate protection against

(1) Constitutive (innate) immunity (resistance) develops as the individual develops. It does not require contact with any parasite for full expression.

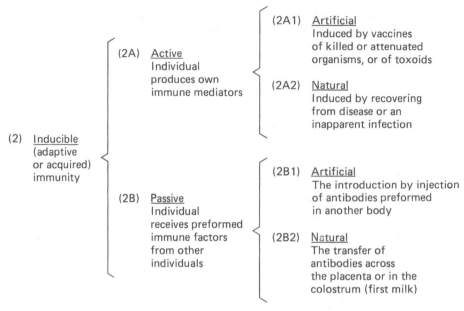

(2) Inducible (adaptive or acquired) immunity

   (2A) Active Individual produces own immune mediators

      (2A1) Artificial Induced by vaccines of killed or attenuated organisms, or of toxoids

      (2A2) Natural Induced by recovering from disease or an inapparent infection

   (2B) Passive Individual receives preformed immune factors from other individuals

      (2B1) Artificial The introduction by injection of antibodies preformed in another body

      (2B2) Natural The transfer of antibodies across the placenta or in the colostrum (first milk)

Figure 1.1. There are a variety of mechanisms by which organisms resist parasitization. The constitutive mechanisms (1) develop as the individual develops. The development is under endogenous control. The inducible mechanisms (2) develop only partially under endogenous stimuli and require contact with the parasite or its products for full development. The inducible mechanisms are commonly classified into active (2A) and passive (2B) forms depending on whether the individual develops its own immune mediators or receives those produced by another. Active and passive immunity may each be further divided into artificial (2A1; 2B1) and natural (2A2; 2B2) types. The artificial types are those that result from intervention by physicians or veterinarians.

disease and decay. We must beware the enemy that breaches them. Pathogens bypass barrier immunity when they enter the body through cuts, are transmitted directly into tissues by a biting insect, or invade cells lining the respiratory or alimentary passages after inhalation or consumption. Once in the body, pathogens encounter the constitutive defense processes that comprise the inflammatory response system. The inflammatory mechanisms of defense are mediated by molecules and cells that activate when they contact damaged body tissues. The molecular basis of the response is similar whether tissue damage is wrought by heat, abrasion, laceration, a biting insect, or a pathogen. The resulting reaction is called an inflammatory response.

The "weal and flare" that results from a minor skin scratch illustrates the speed, potency, and features of an inflammatory response. This reaction is characterized by redness, swelling, heat, and pain. Redness and heat are due to an increase in blood flow to the site of inflammation and result from local vasodilation caused by chemical mediators produced in response to tissue damage. Swelling is due to leakage of blood fluids into the site of inflammation as a result of mediator-induced changes in the permeability of endothelial cells lining local blood ves-

sels. Pain is due to tissue destruction exacerbated by proteolytic enzymes, lipolytic enzymes, and reactive oxygen intermediates released from cells (neutrophils,
macrophages) that are recruited from the blood circulation into the inflammatory
site. Prostaglandin E2 that is produced at the site of inflammation enhances sensitivity of local nerve cells also contributing to pain associated with inflammation. Pain itself is a defense mechanism. It calls attention to the damaged site and
induces behavioral responses aimed at limiting damage and inducing avoidance
of damaging behavior.

The scratch-induced "weal and flare" reaction is short-lived. That is not the case
if the damaged tissues harbor pathogenic organisms, which typically have surface
structures that interact with serum components to amplify production of the chemical mediators of inflammation.

Within an inflammatory site, invading organisms are exposed to damaging enzymes and oxygen radicals and can become coated with a series of serum enzymes
(complement factors) that ultimately punch holes into their surfaces. The organ-
isms can also be coated with fragments of complement such as $\overline{C3b}$ and $\overline{iC3b}$, which
cause them to be engulfed (phagocytosed) and destroyed by cells that are special-
ized for this activity, namely, neutrophils and macrophages. Once microbes are
engulfed by phagocytic cells, they are exposed to a hostile environment comprising proteolytic enzymes, acid pH, reactive oxygen intermediates, nitric oxide, and
antimicrobial peptides called defensins within the phagocytic cells. The majority of
microbes cannot withstand these conditions. Antiviral agents (interferons) produced
by cells participating in the inflammatory response help control viral infections in
neighboring cells and enhance antibacterial activity of macrophages.

Adaptive or Inducible Immunity
Adaptive Immune Responses
Uncontrolled inflammatory responses can sometimes lead to debilitating tissue and
organ damage, but the responses typically subside as organisms that provoke them
are eliminated, and tissue damage is repaired. Elimination of invading pathogens
usually requires the development of pathogen-specific immune responses in addition to the mechanisms of the inflammatory response. These responses take several
days to develop, during which time fragments of invading pathogens are cleared
from inflammatory sites into lymph vessels as a result of increased pressure from
fluid accumulation in the inflamed tissue. They are thenceforth drained to local
lymphoid organs and are captured by specialized cells which in turn stimulate
lymphocytes with appropriate antigen-specific receptors to proliferate and express
antimicrobial functions.

Lymphocytes bear antigen-specific receptors that bind complementary structures
(antigenic epitopes) on pathogens and components of pathogens. Each lymphocyte
is capable of binding only one type of antigenic epitope. There are legions of pathogens in our biological universe which jointly have millions of antigenic epitopes.
These are countered by an army of lymphocytes in which each member is coated
with copies of an antigen-specific receptor capable of binding only one antigenic
epitope, and in which the population has the capability of reacting with most, if not
all, of the antigenic epitopes that are expressed by pathogens. Lymphocytes are
activated by antigen only when the strength of interaction is adequate to ensure
stable association. Receptor and antigen association is mediated by a combination
of charge, and hydrophobic and hydrogen bonding interactions and is affected by

the size, shape, and fit of the interacting surfaces. The few lymphocytes with any particular specificity of receptor necessitates antigen-driven replication to a critical mass, and this, together with a requirement to differentiate before expression of function, accounts for the time taken in development of an adaptive response. Two classes of lymphocytes are noted for participation in adaptive immune responses, namely, B cells and αβ T cells. These cells recognize exclusive sets of antigenic epitopes and have different specialized functions.

B Cells and Antibodies
B cells, when appropriately activated, multiply and eventually differentiate to plasma cells that secrete water soluble copies—called antibodies—of their antigen-specific receptor. This accounts for the direct cause and effect relationship between administration of antigen and production of specific antibodies that form stable complexes with the antigen. Secreted antibodies neutralize pathogens and their products, e.g., bacterial toxins, in blood and tissue fluids and at mucosal surfaces. They can react with the surface of microbes so long as their target antigen is exposed. After binding to the pathogen, or its products, the antibodies recruit a variety of molecules and cells to effect elimination of the pathogen or its products. Reactions include assembly of membrane attack complexes composed of complement factors that make holes in lipid bilayer membranes and the tagging of pathogens for phagocytosis by macrophages and neutrophils. Antibodies are also secreted across mucosal surfaces, thus, helping to eliminate pathogens and their products from the eyes, mouth, gut, and urogenital tract.

T cells, Major Histocompatibility Antigens and Cytokines
The αβ T cells react with plasma membrane components of nucleated self cells that harbor pathogens or have phagocytosed pathogens. The interaction is directed by the antigen-specific receptors on αβ T cells which react with peptide fragments of the pathogen that are exposed on the surface of the host cell as a result of their combination with self components encoded by genes in the major histocompatibility complex (MHC) and called MHC molecules. The antigen-specific receptor of an αβ T cell is not synthesized in a water soluble form nor secreted, but remains bound to the membrane of the T cell. Hence, αβ T cells are specialized to participate in cell contact reactions. Some antigen-activated αβ T cells can kill infected target cells. Stimulated αβ T cells also secrete biologically active polypeptides called cytokines. There is a wide variety of cytokines with distinct biological activities, and different subclasses of αβ T cells produce and secrete different groups of cytokines. Cytokine products of one major group of activated T cells work together with antigen to cause other T cells to proliferate and differentiate, and to activate macrophages, while cytokine products of the other major T cell group work together with antigen to cause B cells to proliferate and differentiate to antibody-secreting cells. Cytokines produced by T cells signal stem cells to produce more lymphocytes and phagocytes.

Vaccination
In addition to maturing to effector cells, B cells and αβ T cells that are exposed to their priming antigen also give rise to progeny cells that, once formed, cease development and remain inactive until they contact the same antigen again. They are thus capable of mounting a "memory" or "recall" response, when they encounter the priming antigen again. Memory lymphocytes retain the same antigen-binding

specificity as their parent cells, but there are more of them and therefore, their response is more rapid and of greater magnitude accounting for the benefit of vaccination in preparing for defense against known pathogens. Because B cell and T cell antigen-specific receptors are clonally distributed, priming of the immune system against one antigen does not diminish its capability to mount a response against other different antigens. This is an important point to grasp because a backlash against vaccination expressed by some members of our society is based on a groundless fear of immune exhaustion. Some resistance to vaccination is also based on the fact that any vaccine may produce an allergic reaction in some individuals, and some vaccines may also cause damage by other means also. The potential harm of a course of action must be balanced against the benefit conferred when making decisions to act in immunization procedures, as in all other decisions for action.

Passive Immunity

Fetal development occurs in a sterile environment whereas newborn mammals are exposed to many environmental pathogens. During the first weeks after birth, newborn mammals are protected by antibodies that are derived from the mother. Human babies receive maternal antibody of the IgG class across the placenta during fetal development and additional classes of antibody in colostrum which accumulates in the mammary gland during the last few weeks of pregnancy. The structure of the placenta in domestic cattle and some other mammal species precludes transfer of IgG to the fetus. Newborn mammals of these species obtain all of their maternal antibodies in the first milk, i.e., colostrum. The newborn digestive system does not degrade the antibodies, and the newborn gut epithelia allow their passage from the gut into the bloodstream. The maternal antibodies protect the newborn mammal from environmental pathogens during maturation and priming of its immune system. Maternal antibodies may also play a subtle role in regulating the antigen-binding specificity of lymphocytes that are maturing in the newborn.

Passive immunity can also be produced by serum or cell transfer. This is a medical procedure in which immune products formed by one individual are transferred to a nonimmune individual. Variations on the theme include the collection of peripheral blood leukocytes from an individual, their stimulation with antigens or tumor cells or cytokines *in vitro*, and reinfusion into the original donor with a view toward enhancing immunity.

HOST AND PATHOGEN INTERACTIONS
Immune Evasion Strategies of Pathogens

Some pathogens are capable of survival and replication in the absence of host species, but other pathogens have an absolute requirement for a host. Survival of the latter organisms requires both host availability and evasion of immune elimination at least until transmission to a new host. Host immune systems and pathogen immune evasion strategies are products of the coevolution of hosts and pathogens and development of both systems is an ongoing process.

Immune responses are not always sufficient to control infections. During evolution pathogens have been selected to express a plethora of methods to prevent development of, or their destruction by, immune responses. Specific examples can be accessed by consulting PubMed at the web address given at the end of this chapter using appropriate search phrases such as "AIDs virus" and "immune evasion." Immune evasion strategies expressed by different pathogens include

(1) The inactivation of constitutive defenses by enzymes that destroy oxygen radicals, inactivate proteolytic enzymes, and prevent assembly of serum complement components that build the membrane attack complex. (2) The subversion of acquired immune responses by acquisition of a coat of host antigens or the induction of immunosuppressive cells. (3) The evasion of acquired antibody responses by the degradation of bound antibodies or surface antigenic variation. (4) The evasion of antibody-mediated destruction by "hiding-out" in cells. Some organisms use host complement factors to expedite their phagocytosis, while others have specialized cell invasion structures. Organisms that are phagocytosed are sometimes able to withstand the antimicrobial activities of the phagocytic cell through inactivation of hydrolytic enzymes and reactive oxygen intermediates in the phagocytic vacuole. Others counter the defense mechanisms of the phagosome and phagolysosome by escaping into the cell cytosol. (5) The subversion of acquired cell mediated immune responses by stealth technology. Some viruses prevent or limit assembly of pathogen-peptide fragments with MHC molecules thereby preventing their display on the cell surface and detection by T cells. (6) The manipulation of immune responses by the generation of molecules that mimic host cytokines or cytokine receptors thus confounding molecular communications within the immune system. (7) The direct suppression of immune function. The AIDS virus lives and replicates in a class of T cells that is involved in regulating responses of other lymphocytes, causing their depletion and subverting host immune competence. (8) The misdirection of immune responses. Some pathogens induce inappropriate immune responses, e.g., stimulate production of large amounts of antibody when efficient development of a T cell-mediated immune response is required for effective control, or vice versa. (9) Manufacture and release of large quantities of parasite capsular material to provide a smoke screen and to tie up host defenses.

Failure of the immune system to control invading pathogens typically results in escalating stimulation of inflammatory and other inappropriate immune responses. In addition, this can lead to self-destruction of the host, e.g., by an unrelenting and overwhelming fever response; or by the acute wasting disease that results from overproduction of some cytokines such as tumor necrosis factor (TNF); or by massive deposition of immune complexes in the kidney causing kidney failure.

Host Selection by Disease
In an endemic disease situation, those individuals who are least affected by disease are most likely to reproduce. In this way, infectious organisms will eventually select for a relatively resistant host population, a process that some people argue actually led to the development of immune systems. Similarly, pathogen selection in resistant hosts leads to propagation of those organisms that are most able to survive and replicate in the face of an efficient immune response and hence can in some way elude elimination by the response. Specific pathogens coevolve with specific hosts and stable pathogen and host relationships reflect subtle checks and balances that have evolved over eons of time. These are worked out through the genetic sculpting of interacting host and pathogen proteins. A pathogen that causes no signs of disease in one host population, or species, may nevertheless cause devastating disease in another due to minor variation in the structure of one or more interacting molecules. This lies at the core of so-called "emerging diseases." Control of such diseases will challenge our ingenuity in upcoming decades as we move

into and attempt to exploit new niches while challenging the carrying capacity of the regions in which we live.

PUBLIC HEALTH MEASURES

Organized societies devote effort to protecting their members from disease exposure. The water and food supplies are monitored for infectious organisms and toxins, and strict standards are enforced. Similarly strict health and safety standards are enforced in stores and restaurants. Permits are required for plant and animal imports and strictly monitored to limit introduction of exotic diseases. Our waste, including human excretory products, is collected and processed to reduce the flow of disease-causing organisms among people and from people into animal and plant species in our habitat. Blood and organ supplies for human clinical use are screened to exclude transmission of disease. Standards are being developed for humanized animal tissues which are being generated by recombinant cloning technologies and are expected to contribute resources for tissue and organ transplants. These standards, when enforced, will help to limit spread of novel diseases from animal organ donors to people. Information is constantly collected on disease incidence and routes of transmission within the community so that members can be advised of safe health practices. Disease spread is also regulated by required vaccination and, on occasion, by isolation. In addition, our disease sleuths scan the globe for emerging infections and track their movements so that provisions can be made to protect the world and local community.

Personal Health Measures

We can assist our immune system in control of pathogens by making use of recommended vaccines and by taking common sense precautions, *e.g.*, avoid touching objects that are handled by large numbers of other people, wash your hands before handling and eating food, avoid conditions that are conducive to transmission of respiratory infections, e.g., crowded places with poor ventilation, avoid contact with and consumption of contaminated water or food, avoid infected vectors of diseases, and avoid sharing of body fluids with people who are carrying blood-borne infectious organisms. These precautions may help to keep you free of disease and consequently, limit the spread of disease within your community.

Impact of Public and Personal Health Measures on Pathogens

Efficient public and personal health measures limit the spread of disease between individuals in a community and can determine the profile of pathogens that circulate in the community. Under these conditions highly pathogenic organisms that kill their hosts before they are transmitted to a new host are selected against. In contrast, less pathogenic organisms that establish chronic infections may continue to be propagated. The circulation of weakly pathogenic organisms within a host community may actually induce immunity that is effective against virulent variants, and therefore suppress the appearance of these variants within the community. When public and personal health practices fail to prevent infection, disease may be controlled by chemotherapeutic agents. However, the treatment regimes that we use to control environmental pathogens also exert selective pressures on those pathogens. Antibiotic-resistant bacteria and drug-resistant parasites have been selected by decades of use of prophylactic and therapeutic agents by ourselves and the world community. This often results from the use of drugs at doses, or in dose regimes, that alleviate disease symptoms but fail to kill all of the causative organisms.

The organisms that cause disease are an unrelenting enemy. Their capacity for change is enormous and unpredictable, and disease-causing organisms do not recognize frontiers. We can never relax our vigilance regarding disease nor cease our efforts to characterize disease-causing organisms and the host responses that they invoke. We must also sustain our efforts to develop vaccines and drugs that alleviate disease.

SUMMARY

The chapter introduces six fundamental concepts. (1) We and other vertebrates require functional immune systems to survive. (2) The constitutive immune responses, i.e., barrier immunity and inflammation, work together with the adaptive immune responses, which are mediated by B cells, T cells, and their products, to control pathogens. (3) The constitutive responses are mediated by molecules and cells that are present before infection and hence, little time is taken in mobilizing this arm of defense. The cells that participate in the constitutive defense mechanisms do not need to replicate or differentiate to express function. The constitutive defenses are activated by tissue damage and surface components of pathogens, result in inflammation, and damage both pathogens and neighboring tissues. (4) Adaptive or inducible immune responses are mounted by B and T lymphocytes, which have clonally restricted antigen-specific receptors, replicate and differentiate in response to pathogens, are functionally specialized, have memory, and eliminate pathogens and their products without much colateral damage of host tissues. (5) Pathogens have evolved numerous ways to evade immune elimination and can cause devastating disease in a nonadapted host. (6) Our public and personal health practices affect the incidence and virulence of pathogens that circulate in our community.

SUGGESTIONS FOR FURTHER READING

Mims, C.A. *The pathogenesis of infectious disease.* 3d ed. Academic Press Inc., 1990. ISBN 0-12-498260-3 and ISBN 0-12-498261-1.

PubMed—*http://www.ncbi.nlm.nih.gov/PubMed/*—This web address directs you to the National Library of Medicines search service for more than 9 millions of citations of abstracts from scientific journals. Use of this free service will greatly enhance your appreciation of ongoing work in the field of immunology.

Silverstein, Arthur M. "The History of Immunology." In. *Fundamental Immunology.* 3d ed. Edited by W.E. Paul. 21–41. Raven Press, 1993. ISBN 0-7817-0022-1.

Tizard, Ian R. "Immunity in the Fetus and Newborn." In *Veterinary Immunology, an Introduction.* 5th ed., 237–250. W.B. Saunders Company, 1996. ISBN 0-7216-5772-9.

Warren, Kenneth S. "The Global Impact of Parasitic Diseases." In. *The Biology of Parasitism.* Edited by Paul T. Englund and Alan Sher, 3–12. Alan R. Liss, Inc. 1988. ISBN 0-8451-2208-8 and ISBN 0-8451-2209-6.

Nesse, R.M. and G.C. Williams. *Why We Get Sick.* Times Books, Random House, 1994. ISBN 0-8129-2224-7.

QUESTIONS

1. What observations support the argument that we need a functional immune system to survive?
2. How are the inflammatory immune responses stimulated, what accounts for their rapid development, and how do they help protect against invasion by pathogens?
3. In what way is the functional specialization of αβ T cells and B cells linked to their antigen-specific receptors?
4. How do pathogens evade immune elimination?
5. How do our public and personal health practices affect the incidence and virulence of pathogens in our environment?

ANSWERS

1. Individuals with defective immune systems typically develop life-threatening disease.
2. Innate immune responses are mediated by phagocytic cells that are rapidly recruited and activated by chemical mediators generated from constitutive serum components upon exposure to damaged tissues and activating sites on pathogens.
3. The antigen-specific receptors of an αβ T cell are made in a membrane-bound form only, detect peptide fragments of pathogens in association with host cell MHC molecules, and hence mediate cell-contact reactions. The antigen-specific receptors of a B cell are made in membrane-bound and water-soluble forms and bind antigenic epitopes that are not associated with any host cell component. B cells and their secreted antibodies can thus react directly with pathogens and their products.
4. Pathogens evade immune elimination by preventing the induction of immune responses, or by evading destruction by immune responses by any of a large number of mechanisms listed in the chapter, or by inducing inappropriate and ineffective immune responses.
5. Poor health practices result in frequent transmission of disease causing organisms from individual to individual within a community. This ensures propagation of the most abundant organisms which are typically those that replicate most rapidly, induce least effective immune responses and consequently are highly virulent.

CHAPTER 2

Host-Parasite Relationships

Julius P. Kreier

INTRODUCTION

TYPES OF HOST-PARASITE
RELATIONSHIPS

THE NORMAL MICROBIAL
POPULATIONS ON AND
IN MULTICELLULAR
ORANISMS

MICROBIAL POPULATIONS
NORMALLY ASSOCIATED
WITH HUMANS
Skin
Mouth
Digestive Tract
Genitourinary Tract

KOCH'S POSTULATES AND
THEIR LIMITATIONS

SUMMARY

SUGGESTIONS FOR
FURTHER READING

QUESTIONS

ANSWERS

INTRODUCTION

Parasitism is a life-style that has been adopted by many types of living things. There are parasitic forms among most groups of multicellular plants and animals, among the fungi, and in most groups of unicellular organisms. All viruses are parasites. There are many species of parasites which inhabit the bodies of plants and animals. Examples of parasitic flowering plants are dodder, indian pipe, and mistletoe. Various species of hookworms, ascarids, and trichinella are common in humans and other animals, and many species of nematode infest the roots of plants. The organism that causes athlete's foot is a parasitic fungus. Unicellular protozoa cause malaria, dysentery and other diseases. A large variety of species of bacteria are parasitic; anthrax, diphtheria, tuberculosis, and brucellosis, for example, are diseases caused by parasitic bacteria (Figure 2.1).

Some of the parasitic organisms cause severe disease. Others draw nourishment from their hosts but do little harm, and some benefit the host while benefiting themselves. The obligatorily parasitic viruses may cause severe disease or may be harmless commensals.

The term *parasite* is used with several meanings. In common medical and veterinary terminology, it may be used to describe a blood-sucking arthropod, such as a flea or louse; a worm inhabiting the digestive tract, such as a hookworm or tapeworm, or a protozoan such as the amoeba that causes amoebic dysentery. In this usage bacteria and viruses are not included among the parasites, and they are not studied in conventional courses on parasitology. In the usage followed in this book, all organisms living in or on the bodies of other organisms and drawing their sustenance from them are considered to be parasites; thus the group includes bacteria and viruses as well as arthropods, worms, and protozoa.

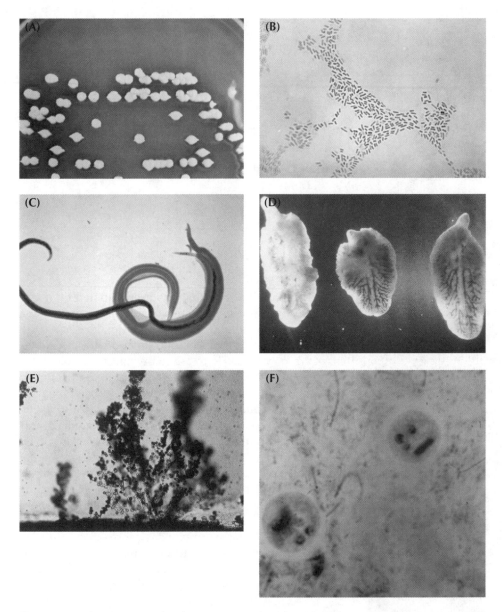

Figure 2.1. Photomicrographs of parasitic organisms. A wide variety of organisms are parasitic. (A) Bacteria form colonies visible with the naked eye when streaked on nutrient agar. (B) Microscopic examination of bacteria streaked out on a microscope slide and stained reveals the individual organisms, in this case bacilli. Worms may also be parasites. Schistosomes (C) and liver flukes (D) cause severe diseases in man and other animals. Many fungi grow on and in the bodies of plants and animals, sometimes as harmless commensals and sometimes as pathogens. *Candida albicans* is a common parasite of humans (E). Protozoa inhabit blood and body cavities. (F) *Entamoeba histolytica* is a common inhabitant of the colons of humans. The cyst form shown here is passed in the feces. The organism may cause moderate to severe diarrhea. (G) *Giardia intestinalis* inhabits the intestines of humans. It causes diarrhea. It is usually spread in contaminated water. (H) *Trypanosoma cruzi* grows in the blood and tissues of humans and other animals causing Chagas' disease. (I) The reduviid bug, a bloodsucking insect, spreads the organism. The trypanosome is a parasite in the parasitic insect that serves as its vector.

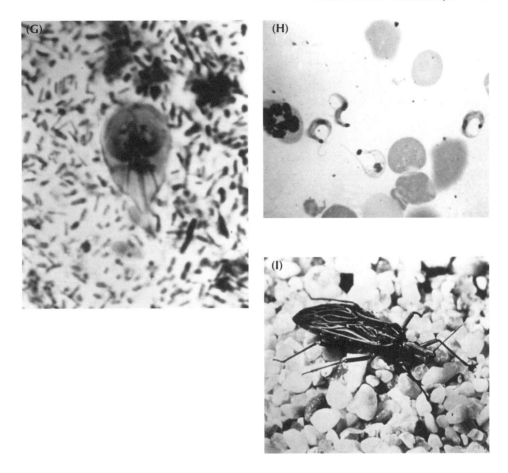

Figure 2.1. *(concluded)*

TYPES OF HOST-PARASITE RELATIONSHIPS

As noted in the previous section, parasites are organisms that live in or on the bodies of another organism, the host, and derive their sustenance from it. It is not generally in the interest of a parasite to seriously harm its host because then the parasite would be in danger of losing its support. In fact, many parasites cause little harm to their hosts. Serious harm usually indicates a poor adaptation of the host and parasite. Some damage to the host may however be a necessary part of the parasite's life cycle, and thus be unavoidable.

Damage associated with parasite entry into the host and migration to its site of development is often associated with a parasitic relationship. Some parasitic worms—the hookworm, for example—penetrate the skin to initiate infection and cause local injury characterized by development of a rash; they may also pass through the lungs during their migration to the digestive tract, thus causing pneumonia.

A variety of parasites cause injury as part of their mechanism of dispersal from one host to another. Most viruses of the respiratory tract, such as the influenza virus, and some bacteria, such as the organisms causing tuberculosis and diphtheria, cause considerable irritation to the mucosa of the respiratory tract. This irritation causes increased fluid release, with coughing and sneezing that facilitate the

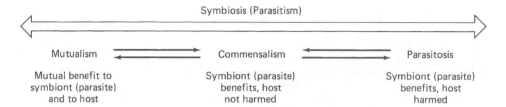

Figure 2.2. Symbiotic relationships may vary over time. Depending on environmental factors such as host resistance, the relationship of a given host-parasite pair may shift between mutually beneficial (mutualism) and harmful to the host (parasitosis). Intermediate stages of toleration (commensalism) may occur.

exit of the parasite from the host. The diarrhea caused by bacteria and viruses infecting the intestines also serves to spread these parasites.

One of the more unique mechanisms for spread of a parasite, and one which is damaging to the host, was developed by the neurotrophic rabies virus. The virus, which grows in the host's brain and its salivary glands, causes changes in the host's behavior so that it attacks other potential hosts, inoculating infected saliva during the attack. In most of the host species of the rabies virus, the damage to the nervous system that causes these changes is finally fatal to the host. However, in bats and skunks, which are probably the hosts in which the rabies virus maintains itself between epidemics, damage is limited and spread is not dependent on changes in the host's behavior. The occurrence of some damage as a result of parasitization does not change the fact that it is usually not in the interest of a parasite to severely damage its host.

Our understanding of host-parasite relationships has developed and changed with the passage of time, as have the terms used to describe them. Originally the term *parasitic* was used for any relationship in which two organisms live together in an intimate association. The term *symbiotic* has come to be used as a general term to describe any relationship in which two organisms live together in an intimate association (Figure 2.2). In this usage symbiotic relationships are considered to be *mutualistic* if both members of the pair benefit, *commensal* if the symbiont benefits, and the host is not harmed, or *parasitic* if the symbiont benefits and the host is harmed to a greater or lesser degree. The term *parasitosis* is sometimes used to designate a parasitic relationship that is particularly harmful to the host.

In practice the categories into which host-parasite relationships have been divided are somewhat arbitrary and grade one into the other. This is as one should expect, as host-parasite relationships are subject to and are the results of evolution, and at any given time transformation from one relationship to another may not be complete. Evolution toward mutual interdependence between host and parasite has been realized to a remarkable degree in some instances. As a result of evolutionary change, for example, some mutualistic relationships have become so intimate that the members of the pair are no longer considered separate individuals. This is the case with chloroplasts and the plant cells in which they occur, and with the mitochondria inhabiting plant and animal cells.

Parasites may be distinguished from predators and from saprophytes. Predators are organisms that hunt, catch, and kill other organisms before eating them. Usually prey and predator are similar in size. The prey may be somewhat smaller than the predator, as is a mouse preyed on by a cat, or larger, as is a deer preyed on by wolves. Parasites, on the other hand, are almost always much smaller than their hosts. Fleas, for example, are much smaller than dogs, and the pneumococcus is much smaller than the human in which it causes pneumonia. The major difference between parasites and predators is not size, however, but behavior. Parasites such as fleas and bacteria do not hunt, catch, and kill their prey before eating it; rather they eat it while it continues to live.

Saprophytes, unlike parasites and predators, neither feed on the still-living nor kill before eating; they eat dead organisms that they did not kill. Animals such as buzzards, which scavenge for their living eating dead animals, are in a sense saprophytes, but in conventional usage, the term *saprophytes* is reserved for micro-organisms such as bacteria, protozoa, and fungi that digest and thus degrade the bodies of dead plants and animals.

As noted earlier, parasites live in or on another organism and gain their sustenance from it. They draw their nourishment from the living bodies of their hosts. The parasitic worms and arthropods that live on the surface of the body or in the lumens of the hollow organs such as the intestines are usually described as *infesting* their hosts.

The implication of the word *infection* is of a generalized invasion of the host's tissues, whereas an *infestation* is more superficial. Parasites that are described as causing infestations are also usually larger than those described as causing infections. The distinction between the terms, however, is not sharp. Dermatomycoses caused by fungi are usually referred to as infections, for example, and parasitization by relatively large worms such as trichinella, which invade the tissues of the body, is usually considered an infection.

Some of the difficulty in the terminology used to describe host-parasite relationships is the result of historical accident. Classical parasitology (the science that deals with the parasitic protozoa, worms and arthropods) developed as a part of zoology. The study of parasitic bacteria and viruses was a province microbiology. As a result of this separate development, separate terminologies developed to describe essentially similar processes.

People studying microbes became aware quite early that infection with some microbes would result in disease, whereas with others infection either did not result in disease or did not occur at all. Failure by a given microorganism to induce disease in a particular organism may be a result of host specificity. Because of host specificity, a microorganism that produces disease in one animal may be totally harmless to another. It may fail to infect or it may infect but produce no disease. The virus that causes canine distemper, for example, is totally incapable of infecting humans, and the bacteria that cause tuberculosis in chickens do not generally infect cattle or humans.

Some degree of host specificity is the rule for most host-parasite interactions. When parasites do succeed in infecting new hosts, the results can be devastating. *Trypanosoma brucei*, a protozoan, exists in many species of antelope in Africa, where it causes little or no harm. In domestic cattle, however, the same organism usually produces a rapidly fatal disease. Some variants of *T. brucei* that normally occur in antelope can produce severe disease when they infect humans.

Microbes capable of causing infections that result in disease are called *pathogens*. Infection even with a potentially pathogenic microorganism, however, does not always result in disease. If we wish to describe the degree of pathogenicity of a microbe, we refer to its virulence. *Virulence* is a quantitative term. Infection of a susceptible animal with a highly virulent pathogen will almost always result in disease, whereas infection with a pathogen of low virulence will often fail to produce disease or produce only a mild disease. One must in any case distinguish between infection and disease. Infection is the successful colonization of a host by a parasite; disease is the disorder that may result from the infection.

There are, of course, many microbes that cannot produce even infection, let alone disease. The great bulk of free-living microbes are of this type. There are many free-living microbes that dwell in soil and water. They may prey on other microbes, as do many of the free-living amoeba, or they may live as saprophytes. Some free-living microbes can, under some circumstances, cause infection and disease. Normally free-living microbes that can opportunistically cause infection are called *facultative parasites*. *Legionella pneumoniae* is an aquatic bacterium. If it is inhaled in an aerosol such as is produced by the cooling towers of some water-cooled air conditioners, it is capable of causing infection in the lungs and severe pneumonia. Another example of a facultative parasite is the aquatic amoeba *Naegleria fowleri* which, if sucked into the nose with the water in which it is growing, may invade the brain through the nasal passages and cause meningitis.

One may contrast the life-style of a free-living organism which may accidentally or only occasionally colonize a host with the life-style of an organism that can live only as a parasite. These latter are called *obligate parasites*. All viruses are obligate parasites, but obligate parasitism occurs among all classes of parasites. Plasmodia that cause malaria are obligately parasitic protozoa, trichinella are obligately parasitic worms, and dodder is an obligately parasitic plant. There are some parasites that are obligate parasites during some stages of their life cycles and are free-living in others. The common flea, for example, is free-living in its larval stage but is parasitic as an adult.

THE NORMAL MICROBIAL POPULATIONS ON AND IN MULTICELLULAR ORGANISMS

If one is to understand host-parasite relationships and the relationship of microbes to disease, one must be aware that microbes normally live on the outer surfaces of plants and animals. In animals they also live throughout the digestive tract, in the upper portions of the respiratory tract, and the lower portions of the reproductive tract. In healthy plants and animals few microbes live within the tissues of the body, and in healthy animals the lungs, bladder, and uterus are normally free of microbes.

The microbes that live on the body's surfaces and in the hollow organs are usually considered to be commensals benefiting from the association. Commensals gain food and shelter for themselves and do little or no harm to their hosts. In some cases these microbes can be shown to benefit their hosts, and the relationship is thus mutualistic. The microbial inhabitants of the lower bowel of humans, for example, benefit their hosts. If they are eliminated by antibiotic treatment, the microbes that then may colonize the region may cause severe diarrhea. The microbes living in the rumen of cattle are clearly mutualistic since they digest cellulose for the host animals.

Many of the microbes normally colonizing the skin and digestive tracts of animals, including those that may be considered commensals or mutualists, may, if circumstances are appropriate, become pathogens. Any break in the skin is usually followed by at least a local infection. The infecting organisms are most commonly

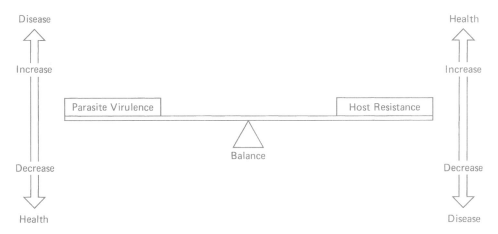

Figure 2.3. The host and parasite exist in a balance. Any decrease in host resistance or increase in parasite virulence can result in development of disease in host-parasite relationships that had previously been innocuous.

ones living on the skin. In a similar way, injury to the bowel is followed by infection in the body cavity by the organisms usually growing in the bowel. In this case organisms that in one situation have a mutualistic relationship to their hosts become disease-causing microorganisms under changed circumstances.

These examples illustrate the role of host resistance in host-parasite relationships. Studies on individuals infected with diseases such as acquired immune deficiency syndrome (AIDS), which weakens or destroys host resistance mechanisms, and of medical treatments that permit graft acceptance or destroy tumors but also weaken the host defense mechanisms has shown clearly the degree to which host-parasite interaction is a dynamic equilibrium. When host resistance is impaired, organisms that are normally present may cause disease (Figure 2.3).

MICROBIAL POPULATIONS NORMALLY ASSOCIATED WITH HUMANS

The symbiotic association of microorganisms with humans (as with other animals and plants) is a normal occurrence. Microorganisms are established on the skin, in the mouth, digestive tract, and genitourinary tract of humans. Not all of the microorganisms normally occurring in association with humans have been described. This is in part because many of them are difficult to grow in culture and thus are difficult to study. Many microorganisms of the normal population inhabit their hosts only sporadically and are therefore referred to as *transient normal flora* or *transient microbial populations*. Those that stay permanently are called *resident microbes*.

Only a small fraction of the many microorganisms in the environment are able to establish themselves and grow in association with the microbes that normally exist in a relationship with humans. The prevention of colonization by microbes not part of the normal population by the ones normally present is called *competitive exclusion*. Often the benefit derived by the host from the resident microbial population is a result of the competitive exclusion of pathogenic microorganisms. Because of competitive exclusion, the most abundant microorganisms among the normal microbial populations colonizing humans play a role in maintaining health. Some microorganisms, however, may directly benefit the host by producing substances useful to the host.

Table 2.1. Microbes commonly living in association with humans.

Location: Tissue/Organ/Site	Microorganism
Skin	Diphtheroids (resemble *C. diphtheriae*)
	Propionibacterium acnes
	Staphylococcus epidermidis
	Pityrosporum (yeast)
Mouth	
Tongue	*Streptococcus salivarius*
Teeth	*S. sanguis*
Mucosa	*S. mitis*
Dental plaque	*Strep. sp., Actinomyces, Nocardia, Bacterionema, Veilonella*
Gingival surfaces	*Bacteriodes sp., Fusobacterium sp.*
Digestive Tract	
Small intestine	*Streptococci, Lactobacilli, Candida albicans*
Large intestine	Anaerobes:
	Bacteroides
	Facultative Anaerobes:
	Lactobacillus, Streptococcus faecalis, Klebsiella, Proteus, Escherichia coli
Urinary Tract	*Streptococcus sp.*
	Mycobacterium
	Bacteriodes
Vaginal Tract	Low pH (in sexually mature females)
	Lactobacilli
	Neutral pH (in immature and postmenopausal females)
	Streptococci mixed with other microbes

Some of the most common microbes normally inhabiting the bodies of humans and their locations in tissues and organs are listed in Table 2.1.

Skin

A wide range of organisms normally live on the skin of humans. The populations include animals such as mites and bacteria such as staphylococci. The microbial populations are large. Estimates based on colony counts usually exceed 200 thousand per cm². The organisms are often found in clusters. Their precise location on and in the skin is determined by many factors. Moist and hairy areas, for example, have more organisms on them than do smooth and dry areas. There are three main types of microbes on the skin. These are diphtheroids, Gram-positive cocci, and yeasts.

Diphtheroids are Gram-positive pleomorphic rods of low virulence. The diphtheroids resident on the skin are similar to but clearly different from *Corynebacterium diphtheriae*, the related organism that is the causative agent of diphtheria. The diphtheroid found in the largest numbers on human skin is *Propionibacterium acnes*, which is anaerobic and grows in the hair follicles. Its growth is enhanced by the oily secretions of the sebaceous glands. *Propionibacterium acnes* has been implicated as a cause of acne. *Propionibacterium acnes* alone does not cause acne, however. Host factors are important contributors. It is well known that acne is most common during adolescence, and thus hormonal factors may be important. Other microbes such as staphylococci, as well as diet, may also be factors in the development of acne.

In addition to the anaerobic *P. acnes*, aerobic diphtheroids are always present in cultures obtained from the skin. The diphtheroids release fatty acids from sebum and thus contribute to the maintenance of the normal level of free fatty acids on the skin. Free fatty acids inhibit the growth of many potentially pathogenic microbes.

The second most abundant group of bacteria on the skin are Gram-positive cocci. Many of these cocci resemble the pathogenic *Staphylococcus aureus*, but differ in that they do not produce coagulase. Coagulase production is a distinguishing feature used to differentiate pathogenic from nonpathogenic staphylococci. The various commensal micrococci and staphylococci that are present probably prevent colonization of the skin by other potentially pathogenic Gram-positive bacteria. The nonpathogenic Gram-positive cocci normally present on the skin are often collectively called *Staphylococcus epidermidis*. The Gram stain reaction and other attributes of bacteria are described in chapter 15. The pathogenic *S. aureus* frequently colonizes the nose and perianal region of healthy people. When this occurs in doctors, nurses, and other health personnel, they may infect patients with whom they have contact.

Yeasts of the genus *Pityrosporum* make up the third-most numerous group of microorganisms on the skin. Extensive growth of these yeasts may result in minor skin diseases that range from scaliness to dandruff.

Mouth

Normally there are 10^9 bacteria in each milliliter of saliva and 10^{11} in each gram of deposit on the teeth. Streptococci of various species are the most common bacteria in the mouth and make up from 30 to 60 percent of the bacteria present. The various species of bacteria in the mouth are each associated with a specific location. The ability of the bacteria to attach to specific tissues governs their site of growth. Bacteria of some species attach to the hard tissue, some to the soft.

The deposits formed by bacteria on the teeth are called *dental plaque*. Organisms in dental plaque are facultative anaerobes and include streptococci, filamentous Gram-positive *Actinomyces*, *Nocardia*, and *Bacterionema*. The Gram-negative microorganism *Veilonella* also is present in plaque. Some pathogens may also be present in dental plaque. For example, *Streptococcus mutans* which is frequently present and releases acid that causes tooth decay. The gingival crevices contain strict anaerobes of the genera *Bacteroides* and *Fusobacterium*.

Digestive Tract

The human stomach is usually sterile. The small intestine contains relatively few bacteria (10^3 to 10^5 per milliliter). Those organisms that are present in the small intestine are facultative anaerobes of the genera *Streptococcus* and *Lactobacillus*. The yeast *Candida albicans* may also be present. The microbial population of the small intestine is quite transient. In individuals with digestive disorders, the microbial population in the small intestine may resemble that in the colon.

In contrast to the small intestine, the large intestine, or colon, contains many bacteria. Feces contain more than 10^{11} bacteria per gram. Up to one-half of the fecal mass may be bacteria. Most of the bacteria in the large intestine are obligate anaerobes of the genus *Bacteroides*. Facultatively anaerobic Gram-negative rods of the genera *Escherichia* and the Gram-positive rods of the genus *Lactobacillus* make up the bulk of the remaining population.

The microbes of the intestine may synthesize vitamins: these include thiamine, niacin, riboflavin, vitamin B_{12}, folic acid, biotin, and vitamin K. It is only if the diet is deficient in these vitamins that the production by microorganisms contributes significantly to the nutrition of humans.

Genitourinary Tract

The kidneys, ureter, and bladder are normally free of bacteria. Infection, however, is common in these sites in humans. This is probably because the urethra opens near the anal orifice and is thus often contaminated with streptococci, *Bacteroides*, and enterobacteria. Infection through sexual activity is also common.

The female genital tract has a normal flora that changes depending on the female's hormonal status and stage of sexual development. The carbohydrate secretions of the vaginal wall vary during the estrus cycle, and this in turn regulates the pH of the vagina because the carbohydrate is fermented to lactic acid by resident lactobacilli. The lactobacilli are predominantly found on the vaginal epithelial cells where they are conveniently located to bring about the fermentation. The vagina has a neutral pH in prepubescent females and those past menopause. During these periods the vaginal wall secretes little carbohydrate. The microbial populations in the vagina of the prepubescent and aged female include streptococci and many other bacteria but few of the carbohydrate-fermenting, lactic acid-producing lactobacilli.

KOCH'S POSTULATES AND THEIR LIMITATIONS

Our knowledge of the relationship of microbes to infection and disease is of relatively recent origin. It was only in the nineteenth century that the science of bacteriology was created. Before that time many explanations for disease were given. Miasmas from swamps and bad air, for example, were considered to be causes of disease. In English the name *malaria*, given to the disease caused by a protozoan and spread by mosquitoes, immortalizes this misconception. Malaria is Italian for *bad air*.

Two individuals who were leaders in the development of the field of medical microbiology and in gaining acceptance for the roles of germs in disease were Louis Pasteur of France and Robert Koch of Germany. Pasteur showed that fermentation of grape juice to wine was a microbial process brought about by yeasts, and that wine spoilage was the result of other fermentations by other organisms. He showed that many off-tastes in wines could be prevented by heating the wine moderately to kill heat-sensitive microbes before bottling it. The process, now called *pasteurization* in his honor, is widely used today. Its use has been extended to products other than wine, milk being perhaps the most familiar. Pasteur considered that illness in humans and animals was analogous to spoilage in wine, and much of his subsequent work and our present understanding of infection and disease stems from this insight.

Robert Koch was among the first to offer convincing scientific proof that germs caused disease when, in 1876, he showed that *Bacillus anthraxis* was the causative agent of anthrax, a fatal disease in cows, sheep, and humans. Robert Koch's major contribution to our present understanding of the role of microbes in disease stemmed, however, from his systemization of techniques for determining which organisms caused which diseases. The systems he developed for cultivation of bacteria in solid media permit ready isolation and growth of bacteria in pure culture.

Table 2.2. Koch's Postulates.

1. The microorganisms must be present in all cases of a disease and not present in the healthy counterparts of the host.
2. The microorganisms must be isolated from the host and grown in pure culture.
3. The disease must be induced by the inoculation of the pure culture of the isolated microorganisms into a suitable experimental animal.
4. The microorganism must be recovered from the experimentally infected host.

When the systems are used, the bacterial cultures obtained are from colonies that develop from single organisms fixed in space in a solid medium. They are thus pure cultures of the organism producing the colony. The use of solid-culture techniques thus permits one type of microbe to be isolated from among the complex and confusing mixtures normally present in the environment.

Koch's formulation of a set of rules, now called Koch's Postulates, systemized the criteria for relating the various microbes that were isolated by the new techniques to the particular disease they cause. Koch's Postulates consist of four rules for determining the relationship of a microbe to a disease (Table 2.2). They are that one must (1) isolate the disease-causing microorganism from all cases of the disease but not from healthy individuals; (2) grow the microorganism in pure culture; (3) induce the disease with the cultured microorganism in some experimental animal; and (4) reisolate the microorganism from the diseased animal.

These rules have both great utility and severe limitations. The limitations can best be understood if one considers the fluidity and variety of host-parasite relationships. Some hints of this fluidity and variety can be seen from our discussion of the normal microbial populations in the preceding sections.

There is little trouble using Koch's Postulates to define the relationship between a highly virulent pathogen and the disease it causes. Such a relationship, however, is the exception and not the rule. Problems arise particularly in application of the rules to microbes of low virulence and to microbes that may be opportunistic pathogens. In the latter groups, one finds many organisms that are a part of the normal microbial population associated with plants and animals.

The association of potentially pathogenic microorganisms with healthy hosts makes application of the second part of the first postulate problematic. In such cases, one cannot show that the pathogen is always absent for healthy individuals. The best-documented examples of the maintenance of a pathogenic microbe in healthy humans are those for *Salmonella typhi, Corynebacterium diphtheriae*, and *Neisseria gonorrhoeae*. A woman named Mary, later known as "Typhoid Mary," was a cook. Wherever she worked, people developed typhoid fever. It was shown that she shed *S. typhi* in large numbers in her feces. She contaminated her hands when cleaning herself and then contaminated the food she handled. No carrier of *C. diphtheriae* or *N. gonorrhoeae* has ever become as famous as Typhoid Mary, but these organisms can be cultured from the mouths and vaginas, respectively, of some healthy people. These healthy carriers are often reservoirs of infection between epidemics. In recognition of this problem, the requirement that the organisms be absent from healthy individuals is commonly deleted when the postulates are stated.

The first part of the first postulate, which requires that the organism always be present in all cases of the disease, may not be true of certain diseases. Some causative organisms, for example, need not themselves be present in the host to cause disease. The ingestion of the toxin of *Clostridium botulinum* with food is sufficient to produce the disease botulism. This makes application of the first part of the first postulate inappropriate for this disease.

The first part of the first postulate may be impossible to fulfill in other cases also. One cannot always expect the same organism to be present in all cases of the disease. To explain this anomaly one must recognize that there are only a limited number of ways in which disease may manifest itself. Infection in the lungs by any of many different organisms may produce pneumonia. Hepatitis may be produced by a variety of viruses as well as by other agents. Diarrheas are also caused by many types of organisms. As a consequence, it may not be possible to isolate the same organism from all cases of a given disease.

The second postulate, requiring not only the isolation of the microorganism but its growth in pure culture, may also be difficult to fulfill. Growth in culture has been particularly difficult for some bacteria such as *Mycobacterium leprae*, the cause of leprosy, and the spirochete that causes syphilis, *Treponema pallidum*. Viruses are a particularly difficult case. They cannot be cultivated apart from living cells. Many other obligate parasites also cannot be cultivated without a host cell. In such cases growth of the organism in association with suitable host cells may be accepted as equivalent to pure culture.

Restriction in host range may be a serious handicap to the study of some human pathogens. The third postulate cannot be fulfilled if no suitable experimental host is available. Until recently, for example, no experimental host could be infected with Hanson's bacillus (*Mycobacterium leprae*). This prevented fulfillment of the third postulate for leprosy. Today it is known that the organism will grow in the armadillo. Even when an experimental host has been found in which an organism may grow, the disease produced may not resemble that in the definitive host. These are a few of the factors limiting the utility of Koch's Postulates, or at least making it necessary to consider their application with some discretion.

SUMMARY

Parasitism is a life-style that has been adopted by a wide range of types of organisms. In the usage of the term followed in this book, *parasitism* is a subdivision of the broad term *symbiosis* which simply means living together. Parasitism in this usage carries an implication of actual or potential harm to one member of the symbiotic pair, the one designated the host.

The degree of damage to the host, or whether damage occurs at all, is a result of the interaction of the parasite's ability to cause damage and the host's ability to resist the actions of the parasite. Some parasites are only occasionally able to cause disease and are thus called facultative or opportunistic parasites. Others are highly virulent and always cause disease when they enter their host.

The importance of the host's ability to resist the production of disease in the host-parasite interplay has been dramatically revealed by the AIDS epidemic, a situation in which the infecting agent destroys certain aspects of the host's disease-controlling mechanisms causing sickness and death in the host by organisms normally, or at least often, present but causing little or no harm.

The relationship of parasites to disease production was first made clear by Louis Pasteur and interestingly grew out of his studies on wine production and wine spoilage. His studies led him to the conclusion that fermentation as in wine spoilage was a microbial process, and he recognized the similarity of microbial spoilage of wine and disease in man and other animals. Robert Koch systemized the study of the relationship of microbial actions to disease and formulated a set of rules (the Koch's Postulates) for concluding that a particular organism caused a particular disease. Perhaps his greatest contribution to the clarification of the relationship of microorganisms to disease was his development of technologies for isolation and culture of microorganisms.

SUGGESTIONS FOR FURTHER READING

1. Burnet, F. MacFarlane and D.O. White. *Natural History of Infectious Diseases*. Cambridge: The University Press, 1972.
2. Kreier, J.P. and J.R. Baker. *Parasitic Protozoa*. London: Allen & Unwin, 1987.
3. Kreier J.P., ed. *Parasitic Protozoa*, 2d ed. San Diego: Academic Press, 1991.
4. Mims, C.A. *The Pathogenesis of Infectious Diseases*. 3d ed. New York/London: Academic Press, 1988.
5. Nesse R.M., and G.C. Williams. *Why We Get Sick*. New York: Times Books, Random House, 1994.
6. Smith H., J.J. Skohal, and M.J. Turner., eds. *The Molcular Basis of Microbial Pathogenicity*. Weinhein, Germany: Verlag Chemie Weinheim, 1980.
7. Trager, W. *Living Together: The Biology of Parasitism.* New York: Plenem Press, 1986.
8. Whitefield P.J. *The Biology of Parasitism.* Baltimore, MD: University Park Press, 1979.

QUESTIONS

1. What types of organisms are parasites?
2. What are the subdivisions in the category symbiosis?
3. How does infection differ from disease?
4. Where in the human body would you expect to find normal microbial colonization and where is sterility the normal condition?
5. List Koch's Postulates and describe their limitations.

ANSWERS

1. Many types of organism are parasites. Multicellular organisms such as worms and insects, syncytial organisms such as some fungi, unicellular forms such as bacteria, fungi, and protozoa, and acellular forms such as the viruses.
2. Symbiotic relationships may be divided into mutualistic ones in which both partners benefit, commensal ones in which one benefits and the other is not harmed, and parasitic in which one—the parasitic partner—is benefitted and the other—the host—is harmed.
3. Infection is the entry into and colonization of a host by a parasite; whereas disease is a disorder that may result from the colonization. Not all infections cause disease and not all diseases are a result of infection.
4. The skin, mouth, colon, nose, lower genital tract and rectum are all heavily colonized by microorganisms. The lungs, bladder, uterus, urethra, kidneys, peritoneal cavity and most tissues are normally sterile.
5. 1. The microorganism must be present in all cases of the disease and absent from healthy persons; 2. The microorganism must be isolated from the diseased individual and grown in pure culture; 3. The disease must be induced by the inoculation

of the pure culture of the isolated organism into a suitable experimental animal; 4. The microorganism must be isolated from the experimental animal in which the disease is produced.

Problems arise in application of the rules to diseases produced by microbes of low or opportunistic virulence. Such organisms are often found in healthy individuals. There are also healthy carriers of organisms normally highly virulent. Some diseases may have more than one cause, pneumonia and hepatitis are examples of such diseases. A suitable experimental animal may not be available for study of the disease as many parasites are quite host-specific and some parasites, including all viruses, cannot be grown in pure culture.

INTRODUCTION
THE EXTERNAL DEFENSE
  SYSTEMS
  The Skin
  The Mucosa
  The Respiratory Tract
  The Mouth
  The Digestive Tract
  The Urogenital Tract
  The Eye
THE INTERNAL DEFENSE
  SYSTEMS
  The Morphology and
    Development of
    Phagocytic Cells
  Chemotaxis
  Phagocytosis
  Opsonization
  Ingestion
  Oxygen-Dependent
    Killing of Microbes
  Oxygen-Independent
  Killing of Microbes
  Destruction of Ingested
  Microorganisms
SUMMARY
SUGGESTIONS FOR
  FURTHER READING
QUESTIONS
ANSWERS

CHAPTER **3**

Constitutive Host Resistance

Cynthia Baldwin

INTRODUCTION

Constitutive, or natural, resistance is the result of the actions of a number of systems. These may be differentiated into external or internal systems. Among the external systems are the skin and mucous membranes which protect by inhibiting entry of microbes into the body, and various antimicrobial substances secreted onto the skin and mucous membranes that inhibit microbial colonization. The internal systems are those which inhibit colonization by microbes which succeed in passing the external systems. These include a variety of antimicrobial substances in the blood and body fluids, and a variety of phagocytic cells. The internal systems come into play following injuries that breach the physical barriers and permit entry of microbes into the body.

The nature of the constitutive resistance systems varies to some extent from species to species and is also affected by the environment. Important factors in determining effectiveness of the constitutive resistance systems include nutritional status, injury, and age.

THE EXTERNAL DEFENSE SYSTEMS

The first lines of defense against infection are the external systems. A major component of the external systems is the mechanical barriers; the effectiveness of which is enhanced by various antimicrobial secretions (Figure 3.1). The mechanical barriers to microbial invasion of animals are formidable.

The Skin

The skin covers most of the external surface of the body. It is continuous with the mucosa at the body's orifices. The mucosa lines the lumens of all of the hollow organs that connect to the body's orifices. The skin is the largest organ

27

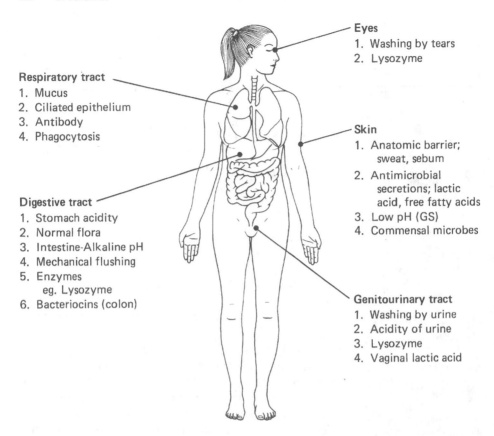

Eyes
1. Washing by tears
2. Lysozyme

Respiratory tract
1. Mucus
2. Ciliated epithelium
3. Antibody
4. Phagocytosis

Skin
1. Anatomic barrier; sweat, sebum
2. Antimicrobial secretions; lactic acid, free fatty acids
3. Low pH (GS)
4. Commensal microbes

Digestive tract
1. Stomach acidity
2. Normal flora
3. Intestine-Alkaline pH
4. Mechanical flushing
5. Enzymes
   eg. Lysozyme
6. Bacteriocins (colon)

Genitourinary tract
1. Washing by urine
2. Acidity of urine
3. Lysozyme
4. Vaginal lactic acid

Figure 3.1.   Many factors mediate natural resistance to penetration of the external surface of humans and other animals by parasites. The physical barriers, the skin and mucous membranes, are of primary importance in this resistance. The lumens of the digestive, respiratory, and genitourinary tracts are considered external since the epithelia lining these organs forms a continuous layer with the skin. Some factors enhancing the effectiveness of the physical barriers are listed in this figure.

in the body, weighing up to 5 kg in adult humans. The skin provides a tough, dry surface that is resistant to penetration. In some areas, hair masses protect the skin from injury. The skin is constantly lubricated by sweat and sebum. These glandular secretions contain lactic acid and free fatty acids which inhibit microbial growth. The low pH (about pH 5.5) of the skin surface, which is in part determined by the lactic acid and free fatty acids, also provides a poor environment for many pathogenic microorganisms.

The skin normally has microbes growing on it. These organisms, which are adapted to life on the skin, may prevent colonization by pathogens by filling up available space and utilizing attachment sites and available nutrients.

The Mucosa
The mucosa lining the lumens of the hollow organs of the body, which connect to the body's orifices, provides a barrier in these locations as the skin does for the external surfaces. Since many essential exchanges, such as gas exchange in the lungs

and nutrient absorption in the intestines, must occur across the mucosa lining hollow organs, these membranes cannot be as effective a barrier as the skin.

The mucosa has several associated systems that aid in preventing microbial colonization and penetration. These include a layer of mucus which is constantly renewed, and in some mucosal surfaces, ciliated cells that move the mucus layer in an ordered fashion to sweep out particles that adhere to it.

The Respiratory Tract

In the respiratory tract, the mucus layer and ciliated cells together are called the ciliary escalator system. Both the upper and lower respiratory tracts are protected from inhaled particles by the ciliary escalator system. The mucus on the mucosa in the nasal cavity traps many inhaled particles. The turbinates, which act as baffles for the airflow, increase the surface for trapping. The cilia in the nasal mucosa keep the film of mucus moving toward the mouth. The particles trapped in the mucus are swallowed when they reach the mouth. Small particles ($\leq$0.5 um) may escape trapping in the nose and are inhaled into the lower tract. They may be trapped in the mucus in the trachea and broncheoles or enter the alveoli of the lungs where they are ingested by phagocytic cells. The particles trapped in the mucus in the trachea and bronchioles, and those ingested by cells in the alveoli, are moved upward within the mucus secretion by the mucociliary escalator. The ciliated cells in the lower tract are similar to those that line the upper respiratory tract. The mucus is swept upward at a rate of about 1 cm per hour to the back of the mouth where it is swallowed. Sneezing and coughing may also aid removal of material from the respiratory system.

The Mouth

The mouth is normally populated with microorganisms. Some adhere to the teeth and some to the cheeks and gums. Saliva constantly enters the mouth. The tongue cleans the teeth, and swallowing removes the saliva and loosened particles as well as the mucus from the respiratory tract. Organisms which do not adhere cannot persist in this environment.

In addition to the mechanical cleaning systems in the mouth, there are chemical ones. Saliva, for example, contains lysozyme, an enzyme that digests the cell walls of bacteria, especially Gram-positive microorganisms, and thus destroys many pathogens.

As noted in the previous section, microorganisms entering the mouth from the respiratory system are cleared by swallowing. Swallowed microorganisms enter the digestive tract.

The Digestive Tract

The human digestive tract is protected from swallowed microbes by the antimicrobial environment of the stomach. The high acidity (pH = 2.0–3.0) of the human stomach is very effective in killing ingested microbes. The small intestine has an alkaline pH but contains abundant proteolytic enzymes that may inhibit microbial growth. The movement of intestinal contents may keep normal populations down by sweeping microbes out of the small intestine. The large intestine, unlike the stomach and small intestine, characteristically contains many bacteria. Gram-negative microorganisms within the normal flora secrete substances called bacteriocins that inhibit growth of many pathogens. They also prevent the establishment of pathogens by competing for food and space. The normal movement of food and feces through the intestinal tract prevents many pathogens from establishing themselves there. Clearance is most effective against organisms that cannot adhere to the mucosa.

The Urinogenital Tract
The urinogenital tract is protected primarily by mechanical barriers and flushing mechanisms. Sterile urine flushes the urinary tract every five or eight hours, removing nonadherent organisms and preventing the adherence of microorganisms to all but the outermost portions.

The vagina has a tough epithelium and during the period of sexual activity the epithelium produces secretions rich in carbohydrates, which support a normal population of lactic acid-producing bacteria. The low pH (pH ~ 5.0) produced within the vagina by the lactic acid-producing bacteria is inhibitory to many pathogens.

The Eye
The conjuctiva, the membrane surrounding the eye, is protected chiefly through the flushing action of tears. Tears continually bathe the eye, and fluid movement is enhanced through the action of blinking. When the eye is irritated, tears are produced in large volumes. This enhances the mechanical flushing of the eye. Tears also contain large amounts of lysozyme which, as noted previously, lyses many bacteria.

THE INTERNAL DEFENSE SYSTEMS
Microbes that by one means or another succeed in passing the external barriers and associated defense systems next encounter the second line of defense, the internal systems. These include, as mentioned earlier, a variety of antimicrobial substances in the blood and body fluids and a variety of phagocytic cells. The phagocytic cells are a major factor in this line of defense.

The Morphology and Development of Phagocytic Cells
In mammals there are two classes of phagocytes, the mononuclear and the polymorphonuclear phagocytes. These cells are part of the leukocyte system, which includes, in addition, the lymphocytes important in the inducible system (Figure 3.2).

The mononuclear and polymorphonuclear phagocytes are produced in the bone marrow from a common stem cell (Figure 3.3). The stem cells committed to produce polymorphonuclear leukocytes differentiate into myeloblasts, and those that will produce mononuclear phagocytes differentiate into monoblasts. The sequence for polymorphonuclear leukocyte differentiation requires four cell divisions; each results in a progressive decrease in cell size and an increase in nuclear compaction. The compact nucleus ultimately assumes the characteristic polymorphonuclear shape. The myeloblast gives rise to promyelocytes that divide to produce first myelocyte I cells, then myelocyte II cells. The myelocyte II cells give rise to metamyelocytes. Following the production of the metamyelocyte, no further cell division occurs. The metamyelocytes develop into band cells that become segmented cells and, finally, mature polymorphonuclear leukocytes as they leave the bone marrow and enter the blood. Under conditions of stress, such as is caused by infection, immature forms such as band cells may enter the blood.

The mononuclear phagocyte is derived from the monoblast. The monoblast pro-

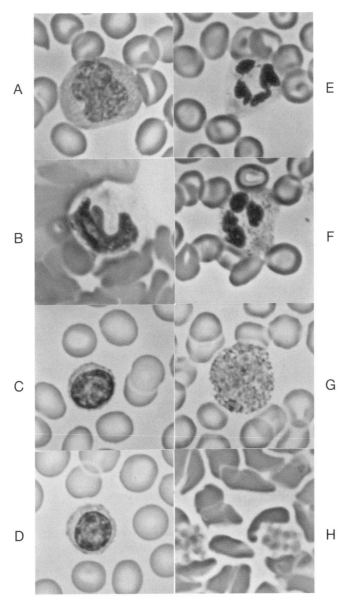

Figure 3.2. Photomicrographs of cells in Giemsa stained blood films. The morphology of the various leukocytes in human blood, including monocytes (A, B), lymphocytes (C, D), poly-morphonuclear neutrophils (E, F), eosinophils (G), and platelets (H), is shown. Monocytes have a relatively large, often bean-shaped nucleus and extensive cytoplasm. Lymphocytes have a small, round, compact nucleus and a thin rim of cytoplasm. Polymorphonuclear neutro-phils have a multilobulated nucleus, the lobes of which are connected by thin strands of nuclear material. They have a poorly staining cytoplasm. Eosinophils have nuclei similar to polymorphonuclear neutrophils, but the cytoplasm is filled with eosinophilic granules which, in the example shown, almost obscure the nucleus. Platelets are anucleate fragments broken off from pseudopods produced by megokaryocytes which reside in the bone marrow. In the photomicrograph shown, there are two clumps of platelets, each containing eight to twelve platelets. The clumping results from handling of the blood during slide preparation. Erythro-cytes, roughly circular anucleate cells that in some cases were grossly distorted when the blood film was prepared, are visible in all of the micrographs.

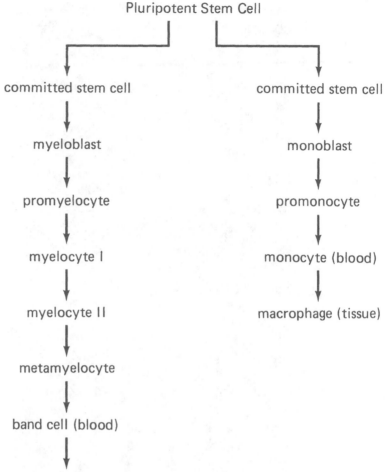

Pluripotent Stem Cell

committed stem cell

myeloblast

promyelocyte

myelocyte I

myelocyte II

metamyelocyte

band cell (blood)

committed stem cell

monoblast

promonocyte

monocyte (blood)

macrophage (tissue)

mature polymorphonuclear leukocyte (blood)

Figure 3.3. Differentiation of polymorphonuclear leukocytes and mononuclear phagocytes. A common stem cell in the bone marrow gives rise to committed stem cells that will form either polymorphonuclear leukocytes or macrophages. When polymorphonuclear leukocytes are produced, the stem cells give rise to myeloblasts that divide and differentiate into promyelocytes, myelocytes I and II, and metamyelocytes. The metamyelocytes mature with no further cell division into band cells, which in turn mature into segmented cells that enter the blood and become mature polymorphonuclear leukocytes. To form macrophages, the committed stem cell will divide and become a monoblast. The monoblasts differentiate into promonocytes. The promonocytes divide three times and differentiate into monocytes that enter the blood. The monocytes may leave the circulation and enter the tissues to become macrophages.

duces promonocytes thus divide three times before becoming monocytes. The maturation of the monocyte into the macrophage requires no further cell division. The monocyte enters the blood and circulates before it enters the tissues to become a macrophage.

Macrophages may be fixed at some site or may be free to wander, they are found throughout the body. Macrophages have a long life span. The maturation of the

Table 3.1. Enzyme content of granules and lysosomes in neutrophils and macrophages.

NEUTROPHILS		MACROPHAGES
Primary granules	*Secondary granules*	*Lysosomes*
acid hydrolases	lysozyme	acid hydrolases
neutral proteases	lactoferrin	neutral proteases
peroxidase		peroxidase
myeloperoxidase		myeloperoxidase
cationic proteins		lysozyme
lysozyme		

macrophage is influenced by the tissue environment, and the macrophages may take on different characteristics, depending on their anatomical location. This attribute of macrophages has resulted in a confusing nomenclature. For example, macrophages in the endothelial lining of the blood vessels of the liver are called *Kupffer cells*; macrophages in the connective tissue are referred to as *histiocytes*; those in the central nervous system are called *microglial cells*; and those in the skin are called *Langerhan's cells*. The phagocytic cells in the peritoneal cavity, lung, spleen and lymph nodes are just referred to as *macrophages* and are distinguished by their anatomical location. Macrophages found in the lung, for example, are called *alveolar macrophages* and those in the abdomen are called *peritoneal macrophages*.

The polymorphonuclear leukocytes are also known as *granulocytes* because of the many granules found in their cytoplasm. The contents of the granules determine the cell's staining properties and help to distinguish the different cells of the granulocytic series. Three types of granulocytes based on staining characteristics have been described. These are neutrophils, eosinophils, and basophils. The stain most commonly used to distinguish the cells is the Giemsa stain, an azure B eosinate. It is prepared by interaction between two basic dyes, azure B and methylene blue, and an acidic dye, eosin. The basophilic, or cationic, components react with the negatively charged molecules of the granules, staining them blue. The acidophilic, or anionic, component reacts with the positively charged molecules, staining them red. The granules of the neutrophil are not ionically charged at physiological pHs and thus do not stain; they assume a grey or neutral tint.

The granules of the neutrophil and eosinophil contain enzymes, whereas those within the basophil contain biologically active amines. The enzymes in the neutrophilic granules are important for the destruction and digestion of microorganisms and other foreign organic materials (Table 3.1). The granules are classified into two types: the primary or azurophilic granules, and the secondary, or specific, granules. The terms *primary* and *secondary* refer to the color or appearance of the granules during differentiation rather than to the importance of the granules. The azurophilic granules contain peroxidase, myeloperoxidase, acid hydrolases, neutral proteases, cationic antimicrobial proteins, and lysozyme. The neutral proteases include elastase, collagenase, and cathepsin G. Enzymes released by neutrophils will activate complement and generate kinins (see chapter 4); the enzymes therefore enhance vascular permeability and chemotaxis indirectly. The specific granules contain lactoferrin and lysozyme.

The polymorphonuclear neutrophil is the most abundant of the white blood cells in humans, comprising about forty-five to seventy percent of the circulating leukocytes. They have a life span of three to five days, are mobile, respond to chemotactic stimuli, and are highly phagocytic. They are among the first cells to accumulate at a site of injury.

The eosinophils play a major role in the defense against helminthic parasites such as *Trichinella* and *Schistosoma*. The basic protein found in the granules of these cells may be the major factor in killing of these parasites. The eosinophils attach to the surfaces of the parasites, probably with the aid of antibody, and discharge their granules against the parasites' surface, where they cause injury to the parasites' membranes. Eosinophils are much less phagocytic than are neutrophils. These cells make up one to two percent of the polymorphonuclear leukocytes.

Basophils function as carriers of inflammatory mediators. The granules of basophils contain histamine and other vasoactive compounds. The release of the contents of the granules serves to amplify the inflammatory response (see chapter 4). Basophils generally account for less than one percent of the granulocytic leukocytes.

Cells of the mononuclear phagocyte lineage initially contain granules; these are lost during differentiation. The mononuclear phagocytes, which comprise from two to eight percent of the circulating leukocytes, contain enzymes similar to those present in neutrophils (Table 3.1). The enzymes are contained within bags bounded by membranes, called *lysosomes*. The mononuclear phagocyte is long-lived and continues to synthesize enzymes throughout its life. The acid hydrolases of mononuclear phagocytes act at acidic pH and cleave phosphate ester bonds that occur in proteins, polysaccharides, lipids, and nucleic acids. The enzymes are distinguished by their substrates and include fucosidase, 5'nucleotidase, galactosidase, arylsulfatase, mannosidase, N-acetyl-glucosaminidase, glucuronidase, and glycerophosphatase. Other enzymes included in this group are responsible for protein hydrolysis and are called cathepsins A, B, and C, and so on. Neutral proteases include cathepsin G, whose substrates are cartilage, proteoglycans, fibrogen, and casein, and the enzymes, elastase and collagenase. The latter two enzymes have been shown to play an important role in the destruction of normal tissues that may occur during an inflammatory response. The peroxidase enzyme catalase protects the phagocytes from the toxic effects of the hydrogen peroxide produced following the binding and phagocytosis of foreign substances.

Chemotaxis
Phagocytic cells are attracted to an area of infection or tissue damage by microbial and by host-derived chemotactic factors. The host-derived chemotactic factors include components of the complement, clotting, fibrinolytic, and kinin systems that are activated either directly, by contact with microbes, or indirectly by the actions of proteolytic enzymes released by the invading microorganisms on damaged cells. The complement component $\overline{C5a}$ is a chemotactic factor.

Phagocytosis
Many of the antimicrobial substances in the blood and body fluids function by facilitating phagocytosis. Some antimicrobial substances, such as those of the complement system, act both by facilitating phagocytosis and by directly inducing damage to the membranes of the microbes. The direct antimicrobial actions of complement will be described fully in chapter 9 in the section entitled *Complement-Mediated Effector Mechanisms*.

Phagocytosis by single-cell animals is a feeding process. In multicellular organisms, the feeding process has increased significance, as it is a function of specialized

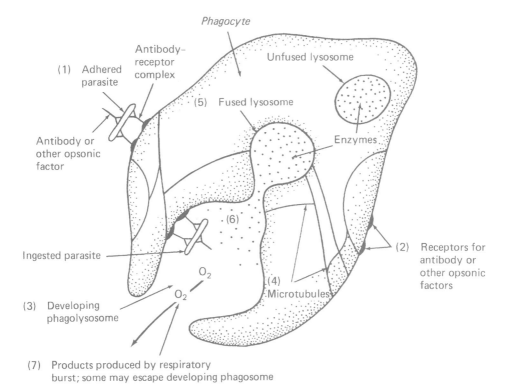

Figure 3.4.   Binding of an opsonized bacterium (1) to receptors on the surface of the phagocyte (2) results in initiation of phagocytosis (3) and the respiratory burst. Ingestion proceeds
with the aid of microtubles (4) by a series of actin-binding reactions. Fusion of the phagosome
with granules and lysosomes (5) results in the release of enzymes into the phagolysosome (6).
Some enzymes and other substances may escape from the developing phagolysosome under
some circumstances (7), as when the particle is too large to be ingested, for example.

cells that protect from infection and remove foreign material from the body. These
specialized cells, or phagocytes, scavenge foreign material, including microbes, that
may enter the body. They do this based on recognition mechanisms in their membranes and with the aid of constitutive and inducible opsonins. In addition to their
role as scavenger cells, the phagocytes participate in the inflammatory response and
initiate and regulate the inducible immune response which develops in vertebrates
following the breaching by parasites of the physical barriers to infection.

Opsonization
Once the phagocytes have arrived, they must bind to the foreign object through
membrane receptors for phagocytosis to occur. The phagocyte may recognize inert
particles through electrostatic bonds and hydrophobic interactions that do not form
with the hydrophilic surfaces of the animal's own cells. Some inert materials, such
as carbon particles, are only ingested following coating with serum proteins. The
specificity for recognition of the particles as foreign in such cases is a function of
the serum protein. These serum proteins also have sites recognized by receptors on
the phagocytes and thus serve as a bridge between the phagocyte and its target
(Figure 3.4).
   The process of preparation of a particle for ingestion by coating with serum pro-

tein is called opsonization. Opsonins are substances in the serum that coat particles and cause them to be engulfed by phagocytic cells. The most important of the opsonins in serum are antibodies, the $\overline{C3b}$ component of the complement system, and fibronectin (see chapter 4).

Antibodies are components of the inducible immune response and will be considered fully in chapter 7. The complement system is involved in both the constitutive and the inducible systems. The complement system is a group of serum proteins which activate each other sequentially following activation of the initial component by contact with permissible surfaces of microbes or other foreign material, or by contact with immune complexes in the body. When involved in the constitutive defense, complement is activated through the alternate pathway. When involved in the inducible response, activation is through the classical pathway. In the latter case, combination of antibody with the microbe or other target initiates activation of C1; in the former, direct binding of the constitutive serum protein—the complement component C3—with the microbe or other target initiates the process (Figure 3.5).

The surfaces of many nonpathogenic microorganisms contain components that initiate the complement cascade by the alternate pathway. It would perhaps be better to say that many microorganisms are nonpathogenic because they activate complement through the alternate pathway and are thus opsonized and phagocytized by constitutive mechanisms.

By definition, pathogenic microorganisms are those that have the ability to evade or negate the various constitutive defense mechanisms. This is illustrated by the case of the pneumococcus. The antiphagocytic components covering the microbe's surface protect it. After antibody is produced as part of the inducible response, it binds the antiphagocytic components. The microbe is thus opsonized and then may be phagocytized. The inducible response thus negates the mechanism used by the microbe to evade the host's constitutive defense. It is probable that complement, acting as a constitutive opsonin following activation by the alternate pathway, is the older mechanism of defense, having evolved earlier than the inducible system.

Fibronectin is a high molecular-weight serum protein that facilitates binding of most particles to phagocytic cells. It is thus an important constitutive opsonin. The opsonic activity of fibronectin is actually an attribute of fragments produced by proteolytic enzymes. These enzymes are active at sites of injury and microbial invasion, and thus activate the opsonic fibronectin system at sites where it is needed. Since the formation of antibody after infection requires time, the constitutive opsonins $\overline{C3b}$ and fibronectin, which are always present in serum, are probably the most important opsonins active soon after injury. Other serum proteins, such as the acute phase reactants, including C-reactive protein, may also be constitutive opsonins.

Ingestion
After attachment of an opsonized particle to the phagocyte, the phagocyte will surround the particle by forming pseudopods. The extent to which the phagocyte surrounds the opsonized particle is directly proportional to the extent of opsonization. The pseudopods move along the particle in a zipper-like fashion from one opsonizing molecule to the next until the particle is completely surrounded by pseudopodia which then fuse.

The exact mechanism by which the pseudopods surround the particle is only

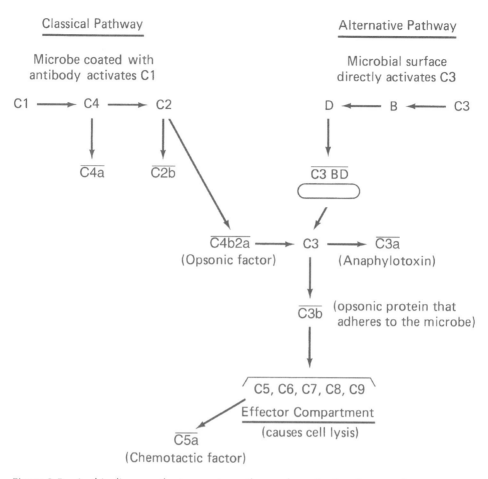

Figure 3.5. In this diagram, the two major pathways for activating the complement system are shown, along with the common components that make up the effector compartment. Factors B and D of the alternative pathway are distinct from C1, C4, and C2 of the classical pathway. C3 is common to both pathways. During activation by the classical pathway, C1 binds to the antibody-coated microbe and activates C4 and C2 simultaneously. The $\overline{C4b2a}$ complex serves as a C3 convertase to activate more C3. In the alternative pathway, C3 binds directly to the microbe's surface as a complex with factor B and is activated. Factor B binds factor D. A complex of factors B, D, and activated $\overline{C3b}$ is thus generated on the microbe's membrane and converts additional C3. $\overline{C3b}$ and $\overline{C4b}$ are opsonic; $\overline{C3a}$ and $\overline{C4a}$ are anaphylatoxins, $\overline{C4b}$ is formed when C4 is activated. The components C5 through C9 are activated in numberical order and form a very large complex of factor C9 that is inserted into the microbe's membranes and results in the lysis of the bacterium or other microbe that has entered the body. One of the products of activation of C5 is $\overline{C5a}$, a strongly chemotactic factor.

partially understood. Nonetheless it is clear that the contact of the particle with the phagocyte's membrane activates actin-binding protein in the cytoplasm. These proteins promote the assembly of actin molecules and gelation of the actin in the cytoplasm underlying the attachment site. Myosin binds to polymerized actin and then the molecules contract, producing movement of the pseudopods around the particle being engulfed. Orientation of the microfilaments and their points of attachment to the cell membrane determine the form and direction of pseudopodial extension. The pseudopod moves around the particle by a series of reactions initiated by additional membrane-particle contact (Figure 3.4). Once a microbe or other particle is within the cell, it is surrounded by the cell membrane that lines the phagocytic vacuole or phagosome.

For protection to result, it is of course not enough for the phagocyte just to ingest a microbe; it must also kill it. The killed microbe or other ingested particle must then be disposed of. The killing of ingested microbes and the destruction of ingested material is carried out by a variety of mechanisms. The mechanisms by which phagocytic cells kill microorganisms can be classified as either oxygen-dependent or oxygen-independent.

Oxygen-Dependent Killing of Microbes

In the oxygen-dependent reactions, adherence of a particle to the phagocyte's surface initiates a series of biochemical changes within the phagocyte that are collectively called the *respiratory burst* (Figure 3.6). The final result of these changes is production of superoxide, singlet oxygen, hydrogen peroxide, and hypochlorite in the phagolysosome; these oxidize proteins and lipids in the microbe, thereby causing its death.

The first event in the series of events which constitute the respiratory burst is the activation of the oxidase that catalyzes the transfer of one or two electrons from NADPH to oxygen and results in the formation of superoxide and hydrogen peroxide. During the course of this reaction, highly reactive oxygen intermediates are formed. These are superoxide ions, peroxide ions and hydroxyl radicals. Singlet oxygen has two unoccupied electron orbits in its outer valence orbit. It is the reduction of oxygen by the acquisition of electrons in this outer valence orbit that produces the superoxide ions and peroxide ions. The hydroxyl radicals are formed by the Haber-Weiss or Fenton reaction when the superoxide ions react with hydrogen peroxide in the presence of iron or copper.

During the course of the reactions involved in the respiratory burst, oxygen is energized and an atomic rearrangement occurs. As a result of this, the valence electrons move from their normal orbits to orbits at a higher energy state. These energized forms of oxygen are unstable, and when their electrons return to the ground state, energy is released as photons, which can be detected as emitted light. The resulting emitted light, or chemoluminescence, is a sensitive indicator of the occurrence of the respiratory burst.

As noted previously, among the metabolites of oxygen that are known to participate in microbial killing are hydrogen peroxide, which occurs in millimolar concentrations within the phagolysosome and hypochlorite. Hydrogen peroxide has only moderate antimicrobial activity by itself, because bacteria make catalase to neutralize hydrogen peroxide, and because a number of substances programmed by stress response genes are used by bacteria to resist the effects of hydrogen peroxide. Without the products produced by these genes, the bacteria may be very susceptible to hydrogen peroxide killing. The major contribution of hydrogen peroxide to microbial killing is indirect. It appears to be through the generation of hypohalites via the myeloperoxidase-halide system. Myeloperoxidase is known to catalyze the reduction by hydrogen peroxide of halide ions to hypohalite. The hypohalites formed are hypochlorite, hypoiodite and hypobromite, depending on the halide ion oxidized (Figure 3.6). These halide compounds may directly affect microorganisms or may further react with hydrogen peroxide to form singlet oxygen, which is also a strong oxidizing agent.

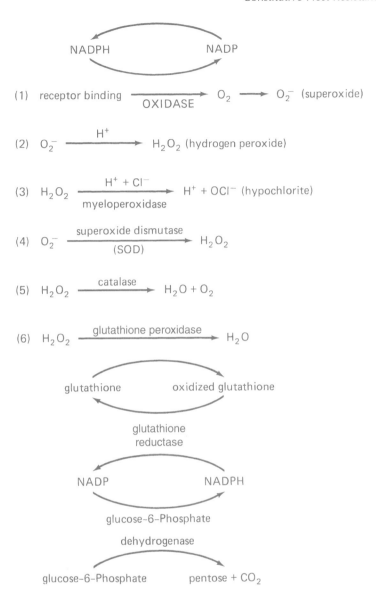

(1) receptor binding $\xrightarrow[\text{OXIDASE}]{}$ $O_2 \longrightarrow O_2^-$ (superoxide)

(2) $O_2^- \xrightarrow{H^+} H_2O_2$ (hydrogen peroxide)

(3) $H_2O_2 \xrightarrow[\text{myeloperoxidase}]{H^+ + Cl^-} H^+ + OCl^-$ (hypochlorite)

(4) $O_2^- \xrightarrow[\text{(SOD)}]{\text{superoxide dismutase}} H_2O_2$

(5) $H_2O_2 \xrightarrow{\text{catalase}} H_2O + O_2$

(6) $H_2O_2 \xrightarrow{\text{glutathione peroxidase}} H_2O$

glutathione ⟶ oxidized glutathione

glutathione
reductase

NADP ⟶ NADPH

glucose-6-Phosphate

dehydrogenase

glucose-6-Phosphate ⟶ pentose + CO_2

Hexose Monophosphate shunt

Figure 3.6. O_2-dependent reactions occur within phagocytes during the respiratory burst. The respiratory burst is initiated by binding of an opsonized particle to a phagocyte. This binding may initiate ingestion and activation of an oxidase enzyme, resulting in the production of superoxide within the developing phagosome; NADPH is converted to NADP in this process: (1) the superoxide is converted to hydrogen peroxide (2) within the phagosome by addition of a hydrogen ion. Fusion of lysosomes or granules with the phagosome introduces myeloperoxidase and halides (I_2, Cl_2, or Br_2) into the phagosome (now called a *phagolysosome*). The introduced enzymes and halides produce a hypohalite, hypochlorite (OCl-), that will cause halogenation of microbial proteins and lipids and will kill the microbe (3). Reactions 4 through 6 are a mechanism to inactivate any H_2O_2 that may escape from the phagolysosome and thus protect the cell. (4) Superoxide is dismutated to H_2O_2, that is acted on by catalase (5) to form H_2O and O_2. Reaction (6) results in inactivation of H_2O_2 by oxidation of glutathione.

Several mechanisms have been proposed for the killing of bacteria and other microbes by products of the myeloperoxidase-halide-hydrogen peroxidase system. These mechanisms include halogenation of microbial proteins, with subsequent loss of structure and function of the protein, the oxidative decarboxylation of amino acids, with the generation of toxic aldehydes, and the oxidation of thiol groups in enzymes, which may result in inactivation of enzymes that are vital to microbial function.

Oxidation or halogenation of carbon bonds present in unsaturated fats and lipids may also occur. Lipids are essential components of the cell walls and membranes of all cells, including those of bacteria. The oxidation of lipids can lead to alterations in membrane structure and function, and can be as serious to microbial survival as is damage to microbial proteins.

Oxygen-Independent Killing of Microbes

The oxygen-independent antimicrobial activities of phagocytes result from the actions of materials from lysosomes and from the components of granules in the phagocyte cytoplasm. Fusion of the phagosome with cytoplasmic granules and lysosomes results in introduction into the phagosome of materials which cause acidification. The result is the lowering of the pH of the phagolysosome containing the microorganisms from neutrality to a pH of from 3.0 to 6.0. Some microorganisms are directly killed by the low pH or by the organic acids in the phagolysosome. The acidification of the phagosome also provides the optimal environment for action of enzymes such as myeloperoxidase and the acid hydrolases that digest microbes.

Another oxygen-independent antimicrobial mechanism acts through lysozyme. Lysozyme acts by attacking the beta 1-4 glycosidic linkage that joins the N-acetyl muramic acid and N-acetyl glucosamine in the bacterial cell wall. In most intact bacteria, these bonds are buried in the cell wall and are not generally accessible to the enzyme. However, the action of a combination of hydrogen peroxide and vitamin C in the acidic environment within the phagolysosome exposes these bonds and facilitates the action of lysozyme.

Many polycationic proteins that have antimicrobial activity have been described. Both large (50,000 daltons) and small polycationic proteins (10,000 to 25,000 daltons) are present in phagolysosomes. These inhibit respiration and the synthesis of protein, DNA, and RNA, and increase the permeability of bacterial cell membranes. The sensitivity of microorganisms to cationic proteins varies with the microbial species.

Lactoferrin, a protein which occurs in the phagocyte's granules, has a strong affinity for iron. It competes with the microorganisms for iron, a growth requirement of bacteria. Lactoferrin is usually secreted by the neutrophil into the extracellular environment, where it acts, and is rarely found in the phagosome. Limiting intracellular iron may be achieved by activating the macrophage with a cytokine interferon-gamma that is produced by types of lymphocytes known as natural killer cells and T lymphocytes. When activated by interferon-gamma, the transferrin receptors on the macrophage membrane are decreased in number thereby decreasing transport of iron into the cell by iron-loaded transferrin.

Phagocytes from some species of animals also contain small antimicrobial molecules called defensins. They are a family of small cytotoxic peptides first identified in rabbit macrophages but also are found in polymorphonuclear neutrophils in other species. These molecules can kill microbes even in a cell-free system suggesting that they may be powerful enough to kill the microbes without assistance from other components of the phogocyte antimicrobial defense. There is evidence that they use multiple mechanisms to kill microbes including permeabilizing the outer and inner cell membranes which changes the protonmotive force of the membrane and exposes it to otherwise membrane impermeant molecules.

Macrophages also produce nitric oxide which is lethal to many microbes including bacteria and protozoan parasites. It is made when the guanido nitrogen of arginine is oxidized which leads to generation of nitric oxide, which is extremely unstable, and its metabolites nitrate and nitrite. The production of nitric oxide is increased when macrophages are activated by interferon-gamma although low levels are constitutively made. Its antimicrobial activities may stem from its ability to scavenge iron from enzymes among other mechanisms.

Destruction of Ingested Microorganisms

The destruction of the microorganisms killed by the various means in the phagocytes and the destruction of other ingested biodegradable material is carried out by enzymes. These enzymes, which are similar to enzymes of the digestive tract, generally are present in the lysosomes of the phagocytes. The fusion of the lysosomes with the phagosomes results in the exposure of the phagocytized material in the vacuole to the enzymes. The fusion of the lysosomes with the phagosome and the subsequent activation of the enzymes only within the phagolysosome protects the phagocyte's cytoplasm from damage by the enzymes. Some of the enzymes may escape from the phagosome through the membrane channel formed when fusion of the pseudopods is occurring, or the enzymes may be liberated as a result of cell death. These extracellular enzymes are probably responsible for the tissue injury that may occur during inflammatory reactions. They may, also as noted previously, activate the fibronectin system.

SUMMARY

The barrier system of immunity is the first component of a host that microbes encounter and must survive in order to infect a host. It includes physical, chemical, microbial, and mechanical components. Following a breach of the barrier system microbes encounter phagocytes, including monocytes, macrophages, and polymorphonuclear neutrophils, which are cells professionally adept at eating (or phagocytosing) microbes. Phagocytosis may be facilitated by opsonins which include antibody molecules and components of complement which serve to "tie" the microbe to the phagocytic cell. Following phagocytosis the microbes must withstand a series of reactive oxygen intermediates, nitric oxide, antimicrobial peptides known as defensins, low pH, limited iron and a series of enzymes in order to survive. Most do not survive and are digested by the phagocyte thus preventing establishment of an infection.

SUGGESTIONS FOR FURTHER READING

1. Bogdan, C. "Of Microbes, Macrophages and Nitric Oxide." *Behring Inst. Mitt.* 99 (1997):58–72.
2. Fearon, D.T., and W. Wong, "Complement Ligand Receptor Interactions that Mediate Biological Responses." *Ann. Rev. Immunol.* 1 (1983):243.
3. Fleming, S.D., and P.A. Campbell, "Some Macrophages Kill *Listeria Monocytogenes* While Others Do Not." *Immunol. Rev.* 158 (1997):69–77.

4. Gallin, J.I., I.M. Goldstein, and R. Snyderman. *Inflammation: Basic Principles and Clinical Correlates*. New York: Raven Press, 1992.
5. Kagan, B.L., T. Ganz, and R.I. Lehrer, "Defensins: A Family of Antimicrobial and Cytotoxic Peptides." *Toxicology* 87 (1994): 131–149.
6. Silverstein, S.C., S. Greenberg, F. DiVirgilio, and T.H. Steinberg. "Phagocytosis." In *Fundamental Immunology*. Edited by W.E. Paul, 703. New York: Raven Press, 1989.
7. Snyderman, R., and M.C. Pike. "Chemoattractant Receptors on Phagocytic Cells." *Ann. Revs. Immunol.* 2 (1984):257.
8. Weinberg, E.D. "Iron Depletion: A Defense Against Intracellular Infection and Neoplasia." *Life Sci.* 50 (1992):1289–1297.
9. Weiss, J. "Leukocyte-Derived Antimicrobial Proteins." *Curr. Opin. Hematol.* 1:78–84, 1994.

QUESTIONS

1. The external system of constitutive immunity has several components. List an example of a physical, a chemical, a microbial, and a mechanical barrier.
2. Why is the constitutive or natural resistance system also referred to as the innate system or as the nonadaptive system?
3. Both macrophages and polymorphonuclear neutrophils are part of the myeloid system and thus have similarities as well as differences. Are they similar or different with regard to:
   a. nuclear morphology.
   b. life span in the blood or tissues after they leave the bone marrow.
   c. phagocytosis.
   d. enzymes in their granules.
4. Since macrophages are the next line of defense following a breach of the barrier or external defense system, where would you expect to find macrophages?
5. Name six general mechanisms used by phagocytes to kill microbes following phagocytosis.

ANSWERS

1. Examples of physical barriers include the skin, the mucous membranes, saliva and mucous; chemical defenses include low pH on the skin and in the vagina and stomach, and lactic acid and fatty acids on the skin, as well as lysozyme in the saliva and tears; the microbial barriers include the normal flora on the skin, in the vagina and in the large intestine; the mechanical barriers include flushing by tears, sweat, and sebam, the ciliary escalator system, sneezing, coughing and intestinal peristalsis.
2. Because it is present at birth, it is the same in all animals of a species and its efficiency does not increase following infection or aging.
3. With regard to nuclear morphology the monocytes or macrophages have large, round or bean-shaped nuclei with extensive cytoplasm while polymorphonuclear neutrophils have a multilobulated nucleus consisting of lobes connected by thin strands of nuclear material. Neutrophils live for three to five days in the blood while monocytes migrate through the blood for a few days and then have a long life span in the tissues they reside in. Both are efficient phagocytic cells. For the enzymes in granules, see Table 3.1 which shows the enzymes in the primary and secondary granules of neutrophils and in the lysosomes of macrophages and you will discover that neutrophils contain additional components not found in macrophages.

4. Macrophages are expected to be under the skin and in tissues underlying the mucous membranes of the upper respiratory track and lungs and the mucosal lining of the gut and the peritoneal cavity. They are actually found there and also throughout the body including in the liver, which cleanses the blood coming from the intestines, and in the central nervous system. Macrophages in the capillary network of the lungs also clean particulate material from the blood passing through the lungs.

5. The general mechanisms include: reactive oxygen intermediates such as hydrogen peroxide, hydroxyl radicals, and hypochlorite; the acidic environment in the phagolysosomes; enzymes that digest microbes including lysozyme, which destroys the cell wall of bacteria; low iron availability resulting in nutritional starvation of the microbe; defensins, which are small antimicrobial peptides that insert themselves into the cell membranes of microbes; and nitric oxide, which interferes with microbial enzymes.

INTRODUCTION
OVERVIEW
LOCAL INFLAMMATORY
    EVENTS
Effects of Vasoactive Amines
    on the Microcirculation in
    the Inflamed Area
Effects of Prostaglandins and
    Leukotrienes on the
    Inflamed Area
Mediation of Inflammation
    by Blood Proteins
Blood Cell Movement into
    the Inflamed Area
SYSTEMIC CONSEQUENCES
    OF THE INFLAMMATORY
    REACTION
Induction of Fever
Stimulation of Production of
    Blood Cells by Colony-
    Stimulating Factor
Induction of Acute Phase
    Reactants
SUMMARY
SUGGESTIONS FOR
    FURTHER READING
QUESTIONS
ANSWERS

CHAPTER 4

The Inflammatory Response: A Bridge Between The Constitutive and Inducible Systems

Samuel J. Black

INTRODUCTION

This chapter describes the molecular and cellular basis of the inflammatory response, a set of parallel reactions that is conserved in all vertebrates and provides rapid but relatively nonspecific defense against microbes. The inflammatory response is initiated by all types of tissue damage and mediates both wound cleansing and healing.

OVERVIEW

Tissue damage elicits a complex series of events jointly called inflammation. This response occurs within minutes after injury and, as indicated in chapter 1, serves two purposes: to seal and repair the site of injury, and create a local environment that limits population expansion of any microbes that are present at the inflammatory site. It does not matter whether the tissue damage results from traumatic injury, a burn, surgery, the bite of an insect or tick, a tunneling worm, or a pocket of replicating microbes, the inflammatory response that arises in each case is the same although its magnitude and duration might differ dependent on the degree of tissue damage and whether or not damage is accompanied by infection.

The molecules that participate in inflammatory responses circulate in an inactive form in the blood and are present at low concentration in tissue fluids. They are activated by components of tissues that only become exposed after damage. The initial response to tissue damage occurs within minutes and is characterized by four cardinal signs: redness, swelling, heat, and pain. These signs result primarily from local change in blood flow, and the leakage of blood plasma into the inflammatory site. Vasoactive molecules generated in response to tissue damage induce local vasodilation, and the elevated

45

blood flow to the damage site results in redness and heat. Exudation of plasma from the blood vessel into the tissues at the inflammatory site causes swelling and pressure on nerve endings, which, together with local generation of prostaglandins, causes pain.

Some components of the inflammatory response, called opsonins, bind to microbes tagging them for engulfment (phagocytosis) and intracellular destruction by neutrophils and macrophages that are recruited to the inflammatory site. Activated neutrophils and macrophages also release a battery of water-soluble molecules some of which amplify the inflammatory response and others that help repair tissue damage by stimulating replication of fibroblasts and the deposition of extracellular matrix. Products of activated macrophages can also cause a fever response and loss of body weight by mechanisms that are discussed below. Some of the soluble mediators of inflammation contribute to the development of the acquired immune response by binding to specific receptors on lymphocytes.

Leakage of plasma at the inflammatory site causes collection of edematous fluid which exerts pressure on local lymphatic vessels. This causes flap valves on the lymphatic vessels to open and the fluid to drain. Fragments of microbes in the edematous fluid are carried with the lymph to a local lymph node where they induce an acquired immune response. The acquired response typically takes several days to develop and when matured, is much more effective than the inflammatory response at eliminating microbes. In some cases, the combination of inflammation and an acquired immune response is unable to clear infection. When pathogen population expansion is restrained so that the microbes do not spread beyond their initial site of invasion, chronic inflammation may ensue leading to formation of an ulcer or a granuloma. In other cases, the host response cannot restrain pathogen population expansion, and the inflammatory response can become amplified so that the afflicted individual might die as a result of unrelenting fever, severe weight loss, and organ failure. Typically, however, the combined assault of the local inflammatory and acquired immune responses eliminates invading microbes, and with their elimination, the inflammatory response subsides and the tissue damage heals. All of the events between the initial damage and the final restoration of the integrity of the tissue may be considered parts of the inflammatory response. The inflammatory response brings to the site of injury and invasion the cells and molecules that affect the adaptive immune response and thus serves as a bridge between the constitutive and adaptive systems of host defense.

LOCAL INFLAMMATORY EVENTS
Effects of Vasoactive Amines on the Microcirculation in the Inflamed Area
There are dramatic changes in both the microcirculation and the distribution of blood cells at sites of tissue damage. The injury itself elicits a neurological response which, within seconds of injury, causes contraction of smooth muscle in blood vessels and a temporary decrease in blood flow to the area. The injury also causes the release of histamine and serotonin from tissue mast cells which store these substances in granules. The stimulus for mast cell degranulation is an influx of Ca^{++} which can result from exposure of the mast cell to complement breakdown fragments $\overline{C5a}$, $\overline{C3a}$, and $\overline{C4a}$, the generation of which is discussed below, or from the binding of antigen to antibody of the IgE class which absorbs onto the surface of mast cells. Production of IgE and its association with mast cells is discussed in a later chapter. Histamine and serotonin are also released from platelets that attach to endothelium lining blood vessels close to the site of tissue damage, and modified by exposure to injury-induced soluble mediators.

Histamine and serotonin are amines that have potent effects on smooth muscle. Within minutes of injury, these substances will cause the smooth muscle of capillaries and arterioles to relax, resulting in increased blood flow which causes the wound temperature to increase by 3 to 5°C and the tissue to become red which is the first visible sign of inflammation.

Dilation of the capillaries and especially the postcapillary venules due to the actions of the vasoactive amines on smooth muscle causes the gaps between the endothelial cells that line the vessels to become enlarged. The enlarged gaps permit leakage not only of plasma, but also of leukocytes. The leukocytes actively emigrate through the openings by a process that is shown in Figure 4.1, and discussed in greater detail below.

Effects of Prostaglandins and Leukotrienes on the Inflamed Area

In addition to the vasoactive amines, histamine and serotonin, there are other vasoactive hormones released at the site of an inflammatory response. They include the prostaglandins and leukotrienes. The prostaglandins and leukotrienes are lipid hormones. They are derived from arachidonic acid which is cleaved from the membrane phospholipids by phospholipase A2 (Figure 4.2). The phospholipase is activated by substances that damage cell membranes. After release, the arachidonic acid is oxygenated by one or the other of two enzyme systems. These are the cyclooxygenase system, the actions of which result in the production of the prostaglandins, and the lipooxygenase system, the actions of which result in the production of the leukotrienes. A large number of different prostaglandins have been described. The major prostaglandins produced are PGE_1, PGE_2, PGF_2a, prostacyclin (PGI_2), and Thromboxane A_2. The leukotrienes produced include LTB_4, LTC_4, LTD_4, LTE_4, and LTF_4.

The prostaglandins were so named because they were originally identified in that portion of human seminal fluid produced by the prostate gland. However, the production of prostaglandins is not limited to reproductive organs. They are produced by most cells, including the phagocytic leukocytes. The leukotrienes derive their name in part from the leukocytes that produce them and in part from their chemical structure which is that of a triene, i.e., a polyunsaturated fat.

One of the important events that occurs during an inflammatory response is the infiltration of leukocytes into the inflamed site. One of the leukotrienes LTB_4 is strongly chemotactic and attracts neutrophils and mononuclear phagocytes. Most of the other leukotrienes are relatively weak chemotactic agents compared to LTB_4.

Prostaglandins and leukotrienes together with the vasoactive amines, histamine, serotonin, and bradykinin, play an important role in causing the pain characteristic of inflammation. They do this in part by inducing swelling that causes pressure on nerve endings but they may act directly also. The vasoactive amines described earlier in this section act synergistically with the prostaglandins to directly induce pain. While prostaglandins of the E series can induce a sensation of pain alone by sensitizing pain receptors, the prostaglandin PGE_2 usually acts together with histamine and bradykinin to intensify the sensation. A combination of various leukotrienes and prostaglandins alone also may elicit pain. Pain is an important factor in our response to injury or infection. It causes us to protect the painful area and to reduce activities that may aggravate the damage. Without pain, use of the affected part may be continued until severe damage occurs.

The synergistic actions of prostaglandins, leukotrienes, and vasoactive amines in the inflamed site not only increase pain, they also affect vascular permeability. The

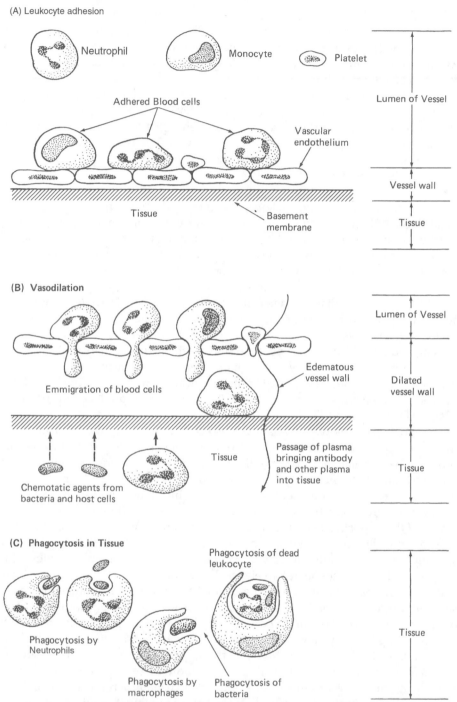

Figure 4.1. Changes within the postcapillary venules at an inflamed site and some of their consequences.

(A) Adherence (margination) of platelets, neutrophils, and monocytes to vascular endothelial cells.

(B) Vasodilation and increased permeability of vascular walls to leukocytes and emigration of neutrophils from the blood into the tissue in response to chemotactic agents.

(C) Clearance of microorganisms and damaged tissue from the inflamed site by phagocytosis.

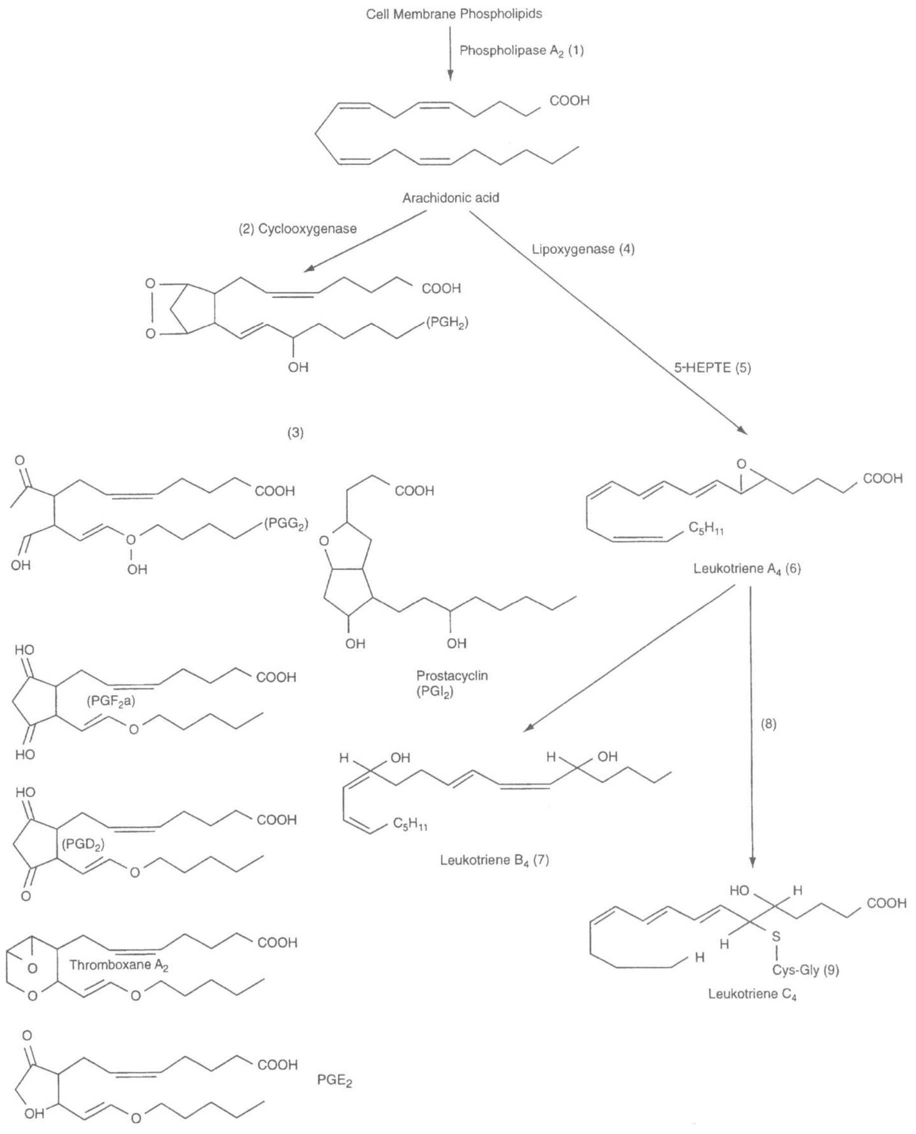

Figure 4.2. This figure outlines the production of arachidonic acid metabolites from cell membrane phospholipids. The arachidonic acid is released from the membrane by action of phospholipase A_2 (1). When the released arachidonic acid is oxygenated by cyclooxygenase, (2) PGH_2 is formed. Prostaglandins PGG_2, PGF_2a, PGD_2, Thromboxane A_2, PGE_2, and PGI_2 are formed by enzymatic reactions from PGH_2 (3). When the arachidonic acid is oxidized by lipoxygenase (4), 5-HPETE is formed (5). The leukotrienes are derived from 5-HPETE which serves as the precursor for leukotriene A_4 (6). Leukotriene B_4 (7) is formed from A_4 by a different enzymatic reaction than that which converts A_4 to C_4 (8). Leukotriene C_4 is formed by the addition of glutathione. Leukotriene D_4, E_4, and F_4 are formed by a series of reactions that only affect the amino acid substitution on the Cys-Gly residue (9). Slow-reacting substance-A is another name for a mixture of the leukotrienes C_4, D_4, and E_4.

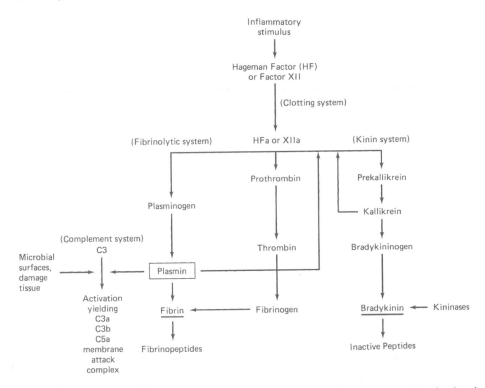

Figure 4.3. This figure shows the relationships between the four protein systems involved in the inflammatory response. The systems are identified in the figure by placing their names in parenthesis in the appropriate locations. A small "a" after the name identifies an activated factor or product. Only the major reactants are shown. Fibrin and bradykinin are the major products of the clotting and kinin systems. Plasmin is an important product of the fibrinolytic system because it not only lyses fibrin clots but also contributes to activation of the various other systems. The complement system releases chemotactic substances (C3a, C5a), opsonins (C3b, C4b), vasodilators (C2b, C4a, C3a, C5a), and the membrane attack complex (C5-9) which causes lysis of membranes to which it attaches. The clotting system yields fibrin for formation of clots to limit bleeding and stop spread of infection. When acted on by plasmin of the fibrinolytic system, the clots yield fibrinopeptides which are vasodilators. The kinin system yields bradykinin which is a vasodilator and is chemotactic and kininases that inactivate bradykinin.

effects on vascular permeability may be different depending on which prostaglandins and leukotrienes are present.

The synergistic interactions between PGE_2, PGI_2, and histamine increase vascular permeability during inflammation. The leukotrienes LTC_4 and prostaglandin OGE_2 acting jointly also increase vascular permeability. The leukotrienes LTC_4 and LTD_4 produce vasoconstriction. The enhancement of permeability by the combined actions of prostaglandins, leukotrienes, and vasoactive amines results in great enhancement of the inflammatory response with increase in infiltration of plasma and leukocytes into the site of tissue damage. The vasoconstriction on the other hand reduces the inflammation. As the degree of inflammation produced depends in part on the relative concentration and the types of prostaglandins and leukotrienes at the sites of inflammation, these hormones play a significant role in the regulation of the response.

Table 4.1. Important mediators of inflammatory events that are generated from blood protein.

Mediator	Source	Increased vascular permeability	Chemotactic for Phagocytes
Bradykinin	Kinin system	+	+
Kallikrein	Kinin system	–	+
Fibrinopeptides (fibrin split products)	Fibrinolytic system	+	+
C3a	Complement system	+	+
C5a	Complement system	+	+

Mediation of Inflammation by Blood Proteins

There are several major blood protein systems, the activation of which is triggered by injury and which contribute to inflammation. The activation of components of each system results in a cascade of chemical reactions that generate the soluble mediators of inflammation. These systems include the kinin system, the complement system, the clotting system, and the fibrinolytic system (Figure 4.3). Each cascade consists of a set of reactions which develop in an ordered sequence. The components of the systems are plasma proteins. Some of the components are enzymes and have as their substrates the next component within the series. The purpose of these cascades is to amplify the local response and to initiate events further from the site. The local events include all those already described as characteristic of inflammation; an increase in blood flow to the site of inflammation, the attraction of leukocytes, and an increase in blood vessel permeability (Table 4.1). These systems not only generate products that enhance inflammation, but also generate products that serve as feedback inhibitors to control the extent of activation. This is necessary to prevent the reactions from becoming too extensive.

The mediators of inflammation are all present in the blood plasma in inactive form. The initial event triggering activation is common for the clotting system, the kinin system and the fibrinolytic system but not for the complement system. When plasma enters damaged tissue, the first component of these blood-borne systems to be activated is Hageman Factor. Activation results from contact with and binding to collagen in the damaged tissue. Collagen is present throughout the body as collagen fibers make up the matrix of the body's tissues. It is typically covered by other components of the extracellular matrix, namely, fibrinonectin and proteoglycans, which are stripped from it by the injury that initiates inflammation.

Hageman Factor is usually described as the first component (Factor XII) of the clotting system, but as activated Hageman Factor (HFa) also initiates the activation of the kinin and the fibrinolytic systems, it could be considered the first component of these systems also.

The clotting cascade which results in the formation of clots consists of a sequence of reactions that convert prothrombin into thrombin which then converts fibrinogen into fibrin forming the dense mesh or web of stable fibers characteristic of clots. This fiber web traps platelets and other blood cells and microorganisms inhibiting bleeding and the spread of microorganisms from the site of injury.

For proper healing to occur, clots must be removed. This is done by enzymatic digestion. An important enzyme in this process is plasmin. Plasmin exists in the plasma in its inactive form plasminogen. Plasminogen is activated in inflamed tis-

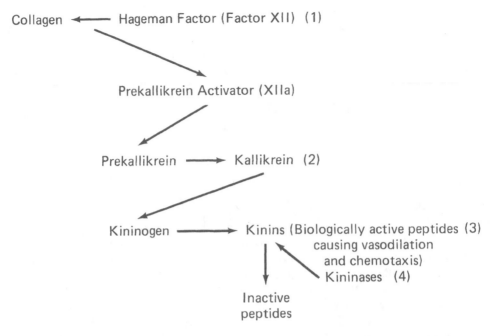

Figure 4.4. The Kinin System.
When Hageman Factor in the plasma comes in contact with collagen in the tissue, it becomes activated (1). Following a series of subsequent interactions (2), kinins, including bradykinin (3), are produced. These hormones are released in the tissues and cause further vasodilation and transvasation of more plasma. The chemotactic characteristics of bradykinin cause leukocytes to enter the inflamed tissue. The kininases (4) are enzymes that degrade kinins and thus reduce inflammation. Regulation of inflammation is a result of a shifting balance between production and destruction of the various agents that mediate inflammation.

sue by products of the kinin system; it in turn activates the complement system and Hageman Factor.

As noted above, plasmin is a proteolytic enzyme, one function of which is to lyse clots. Plasmin slowly degrades the fibrin network that is the result of the clotting reaction and thus allows access of phagocytic cells to the microbes trapped in the clot and paves the way for replacement of the clot by scar tissue or cells. Some of the products of plasmin digestion of fibrin are short polypeptides called fibrinopeptides. These are vasodilators and thus bring more plasma and leukocytes into the area while the clot is being resolved. When plasmin acts on Hageman Factor, it converts it to a prekallikrein activator. The latter protease converts prekallikrein into kallikrein, which in turn converts the precursor protein kininogen into bradykinin. Bradykinin is an extremely potent vasodilator and also is chemotactic for phagocytic cells and thus further amplifies the reaction. Various kininases are also produced as the inflammatory reaction progresses. These break bradykinin down to inactive peptides and thus control the extent of activation by this pathway (Figure 4.4).

Components of the complement system enter the tissues with the infiltrating plasma. The complement components make up ten percent of the globulin fraction of the serum. The complement system is a multicomponent system consisting of many enzymes and binding proteins. There are three distinct pathways for activation of the complement system, one is called the classical pathway and consists of

Table 4.2   Biologically active components generated by activation of the complement system.

Complement component	Activity
$\overline{C2b}$	Vasodilation
$\overline{C4a}$	Causes release of vasodilating amines (anaphylatoxin) from granulocytes
$\overline{C4b}$	Opsonization (causes adherence of microbes to leukocytes)
$\overline{C3a}$	Causes release of vasoactive amines from granulocytes (anaphylatoxin), induces chemotaxis
$\overline{C3b}$	Opsonization (causes adherence of microbes to leukocytes)
$\overline{C5a}$	Causes release of vasoactive amines from granulocytes (anaphylatoxin), induces chemotaxis

nine numbered components, of which the first (C1) is triggered by binding to antibody when it is present in an immune complex. The second pathway is the alternative pathway which is triggered by the binding of the third component (C3) of complement to a variety of membranes or membrane-bound substances, including carbohydrates on cell walls of many bacteria and the damaged tissue found at inflammatory sites. As antibody is not generated for several days after infection and is thus not available to form complexes immediately, the complement activation that occurs early in the inflammatory reaction is through the alternative pathway.

A third pathway is activated by binding of mannose binding lectin (MBL) to mannose residues on micro-organisms. MBL is produced by liver cells as a rapid response to inflammation. Binding of MBL to micro-organisms allows subsequent binding and activation of a serum serine protease that can cleave and activate complement factor 4. This facilitates the activation of downstream components of the complement cascade. The alternative and MBL-activated pathways of complement activation are important constituents of innate immunity.

The activation of the complement cascade results in the generation of mediators of inflammation, some identical and some distinct, from those of other systems (Table 4.2). The system provides a number of proteins that can facilitate the phagocytosis of microbes and thus enhance immunity. The effector compartment of the complement cascade begins with the deposition of C3 onto cell membranes in the form of a split product of C3, designated $\overline{C3b}$. When $\overline{C3b}$ is deposited on the membrane of a microbe, the microbe's susceptibility to ingestion by phagocytic cells is enhanced. The small molecules split from complement components during activation—$\overline{C4a}$, $\overline{C3a}$, $\overline{C5a}$—are all anaphylatoxins, which means they cause the release of histamine from cells and as a result, smooth muscle contraction. Histamine, as noted earlier, increases vessel permeability. The small split component of $\overline{C5}$, C5a, is a very potent chemotactic factor for polymorphonuclear leukocytes and macrophages. The mechanism whereby the complement components interact and activate each other will be described in detail in the context of activation of complement by immune complexes in chapter 9.

That the actions of the complement system are important among the protective mechanisms invoked during inflammation is apparent as individuals lacking complement are more susceptible to infection, particularly with Gram – negative bacteria and to immune complex disease, than are normal people.

The kinin and complement cascades are considered to be more important in host defense than the clotting and fibrinolytic systems. The latter are considered to be more important as homeostatic mechanisms than host protective mechanisms. One must consider, however, that formation of clots may contribute to host defense by the development of the fibrin barrier to the spread of microbes. This fibrin barrier may be greatly strengthened by subsequent transformation into scar tissue. The actions of fibrinolytic factors such as plasmin may dissolve the clot. Further enzymatic action may result in liquidation of the injured tissue. The liquified material is called pus if it contains many infiltrated leukocytes. Pus may be either resorbed or discharged to the outside. If pus formation occurs inside an area walled off by fibrosis, the result is formation of an abscess. Microbes may survive inside an abscess but at least their effects are then only local. Infection with some microorganisms, such as staphylococci, commonly results in formation of abscesses. Infection with others, such as streptococci, commonly results in spreading infection with little tendency to abscess formation.

Blood Cell Movement into the Inflamed Area

In the inflamed area, the endothelial linings of the capillaries and venules change under the influence of the various soluble mediators in such a way as to promote the adherence of platelets, polymorphonuclear neutrophils, and monocytes. Platelet adherence to the endothelial lining of the altered capillary or venule is prominent early in the response. Platelet adherence requires thrombin (a clotting system factor) and divalent cations (Mg^{++}, Ca^{++}). The first platelets to adhere release adenosine diphosphate which causes other platelets to attach, aggregate with each other, and release serotonin and histamine, factors that promote clotting. Clotting takes place both within the vessels and outside of the circulation at the inflamed site. If platelets are depleted from a laboratory animal, the inflammatory response is greatly diminished.

The inflammatory response causes circulating phagocytic cells, called neutrophils, to home into the site of tissue injury. Neutrophils belong to a class of cells named polymorphonuclear leukocytes after the morphology of the nucleus in the mature cell. Inactive neutrophils survive for less than a day and in people about a hundred million of these cells die and are replaced each day. Neutrophils are armed to the teeth with weapons of biological destruction that include granules filled with acid hydrolases, myeloperoxidase, lysozyme and collagenase. Their surface is equipped with sensors (receptors) for opsonins, which are a class of molecules deposited on microbes during inflammatory and acquired immune responses, that tag them for phagocytosis. Opsonin-coated microbes are engulfed by neutrophils and taken into their cytoplasm (phagocytosed) within a bilayer lipid membrane derived from the neutrophil plasma membrane. Enzyme-filled sacs (lysosomes) within the cytoplasm of the neutrophil fuse to the phagocytic vesicle releasing their contents into the vesicle and damaging the engulfed microbe. Phagocytosis also causes the assembly of a powerful oxidase, NADPH oxidase, on the inner side of the plasma membrane of neutrophils adjacent to the site of phagocytosis. This oxidase remains associated with the phagocytic vesicle and generates superoxide anion which is converted to hydrogen peroxide within the phagocytic vesicle. The hydrogen peroxide is in turn coverted to hydroxyl radicals and hypohalides within the phagocytic vesicle, both of which contribute to the destruction of engulfed microbes.

Neutrophils have surface receptors for molecules, called selectins that are typically stored inside endothelial cells lining blood vessels, but are placed on the surface of the endothelium in response to vasoactive material generated by damaged tissue. Binding of neutrophils to the selectins is transitory and slows them down, causing them to roll along the surface of the endothelium and to receive short range signals including platelet-activating factor that enhance their expression of another surface receptor, an integrin, that allows high affinity binding to an adhesion molecule (ICAM-1) on the endothelium. The engagement of the neutrophil integrin and endothelial cell ICAM-1 causes the rolling neutrophils to adhere to the surface of the endothelum. The immobilized neutrophils subsequently uncouple from the endothelium, squeeze between endothelial cells and pass through the basement membrane into the site of tissue damage in response to chemotactic stimuli from the complement fragments $\overline{C5a}$, $\overline{C3a}$, and $\overline{C4a}$ as well as platelet-activating factor and leukotriene B4 (LTB4). The process of neutrophil arrest on inflammatory endothelium is called margination and the activity of squeezing between endothelial cells and into the inflamed tissue in response to a chemotactic stimulus is called diapedesis. Neutrophils that are recruited into the inflammatory site live longer than inactive neutrophils, and become more actively phagocytic. When exposed to high concentrations of $\overline{C5a}$, $\overline{C4a}$ and $\overline{C3a}$, neutrophils degranulate and enzymes released from the granules cause extensive extracellular damage.

Blood monocytes are recruited in a similar way to the neutrophils. However, these cells move more slowly than neutrophils and arrive later into the inflammatory site. Monocytes are immature forms of tissue macrophages, phagocytic cells that possess surface receptors for the opsonic complement fragments $\overline{C3b}$ and $\overline{iC3b}$ as well as receptors for some antibody and antigen complexes. Monocytes that are recruited to the inflammatory site mature to macrophages, which can phagocytose and destroy opsonized microbes and engage T lymphocytes in immune responses by presenting processed peptide on their surface together with major histocompatibility antigens. This process is referred to in chapter 1 and discussed in detail in a later chapter. Macrophages also release a variety of proinflammatory molecules including hydrolytic enzymes and reactive oxygen intermediates.

Although inflammation may result in tissue destruction, the final result is healing with the formation of new connective tissue. This is accomplished by enzymatic digestion of dead tissue, phagocytic removal of microbes and dead cells, the growth of capillaries into the damaged site, synthesis of collagen by fibroblasts, and regeneration of cells including mucosal and epithelial cells.

SYSTEMIC CONSEQUENCES OF THE INFLAMMATORY REACTION
Induction of Fever
Several important consequences of the inflammatory response are systemic. Fever is one hallmark of the systemic inflammatory response. During the localized inflammatory response, macrophages release a pyrogenic (fever-inducing) substance called endogenous pyrogen that acts on the portion of the hypothalamic region of the brain that controls body temperature. An elevated temperature can have a deleterious effect on microbes and on host cells that are harboring pathogens, and is an important component of the constitutive host defense. Endogenous pyrogen is a hormone or a mixture of hormones and is very closely related to the macrophage product called interleukin-1 (IL-1), which acts on lymphocytes to augment specific immune responses. IL-1 was one of the first products of macrophages to be shown to augment specific immune responses and to induce fever. IL-6 and tumor necrosis factor alpha (TNF α) which are secreted by activated macrophages are also components of endogenous pryogen. TNF α has a wide range of biological activities that include the induction of cachexia, a severe infection-induced loss of weight resulting from a change in fat cell metabolism caused by TNF α.

Another group of hormones generated during inflammation and which induce

Table 4.3. Acute phase reactants induced by inflammation and their biological activities.

Acute phase reactant	Inflammatory activity
C3	Anaphylatoxin, opsonin
a_1-antitrypsin	Inhibits trypsin and thus reduces tissue damage
a_1-antichymotrypsin	Inhibits chymotrypsin and thus reduces tissue damage
Haptoglobulin	Salvages iron from hemoglobulin
Transferrin	Blocks use of iron by microbes
Fibrinogen	Causes clotting
C-reactive protein	Activates the complement system, opsonin

fever are the prostaglandins discussed earlier. The relationship of prostaglandins to fever was first suspected when it was discovered that fever-reducing drugs, such as aspirin, inhibited prostaglandin production. Later it was shown that the injection of PGE_1 or PGE_2 causes fever. Like IL-1, prostaglandins of the E series appear to work through the hypothalamic region of the brain to raise body temperature.

Stimulation of Production of Blood Cells by Colony-Stimulating Factor

During an acute inflammatory reaction, in addition to production of Il-1, prostaglandins, leukotrienes and vasoactive amines, there is a greatly increased production of a group of substances, termed colony-stimulating factor (CSF), which are required for the production of granulocytes or monocytes from bone marrow precursor cells. The increase in CSF in serum during inflammation presumably initiates production of the polymorphonuclear leukocytes and monocytes needed to replenish losses which occur during the inflammatory response.

Induction of Acute Phase Reactants

Within six to twelve hours of the initiation of an inflammatory response, there is a marked increase in the synthesis by liver hepatocytes of a group of plasma proteins that are called acute-phase reactants. This diverse group of plasma proteins includes some that are substrates of the local inflammatory response (e.g., C3, and fibrinogen) and others such as $\alpha1$- antitrypsin that serve as protease inhibitors to limit tissue damage. C-reactive protein (CRP) is the prototype acute phase reactant of humans and displays Ca^{++}-dependent binding to some bacteria (for example, pneumococci) and to damaged membranes. The binding of CRP to a bacterium facilitates its phagocytosis by macrophages and polymorphonuclear leukocytes. CRP also activates complement by the classical pathway, but inhibits its activation by the alternative pathway. Since "CRP-like" proteins are widely distributed among both invertebrates and vertebrates, it is probable that these proteins represent the forerunners of the recognition structures that evolved into antibody molecules. CRP and some related proteins have been retained by vertebrates through evolution. They probably serve as nonspecific host resistance factors and may also function to aid tissue repair. Table 4.3 lists several acute phase proteins.

SUMMARY

This chapter makes six main points:

(1) *Inflammation is initiated by damaged tissue in four main ways,* (a) through the activity of membrane phospholipase which makes arachidonic acid available for cleavage by cycloxygenase and lipoxygenase which yield respectively vasoactive

prostaglandins and leukotrienes, (b) by exposing surfaces that can support the alternative pathway of complement activation which results in the generation of $\overline{C5a}$ and $\overline{C3a}$, anaphylatoxins that cause mast cells to degranulate and release vasoactive serotonin and histamine, and that are chemotactic for neutrophils and monocytes, (c) by stripping extracellular matrix from collagen thus allowing activation of the kinin, clotting and fibrinolytic systems, and (d) by changing local vascular endothelium so that platelets bind and degranulate releasing vasoactive serotonin and histamine, as well as chemotactic platelet activating factor.

(2) *The purpose of the inflammatory response is to enhance tissue defense* i.e., to limit replication of, or destroy, invading organisms, *as well as to promote tissue repair*. Destruction of microbes results from opsonization or lysis by complement factors, their phagocytosis by neutrophils and macrophages and degradation in phagolysosomes, or their exposure to extracellular enzymes and reactive oxygen intermediates that are released by activated neutrophils and macrophages.

(3) *The four cardinal signs of inflammation are redness, heat, swelling, and pain.* Redness and heat result from relaxation of smooth muscle which causes dilation of local blood vessels and increased local blood flow. Relaxation of smooth muscle results from the action of serotonin, histamine, prostaglandins, and leukotrienes. Swelling is due to local edema. This is caused by the leakage of plasma proteins and fluids through the enlarged gaps between vascular endothelium brought about by vasodilation. Pain results from the effects of tissue swelling and from the direct action of some of the mediators of inflammation such as the prostaglandins.

(4) *Recruitment of neutrophils and macrophages into the inflammatory site is mediated by two separate processes brought about by vasoactive and chemotactic molecules.* Firstly, exposure of vascular endotheium to vasoactive amines, prostaglandins, and leukotrienes causes a change in their expression of surface adhesins that result in the binding of circulating neutrophils and monocytes, a process that is called margination. Secondly, chemotactic stimuli which include $\overline{C5a}$, $\overline{C3a}$, $\overline{C4a}$, and leukotriene B4 cause the bound cells to squeeze through gaps between endothelium that lines capillaries at the inflammatory site and to enter the inflammatory site by a process called diapedesis.

(5) *Neutrophils and macrophages at the site of inflammation release three categories of factors,* those that amplify local inflammation (e.g., proteolytic enzymes, reactive oxygen intermediates, complement factors), those that facilitate wound repair (e.g., $\alpha1$ anti-trypsin, histaminase, protein kinase inhibitor), and those that induce systemic aspects of inflammation, namely, endogenous pyrogen (IL-1, IL-6, TNFα) and cachectin (TNFα).

(6) *Inflammatory responses subside when the agent that provokes inflammation is eliminated,* but can amplify until death of the affected individual or animal if the proinflammatory agent is sustained. The inflammatory response does not have a memory component.

SUGGESTIONS FOR FURTHER READING

1. Davies, P., P.J. Bailey, M.M. Goldenberg, and A.W. Ford-Hutchinson, "The role of arachidonic acid oxygenation products in pain and inflammation," *Ann. Rev. of Immunol.* 2 (1984):335.
2. Diaz-Gonzalez, F., and F. Sanchez-Madrid. "Inhibition of Leukocyte Adhesion: An Alternative Mechanism of Action for Anti-Inflammatory Drugs." *Immunology Today* 19 (1998):169.

3. Larsen, G.L., and P.M. Henson, "Mediators of Inflammation," *Ann. Revs. Immunol.* 1 (1983):335.
4. Gallin, J.I. "Inflammation." In *Fundamental Immunology*. 3d ed. Edited by W.E. Paul, 1015. New York: Raven Press, 1993.

QUESTIONS

1. What induces an inflammatory response and how quickly does it develop?
2. In what way does the inflammatory response help in defense against disease causing organisms?
3. What is the molecular basis of the pain response during inflammation and what is the biological advantage of this response?
4. How are circulating neutrophils and monocytes recruited into the inflammatory site?
5. What roles do: mast cells, platelets, anaphylatoxins, kinin-, clotting-, fibrinolytic- and complement-systems play in the inflammatory response?

ANSWERS

1. An inflammatory response can be initiated by any type of tissue damage that; (a) activates membrane phospholipase leading to the generation of prostaglandins and leukotrienes, (b) exposes collagen leading to the activation of kinin, clotting and fibrinolytic systems, (c) modifies the surface of vascular endothelium so that it binds and activates platelets, and (d) supports the alternative pathway of complement activation leading to production of anaphylatoxins. Inflammatory responses are exacerbated by the presence of microbes at the site of injury mainly as a result of complement activation. Signs of an inflammatory reaction can be detected within minutes of injury including increased redness, heat, swelling, and pain at the inflammatory site. However, the inflammatory response continues to develop until the tissue injury is repaired and associated microbes eliminated. Fever and weight loss (cachexia) are systemic consequences of an acute inflammatory response which may result from catastrophic injury, or an infection and consequently may take hours to days to develop.

2. Several aspects of the inflammatory response affect disease-causing organisms. Firstly, the increased temperature at the inflammatory site affects biochemical pathways that support cell function and can inhibit growth of some microbes. Secondly, clot and scar tissue formation can limit the spread of organisms out of the inflammatory site. Thirdly, opsonization of organisms leads to their phagocytosis by neutrophils and macrophages and exposure to proteolytic enzymes and damaging reactive oxygen intermediates (superoxide anion and hydrogen peroxide) in the endosomal system of these cells. Fourthly, complement activation by the alternative pathway on the surface of microbes can result in formation of a membrane attack complex that can cause cell lysis. Lastly, extracellular deposition of neutrophil granule contents and secretory products of macrophages exposes microbes to a variety of damaging enzymes and reactive oxygen intermediates.

3. Prostaglandins, leukotriene, and vasoactive amines induce leakage of blood fluids into the inflammatory site causing swelling and pressure on nerve endings. These agents also have direct effects on nerve endings. Prostaglandins act by sensitizing pain receptors. Various combinations of leukotrienes and prostaglandins, and of prostaglandins, serotonin, and bradykinin cause pain. Pain is a behavior modifier. It

causes the affected animal or individual to reduce activities that may aggravate damage. It also alerts us to take steps to alleviate the pain, to repair any damage that has been done, and to avoid behavior that will lead to damage.

4. Within the bloodstream, neutrophils and monocytes are tumbled along blood vessel walls making periodic contact with the endothelium. Neutrophils and monocytes have receptors (L selectin) for molecules (P and E selectins) that are stored in vesicles within normal vascular endothelium and exposed on the endothelial cell surface in response to agents produced early in inflammatory responses. Neutrophils and monocytes bind transitorily to exposed selectins on vascular endothelium. This binding converts their tumbling motion to a slow roll and allows short range communication molecules to pass between the endothelium and the phagocytic cells. These include platelet activating factor which when perceived by the neutrophils and monocytes elevates their surface expression of integral membrane proteins called integrins. Binding of the neutrophil and monocyte integrins to ICAM-1 that is expressed on the endothelium completely arrests the rolling motion of the neutrophils and monocytes. Receptors on the surface of the neutrophils and monocytes allow them to detect chemotactic C5a, C3a, C4a and leukotriene B4 that diffuse from the inflammatory site, which cause them to squeeze through gaps between endothelial cells, pass through the extracellular matrix that forms the basement membrane and enter the inflammatory site.

5. Mast cells are distributed throughout tissues and contain vasoactive serotonin and histamine within granules stored in their cytoplasm. The anaphylatoxins C5a and C3a induce an influx of Ca^{++} into mast cells, as does binding of antigen to IgE absorbed on the mast cell surface. The increase in intracellular Ca^{++} alters the structure of the mast cell actin cytoskeleton which allows cytoplasmic granules to fuse to the mast cell plasma membrane, and the granule contents to be spilled to the extracellular space. Released histamine and serotonin relax blood vessel smooth muscle causing dilation of the blood vessel, increased local blood flow and increased leakage of plasma proteins into the inflammatory site.

The Inducible System: History of Development of Immunology as a Component of Host-Parasite Interactions

Ralph A. Sorensen

INTRODUCTION
IMMUNIZATION
THE NATURE OF INDUC-
   IBLE IMMUNITY
THEORIES TO EXPLAIN
   INDUCIBLE IMMUNITY
SELF-RECOGNITION IN
   IMMUNOLOGY
THE STRUCTURE AND
   BEHAVIOR OF
   ANTIBODIES
MONOCLONAL ANTI-
   BODIES
THE GENETICS OF THE
   IMMUNE RESPONSE
HORMONAL SUBSTANCES
   INDUCED IN IMMUNITY
SUMMARY
SUGGESTIONS FOR
   FURTHER READING
QUESTIONS
ANSWERS

INTRODUCTION

In the fields of human and veterinary medicine, the study of how parasites induce a specific immune response in their hosts has overshadowed the study of all other aspects of host-parasite interactions. This is due in large measure to the dramatic effects in disease prevention and treatment which have resulted from the manipulation with vaccines of the immune systems of man and domestic animals. The most dramatic example of this has been the successful elimination of the scourge of small pox from the human population in the mid 1970s by a massive immunization program.

IMMUNIZATION

One of the earliest immunization procedures, probably developed in China, was termed "variolation." People were deliberately inoculated with infectious material from persons with mild cases of smallpox. After recovery, these people were immune to subsequent infection by the smallpox virus. This dangerous procedure was based on the common observation that people who had recovered from even a mild case of smallpox were seldom infected a second time. Immunity was specific, and a person immune to small pox remained susceptible to infection by other pathogenic organisms.

In 1796, the Englishman Edward Jenner discovered that infection with the vaccinia virus, which causes the disease of cowpox in cows but is only mildly pathogenic in humans, provided lasting immunity against smallpox. Jenner's discovery demonstrated that an immune response could react against two closely related viruses. The concept of cross-reactivity was an important exception to the rule of immune specificity.

With the identification of pathogenic bacteria as causative agents of specific diseases in the 1880s by Louis Pasteur in France and Robert Koch in Germany, the stage was set for the rational development of immunization procedures. Quite soon after the identification and isolation of pathogenic organisms, attempts were made to use them to develop vaccines against infectious diseases. Pasteur recognized the necessity of selecting weakly or nonpathogenic strains of the pathogens for use as safe immunizing agents. Such nonpathogenic but immunogenic varieties of pathogenic microorganisms are said to be "attenuated." Pasteur successfully immunized chickens against chicken cholera in 1880 with living but nonpathogenic bacteria. Pasteur also developed vaccines against anthrax (1881) and rabies (1885) using attenuated microorganisms. The induction of immunity by infection with attenuated pathogens was a process similar to that which Jenner developed when he used the cowpox virus to immunize against smallpox. The Latin word for cow is *vacca* and Pasteur called this process "vaccination" in honor of Jenner's achievement.

Not all of the early attempts to immunize against disease were successful. In 1882, Robert Koch identified the bacillus *Mycobacterium tuberculosis* as the causative agent of tuberculosis. He attempted to immunize individuals by injecting them with spent medium from cultures of human tubercle bacilli. No immunity resulted from the injection, but a febrile reaction and swelling at the site of the injection occurred twenty-four to forty-eight hours later in people who were harboring the tubercle bacillus. This reaction was later shown to be diagnostic for tuberculosis and it is still widely used today. The type of material Koch used is now called "old tuberculin." Today we use an extract of old tuberculin called "purified protein derivative" (PPD) to test for tuberculosis. In Koch's honor the tuberculin reaction was called the Koch phenomenon.

Later attempts to immunize against tuberculosis using attenuated strains of the organism met with little success. Thus, the failure to induce immunity was not that Koch used a nonliving preparation as the immunogen. Koch's observations were the first bit of experimental evidence to suggest that fundamentally different types of immune responses can occur. The Koch phenomenon is an example of one of them, delayed-type hypersensitivity, a cell-mediated (as opposed to humoral) immune response.

THE NATURE OF INDUCIBLE IMMUNITY

With the demonstration that immunity could be induced by infection, many scientists became interested in determining how hosts fought infection and how immunity was generated. Some scientists believed that immunity was largely cell-based while others considered humoral factors to be of prime importance. Today we understand that both cellular and humoral immune reactions serve to control infection and establish immunity (Table 5.1).

The Russian zoologist Elie Metchnikoff was a strong advocate of the cellular theory of immunity. He suggested as early as 1884 that leukocytes, through their phagocytic abilities, played a major role in disease resistance. He made this claim on the basis of his experiments with starfish larvae in which he observed phagocytic cells surrounding splinters which he had introduced into the transparent bodies of the animals. Pasteur invited Metchnikoff to the Pasteur Institute in Paris where for the next twenty-eight years he worked to verify his cellular theory of immunity.

The field of cellular immunology has changed dramatically since Metchnikoff worked to elucidate the role of the phagocytic cells in the cellular response. These

Table 5.1. Classification of defense reactions.

Effector Mechanism*	Type of Response	Outcome of Defense Response
Cellular	Engulfment	Uptake of foreign material (phagocytosis)
	Cytotoxic	Destruction of infected or nonself cells by contact
Humoral	Agglutination	Clumping of organisms followed by phagocytosis
	Precipitation	Clumping of soluble molecules followed by phagocytosis
	Neutralization	(a) Inactivation of toxins (b) Blocking of infection by viruses and other intracellular parasites
	Complement fixation	(a) Lysis of parasites (b) Phagocytosis of parasites

*Some cellular and some humoral responses are noninducible, and some are inducible. If noninducible, there is no increase in the response following exposure to antigen; if inducible, there is an increased response.

Table 5.2. Major discoveries in cellular immunology.

Year	Scientist(s)	Discovery
1884	Metchnikoff	Phagocytosis/Cellular Theory of Immunity
1942	Landsteiner & Chase	Transfer of Hypersensitivity by Cells
1944	Burnet & Medawar	Graft Rejection (Cellular)
1948	Snell	Inbred and Congenic Mouse Strains
1953	Billingham, Brent, & Medawar	Immune Tolerance
1955–1959	Jerne, Burnet, Lederberg, & Talmadge	Clonal Selection Theory
1961–1962	Miller, Good	Role of the Thymus in Immunity
1967–1968	Claman, Davies, Miller, & Mitchell	T cell, B cell Interaction
1968–1972	Benacerraf & McDevitt	Immune Response Genes
1970	Gershon	Suppressor T cells
1971	Jerne	Idiotype Network Theory
1974	Zinkernagel & Doherty	Restriction of Antigen Recognition by Major Histocompatibility Complex
1976–1980	Gallo, Smith, Gillis, Waksman, & Oppenheim	Cytokines
1984	Mak, Davis, Marrack, & Kappler	T cell Receptor Structure
1987	Bjorkman, Wiley, & Strominger	Class I MHC Protein Structure

developments have provided a rational explanation for many previously unexplained immunological phenomena (Table 5.2). Karl Landsteiner and his student Merrill Chase, for example, established in 1942 that hypersensitivity to tuberculin and to skin sensitizing chemicals such as the oils in poison ivy could only be transferred from one organism to another by immune cells, not by serum. The cells that successfully transferred immunity were lymphocytes, not macrophages, extending the scope of cellular immunology to another cell type. Our understanding of cellular immunology was further advanced in the 1950s and 1960s when it was shown that lymphocytes were also largely responsible for organ graft rejection.

In 1890, at the same time Metchnikoff was working on phagocytosis, Emil von Behring demonstrated that immunity gave rise to antimicrobial activity in the blood serum. Using serum from a horse immunized with attenuated *Corynebacterium*, he

Table 5.3. Major Discoveries in Humoral Immunity

Year	Scientist(s)	Discovery
1890	Von Behring & Kitasato	Antimicrobial Activity of Immune Serum
1897	Ehrlich	Side Chain Theory
1901	Landsteiner	ABO Human Blood Groups
1917	Landsteiner	Hapten-Carrier Antigens
1930	Heidelberger	Quantitative Immune Response
1934	Marrack	Lattice Theory of Immunoprecipitation
1939	Kabat & Tiselius	Antibody is a Gammaglobulin
1959	Porter, Edelman	Structure of Antibody
1965	Yallow & Berson	Radioimmunoassays
1975	Kohler & Milstein	Hybridomas and Monoclonal Antibody
1977–1982	Tonegawa, Hood, Leder, Baltimore, & Honjo	Antibody Gene Expression

developed an effective therapy for the treatment of diphtheria. The immune serum, injected into sick children, neutralized the toxicity of the diphtheria toxin.
These observations formed the basis of the humoral theory of immunity in which
the term "humor" refers to the blood serum. Since this activity was present in the
blood serum, it was independent of intact cells. The great German chemist Paul
Ehrlich was the most outspoken proponent of the humoral theory of immunity. He
coined the term "antibody" to describe this antimicrobial activity in the immune
serum. Today we understand antibodies to be proteins secreted by lymphocytes.
Many of the important discoveries in the field of humoral immunity are listed in
Table 5.3.

Study of the antimicrobial activity of immune serum led to the discovery of a
normal serum component now called "complement." Pfeiffer observed in 1894 that
the antibacterial action of immune serum was reduced by heating the serum to
56°C for thirty minutes; the activity was reestablished by addition of unheated *normal* serum. Pfeiffer called the heat labile antibacterial component of serum "alexin."
We now call it "complement" because it complements the action of antibodies on
microorganisms. The demonstration of the enhancement of the antibacterial capacity of antibody by a component in normal serum drew much attention to humoral
immunity.

THEORIES TO EXPLAIN INDUCIBLE IMMUNITY
In the course of his studies on the neutralizing activity of antibodies, Paul Ehrlich
proposed the "side chain" theory of immunity to explain antibody production
during an immune response. Publishing his theory in 1897, Ehrlich argued that
antibodies are naturally occurring toxin receptors, or "side chains," found on the
surface of blood cells. After the surface receptors neutralize the toxins to which
they bind, more receptors are produced and shed into the blood as antibody
(Figure 5.1).

When one considers the state of knowledge of cell biology in the late 1800s, it is
remarkable how much of this imaginative theory is correct. Today we recognize the
side chains to be surface antibodies. While the surface antibodies are not the antibodies that are secreted, their specificity is identical since they are encoded by the
same genes. It is also important to remember that, at the time, the only antibodies
known were antitoxins. It seemed reasonable to assume that the immune response
was preprogrammed to respond to a limited number of toxins in the environment

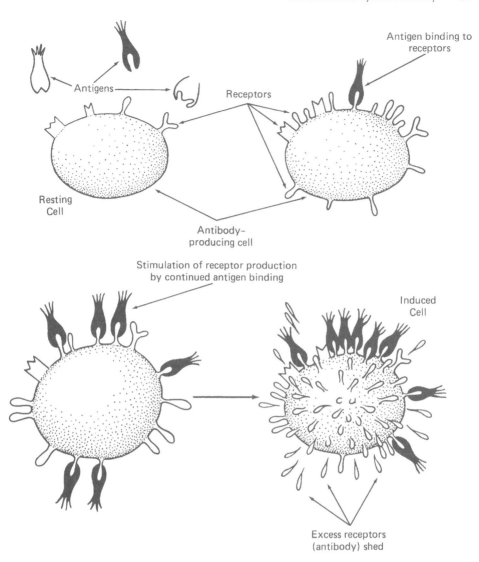

Figure 5.1. The side chain theory of antibody formation from the drawings in the original paper by Paul Ehrlich (1897). The antigen (toxin) binds to a specific side chain (receptor) on the cell surface and stimulates the production and release of more receptors into the blood. The theory correctly predicted the binding of antigen to the antibody-like receptors on the surface of lymphocytes.

rather than an astronomical array of potential antigens. The important conceptual contribution of Ehrlich's idea was that the specific antibody preexisted the matching antigen and that the cell capable of making this specific antibody is thereby selected. Ehrlich's "side chain" theory presaged the clonal selection theory of antibody formation by sixty years.

At the turn of the last century, these apparently opposing theories, cell-mediated and humoral immunity, competed with one another to explain how hosts controlled infection and developed immunity. Although adherents of each theory continued to gather experimental data to support their viewpoint, the obvious truth was that both theories were correct. In 1908 the Nobel prize in Medicine was jointly awarded to Metchnikoff and Ehrlich in recognition of their contributions. The joint award shows clearly the early recognition that the cellular and humoral components of the immune response are simply separate manifestations of one system.

The demonstration that infection resulted in the production of a serum factor, called "antibody" by Ehrlich, which increased the ability of a host to control infection, generated acute interest in the cellular basis of antibody synthesis. Early studies indicated that antibody synthesizing cells were found in both the lymph nodes and the spleens of immunized animals, but whether or not these cells were Metchnikoff's phagocytes or lymphocytes, another cell type prominent in those tissues, was not known. Attempts to induce antibody synthesis *in vitro* by culturing lymphocytes with antigen were unsuccessful. It was not until the mid 1960s that experiments showed that an *in vitro* response required the participation of both cell types. Sidney Raffel's text *Immunity*, written in 1960, summarized this confused state of affairs at the time:

> Cells of the reticuloendothelial system [macrophages and their ilk] are probably not involved in the process—this despite the fact that they come very naturally to the minds of immunologists as possible antibody producers because of their propensity for taking up foreign substances introduced into the body. Lymphocytes have a better claim to some role in the process of antibody formation, if not the central one of actual synthesis. If this turns out to be a valid conclusion, it would be doubly welcome, first for clarifying the mystery of antibody origin and second for answering the question as to what useful purpose these ubiquitous cells serve.

In the ten years after 1960, the specialized roles of different cell types began to be unraveled. The realization that a variety of types of lymphocytes contribute to the immune response was derived from experiments that indicated that lymphocytes from both the bone marrow and the thymus were required for antibody synthesis. One class of lymphocytes, the so-called B cells (signifying bone marrow, but actually named after the Bursa of Fabricius where they are formed in birds) synthesized antibody. Another class of lymphocytes, named T cells (for thymus-derived) that contribute to the development of immunity in other ways, were identified. Additional experiments indicated that macrophages were also required to initiate antibody production but did not themselves produce it.

By the end of the 1960s, it was accepted that B lymphocytes differentiated into plasma cells, the cells that secrete antibody. There was, however, no satisfactory answer to the question of how these cells could make antibody against the vast array of antigenic determinants to which the system was capable of responding. Most antigens are complex and have many determinants on their surfaces. A determinant or "epitope" is the site on an antigen to which antibody binds. The immune response may be directed toward one or all of the determinants on an antigen. The nature of antigens is described in more detail in chapter 6.

On the basis of ideas described by Jerne as early as 1955, both Burnet and Talmadge in 1957 separately proposed the clonal selection theory. This theory states that an organism contains many different clones of lymphocytes, each clone derived from a single parent cell. The lymphocytes that comprise a clone each display surface

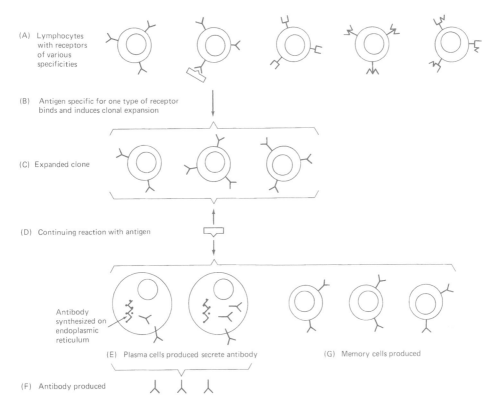

(A) Lymphocytes
with receptors
of various
specificities

(B) Antigen specific for one type of receptor
binds and induces clonal expansion

(C) Expanded clone

(D) Continuing reaction with antigen

Antibody
synthesized on
endoplasmic
reticulum

(E) Plasma cells produced secrete antibody

(G) Memory cells produced

(F) Antibody produced

Figure 5.2. The clonal selection theory of antibody production. A pool of B lymphocytes with surface receptors specific for different antigens exist in lymphoid tissue and in the circulation (A). Antigen specific for one type of receptor (B) induces the expansion of a clone of lymphocytes with identical receptors (C). The continued binding to the antigen (D) induces proliferation of plasma cells rich in endoplasmic reticulum (E) and memory cells (F). The plasma cells secrete antibody (G) and the memory cells are ready to differentiate into plasma cells if antigen is encountered again.

receptors for a single antigenic determinant. Binding of the appropriate determinant to their receptors triggers the proliferation and differentiation of B cells into antibody-secreting plasma cells. The antibody produced has the same specificity as the receptor (Figure 5.2). The central conceptual point of this theory, essentially identical to that described by Ehrlich, is that the antigen induces proliferation of a subset of preexisting lymphocytes from among a large repertoire of lymphocytes in the organism. As with Darwin's natural selection, the antigen "selects" a matching lymphocyte. The matching lymphocyte responds by proliferation and differentiation. The differentiation of the lymphocyte into an antibody-producing plasma cell is the result of interaction with many other cells, but the initial event is the binding of a specific antigenic determinant (epitope) to receptors on specific lymphocytes (Figure 5.3).

As evidence accumulated that lymphocytes were not all of one class, some maturing in the thymus and others in the bone marrow, the clonal selection theory was extended. Burnet proposed that the various clones were developed during the fetal period, and that their production was the result of somatic mutation of the

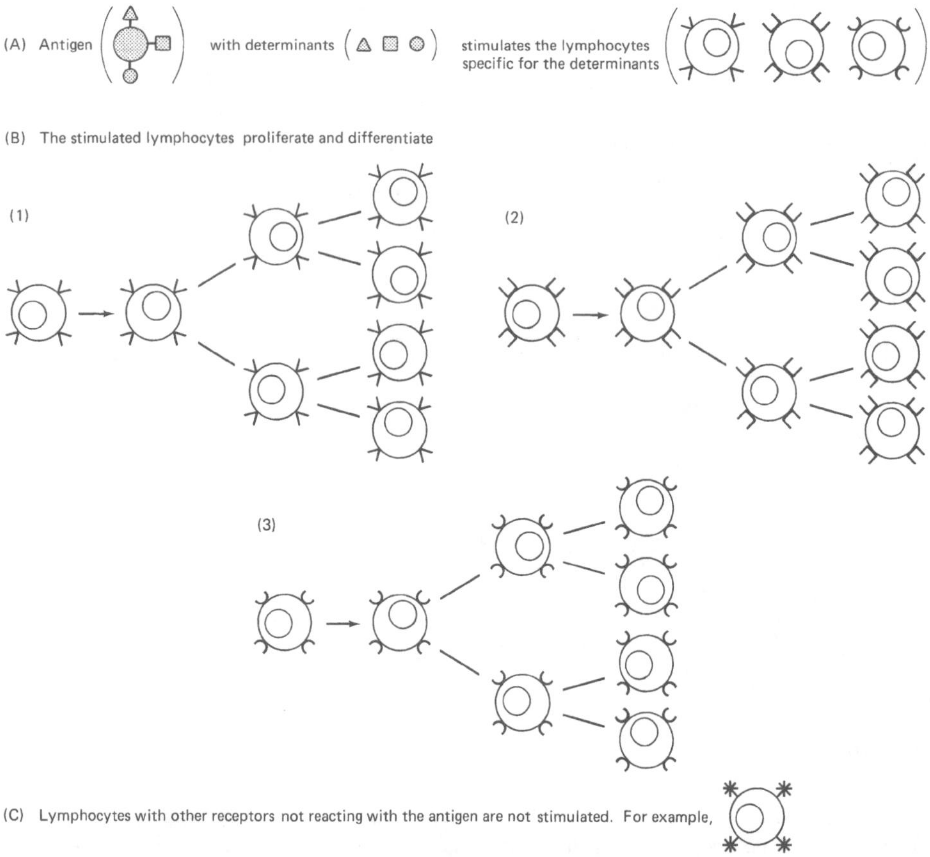

Figure 5.3. The selection of B lymphocyte clones by multiple antigenic determinants on a single antigen. The distinct determinants (A) each stimulate clones with receptors specific for only one of the determinants (B). The response eventually results in the elaboration of polyclonal antibodies to the antigen that can be recovered from the serum of the organism. The unselected clones (C) remain dormant.

lymphocytes' DNA. He also proposed that clones specific for self antigens developed, but were deleted by the host. The deletion of self-reactive clones would protect the host against self-destruction. Burnet and others showed that if the developing fetus was exposed to nonself antigens, the immune system failed to respond to these foreign antigens upon maturation. At present, a variety of explanations are offered for self-tolerance including the deletion or suppression (anergy) of self-clones in the thymus and their suppression in the periphery by suppressor T cells. The fact of autoimmune diseases suggests that not all self-reactive clones are deleted or suppressed permanently.

While the clonal selection theory has gained general acceptance as the mechanism for the specificity of the immune response, a historically important competing theory should be mentioned. Unable to account for the large amount of variability in the immune response, some scientists proposed instructional models for the generation of antibody diversity. As championed by chemist Linus Pauling in the 1940s, polypeptide chains were thought to fold around an antigen, thus forming a perfect match to the antigen (Figure 5.4). The fact that antibody specificity

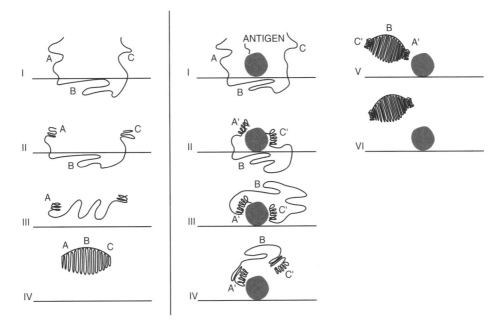

Figure 5.4. Illustration of the instructional model of antibody formation from drawings in the original paper by Linus Pauling (1940). In the series on the left (I–IV), a polypeptide folds spontaneously into a normal serum globulin. In the series on the right (I–VI), the folding process is altered by the antigen such that the globulin (antibody) can bind to the antigen that guided its folding. A' and C' represent those portions of the antibody molecule that bind antigen specifically. (Pauling, L. "A Theory of the Structure and Process of Formation of Antibodies." Figure 1, page 2645. Reprinted with permission from *J. Amer. Chem. Soc* 62 : 2643–2657. Copyright 1940. American Chemical Society.)

was determined by the amino acid sequence in the antibody receptor region put to rest permanently the instructive theories of antibody formation which proposed that antigens directly determined antibody specificity by controlling the precise folding of the antibody molecule.

SELF-RECOGNITION IN IMMUNOLOGY

The concept that antigen is recognized in the "context of self" was an important advance in the clonal selection theory. What this means is that foreign antigens are only recognized if there is also self-recognition. The first and most dramatic demonstration of this phenomenon was reported by Zinkernagel and Doherty in 1974. They found that cytotoxic lymphocytes (T lymphocytes capable of actively killing foreign or virally infected self cells) from mice immunized with a virus only recognized viral antigens expressed on the surfaces of cells obtained from mice of the same genetic strain (Figure 5.5). The cytotoxic T cells were, therefore, "restricted" as to the types of cells against which they could react. Initially, the restriction was seen as simply with regards to self. Genetic analysis revealed that the restriction was actually to a group of cell surface proteins whose genes mapped to a region of DNA called the "major histocompatibility complex (MHC)." Thus the phenomenon of self-restriction was renamed "MHC restriction."

The response to an antigen has now been shown to begin when an appropriate

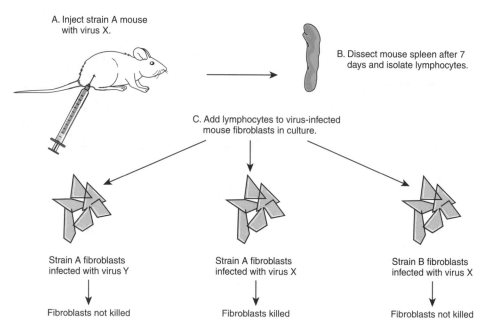

A. Inject strain A mouse with virus X.

B. Dissect mouse spleen after 7 days and isolate lymphocytes.

C. Add lymphocytes to virus-infected mouse fibroblasts in culture.

Strain A fibroblasts infected with virus Y

Fibroblasts not killed

Strain A fibroblasts infected with virus X

Fibroblasts killed

Strain B fibroblasts infected with virus X

Fibroblasts not killed

Figure 5.5. The Zinkernagel and Doherty experiment (1974). Mice of strain A were injected with virus of strain X. Cytotoxic T lymphocytes (CTLs) from the mice were then tested *in vitro* for their ability to kill virus-infected fibroblasts. It was discovered that these CTLs could kill the infected fibroblasts only if two conditions were met. Both the virus and the fibroblasts had to be of the same strain. By using congenic mice, the precise genetic requirement of the mouse strain was pinned down to the major histocompatibility complex (class I MHC).

thymus-derived lymphocyte (T cell) encounters antigen that has been presented on the surface of an antigen-presenting cell. There are several types of antigen-presenting cells including the macrophage and several types of dendritic cells within lymphoid tissues (the spleen, tonsils, lymph nodes, appendix, and diffuse lymphatic tissue in the gut). What is common about these cells is their intense phagocytic activity. The antigens are engulfed by the cell, "processed" within the cell, "presented" on the cell surface where they are then recognized by receptors on the T cells (Figure 5.6). The presentation involves the attachment of an antigen fragment to a surface MHC protein. A fragment of the antigen nestles in a groove on the surface of the MHC protein (Figure 5.7). The antigen receptor on the thymic lymphocyte (the T cell receptor or TCR) can only recognize the antigen fragment when it is presented in this manner. Moreover, the recognition is not only of the antigen, but also of the MHC protein (Figure 5.8). The absolute requirement of the T cell receptor is that the MHC must be a "self" MHC. This is the basis for self-recognition, the simultaneous recognition of self and nonself antigens. Graft rejection is an exception to the rule that foreign antigens are recognized by cytotoxic T lymphocytes only with simultaneous recognition of self MHC antigen. Individuals will reject grafts which have only nonself MHC antigens. The reason for this surprising phenomenon seems to be that the nonself MHC protein looks to the host like a nonself protein presented by a self-MHC.

The term histocompatibility gene was coined in 1948 by George Snell of the Jackson Laboratory in Bar Harbor, Maine. Working with Peter Gorer, Snell developed a

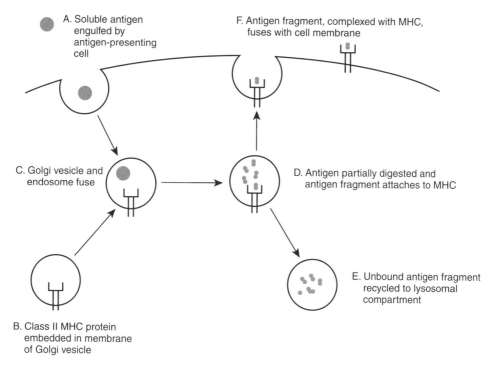

A. Soluble antigen engulfed by antigen-presenting cell

F. Antigen fragment, complexed with MHC, fuses with cell membrane

C. Golgi vesicle and endosome fuse

D. Antigen partially digested and antigen fragment attaches to MHC

E. Unbound antigen fragment recycled to lysosomal compartment

B. Class II MHC protein embedded in membrane of Golgi vesicle

Figure 5.6. The processing of an extracellular protein antigen for presentation to a helper T cell. Soluble antigen is engulfed by an antigen presenting cell (A). The endosome fuses with a Golgi vesicle containing an MHC protein (class II) (B-C). The antigen is partially-digested and an antigen fragment binds to a class II MHC protein embedded in the endosome membrane (D). The peptide-MHC complex is then returned to the cell surface (F) where it is recognized by a helper T cell via its T cell receptor (TCR). Antigen fragments that fail to bind to the MHC protein are recycled to the lysosomal compartment of the cell (E).

method for the construction of mice which differed only at defined genetic regions of the chromosomes. Inbred mice of two different strains (say, A and B) were crossed, and their offspring were backcrossed to one of the parental strains (A, for example). The offspring of the backcross which possessed strain B histocompatibility antigens (as shown by the rejection of transplants to strain A) were selected and again backcrossed to strain A mice. This process was repeated for numerous generations until the only essential difference between the offspring and the parental A strain was the ability to reject the allograft (Figure 5.9). Therefore, the genetic difference was that region of the genome coding for the transplantation antigens. These two types of true-breeding mice are called "congenic."

By studying skin graft rejection in congenic mice, Snell and Gorer described upwards of forty different genes which control transplant rejection. Those which caused a rapid rate of rejection were found to be on a single chromosome (chromosome 17 in mice). They were called the "major histocompatibility antigens." Those which caused slower rejection were called "minor histocompatibility antigens" and were found at many locations in the genome. One of the strongest antigens was Gorer's antigen II. As an homage, Snell named the major histocompatibility gene complex in mice H-2. In humans, the homologous gene complex is called "HLA" for human leukocyte antigens."

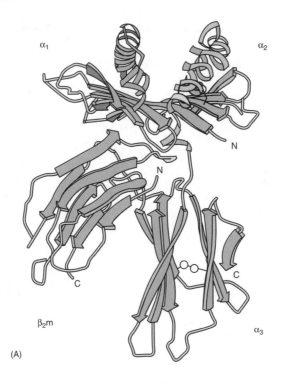

(A)

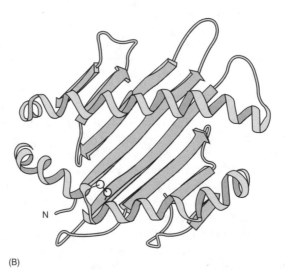

(B)

Figure 5.7.   The structure of a class I MHC protein. The molecule is composed of three distinct domains (α1, α2, and α3). The carboxyl-end of the protein (c) is connected to a region of
α-helix embedded in the cell membrane (not shown). The α1 and α2 domains form an antigen-binding groove to which an antigen peptide binds. A small protein, β-2 microglobin (β2m),
also binds to the MHC protein. (A) A side view of the MHC-β-2 microglobin complex. (B) A top
view of the antigen-binding groove (α1 and α2) bounded by two α-helix walls and a β-pleated
sheet floor. (From P. J. Bjorkman, M. A. Saper. B. Samraoui, W. S. Bennett, J. I. Strominger, and
D. C. Wiley. "Structure of the Human Class I Histocompatability Anitgen, HLA-A2." Figures
2a–2b, pages 508–509. 1987. *Nature* 329: 506–512).

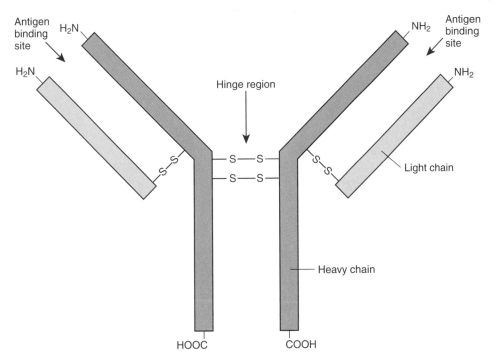

Figure 5.10. A schematic drawing of an antibody molecule. The antibody is composed of two heavy and two light chains held together by disulfide bridges. There are two identical antigen binding sites that can move relative to each other by bending at the hinge region.

cussed in chapter 7. For the time being, our discussion will ignore the issue of antibody classes or isotypes.

The T cell receptor (TCR) is similar to the antibody molecule in that it is a complex protein molecule than can recognize antigen with great specificity. At the same time, there are several key differences. Unlike the antibody molecule, the TCR is not secreted. Instead it is always found on the surface of T cells. The TCR is also composed of only two protein chains, called α and β. The ends of the chains that bind antigen are, like antibody, variable while the ends attached to the cell surface are constant (Figure 5.11). The most significant difference is that the TCR can only recognize antigen when it is associated with self class I or class II MHC proteins on the surface of an antigen presenting cell.

The development of immunochemistry contributed to the development of the understanding of immunology in other ways than through the elucidation of the nature of antibody. It also put immunology on a firm experimental basis through the development of methods for the precise quantitative analysis of antigens and antibodies. Experimentation at the Rockefeller Institute in the 1930s led to the development of quantitative precipitation methods for measuring antigen and antibody, and to the discovery that carbohydrates, as well as proteins, are antigenic. At the same time, scientists at the Rockefeller Institute discovered how antigen and antibody react to form insoluble lattice-like complexes (Figure 5.12).

MONOCLONAL ANTIBODIES
In the course of an immune reaction, many different specific B cell clones are acti-

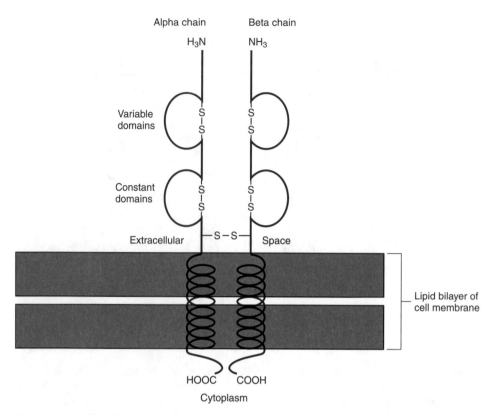

Figure 5.11. The T cell receptor is composed of two simple proteins, the alpha and beta chains, that are held together by disulfide bridges. Alpha helices at the carboxyl end of each chain are embedded in the membrane of the T cell. The variable and constant domains extend into the extracellular space.

vated and many antibodies are produced, each with a different specificity. This is because most pathogens are composed of many different molecules, each with many different antigenic determinants. These antigenic molecules have many different antigenic determinants because they have a welter of different shapes (epitopes) on their surface, each of which will trigger the production of at least one antibody. Since each antibody is produced by a distinct clone of B lymphocytes, the resultant antibody population in the serum is polyclonal and quite heterogeneous.

While polyclonal antibodies are useful in many research and therapeutic applications, such as the treatment of diphtheria with von Behring's antitoxin, they are not as valuable in many uses as are monoclonal antibodies. Monoclonal antibodies are homogeneous and, thus, highly specific and the antigen to which a monoclonal antibody can bind may be known.

Myeloma proteins are monoclonal antibodies: they are the products of the progeny of a single lymphocyte that became cancerous and multiplied to form a tumor (the tumor is a clone). The problem with the use of myeloma proteins in research is that the antigens to which the antibody binds are not known since the original cell giving rise to the clone was induced by the cancerous transformation, not by an antigen.

Georges Kohler and Cesar Milstein developed a technique for producing

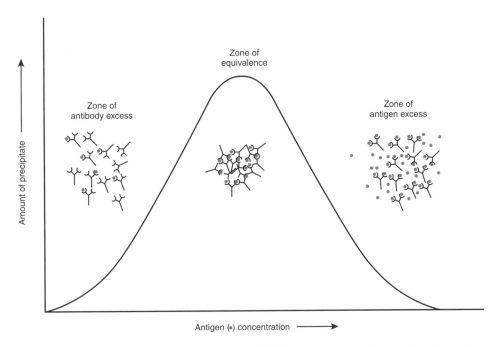

Figure 5.12.   Antigen and antibody form an insoluble lattice structure when both are in roughly equimolar concentrations. Outside of this zone of equivalence, when either antigen or antibody is in excess, precipitation does not occur.

monoclonal antibodies against a known antigen. Antibody secreting plasma cells, unless they are transformed to be cancerous, do not divide. Therefore one cannot pick out a plasma cell that is secreting an antibody of interest and clone it in culture because the plasma cell will not divide. Plasma cells can be coerced into dividing, however, by fusing them with cancerous myeloma cells. Plasma cells from a mouse that has been injected with a known antigen are recovered from the spleen of the mouse and mixed with mouse myeloma cells. The membranes of the two types of cells will fuse together if a "fusagen" is used, the most common being the lipid-dissolving chemical polyethylene glycol. If the myeloma cells have lost the ability to make antibodies, the resultant "hybridomas" (-*oma* is a suffix meaning *tumor*) divide and secrete antibodies against the antigen that was used to produce the plasma cell. Hybridoma cells can be stored frozen and thawed out whenever supplies of a particular monoclonal antibody are needed. Kohler and Milstein shared the 1984 Nobel prize for this technological *tour de force*. But the feat was more than technological. It has opened up a whole new world of research and therapeutic applications.

THE GENETICS OF THE IMMUNE RESPONSE
The clonal selection theory states that antibody specificity is genetically determined. The period of 1976 to 1982 saw the partial resolution of the problem of how an animal can maintain in its genome the huge repertoire of genes which are required to program recognition of all the different antigen epitopes that the system has the capacity to recognize. Scientists in several laboratories using the analytical techniques of molecular genetics have shown that, with gene recombination and so-

matic mutation during development, the number of genes available is quite sufficient to permit development of the multitude of clones of lymphocytes necessary for the production of the vast array of antibodies synthesized by an individual. The same story of gene recombination and somatic mutation is true for the T cell receptor.

One would expect the chromosome regions coding for the variable and constant regions of the light or heavy chain to be adjacent to one another in the immunoglobulin genes. If DNA sequences coding for the constant and variable regions are next to one another in each antibody gene in the germ line, a thorny evolutionary problem must be confronted. In the course of the evolution of the antibody repertoire, it is obvious that the variable portions of the antibodies have diverged dramatically. But the constant portions have not changed. It is hard to imagine a genetic mechanism that would allow one portion of a gene to mutate wildly while the adjacent portion remains unchanged. There is no obvious mechanism or selective pressure that would keep all of the constant region genes identical to one another. Yet, the constant portion of the antibody molecule is in fact just that — constant.

As significantly, immunoglobulin genes segregate during reproduction as a single Mendelian trait. Individuals possess no more than two immunologically detectable characteristics for each antibody class or isotype. These allotypic determinants (referring to their ability to trigger a specific immune response when they are themselves treated as antigens) represent the two alleles of the constant genes of each antibody class. The fact that only one allotype is passed on to the next generation suggested that there is only one gene (represented by two alleles) for the constant region.

The truth about antibody gene structure was, therefore, quite confusing. Any theory about their structure was torn between one set of data that showed multiple variable genes and another which argued for single constant genes. How could these two opposing views of the antibody gene be reconciled?

A radical solution to this problem was proposed in a 1965 paper by Dreyer and Bennett. They hypothesized that there were many different variable (V) genes and *only one* constant (C) gene in the germ line (actually two since the organism is diploid). The process of lymphocyte proliferation and differentiation would be accompanied by the recombination of the DNA such that one (and only one) variable gene would be joined to the single constant gene on the same chromosome to form a new gene different in every lymphocyte. The definitive gene (V_n + C) for the antigen binding protein would be formed by recombination of genes not immediately next to one another in the germ line (Figure 5.13).

This would mean not only that the genes for antigen binding proteins in the germ line would be different from the genes in mature lymphocytes, but also that the genes in different lymphocyte clones would be different from one another. The new techniques of molecular genetics, as used by Tonegawa and others, confirmed this solution to the enigma of antibody diversity. The concept was considered radical since it was at odds with the generally accepted idea that the DNA (the genome) is the same in every cell of an individual. Lymphocytes were, perhaps, the proverbial exception that proved the rule.

HORMONAL SUBSTANCES INDUCED IN IMMUNITY

Among the more exciting developments of recent years was the discovery that lymphocytes and macrophages secrete hormones which allow them to communicate with nearby cells. "Cytokines" (from the Greek *kytos*, the cell, and *kinein*, to

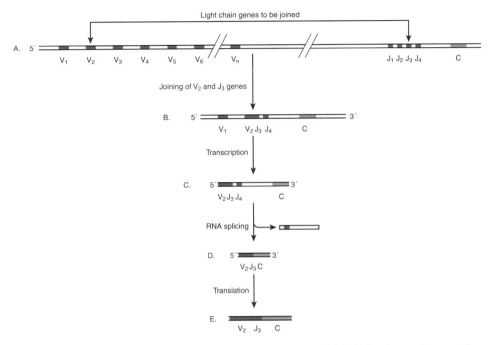

Figure 5.13. Gene recombination in the formation of an antibody light chain. The germ line DNA consists of many copies of V and J genes arranged in tandem (A). During B cell differentiation, one V and one J gene are recombined at random (B). After transcription of the recombined gene (C), the RNA is spliced to remove the intervening sequence of nucleotides separating the variable (V-J) gene from the constant gene (D). The fully processed messenger RNA is then translated into a light-chain protein (E).

move) are small glycoproteins secreted primarily by T cells and macrophages. Cytokines "move" their target cells by way of an elaborate regulatory network of signals within the cytoplasm of the responding cell. This network ties together the beginning (the binding, processing, presentation, and recognition of antigen) and the end (the multiple cellular responses) of immune responses. Cytokines usually, but not always, function locally, affecting the behavior of the cells involved in the immune response. Cytokines usually, but not always, work in concert with other cytokines. The target cell, therefore, has as many different types of cytokine receptors as there are cytokines to which the cell can respond. Each receptor is linked to a cytoplasmic signaling pathway.

As all good protein hormones do, cytokines bind to receptors on the surface of their target cells. After the hormonal message is transmitted to the cytoplasm, the target cells respond predictably. They may become activated, divide, or differentiate. The result of all of this is the elimination of antigen and a return (approximately) to initial conditions.

The discovery that the immune response is mediated by hormones constituted a revolution in immunobiology. For years this truth was obscured by the dominant belief that lymphocyte proliferation and differentiation were driven by antigen alone. Whatever the mechanisms whereby antigen had this effect, it was thought that these mechanisms were unique to the immune system. With the elucidation of the role of cytokines, however, the study of the immune response rejoined the biological fold. More established disciplines were brought to bear on the study of the immune response. Immunobiologists began to communicate with scientists trained in the more traditional fields of endocrinology, enzymology, and pharmacology. Very fruitful research data was gathered as immunobiologists tapped the treasure trove of techniques and knowledge gained from the study of these nonimmunobiological systems. As a result, we understand the immune response much more clearly than we did only a few years ago. Indeed, the interaction of cytokines with lymphocytes is rapidly becoming a model system for the study of how cells respond generally to external chemical signals.

There are many different cytokines involved in the regulation of an immune response to antigen. Learning these cytokines by name and by function is a daunting task for any student! Moreover, many of the names of cytokines are confusing. Confusing names are a common result of the historical development of a science. When a variety of factors are discovered at different times by people in different laboratories using different species and means of measurement, a chaotic nomenclature is inevitable.

The task is made easier if we attempt to sort these cytokines into groups. The foremost category consists of cytokines which regulate the activation, proliferation, and differentiation of lymphocytes. These are the cytokines which directly regulate antigen-specific immune responses. Specific responses include the clonal expansion of T and B cells, and the differentiation of antibody secreting B cells, helper T cells, and cytotoxic T cells.

Second are the cytokines that control inflammation. This category includes cytokines released either by macrophages in nonspecific immune responses or by T cells or macrophages (stimulated by T cells) in antigen-specific responses. T cell cytokines may also have an indirect inflammatory effect by stimulating granulocytes in antigen-specific responses. The nonspecific and specific immune responses are not independent of one another. Acute nonspecific inflammation is a rapid response that holds the fort until a specific immune response, with its chronic inflammatory arm, is mounted.

The last category includes cytokines which stimulate the growth and differentiation of immature leukocytes. These cytokines regulate the proliferation of each of the leukocyte lineages in the bone marrow. As such, they are responsible for the number of leukocytes present and available for action in an immune response.

The first hints at the existence of hormones mediating the immune response to antigen came in the mid 1960s. Experiments demonstrated that conditioned medium (medium in which lymphocytes had been stimulated to divide) was mitogenic. When conditioned medium was added to a culture of T lymphocytes, they were stimulated to divide. Since the responding cells were T cells, the term T cell growth factor (TCGF) was coined to describe this activity. Since lymphocytes were the source of this mitogenic activity, the more general term lymphokine was used to describe the class of molecule.

When it was discovered that medium conditioned by macrophages would also stimulate T cell division, lymphokine became an obsolete term. The macrophage-produced activity was called lymphocyte-activating factor (LAF). Since LAF was not, etymologically speaking, a lymphokine, the term "monokine" (from *mono*cyte, the macrophage precursor) was proposed. Finally, the term "cytokine" was coined to cover both types of molecule. This term is consistent with the fact that some cytokines are produced by nonleukocytes (endothelial cells and bone marrow stroma, for example). Cytokine is the appropriate term for all of the hormones involved in the regulation of immune and inflammatory responses. This term subsumes the older terms, although lymphokine and monokine are still found in the scientific literature.

The mitogenic activity of LAF was, however, limited. Further study made it clear that LAF only potentiated the proliferation of T cells, serving (with TCGF) as a costimulator of T cell growth. Macrophage LAF stimulates T cells to secrete TCGF. In turn, TCGF stimulates T cell division. TCGF is an autocrine hormone; it stimulates the division of the same T cells that produce it.

The discovery of these interactions between macrophage and lymphocyte cytokines gave rise to the descriptive term interleukin (literally, *between leukocytes*). LAF became known as interleukin 1 (IL-1), TCGF as interleukin 2 (IL-2). These terms have turned out to be more appropriate than LAF and TCGF, since their effects are much more numerous than lymphocyte activation and T cell growth stimulation. To date, twenty interleukins (IL-1 to IL-20) have been identified and named.

To add to the confusion, there are cytokines which did not inherit the interleukin handle (tumor necrosis factors, the interferons, and the colony-stimulating factors). These names have persisted despite the fact that these descriptive terms make no mention of their other effects. To make the confusion total, there are also subsets of the originally described interleukins (IL-1α and IL-1β, for example) which have been named after closer biochemical scrutiny.

SUMMARY

The dramatic success of immunization against a large number of bacterial and viral infections has led scientists to try to understand the cellular and molecular bases for the inducible immune response. Inducible immunity was originally thought to be either a cellular phenomenon, as observed in the intense phagocytic activity of macrophages, or a humoral phenomenon, as observed by the presence of antibodies in the serum of immunized animals. Today we understand that both cell-mediated and humoral immunity operate in the inducible immune response.

Antibodies are protein molecules secreted by B lymphocytes after they have encountered antigen. Each lymphocyte and its clonal descendants are capable of secreting only one type of specific antibody. The invading antigen "selects" the matching clone which then proliferates and differentiates into antibody-secreting plasma cells. Elucidation of the structure of the antibody molecule by analytical chemistry and use of the techniques of molecular biology to study the genome led to the discovery that genes undergo extensive recombination of their DNA in order to generate the remarkable antibody diversity that B lymphocytes possess. Since antigens are complex, many different clones are activated and many different antibodies are produced in an immune response to any antigenic exposure. The artificial production of hybridomas, however, allows for the production of monoclonal antibodies.

B lymphocytes rarely respond to antigen alone. They require a precise interaction with helper T cells that trigger B cell proliferation and differentiation. T cells mature in the thymus. Unlike their close cousins, T cells do not secrete antibodies. They do, however, bind antigen through a protein molecule on their surface, the T cell receptor (TCR). The binding of helper T cells to properly presented antigens triggers the T cell's activation. Helper T cells secrete a number of small proteins, called cytokines. Cytokines are the hormones of the immune system. They have a wide variety of effects on many other cells of the immune system and other tissues of the body. Among other activities, cytokines trigger B cells to divide, activate macrophages, and participate in inflammation reactions. The other major subclass of T cells are the killer T cells, also known as cytotoxic T cells (CTLs). CTLs recognize foreign antigen on the surface of other cells and kill that cell. The logic of this reaction is that the foreign protein on the cell surface is commonly a budding virus particle or the protein signature of a cancer cell. Death of the cell terminates the spread of a viral infection or ends the proliferation of cancer cells. The proper presentation of antigen to helper T cells (and the presentation of viral particles on infected cells) requires that antigen fragments be displayed by a group of cell proteins coded for by a region of DNA called the major histocompatibility complex. In order for a response to occur, the MHC proteins must be from the host, a phenomenon known as self-restriction. Presentation of antigen to the helper T cell is accomplished by antigen-presenting cells, including the macrophage. These discoveries finally brought together the cell-mediated and humoral arms of the inducible immune response.

As a result of the developments described, the study of the immunological aspects of the host parasite interaction now has a firm biochemical, genetic, and cellular base. We now know more about the nature of the immunological changes induced in vertebrates by infection than we do about the mechanisms controlling host-parasite interaction in the nonimmune host.

SUGGESTIONS FOR FURTHER READING

1. Alperts, B., D. Bray, J. Lewis, M. Raff, K. Roberts, and J.D. Watson. *Molecular Biology of the Cell*. 3d ed. New York/London: Garland Publishing, Inc., 1994.
2. Bulloch, W. *The History of Bacteriology*. London: Oxford University Press, 1938.
3. Burnet F.M. *The Clonal Selection Theory of Acquired Immunity*. Cambridge: The University Press, 1959.
4. Clark W.R. *The Experimental Foundations of Modern Immunology*. 3d ed. New York: Wiley, 1986.
5. Ehrlich, P. *Collected Papers of Paul Ehrlich*, vol. 2, New York: Pergamon, 1957.
6. Kindt, T.J., and J.D. Capra. *The Antibody Enigma*. New York: Plenum Press, 1984.
7. Landsteiner, K. *The Specificity of Serological Reactions*. Boston: Harvard University Press, 1945.
8. Metchnikoff, E. *Immunity in the Infectious Diseases*. New York: Macmillan, 1905.
9. Silverstein, A.M. *A History of Immunology*. San Diego: Academic Press, 1989.

QUESTIONS

1. What is immunization and why did its discovery lead to the development of immunology as a modern science?
2. What is the difference between innate and inducible immunity? What are the relative advantages and disadvantages of each?
3. Explain the similarities and differences between Ehrlich's side chain theory of antibody production and the clonal selection theory.
4. What does it mean to say that cell-mediated and humoral immunity are "separate manifestations of one system?"

5 Why is necessary for an organism to suppress or eliminate self-reactive clones of lymphocytes?

6 Why did Zinkernagel and Doherty use congenic mice in their experiments?

7 Why is the fact that the antibody molecule has two binding sites important to the precipitation of antigen?

8 How are the T cell receptor and the antibody molecule both similar and different?

9 How are cytokines similar to and different from endocrine hormones such as insulin or growth hormone?

ANSWERS

1 Immunization is the medical procedure whereby a person is rendered immune to infection by the intentional administration of a specific pathogen. This can be accomplished by the infection of an individual with a related but nonpathogenic strain of the organism, by infection with a strain that has lost the ability to multiply in the host, or by the injection of cell-free antigens isolated from the pathogen. The immune response of the host includes the development of immunological memory which makes the treated individual immune to infection by the same pathogen. Since infectious disease was (and still is) a leading killer in human society, the development of effective immunization for diseases such as small pox, rabies, and diphtheria was a tremendous medical advance. The desire to understand how immunity was achieved in the vertebrate organism stimulated scientific efforts to learn how the immune system works.

2 Innate immunity does not require that the individual has had prior exposure to the pathogenic organism. It operates immediately, but it is nonspecific. Inducible immunity is induced by exposure to the pathogen. Innate immunity provides immediate protection and thus time for the inducible immune response to generate activated lymphocytes. The inducible response is very specific and also demonstrates memory, leading to long-term immunity.

3 Both theories have as a fundamental premise the existence of specific antibodies prior to exposure to antigen. Clonal selection adds the important feature that cells proliferate in response to antigen stimulation before differentiating into antibody-producing cells.

4 While it is convenient to divide the immune system into these two separate components, they are in fact quite interrelated and a typical immune response includes both cell-mediated and humoral responses. As an example, the production of helper T cells (a cell-mediated response) leads to the proliferation and differentiation of B cells (a humoral response).

5 The immune response, turned upon the organism that produces it, can be very destructive. Numerous autoimmune diseases such a systemic lupus erythromatosis, myasthenia gravis, and rheumatoid arthritis are cases in point.

6 Congenic mice are genetically identical except for the major histocomptability genes. By using congenic mice with different MHC haplotypes, Zinkernagel and Doherty were able to pinpoint the MHC as the locus of self-restriction.

7 To form a lattice, it is necessary for the antibody to cross-link the precipitated antigen. This requires two antigen receptor sites.

8 They are similar in that they are both capable of specifically binding to antigen. Indeed, they are both members of the same gene family. But there are very important differences. While antibodies bind to the epitopes on free antigens, TCRs bind

only to antigen fragments presented by MHC proteins. Whereas both TCRs and antibodies are found on the surface of B and T cells, respectively, only antibodies are secreted. Structurally, TCRs are composed of two chains, α and β, and antibodies are composed of two light and two heavy chains. Both are produced from genes that undergo genetic recombination to bring the constant and variable genes together in multiple combinations.

9 While both are glycoproteins (there are, however, steroid endocrine hormones as well), endocrine hormones circulate in the blood and have their effects far from the site of production. Cytokines tend to act locally and, as such, are paracrine hormones. As protein hormones, both types fail to enter their target cell but, rather, stimulate specific hormone receptors on the target cell's surface.

INTRODUCTION
CHARACTERISTICS OF
  ANTIGENS
  Foreignness
  Biodegradability
  Molecular Weight and
    Complexity
THE HAPTEN-CARRIER
  CONCEPT
SITES ON ANTIGENS
  RECOGNIZED BY
  ANTIBODIES
MAPPING EPITOPES AND
  ANTIGEN-BINDING
  SITES
THE STRENGTH OF
  ANTIGEN BINDING
CROSS REACTIVITY OF
  ANTIGENS
  Complex Antigens
  Shared Epitopes
  Similarity of Epitopes
THE GENOTYPE OF THE
  RESPONDING ANIMAL
SUPERANTIGENS
ROUTES OF ANTIGEN
  ADMINISTRATION
ADJUVANTS
SUMMARY
SUGGESTIONS FOR
  FURTHER READING
QUESTIONS
ANSWERS

The Inducible System: Antigens

Ralph A. Sorensen

INTRODUCTION

An antigen was originally considered simply to be any substance capable of inducing the generation of antibody. In fact, the word *antigen* was coined from the words "antibody" and "generator." A more complete immunological definition of an antigen is that it is any substance which, when introduced into an immunocompetent animal, induces an immunological response. This definition broadens the meaning of the word to include cell-mediated immune reactions induced by antigens. A complete definition of antigen also includes the fact that antigens interact with the products of the immune response in some observable way. This may include the formation of an antigen-antibody complex or the interaction of an antigen with a T cell receptor (TCR). In the latter case, however, the issue is more complicated since the TCR can only recognize a protein antigen after it has been processed and presented by an MHC protein.

The definition above is operational: antigens are defined strictly in terms of what they *do*. The definition says nothing about what antigens *are*. Our present knowledge of what antigens are is derived from the study of the characteristics of substances shown to be antigenic by the fact that they induce an immune response. Analysis of these substances has shown most of them to be proteins or complex carbohydrates. Lipids and nucleic acids as well as many small molecules such as various drugs and poisons may also stimulate an immune response if they are complexed with proteins or carbohydrates. Proteins are the molecules capable of stimulating a cell-mediated immune response. Chemicals such as picric acid and the lipids of poison ivy will also induce such a response after coupling with a protein, even one which is a component of the exposed individual. As the macromolecular structures of living organisms are made up of proteins, carbohydrates, lipids, and nucleic acids, all of the components of living systems are potential antigens.

An *antigenic determinant* is defined as a region of an antigenic molecule that fits into the combining site of an antibody. It comprises only a small part of the invading pathogen or molecule to which the immune system of the host has responded. The word *determinant* is usually used synonymously with the term *epitope* which literally means "surface shape" and refers to the site on the surface of the molecule to which the antibody binds. Short segments (i.e., polypeptides) of proteins or of polysaccharides may also serve as epitopes. Complex molecules such as proteins and polysaccharides may, therefore, have multiple determinants. The number of epitopes to which an animal responds, however, is usually fewer than the total number of potential epitopes of any protein or carbohydrate. At the same time, some epitopes are *immunodominant* and produce a stronger immune response than other epitopes on the same protein.

Antigenic determinants, if chemically separated from the antigenic molecule, do not induce antibody formation by themselves. They are relatively small portions of a larger molecule that does. Such separated antigenic determinants are called *haptens*. Haptens can react with the products of an immune response, but cannot induce an immune response. To do this they require the rest of the antigenic molecule, referred to as the *carrier*. Some authors prefer the term *immunogen* to distinguish larger antigens (complete) that induce an immune response from smaller antigens (haptens) that do not. In this usage, haptens are antigens, but they are not immunogens.

CHARACTERISTICS OF ANTIGENS

As noted above an antigen is any material which, when introduced into the tissue of an immunocompetent animal, will induce an immunological response and which can be shown to react with the products of that response in some detectable way. A description of the characteristics of antigens is, therefore, a summary of the characteristics of a fairly heterogeneous population of substances.

Foreignness

The essential function of the immunological system of vertebrate animals is protection of the animal from invasion by another living organism. The purpose of this invasion (from the standpoint of the invader) is survival: to survive, the invader must be able to utilize the resources of the invaded host. In general, it is best for the parasite not to kill the host, as then it loses its source of nutrients. In turn, the invaded, or to use the medical term, *infected*, animal must try to minimize any injury to itself resulting from the invasion. To protect itself, the host must be able to recognize and destroy the invader or, if it cannot destroy it totally, at least limit its growth and its spread through the body.

Vertebrates are large, complex multicellular animals. They are colonies of cells, the individual cells of which are highly integrated and tightly controlled. The defense against an invader can only occur if this system of cells can distinguish the invader from itself. The ability to distinguish between self and the invader and then to take action against the foreign agent alone is the measure of immunocompetence. As parasites are constructed of proteins, lipids, carbohydrates, and nucleic acids, just like their hosts, recognition of the parasite as foreign depends on the recognition of fine points of difference between the molecules of the parasite and the host.

Self-tolerance, defined as the failure of the immunological system to respond to self, develops during fetal life. In 1953, Billingham, Brent, and Medawar injected cells from adult mice of the genetic strain A into fifteen-day-old mouse fetuses of the CBA strain. When these animals reached maturity, they were given skin grafts from the A mice. Normally, skin grafts from a different genetic strain would be rapidly rejected. In this case they were not. Self-tolerance had been actively acquired. Tolerance of self was, therefore, learned in some way rather than programmed into the animal.

For the present discussion, it is sufficient to realize that for a molecule to be immunogenic, it must differ in some respect from all the molecules of the immunocompetent animal into which it is introduced. Thus, a molecule that is not normally an antigen to the animal from which it is derived may well be an antigen in another animal. In general, the more distantly related species are, the more differences their molecules will have and the more strongly they will react to the introduction of molecules of the other species. On the other hand, molecules, with structures which have been highly conserved in evolution, make poor antigens.

Still, tissues cannot be freely transferred from one member of a species to another member of the same species. Molecules of one individual of a species which are antigenic in another member of the same species are called *isoantigens* and the antibodies that are produced are called *isoantibodies*. A well-studied example of such antigens is the ABO blood group system in humans. These blood groups are defined by the presence or absence of different glycoproteins on the surfaces of red blood cells. Groups A and B differ only in one sugar: group A glycoproteins have a terminal N-acetyl galactosamine amine and group B glycoproteins have galactosamine. The genes that determine these blood groups encode the transferases responsible for synthesis of the oligosaccharide portion of the glycoprotein. If an individual lacks the gene for the A transferase, he will develop antibodies to A in his blood serum from exposure to similar bacterial antigenic determinants. If the blood of this individual is transfused to someone with type A blood, these isoantibodies will clump and destroy the red blood cells of the recipient. For this reason, careful blood typing is standard procedure before blood transfusion.

The histocompatibility system, of which the blood group system is a special case, prevents the ready transfer of organs such as hearts, kidneys, and skin among individuals of the same species. A moment's reflection makes it obvious that histocompatibility did not arise to prevent tissue transfer among members of the same species. Instead, the development and maintenance of the complex histocompatibility system is the result of selection for the ability to control infection. Histocompatibility is determined by protein molecules present on the surface of animal cells. The primary system that controls tissue transplantation is at a distinct genetic locus called the *major histocompatibility complex* (MHC). In mice this locus is called *H-2*. Immune responses to leukocytes in blood given during therapeutic transfusions provided a means for the study of histocompatibility in humans. Thus the homologous system in humans is called the *human leukocyte antigen* (HLA) system. The normal function of these proteins is to present antigen to responding receptors on T cells.

The presence of a number of genes in the population, each of which has multiple alleles that are reassorted during sexual reproduction, assures a unique histocompatibility display in each individual of the species (see chapter 11). Because this system assures that each individual has a unique pattern of self-markers determined by random segregation during gamete production and gamete fusion, no parasite can evolve a molecular configuration identical to the histocompatibility display of all individuals of the species. This is an important safeguard for the species since no parasite can evade recognition as foreign by *all* members of that species.

While it is generally the case that immunocompetent individuals do not respond to their own molecular structures, it is, unfortunately, not always true. Complex systems can be expected to fail on occasion. A pathological response to self-antigens is called *autoimmunity,* and the self-materials to which the response occurs are called *autoantigens.* The danger of autoimmune disease clearly led to the evolution of self-tolerance. In the very early 1900s, Ehrlich and Morgenroth proposed the existence of a "regulating contrivance" for the development of self-tolerance, an avoidance of self-reaction they called *horror autotoxicus.* Chapter 10 is specifically concerned with autoimmunity.

Development of self-tolerance occurs during fetal life by exposure of the self-molecules to the developing immune system. Some self-materials to which an individual may respond are developed in isolation during embryogenesis and thus escape the development of self-tolerance. These materials do not normally leave their sites of synthesis during the life of the individual. The lens of the eye and much of the brain tissue are in this category. If, as a result of injury, molecules are released from these normally sequestered tissues, the individual may respond to them as foreign since the immune system did not encounter them during the time when self-tolerance was developed.

Slightly altered self-molecules may also be treated as foreign. The subsequent response to these altered self-molecules may produce antibodies that also react with the unaltered molecules. Some therapeutic drugs may initiate autoimmune responses by this mechanism. Blackwater fever, a response to one's own red cells in persons repeatedly infected with malaria and treated with quinine, is such a condition. Streptococcal infection may, by a similar mechanism, bring about rheumatic fever, a consequence of an autoimmune reaction to heart tissue.

Insulin is a protein hormone produced by the pancreas. Individuals with type I, or juvenile-onset diabetes fail to make sufficient insulin due to the autoimmune destruction of the insulin-producing cells. The medical management of this disease therefore requires the frequent injection of insulin. Porcine insulin, which differs from human insulin in only three amino acids, will sometimes cause an immune response in diabetics. This problem can be avoided by use of human insulin produced by genetically modified bacteria. Human insulin is identical in all humans and is thus always treated as self.

Biodegradability
Phagocytosis and subsequent digestion of invading microorganisms evolved early in multicellular animals as a defense against infection. The more sophisticated inducible immune system of higher vertebrates is built upon these primitive systems and is shaped by their nature. Nonbiodegradable materials may be walled off and isolated by the formation of a calcified connective tissue capsule, but phagocytes cannot process indigestible materials and initiate an immune response with them. The requirement for biodegradability is a result of the fact that the antigen present-

ing cells, which are responsible for initiation of most immune responses, can only initiate a response if they can present partially digested fragments of the antigenic molecules to other cells involved in the system. A few *T-independent antigens* do not require processing by antigen presenting cells, but these are few in number and represent a special case.

Molecular Weight and Complexity

It is clear from empirical observation that molecules must be fairly large to be immunogenic. One of the smallest proteins shown to be immunogenic in rabbits is human glucagon. It has a molecular weight of 3500 daltons and is a straight chain polypeptide of twenty-nine amino acids. But this is unusual and, speaking generally, the larger the molecule, the greater the immunogenicity.

Complexity is also important for a molecule to be immunogenic. Synthetic amino acid homopolymers, composed of a single amino acid, are notoriously poor immunogens regardless of their size. The addition of different amino acid types (aromatic, basic, acidic) increases a synthetic polymer's immunogenicity. Since the topology of a protein defines the number of potential epitopes, the greater the structural complexity of a protein, the greater its immunogenicity. Thus, a protein with a complex tertiary or quaternary structure produces a stronger immune response than a protein with a simple repeating structure.

THE HAPTEN-CARRIER CONCEPT

Immunological reactions are very sensitive tests for the detection of molecular structure. Prior to the elucidation of the structure of antibodies, important details were discovered about the way they bind antigen. The exquisite specificity of antibodies was uncovered in a series of pioneering experiments by Karl Landsteiner (1868 to 1943).

Landsteiner approached the problem of how antibody binds antigen from the point of view of the antigen. His strategy was to make subtle modifications in a simple antigenic molecule and to observe the consequences of the changes to antibody recognition. He used standard chemical techniques to covalently bond different small molecules to carrier proteins (Figure 6.1).

By itself, aminobenzene is not immunogenic. But if this small organic molecule is covalently linked to an immunogenic protein, such as serum albumin, it could then cause an immune response. Landsteiner called the small organic molecule a *hapten* and the protein molecule the *carrier.* The immunization of a rabbit with bovine or equine serum albumin to which aminobenzoic acid had been conjugated resulted in the production of antibodies specific for aminobenzoic acid as well as for various epitopes on the carrier molecule. Absorption of the immune serum with the carrier molecule alone removed the antibodies specific for the carrier, leaving a solution of antibodies specific for the hapten.

In one critical series of experiments, he used the simple organic molecule aminobenzene substituted with different acidic functional groups (carboxyl, SO_3H, or AsO_3H_2). Aminobenzene is a six-carbon ring with an amino group attached to one of the carbons. The substituent groups could be added to carbons at different positions around the ring. These positions were named *ortho, meta, and para*, referring to the position of the amino group on the ring. He then linked these subtly different haptens to a carrier and injected the hapten-carrier complexes into rabbits and tested the antisera the rabbits produced.

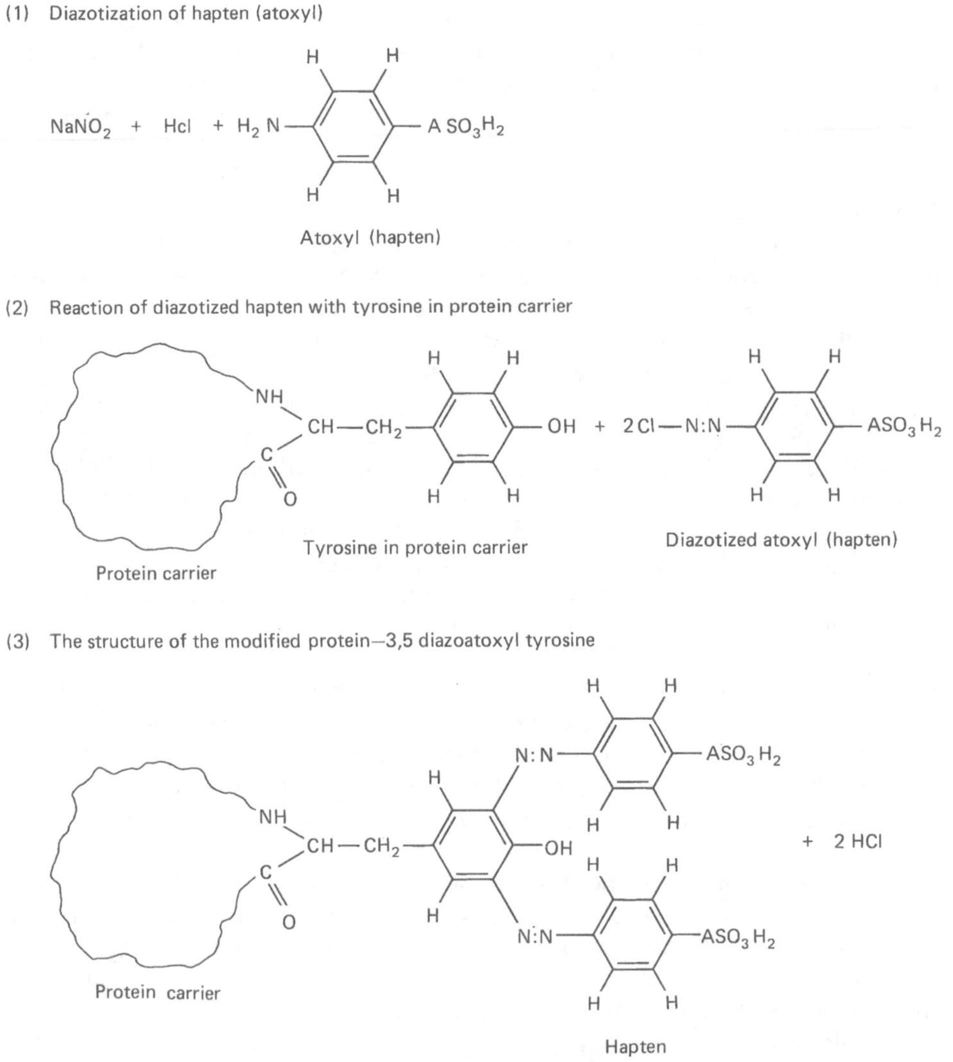

(1) Diazotization of hapten (atoxyl)

Atoxyl (hapten)

(2) Reaction of diazotized hapten with tyrosine in protein carrier

Tyrosine in protein carrier

Diazotized atoxyl (hapten)

Protein carrier

(3) The structure of the modified protein—3,5 diazoatoxyl tyrosine

Protein carrier

Hapten

Figure 6.1.   A common method of attaching haptens to a carrier molecule is by diazotization. In this process the hapten is first modified by reaction with $NaNO_2$ in HCl (1). As a result, a reactive diazo group replaces an NH_2 group on the hapten. The diazotized hapten reacts with the aromatic ring of any tyrosine residues in the protein (2), yielding the modified protein (3).

The results of his experiment are shown in Table 6.1. The clear conclusion is that antibodies can distinguish between the ortho-, meta-, and para- isomers of the same molecule. This suggested that antibodies recognize subtle differences in the shape of an epitope on an antigen: they interact with antigens not because of the antigen's chemistry (each is an isomer of the same molecule), but with the antigen's shape.

In 1930, Landsteiner was awarded the Nobel Prize for his discovery of human blood group antibodies — a contribution of immense medical importance. Nonetheless, Landsteiner regarded his work on antibody specificity to be of more fundamental importance and reported to others that he felt he had been rewarded for the wrong thing!

Table 6.1. Landsteiner's data on the specificity of antigen-antibody reactions. Immune serum was raised against *meta*-aminobenzene sulfonic acid (and two other acidic substituents) and the ability of this antisera to precipitate the antigenic compound and closely related isomers was measured. (From K. Landsteiner, *The Specificity of Serological Reactions*, Revised edition, page 169, Dover Publications, New York, 1962).

Antigens	NH_2, R ortho-	NH_2, R meta-	NH_2, R para-
Aminobenzene sulfonic acid	$+\pm$	$++\pm$	$\pm$
Aminobenzene arsenic acid	o	$+$	o
Aminobenzoic acid	o	$\pm$	o

R designates the acid groups (COOH or SO_3H or AsO_3H_2).

There is no real difference between an aromatic ring attached to a protein by a chemist and the same aromatic ring that is a part of an amino acid on a protein. Any site on an antigen to which an antibody reacts can be considered to be a haptenic site. In the case of the ABO blood groups, the N-acetyl galactosamine of group A and the galactosamine of group B are distinct haptens on red blood cell antigens.

Antibodies specific for virtually any small molecule can be produced if they are attached to a suitable carrier molecule. Antibodies raised in this way are used today for detection and quantization of many hormones and drugs which, by themselves, are not immunogenic.

Antibodies to a hapten will bind tightly to haptens in solution, but since free haptens have just one antibody combining site, no cross-linking and thus no precipitation will occur. The combining sites of the antibodies will, however, be blocked by bound hapten and the antibodies will not be able to react with haptens on a carrier molecule. Thus haptens can be detected by ability of the free hapten to block precipitation of the hapten-carrier complexes (Figure 6.2).

SITES ON ANTIGENS RECOGNIZED BY ANTIBODIES

The sites on an antigen that are recognized by antibodies (epitopes) may be conformational or sequential (Figure 6.3). A conformational site is any surface shape determined by the complex folding of the molecule. The conformational site is analogous to a mountain range on the surface of the earth which results from continental drift and the crushing together of rock strata. The conformational sites of proteins may be determined by widely separated stretches of amino acid sequences that are brought into proximity by the folding of the polypeptide. Thus, conformational sites are lost with denaturation of molecules, a process which destroys secondary and tertiary structure.

Sequential sites are sites determined by the sequences of the monomers in the polymeric chain that make up organic macromolecules. In antigenic proteins these sites are sequences of amino acids; in carbohydrates they are sequences of sugars. Sequential sites are not much affected by denaturation since there is little secondary or tertiary structure in a short contiguous sequence in a short chain.

Western blotting is a popular and powerful biochemical technique whereby proteins are denatured, separated by electrophoresis, and transferred (blotted) to a

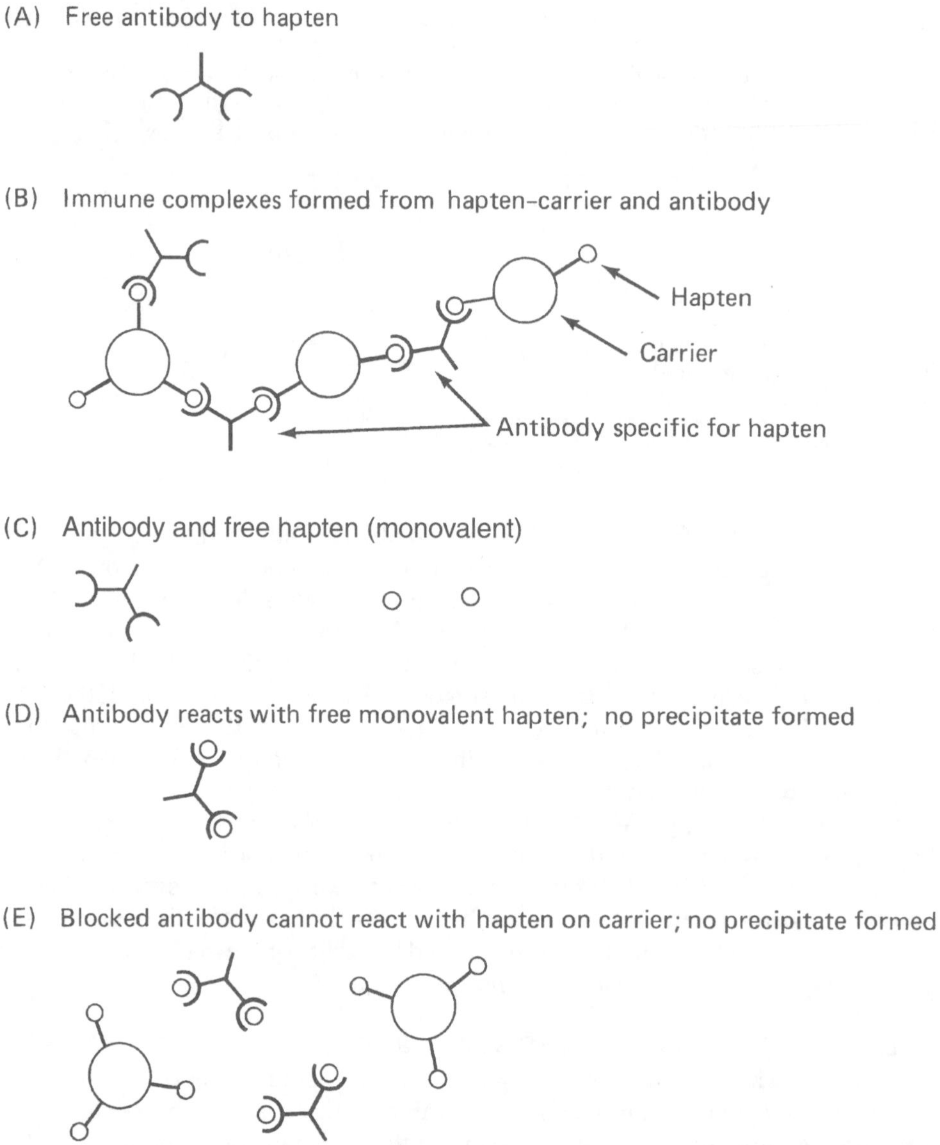

(A) Free antibody to hapten

(B) Immune complexes formed from hapten–carrier and antibody

Hapten

Carrier

Antibody specific for hapten

(C) Antibody and free hapten (monovalent)

(D) Antibody reacts with free monovalent hapten; no precipitate formed

(E) Blocked antibody cannot react with hapten on carrier; no precipitate formed

Figure 6.2.   The reaction of haptens with antibody can be detected by using free haptens to block the reaction of the antibody with the hapten-carrier complex. Antibody (A) to the hapten will react with the hapten-carrier complex to form a lattice, yielding a visible precipitate (B). If the antibody first reacts with free monovalent hapten molecules (C), then the reactive sites on the antibody are filled (D), and the antibody cannot react (E) with the multivalent hapten-carrier to produce a visible precipitate.

piece of nitrocellulose. Antigens on the blot are then probed by an antibody labeled with a radioactive isotope, an enzyme, or a fluorescent dye. Since the antigen is denatured by this procedure, antibodies to conformational sites may not be detected by this technique. Western blotting does, however, detect epitopes which are formed of sequences of amino acids or sugars in large polymers.

   The T cell receptor recognizes fragments of protein antigens which are nestled in a

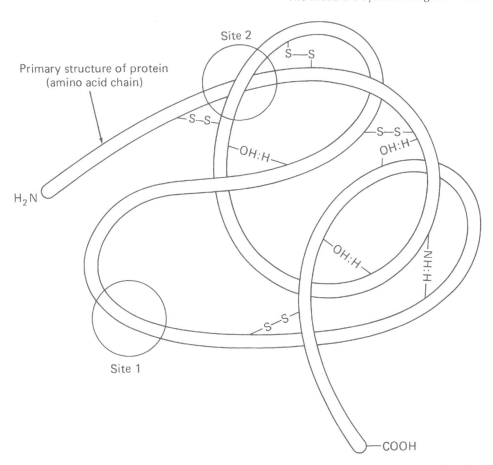

Figure 6.3.   The nature of conformational and sequential epitopes on antigenic molecules. The amino acid chains composing proteins are wound back upon themselves like balled string. The epitope may be a section of the chain not involving amino acids in adjacent chains (site 1). This is a *sequential epitope*. The site may be formed by areas where a portion of the chain is linked to adjacent portions of the chain (site 2) A site formed in this way depends on the folding of the polypeptide chain and is thus called a *conformational epitope*. Since conformation epitopes depend on the folding of the chain, they are lost if the molecule is unfolded. Unfolding is one type of denaturation, a process in which the conformation of the molecule is lost. The chains may be held together by covalent disulfide (—S—S—) bonds, hydrogen bonds, and other noncovalent types of bonds.

surface groove on the MHC protein on the membrane of an antigen-presenting cell. These peptides are created in the cytoplasm of the antigen-presenting cell by protein-digesting organelles called *proteosomes*. The peptides bound to class I MHC proteins are eight to ten amino acids in length and approximately thirteen amino acids in length for those bound to class II MHC proteins. These sequences are too short to have any secondary or tertiary structure. The TCR is specific for both the conformation of the MHC protein and the primary structure of the antigen fragment. Because of this characteristic of the T cell receptor, cell mediated immunity is limited to responses to sequential antigenic sites. B cell receptors and the humoral immune response, on the other hand, may be induced by both sequential and conformational epitopes.

MAPPING EPITOPES AND ANTIGEN-BINDING SITES

It is possible to cut up polymeric antigens using enzymes and to use the fragments as haptens by attaching them to carrier molecules. Antibodies raised to such "antigen fragments" (haptens) have provided material for the study of many aspects of antigenicity including the size of the epitope. The size of a sequential epitope may be estimated by determining the minimum size of the polypeptide or polysaccharide that most efficiently blocks the binding of the antibody to the intact antigen. Studies of this nature indicate that sequential epitopes of carbohydrates consist of about five sugars and proteins of about six to ten amino acids.

When an immunocompetent animal is injected with an antigenic substance, the immune serum contains a variety of antibodies directed against the various epitopes present on the various molecules in the preparation. They are produced by lymphocytes derived from a number of lymphocyte clones. Such antisera are described as *polyspecific* or *polyclonal*. It is now a common procedure to produce *monospecific* or *monoclonal* antibodies. A given plasma cell secretes antibody specific for only a single epitope. In 1975, Drs. Kohler and Milstein developed a hybrid cell technology that permits selection of a single antibody secreting cell and production of a clonal population from the selected cell (see chapter 20). These monospecific clones secrete antibodies which are directed against a single epitope. The presence of many distinct epitopes on a molecule can be shown by raising many monoclonal antibodies to a single complex and determining if they block each other's binding. Studies of this type are called *epitope mapping studies*.

In these studies one of the antibodies is labeled with a radioisotope. The antigen may be fixed on the walls of a test tube. The unlabeled antibody and the labeled one are allowed to react singly or in combination with the antigen in the test tubes. If the unlabeled antibody binds to the same epitope as the labeled one, then in mixtures, the unlabeled antibody will compete for binding to the epitope and less radioactivity will be bound than if the two antibodies bind to separate sites (Figure 6.4). By using several monoclonal antibodies specific for polypeptides of known sequence, one can map the amino acid sequence of antigen epitopes by determining which monoclonal antibodies bind to the antigen.

For conformational epitopes one can assume that the size of the epitope is approximately the size of the antigen binding region on the antibody molecule. Although the precise size differs from antibody to antibody, it has been estimated to be 15 to 20 nm long by 6 to 15 nm wide. For comparison a human red cell is about 7 μm in diameter and a *Staphylococcus* about 1 μm in diameter. There are 1000 nm in a μm.

To get a better look at the antigen binding site on antibody molecules, the technique of *affinity labeling* has been developed to analyze the detailed nature of the antigen-antibody interaction. In affinity labeling, a hapten is used to *probe* the antigen binding site of the antibody molecule. As an example, the haptens dinitrophenol (DNP) and an analog of DNP, diazonium derivative *m*-nitrobenzenediazonium fluoroborate, or MNBDF, are used (Figure 6.5A). MNBDF is similar enough in shape to DNP that it is recognized by anti-DNP antibodies. The reason for using MNBDF as the epitope is the presence of several reactive groups which will covalently bind to tyrosine. Antibodies normally bind to their antigen epitope noncovalently. When MNBDF binds to the DNP-specific antigen binding site of the IgG molecule, a covalent bond is formed between the diazonium group of the MNBDF and any nearby tyrosine residues on the antibody. By breaking the IgG molecules which have bound MNBDF into pieces and sequencing these pieces, the positions of the tyrosine

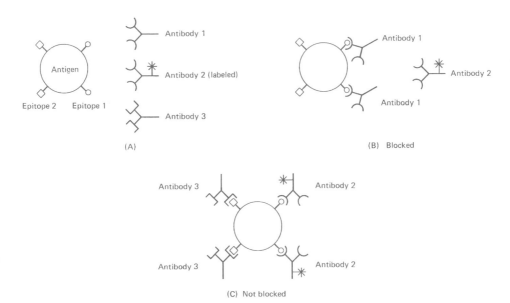

Figure 6.4. Competitive inhibition is used to determine if monoclonal antibodies are directed against the same or different epitopes. In this example, the antigen contains two types of epitopes (A). Unlabeled antibody 1 is specific for the same epitope as labeled antibody 2 and will block reactions of antibody 2 with its epitope (B). Antibody 3 is specific for a different epitope on the antigen and does not interfere with the reaction of antibody 2 with the antigen.

residues can be located since the MNBDF remains bound to them. This information helps define the antigen-binding site.

Another type of hapten used in affinity-labeling antigen is NAP-lysine (Figure 6.5B). When exposed to light, the NAP-lysine hapten in an NAP-lysine-carrier complex will react with all the amino acids in the vicinity and thus identify the antibodies in the antigen-binding site that make contact with the epitope.

Recent progress in NMR (nuclear magnetic resonance) spectroscopy has allowed an even more precise resolution of antigen-antibody complexes. To resolve those parts of the antibody molecule that contact the antigen, the NMR analysis is combined with a technique called hydrogen-deuterium exchange. In this procedure, the antigen-antibody complex is suspended in heavy water [(D_2O), in which the D stands for the hydrogen isotope deuterium]. The hydrogens of the antigen molecule are gradually replaced by deuterium atoms with the exception of those hydrogens that are in regions protected from hydrogen exchange by the bound antibody. NMR analysis of the antigen after the antigen is separated from the antibody reveals which of the amino acids were in contact with the antibody since they did not undergo hydrogen exchange.

THE STRENGTH OF ANTIGEN BINDING

The hold that the antibody has on the antigen is made possible by various types of close contacts. Atoms brought into proximity may be held together by a collection of weak forces: ionic bonds, hydrogen bonds, hydrophobic interactions, and van der Waals forces (produced by the localized induction of partial charges). These weak forces sum up over the surface of the contact. The greater the number and closeness of these contacts, the greater the total binding force. The empirical and

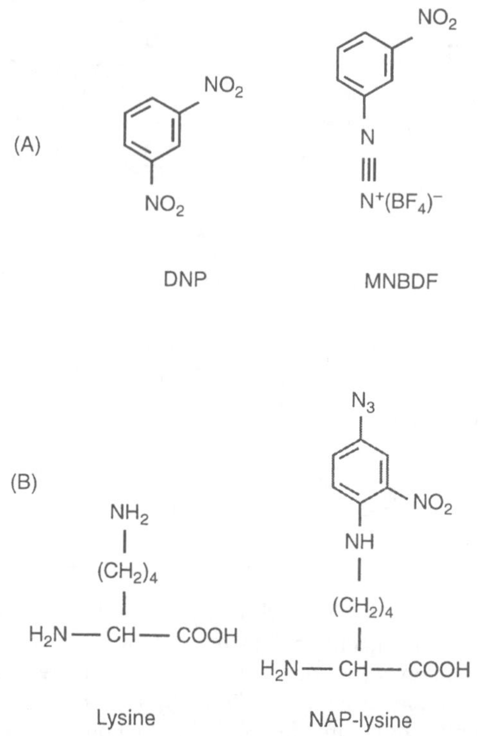

Figure 6.5. Molecular structures of haptens used in affinity labeling studies. (A) Dinitroph-enol (DNP) and its analog *m*-nitrobenzenediazonium fluoroborate, and (B) Lysine and its ana-log NAP-lysine.

mathematically expressed measure of the strength of the total force is called *affinity*. The affinity of an antibody for a given antigen is an important measure used in the study of the workings of the immune system.

Affinity is a factor in determining the equilibrium between the antigen-antibody complex and free antibody and antigen in a mixture since binding is a reversible chemical reaction. In a reversible chemical reaction

$$A + B \rightleftharpoons C + D$$

the concentrations of reactants $(A + B)$ and products $(C + D)$ change until a constant concentration of each is attained. At this point, the rate of product formation (the forward reaction) equals the rate of reactant formation (the reverse reaction). The result is called *chemical equilibrium*. There is no net change in the concentrations of the reactants at equilibrium unless product is removed. This equilibrium is, there-fore, *dynamic*. If some product is removed, the forward reaction replaces it, reestab-lishing the equilibrium. The equilibrium point is a constant for any reaction.

The binding of an antigen by an antibody is a chemical reaction of this type and can be represented by the following expression.

$$Ag + Ab \rightleftharpoons Ag \cdot Ab$$

At equilibrium, the rate of the forward reaction $(Ag + Ab \rightarrow Ag \cdot Ab)$ equals the rate of the reverse reaction $(Ag \cdot Ab \rightarrow Ag + Ab)$. The relative concentrations of free and bound antigen are measured by the *equilibrium constant* (K_{eq}). Mathematically, K_{eq} is equal to:

$$\frac{[Ag \cdot Ab]}{[Ag] + [Ab]}$$

The brackets symbolize the molar concentrations (the number of molecules per unit volume). By examination, it can be seen that the higher the K_{eq}, the higher is the concentration of the antigen-antibody complex at equilibrium. Looked at in another way, the higher the K_{eq}, the higher is the affinity of the antibody for the antigen. For this reason, the K_{eq} of an antigen binding reaction is called the *affinity* or *association constant* (K_a). Affinity constants for antibodies and their antigens vary between 10^4 and 10^{14} M^{-1}. The common sense meaning of this large number is that at equilibrium the large preponderance of antigen is attached to antibody, not free in solution. Stated simply, antibodies bind their matching antigens very strongly.

CROSS REACTIVITY OF ANTIGENS
A given antibody will, of course, bind to an antigen that was used to induce the immune response. Antibodies, however, will also bind to other antigens that are structurally similar to the antibody-generating antigen. Such *cross-reactivity* may have a number of different causes.

Complex Antigens
Antigens used for immunization may actually be complex mixtures of many antigenic molecules. Such is the case if the antigen consists of a preparation of microbes, for example. Immune sera raised to preparations of one species of *Salmonella* will often react, usually to a lesser degree, with preparations of other species of *Salmonella* and even to preparations of more distantly related enterobacteria. In such cases it can be shown that some of the molecules in the different species of organism are identical while some differ. The immune serum raised contains a mixture of antibodies with specificity for the various molecules in the organisms. Cross-reactivity may thus be the result of the presence of common molecules in complex antigens of related species.

In some cases cross-reactivity may occur between antigen preparations from distantly related or unrelated species. For example, antiserum raised to Rickettsia will agglutinate a strain of *Proteus vulgaris* (X19). As *Proteus* are easier to obtain than Rickettsia, *Proteus* preparations are used as antigens in serological tests to detect Rickettsial infections. The test, named after its discoverers, is called the Weil-Felix reaction.

Another reaction of this type is the Forssman reaction. An antigen in guinea pig kidney induces production in rabbits of an antibody that agglutinates sheep erythrocytes. Sera of people with infectious mononucleosis also contain agglutinins for sheep red cells as well as agglutinins for bovine red cells. Adsorption of sera from people with infectious mononucleosis with guinea pig kidney removes agglutinins from sheep erythrocytes but not those for bovine erythrocytes. These reactions are used in the diagnosis of infectious mononucleosis. These reactions are called heterophile reactions and are examples of a fairly common class of cross-reactions. A heterophile antigen is thus defined as an antigen common to members of unrelated species.

Shared Epitopes
In complex antigens, such as preparations of microbes, cross-reactivity may result from the presence of a variety of molecules in the preparation some of which are shared. Immunological reactivity, however, is directed against small regions of

(A) Haptens

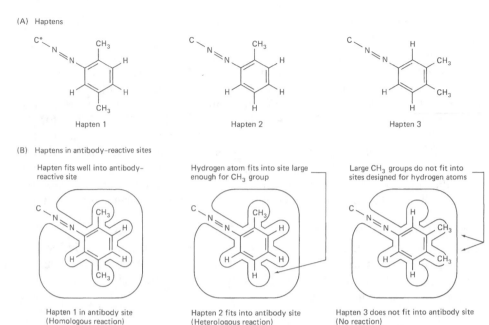

(B) Haptens in antibody-reactive sites

Hapten fits well into antibody-reactive site

Hydrogen atom fits into site large enough for CH₃ group

Large CH₃ groups do not fit into sites designed for hydrogen atoms

Hapten 1 in antibody site (Homologous reaction)

Hapten 2 fits into antibody site (Heterologous reaction)

Hapten 3 does not fit into antibody site (No reaction)

Figure 6.6. Serologic cross-reactions may be based on the similarity of epitopes. The absence of the bulky CH_3 group on hapten 2 does not interfere with entry of the hapten into the site specific for hapten 1. The presence of two bulky CH_3 groups prevent hapten 3 from fitting into the antibody site complementary to hapten 1.

molecules, epitopes, not against the whole molecule. Cross-reactivity may, therefore, also occur because some epitopes on a given molecule may be structurally similar. By this mechanism, immune sera raised to a preparation containing only a single type of molecule may react with preparations of different molecules if some epitopes are shared. Much observable cross-reactivity can, therefore, be explained in terms of the presence of a variety of epitopes in antigen preparations, either on different molecules in the antigen preparation or on the same molecule.

Similarity of Epitopes

Karl Landsteiner demonstrated that antibody preparations reactive with a single hapten would sometimes react with structurally similar haptens. In Landsteiner's day the technology for production of monoclonal antibodies had not been developed. He produced relatively monospecific polyclonal antibodies by absorption of polyclonal serum with related antigens. As described earlier, Landsteiner showed that such antibodies could discriminate between different isomers of aminobenzoic acid. Although some cross-reactivity occurred in most cases, reactions with the homologous system were always the strongest. (In chemical terms, the affinity constants for the several antigen-antibody complexes differed). Landsteiner also demonstrated that a variety of different groups could be deleted and antibody binding (albeit with different affinities) would still occur (Figure 6.6). This type of reaction can be thought of in terms of a hand in a glove. The absence of a finger interferes less with putting on a glove than having the fingers placed in odd positions.

Some microorganisms may produce molecules similar to those of the host but sufficiently different to be treated as foreign. Here too the antibody products of the immune response may react with the related host molecules. Rheumatic fever is probably initiated by infection with streptococci. The autoimmune reaction against heart and joint tissue which follows is a result of similarity of molecules in the parasite and the tissue.

THE GENOTYPE OF THE RESPONDING ANIMAL

Scientists first setting out to study the immune response in vertebrate organisms asked a quite logical question. Was the degree of an immune response to a specific antigen under genetic control? Could strain A respond more or less strongly to antigen B than, say, strain C?

Early workers selectively bred guinea pigs on the basis of their responsiveness to diphtheria toxoid. They discovered that some strains responded significantly better than others. The strains were called *high responders* and the *low responders*. Clearly, immune responsiveness was under genetic control. This result was no surprise. The interesting questions that it raised, of course, concerned the genes that controlled immune responsiveness. What were they and how did they work?

A problem with this type of research is the nature of the antigen. Complex protein antigens are covered with many different epitopes or antigenic determinants, each of which stimulates one or more B cell clones. With this complex response, it was difficult to pin down the putative *immune response genes*.

Hugh McDevitt, working initially in the laboratory of Michael Sela in Israel, used a series of synthetic peptides to explore the problem. The advantage of using these antigens was the fact that they only possessed a few defined epitopes. McDevitt precisely measured the amount of IgG produced on secondary exposure to these defined antigenic determinants.

By pursuing this work with the newly developed strains of congenic mice, McDevitt demonstrated that MHC haplotypes controlled immune responsiveness. Whatever the rest of the genetic background, immune responsiveness correlated with the MHC (H–2) haplotype. For example, genetic strains C3H, CBA, and AKR each responded well to the antigenic determinant (H,G)–AL[1] and poorly to (T,G)–AL *if* they were congenic for the H–2 haplotype k. Strains C57Bl and B10 congenic for H–2^b, by contrast, responded oppositely to these antigens (poorly to (H,G)–AL and well to (T,G)–AL). If, by careful breeding, the H-2^k haplotype was inserted onto the C57Bl background, this strain responded well to (H,G)–AL and poorly to (T,G)–AL.

The conclusion was inescapable. The MHC in mice controls not only the compatibility of surgical grafts (for which the complex was named), but also the degree of an immunoglobulin response to a particular antigen. The explanation of the dual function of the MHC, of course, is that the MHC codes for two types of protein, the class I and class II proteins. These proteins are involved in antigen presentation in both the humoral and cell-mediated immune reactions. It is, therefore, to be expected that graft compatibility and immune responsiveness should be affected by the workings of the antigen presentation mechanisms.

SUPERANTIGENS

The "standard" way for antigens to activate T cells involves, as the first step, the

---

1 This is biochemical shorthand for the sequence of amino acids in a peptide. (H,G)–AL refers to a tripeptide, the first amino acid of which may either be histidine (H) or glycine (G). The second and third amino acids are alanine (A) and leucine (L).

binding of the T cell to a processed antigen fragment nestled in the binding site of a class II MHC protein of an antigen presenting cell. Binding occurs through the antigen-specific T cell receptor. The stimulation of the TCR starts the ball rolling. A cascade of intracellular signals, triggered by TCR binding and augmented by the release of cytokines, results in the clonal expansion of T-helper cells.

The number of different resting T cells activated in this manner is much fewer than one in ten thousand (< 0.01 percent) cells. Although small, this number is larger than the number of B cells activated in a humoral immune response. This is presumably due to the straightforward fact that in T cell activation only the primary structure of an antigen fragment is presented and not the complex (and therefore more rare) tertiary structure of the epitopes recognized by the surface immunoglobulins of B cells.

It is quite surprising, then, that a group of protein antigens has been discovered that will stimulate as many as one in five (20 percent) T cells. Known as "superantigens," these proteins include some bacterial toxins. Among these toxins are the enterotoxins of *Staphylococcus aureus*, responsible for food poisoning and tampon-related toxic shock syndrome in humans, and the exotoxin of *Streptococcus pyogenes*, responsible for the high fever accompanying streptococcal throat infections (strep throat).

Superantigens bind very tightly to the MHC of the antigen presenting cell. The binding site for superantigens, unlike a processed antigen fragment, is *outside* the antigen-binding site of the MHC. Superantigens, therefore, are not processed and are not presented by the APC in standard fashion.

At least two lines of evidence support this contention. First, the stimulatory effect of a superantigen on T cells is not affected by amino acid substitutions in the antigen-binding groove of the MHC protein. The ability of conventional antigens to activate T cells is affected, however, because the processed antigen is bound within this groove. Second, proteolysis of superantigens destroys their ability to stimulate T cells whereas antigen presentation by an MHC protein *requires* the enzymatic breakdown of the protein antigen into smaller fragments.

It is likely that the ability of superantigens to activate T cells is due to their ability to bring the APC and the T cell together. Unlike conventional T cell activation, in which the processed antigen serves as a *bridge* between the binding site of the T cell receptor and the class II MHC, a superantigen serves as a *clamp* between the apposed MHC of the APC and TCR of the T cell (Figure 6.7).

The effect of bringing the APC and T cell together is the activation and proliferation of the T cells. Since superantigens bind APCs outside the MHC antigen-binding site, they will activate all T cells expressing a particular TCR V_β allele. Therefore, superantigens are much less specific than the antigens which are processed and presented in the standard way. Superantigens are *polyclonal activators* of T cells.

The toxicity of bacterial superantigens may be related to their ability to activate so many T cells. The activation of T cells and their subsequent proliferation and differentiation leads to the release of cytokines (chapters 8 and 9). While small amounts of these cytokines are part and parcel of the immune response, the release of large quantities from many expanded clones can be toxic to the host.

ROUTES OF ANTIGEN ADMINISTRATION

To manifest immunogenicity, the potential antigen must enter the tissues of the immunocompetent animal. This may occur by artificial means or natural ones. Injection by subcutaneous, intramuscular, intravenous, or intraperitoneal (into the

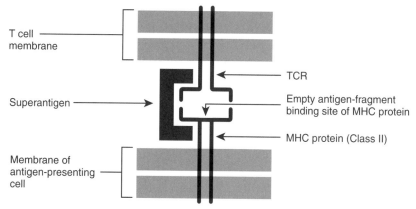

T cell membrane

Superantigen

Membrane of antigen-presenting cell

TCR

Empty antigen-fragment binding site of MHC protein

MHC protein (Class II)

Figure 6.7. Hypothetical structure for the complex of class II MHC, T cell receptor, and staphylococcal enterotoxin. The diagram shows a class II MHC protein in contact with a T cell receptor and a staphylococcal enterotoxin. The site to which a conventional antigen fragment would bind is empty.

peritoneal cavity) routes all serve to introduce antigenic materials into the body. Intravenous injection carries the antigen first to the spleen whereas injections into the tissues carries the antigen by the lymphatic circulation to the nearest lymph nodes. Natural routes of entry usually involve infection. A microorganism invades the tissue, grows there, and thus introduces its components into the tissue. This is the most common natural route of entry of antigens into the body.

Antigens may enter the body by inhalation and rarely by ingestion. Most of our foods are potentially antigenic. If they are injected into tissues, they certainly invoke an immune response. Digestion precedes the assimilation of most foods. Proteins and polysaccharides are reduced to their constituent monomers before they can be absorbed by the gut. These small molecular weight digestion products are not antigenic. It also appears that there are mechanisms in the digestive tract that prevent many potentially antigenic foods from causing an immune response if they do enter the body through the gut wall. The mechanisms sometimes fail and we develop food allergies.

ADJUVANTS

Adjuvants (from the Latin *adjuvare*, meaning *to help*) are substances added to antigen preparations to enhance their immunogenicity. This type of help is important if the antigen is not very immunogenic or in short supply. Adjuvants may or may not be immunogenic in themselves. They are frequently irritating and cause mild inflammation, thus activating cells of the immune system and attracting them to the site of antigen deposition. Some adjuvants bind the antigen tightly and release it slowly after injection, thus prolonging the antigenic stimulation. Most vaccines used in human and veterinary medicine contain adjuvants. Alum (aluminum potassium sulfate) is the most commonly used adjuvant in human medicine. In addition to delaying the release of the antigen, the high salt concentration precipitates the antigen, making it a larger target for phagocytosis by antigen presenting cells.

SUMMARY

Any molecule that will induce an immune response and interact specifically with the products of the induced immune response is an *antigen*. *Immunogen* is another term preferred by some for molecules that will induce such a response. Classically, antigens have been considered to consist of a hapten, which cannot induce an immune response by itself, and a carrier protein which will induce a response. An antigenic determinant, or epitope, is the site on an antigen to which the antibody binds. The three-dimensional shape, amino acid sequence, and ionic charge of the antigen are all crucial to antibody binding. T cell receptors bind to protein fragments presented on the surface of MHC proteins. Therefore, the TCR recognizes two molecules at once: the MHC protein and the presented antigen-fragment.

The best immunogens are proteins or carbohydrates. Lipids or nucleic acids conjugated to proteins are also antigenic. To induce a response, immunogens must be foreign to the responding organism since organisms usually learn in fetal life to tolerate all self-antigens. Because proteins must be processed by antigen presenting cells and attached to MHC proteins before they can be recognized by T cells, biodegradability is another important feature of antigens. Polysaccharides, possibly because they have multiple, repeating antigenic determinants, tend to induce immune responses independent of T cells and need not, therefore, be processed and presented.

The use of chemically defined haptens has allowed a detailed exploration of the antigen binding sites on antibodies. Antibodies bind antigen to which they form a good fit via a number of noncovalent bonds. The goodness-of-fit is measured as the strength of binding, the equilibrium (or affinity) constant of the antigen binding reaction. Since many antigenic determinants have similar shapes and charges, several antigens may cross-react with the same antibody.

The immunogenicity of a molecule is also determined by the genotype of the responding organism. The study of these immune responsiveness traits led to the discovery of the MHC complex and the role of the encoded proteins in the induction of the immune response.

Superantigens are a group of molecules that function very differently from traditional immunogens. By clamping a TCR to an MHC in a unique way, they serve as polyclonal activators of T cells.

In order for an immunogen to induce a strong response, it must physically enter the responding organism. The route of entry, whether by contact, injection, or inhalation, can influence the type and degree of an immune response. Adjuvants are substances that can be included with injected antigens to heighten the immune response.

SUGGESTIONS FOR FURTHER READING

1. Benacerraf, B. "Studies of Antigenicity with Artificial Antigens." Chapter IV in *Regulation of the Antibody Response*. Edited by B. Cinander. Springfield, IL: Charles C. Thomas, 1971.
2. Berzofsky, J.A. and I.J. Berkower. "Immunogenicity and Antigen Structure." Chapter 8 in *Fundamental Immunology*. 2d ed. Edited by W.E. Paul. New York: Raven Press, 1989.
3. Colman, P.M., J.N. Varghese, and W.G. Laver. "Structure of the Catalytic and Antigenic Sites in Influenza Virus Neuraminidase," *Nature* 303 (1983):41–44.
4. Golub, E.S., and D.R. Green. "The Nature of Antigens." Chapter 2 in *Immunology, a Synthesis*. 2d ed. Sunderland, MA: Sinauer Associates, 1991.
5. Johnson, H.M., J.K. Russell, and CH Pontzer. "Superantigens in Human Disease," *Scientific American* (April 1992): 92–101.

6. Kabat, E.A. *Structural Concepts in Immunology and Immunochemistry.* New York: Holt, Rinehart, and Winston, 1968.
7. Kuby, J. "Antigens." Chapter 4 in *Immunology.* 3d ed. New York: W.H. Freeman and Company, 1997.
8. Landsteiner, K. *The Specificity of Serological Reactions.* Rev. ed. New York: Dover Publications, 1962.
9. Paterson, Y., S.W. Englander, and H. Roder. "An Antibody Binding Site on Cytochrome c Defined by Hydrogen Exchange and Two-Dimensional NMR." *Science* 249 (1990):755–759.
10. Sela, M. "Overview: Antigens." Chapter 1 in *Immunochemistry.* Edited by D.M. Weir. London: Blackwell Scientific Publications, 1986.
11. Unanue, E.R., and B. Benacerraf. "Antigens." Chapter 2 in *Textbook of Immunology.* Baltimore, MD: Williams and Wilkins, 1984.

QUESTIONS

1. What is the difference between a hapten and carrier?
2. What is self-tolerance and why is it important for an organism?
3. Why are large and complex macromolecules more immunogenic than small and simple ones?
4. What is the importance of Landsteiner's discovery that antibodies could recognize different isomers of aminobenzoic acid?
5. How is the strength of antigen-antibody binding represented?
6. How can a monoclonal antibody react with more than one epitope?

ANSWERS

1 A hapten is a small fragment of an antigen, too small to be immunogenic. A hapten can be made antigenic by linking it to a larger and more complex molecule, a carrier protein. All of the antigenic sites on the carrier protein can be considered to be haptens.
2 An animal does not normally produce an immune response to molecules in its own body that are, in other circumstances, immunogenic. This self-tolerance is learned by the animal during fetal life. This is vital to the survival of the animal since autoimmune reactions can be quite serious and life-threatening.
3 The larger and more complex a macromolecule, the more antigenic determinants it has on its surface. In the case of proteins, it is necessary for the protein to be phagocytosed by an antigen presenting cell, digested, and displayed on a MHC protein in order for a T cell to respond to it. Larger size increases the likelihood of phagocytosis.
4 Since each of these haptens in chemically identical, this demonstration showed that antibodies recognize the conformation of an antigen, not the chemical composition.
5 The binding of an antibody to an antigen is a chemical reaction with a precise equilibrium point. The equilibrium (or affinity) constant of an antigen-antibody reaction is directly proportional to the strength of binding.
6 A single antigen binding site on an antibody can recognize numerous epitopes if they are similar to the epitope that served as the immunogen. Different antibodies will, however, bind each antigen with a different affinity.

CHAPTER 7

INTRODUCTION
NATURE OF ANTIBODIES
STRUCTURE OF ANTI-
  BODIES
  The Basic Structure
  The Variable Regions
  The Constant Regions
  The Hinge
  Fab, Fc, and F(ab')$_2$
    Molecules
THE B CELL RECEPTOR
  (BCR)
ANTIBODY DIVERSITY
CHANGES IN THE AFFINITY
  AND CLASS OF ANTI-
  BODIES DURING THE
  COURSE OF THE
  IMMUNE RESPONSE
FUNCTIONS OF IMMU-
  NOGLOBULIN CLASSES
DETECTION OF ANTI-
  BODIES: BASIC PRINCI-
  PLES AND CONCEPTS
  BEHIND SEROLOGICAL
  ASSAYS
SUMMARY
SUGGESTIONS FOR
  FURTHER READING
QUESTIONS
ANSWERS

The Inducible Defense System: Antibody Molecules and Antigen-Antibody Reactions

Diane Wallace Taylor

INTRODUCTION

The material in the last two chapters should help us gain an appreciation of the important role of antibodies in the inducible immune response. From the discussion of the Clonal Selection Theory in chapter 5, we should have learned that antibodies are produced by B cells, and that each B cell expresses a unique antibody molecule on its surface that is capable of interaction with a single epitope of an antigen (Figure 7.1). In response to an invading pathogen, only those B cells with receptors complementary to a particular epitope on the antigen become activated. These "selected" B cells undergo cell division and produce a number of identical daughter cells, some of which develop into *plasma cells* that secrete antibodies. These antibodies then interact with the foreign antigen or pathogen and aid in its elimination from the body. Thus, antibodies function both as unique antigen-specific receptors on B cells and as soluble mediators of protection.

Antibodies circulate throughout the body. Those found in the blood and tissue fluids are called *humoral* antibodies. When antigens and pathogens are present in the tissues, humoral antibodies agglutinate or aggregate them and prevent their spread to other parts of the body. Antibodies also bind to receptors on viruses and toxins and prevent them from entering cells (i.e., neutralize them). Some antibodies may specifically interact both with microbes and receptors on white blood cells (e.g., macrophages and polymorphonuclear leukocytes), thereby facilitating phagocytosis and the killing of pathogens. Other antibodies also bind to mast cells where they cause hypersensitivity reactions including allergies. Such antibodies are often referred to as *cell-bound antibodies*.

105

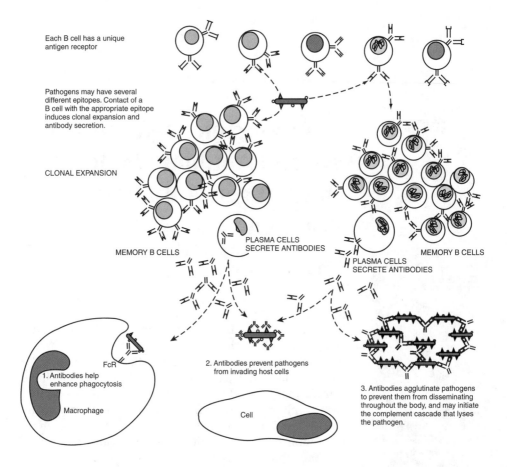

Each B cell has a unique antigen receptor

Pathogens may have several different epitopes. Contact of a B cell with the appropriate epitope induces clonal expansion and antibody secretion.

CLONAL EXPANSION

MEMORY B CELLS

PLASMA CELLS SECRETE ANTIBODIES

PLASMA CELLS SECRETE ANTIBODIES

MEMORY B CELLS

FcR

1. Antibodies help enhance phagocytosis

Macrophage

2. Antibodies prevent pathogens from invading host cells

Cell

3. Antibodies agglutinate pathogens to prevent them from disseminating throughout the body, and may initiate the complement cascade that lyses the pathogen.

Figure 7.1. The clonal selection theory, B cells and antibodies. During an infection, B cells with receptors complementary to pathogens undergo cell division, develop into plasma cells and secrete antibody. Antibodies aid in removing pathogens from the body by either 1) making them easy to phagocytose, 2) blocking key receptors and thus preventing them from invading cells, 3) agglutinating the pathogens to keep them from disseminating throughout the body, or activating complement-mediated lysis of the pathogens.

Antibodies are not only present in blood, but are also found in other body secretions, such as tears, saliva, and colostrum, and in the intestinal tract. Throughout the body antibodies help prevent pathogens and their products from damaging the body.

NATURE OF ANTIBODIES

Human blood contains erythrocytes and leukocytes (white blood cells) suspended in a fluid phase, called *serum* (pl., *sera*). Serum consists of water, salts, and many proteins. When serum proteins are subjected to electrophoresis, they separate into the five fractions, namely, albumin and the alpha 1, alpha 2, beta and *gamma globulins* (Figure 7.2). Antibodies are part of the gamma-globulin fraction of serum, and thus, they are often referred to as *immunoglobulins*.

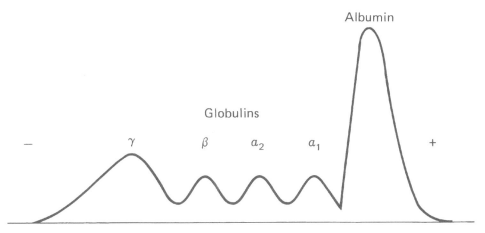

Figure 7.2. Separation of proteins in serum by electrophoresis. Proteins in serum can be separated based on their net charge. In an electrophoretic field, albumin migrates more quickly than the globulins toward the positive pole (anode). Among the globulins, the alpha and beta globulins migrate faster than gamma globulins. Antibodies are found in the gamma globulin fraction of serum.

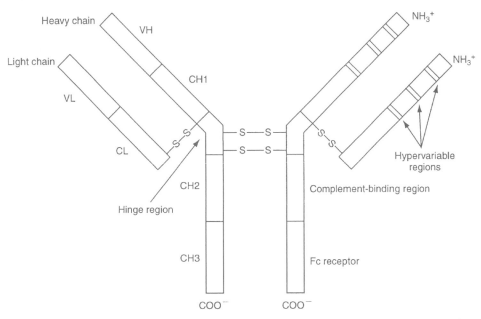

Figure 7.3. The basic structure of antibody molecules. Antibodies are composed of two identical heavy and two identical light chains. Heavy chains (H) consist of a variable (V) domain and 3 to 4 constant (C) region domains. Light chains consist of one variable (V) and a single constant domain. The chains are held together, in part, by disulfide bonds (—S—S—).

STRUCTURE OF ANTIBODIES

The Basic Structure

Immunoglobulins are glycoproteins consisting of four polypeptide chains. The basic structure of antibody molecules is shown in Figure 7.3. There are two identical heavy (H) chains and two identical light (L) chains in each molecule. The H and L chains are held together by covalent disulfide bonds and by noncovalent hydro-

Table 7.1. Characteristics of human immunoglobulins.

Class	IgG	IgM	IgA	IgE	IgD
Molecular formulation	κ2 γ2 or λ2 γ2	(κ2μ2)$_n$ or (λ2μ2)$_n$ n = 1 or 5	(κ2α2)$_n$ or (λ2α2)$_n$ n = 1,2,3 or 4	κ2 ε2 or λ2 ε2	κ2 δ2 or λ2 δ2
Molecular weight	150,000	900,000	160,000 or 500,000	190,000 to 200,000	150,000 to 200,000
Valency of Ag binding	2	10	2 or 4	2	2
Carbohydrate content	3%	12%	7-8%	12%	12-13%
Heavy chain					
Class	γ	μ	μ	ε	δ
Subclasses	4	1–2	2	–	–
Molecular weight	53,000	70,000	58,000	72,000	65,000
Light chain					
Type	κ or λ	κ or λ	κ or λ	κ or λ	κ or λ
Mol weight	22,500	22,500	22,500	22,500	22,500
Allotypes	Km(Inv)	Km(Inv)	Km(Inv)	Km(Inv)	Km(Inv)
J chain	–	present	present	–	–
Secretory component	–	–	present	–	–
Present in epithelial					
secretions	no	no	yes	no	no
Serum level (mg/dl)	600 to 800	50 to 210	70 to 500	0.01 to 0.9	0.1 to 4.0
% of total Ig	70-80	5-10	10-15	0.01	1
Half-live (days)	21-35	5-8	6-11	2-3	2-3
Synthesis (mg/kg					
Body weight/day)	20-40	3-17	3-55	?	0.4
% intravascular	45	76	42	52	75
Placental passage	yes	no	no	no	no
Complement fixation					
Classic	++[a]	+++	–	–	–
Alternate	–	–	+	–	–
Binding to macrophage					
FcR	+++	–	–	–	–
Binding to mast					
cells/basophils	–	–	–	+	–

[a]-The numbers of plus signs indicate relative extent of each pathway.

phobic bonds. H chains are composed of 446 or more amino acids (M.W. 50,000 to 75,000 daltons), while L chains have 213 or 214 amino acids (M.W. 20,000 to 25,000 daltons). The two H and two L chains are assembled into an antibody molecule in the endoplasmic reticulum. The heavy chain is glycosylated as the newly formed antibody molecule moves through the Golgi on its way to the cell surface.

Each H or L chain has a variable (V) region at the amino-terminal end and a constant or (C) region at the carboxyl-terminal end (Figure 7.3). As the name implies, the amino acid sequences in the variable regions differ more than the amino acid sequences in the constant regions. The two regions of the immunoglobulin molecule, variable and constant, are produced by different DNA (gene) segments (see below).

There are differences in the basic four-chain structure of antibodies. These include variation in chain length, amino acid sequence, and carbohydrate content (Table 7.1). These changes affect both the antigen binding-specificity and the biological functions of antibodies. Changes which affect the chemical, physical and

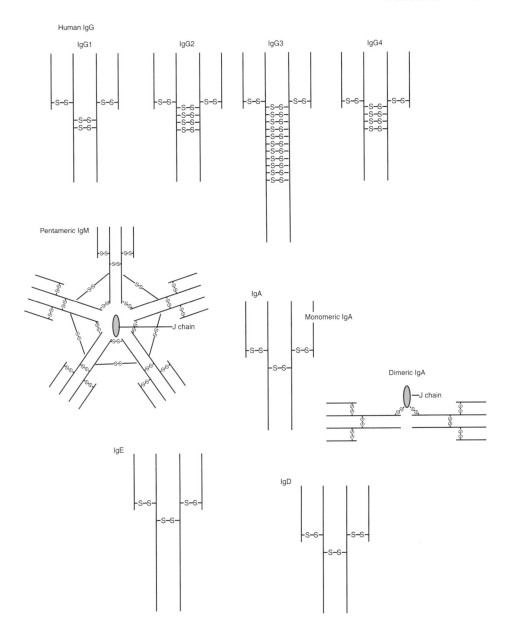

Figure 7.4.   Antibodies consist of monomers or multimers of the basic four-chain plan. There are four subclasses of human IgG. IgM may be monomeric but is usually pentameric. IgA is usually present as a monomer is serum, but is released into secretions in a dimeric form. IgE and IgD are monomeric.

biologic properties of immunoglobulins are found primarily in the heavy chains and are used to categorize the five major *classes*, or *isotypes*, of immunoglobulins: IgG, IgM, IgA, IgD, and IgE (Figure 7.4). The heavy chains of the immunoglobulin (Ig) molecules are designated by Greek letters as gamma (γ), mu (μ), alpha (α), delta (δ), and epsilon (ε), respectively. Some antibody molecules exist as monomers (e.g., IgG), whereas others are composed of more than one of these basic structural

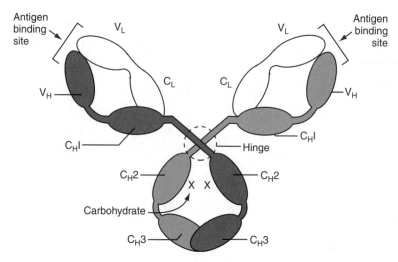

Figure 7.5. Diagrammatic representation of the three-dimensional structure of a typical antibody molecule. Each of the globular domains in the molecule contains about 100 amino acids
and is referred to as an Ig-superfamily domain.

units (e.g., IgM and IgA). Within some of the classes, subclasses with distinctive
heavy chains and differing functional properties occur; there are four subclasses of
IgG and two of IgA (Figure 7.4). There are two immunologically distinct types of
light chains, which differ only in their amino acid sequence. The forms of the light
chain are common to all classes of immunoglobulins and are referred to as *kappa* (κ)
and *lambda* (λ). Any given antibody molecule always contains either kappa or lambda
chains but never a mixture of the two.

The H and L polypeptide chains do not simply remain a linear array of amino
acids after synthesis, but are folded together in a very systematic way determined
by the nature of the component amino acids in the chain (Figure 7.5). The folding
produces compact globular regions known as *Ig-superfamily domains*. Each domain
consists of approximately 100 amino acids. The L chains have two Ig-superfamily
domains, one variable and one constant, labeled VL and CL, respectively. The domains of the H chains of IgG, IgA, and IgD include a variable region designated
VH and three constant region domains, designated CH1, CH2, and CH3. IgM and
IgE have a fourth domain in the constant region, CH4.

The Variable Regions
The ability of the antibody molecule to bind to a single epitope is created by the
"shape" produced by the interaction of the VL and VH domains (Figure 7.6A).
Within the V region of the L and H chains there are areas that are quite constant
from molecule to molecule in amino acid composition. These regions are "conserved" so the molecule can fold properly into the Ig-superfamily domain configuration, and are therefore called the *framework regions* (Figure 7.6B). Within the V
region of the L and H chains, (Figure 7.6B) there are also three regions that are
highly variable and are therefore called the *hypervariable regions*. Each such region
is five to ten amino acids in length. When the molecule folds together, the three VH
and three VL hypervariable regions become located near each other on the outer
surface of the antibody molecule (Figure 7.6B). These regions give the antibody

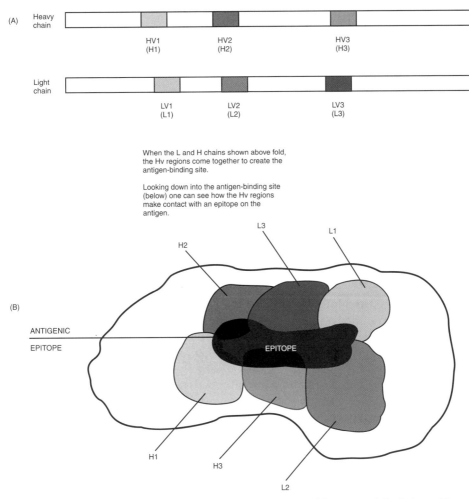

Figure 7.6. The antibody binding site is composed of the variable region of the light and heavy chains. The viable regions of the L and H chains contain ~100 to 110 amino acids. (A) Within the variable regions, there are three regions (each ~5 to 10 amino acids long) where the sequences are highly variable. In between these regions, there are four framework regions where the sequence varies little and which assures that the molecule folds properly. (B) When the molecule folds, these regions, known as the hypervariable regions (Hv) or the complementarity determining regions (CDR), come together on the outer surface of the molecule to create the site that interacts with the antigen.

molecule its "unique" shape. Because one or more of these regions makes contact with the epitope on the antigen, they are also known as the *complementarity determining regions* (CDR). Differences in amino acid sequences in the CDRs are responsible for the large number of unique antigen-binding sites which exist. Because the three-dimensional shape of the variable region is "unique," the shape is referred to as the *idiotype* (*idio* means unique to each individual), and the binding site is the *idiotypic* region. Since the variable region itself has a unique shape, it may serve as an antigen in some situations.

The ability of an antibody to interact with an epitope depends not only upon its complementary physical structure but also upon its charge and charge distribution. The two sites not only must fit together well to permit close approximation of their structures, but the complementary charge patterns must match in order for them to interact.

The Constant Regions

Different biological functions are associated with each of the domains of the H chain constant region. For example, the CH1 domain aids in orienting the variable regions for combining with antigen, and the CH2 domain contains the binding site for the first component of the complement cascade. The interaction between the CH2 domain and the first component of complement activates the Classical Complement Pathway. Finally, the CH3 domain binds to Fc receptors located on phagocytic cells such as macrophages. Although structurally very similar, each domain has a different role in the humoral immune response.

Within a single isotype, i.e., IgG1, there may be some variation in the amino acid sequence of the C region among individuals in the population. These differences are inherited genetically and determine Ig *allotypes* (i.e., differences among individuals of the same species). The areas with different amino acids are called *allotypic markers*. The markers in humans which have been defined are Gm on gamma heavy chains, Am on alpha heavy chains, and Km (or InV) on the K light chains. Three Km (on IgD and IgE), two Am (on IgA), and over twenty Gm (on IgG) allotypes have been defined. Inheritance of these markers is autosomally controlled. In some cases the molecular structure of the allotype marker is known. For example, the KM(1,2) allotype, has leucine at position 191 in the CL domain of the kappa light chain, while Km(3) allotype has valine at this position. These allotypic markers are isoantigens. They are among the epitopes that are recognized by individuals who mount an antibody response to an immunoglobulin from another individual. These allotypic markers were used in paternity testing and in studies of population genetics prior to the development of DNA-based methods.

The Hinge

The *hinge* region is located between the first and second C region domains in the H chain of IgG, IgA, and IgD. This region, which has numerous proline residues and contains inter-H chain disulfide bonds, allows the Ig molecule to flex into various shapes to permit contact of its antigen-combining sites to identical epitopes on separate antigens. It is thought that the molecule maintains a T-shape while uncombined with antigen (to maximize its ability to contact antigen) but assumes a Y-shape after contacting antigen. The length of the hinge region differs among IgG isotypes, thereby allowing some IgG molecules to be more flexible than others.

Fab, Fc, and F(ab')₂ Molecules

The hinge region of the antibody molecule is particularly susceptible to the action of enzymes and chemicals. Enzymatic treatment with papain breaks the H chain at the amino-terminal side of the inter-heavy chain disulfide bonds, yielding three pieces of nearly equal size: two identical antigen-binding *Fab* fragments and one constant or crystalline *Fc* fragment (Figure 7.7). Each of the two Fab fragments consists of an intact light chain and the amino-terminal half of the heavy chain linked by a single interchain disulfide bond. The Fc fragment contains portions of the constant regions of the heavy chains.

The Fab and Fc fragments of the Ig molecule differ in their attributes. The Fab fragment binds to antigen because it contains the antibody's binding site. Fab frag-

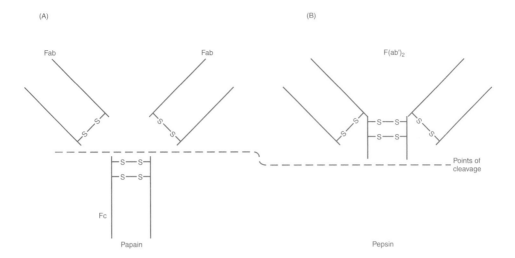

Figure 7.7. Structure of Fab, Fc and F(ab)'$_2$ fragments of antibodies. Enzyme cleavage with papain splits the antibody molecule into two Fab portions and one Fc portion. Each Fab fragment maintains the ability to bind antigen. Treatment with pepsin produced a single molecule called F(ab)'$_2$. The Fc region is degraded.

ments can combine with antigen to form soluble complexes, but they cannot precipitate antigens, as there is only one binding site on each fragment (Figure 7.7). The Fc portion does not bind to antigen but can be crystallized.

Pepsin, in contrast to papain, cleaves the Ig molecule on the carboxyl-terminal side of the inter-heavy chain disulfide bonds, yielding a single bivalent fragment called *F(ab')*$_2$ (M.W. 110,000 daltons); the remainder of the molecule is digested into smaller fragments. The F(ab')$_2$ fragment has the capability of combining with antigen and precipitating them but cannot activate complement or enhance phagocytosis, as these capabilities are on the Fc fragment (Figure 7.7). Thus, neither Fab nor F(ab')$_2$ fragments have all of the biologic properties of intact antibody molecules.

THE B CELL RECEPTOR (BCR)

Each B cell expresses multiple copies of the same antigen-specific receptor on its cell surface. These structures are commonly called *B cell Receptors* (BCR). The receptor has the basic immunoglobulin structure, consisting of two L chains paired with either two μ chains (IgM) or two δ chains (IgD) (Figure 7.8). Both types of BCR on a given cell have the same H and L variable (V) region and thus the same antigen-specificity. Since the BCR is composed of immunoglobulin, it is also often referred to as *surface Ig* (sIg). The receptor has a transmembrane domain that anchors it to the cell surface. In addition, there are proteins associated with the BCR, called Igα and Igβ, that are involved in transmembrane cell signaling. The binding of the BCR with an epitope along with other costimulatory molecules signals the B cell to begin clonal expansion. Some of the daughter cells resulting from this expansion develop into plasma cells. Antibodies secreted by these plasma cells have the same specificity as the BCR on the original B cell.

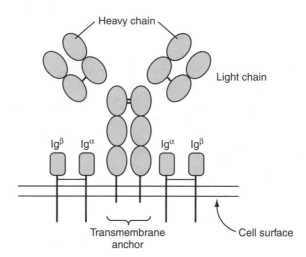

Figure 7.8. The B cell and its receptor for antigen. The BCR has the basic four-chain structure found in IgM and IgD. In addition, there is a transmembrane domain that anchors it to the cell surface. Proteins called Igα and Igβ are associated with the BCR.

ANTIBODY DIVERSITY

Humans can make millions of B cells, each with the ability to secrete antibody with a unique specificity. Since antibodies are proteins, they are coded for by DNA. If each antibody were coded for by a separate gene, then a huge amount of the human genome would be needed to code for antibodies capable of binding to millions of different epitopes. There is in fact not a gene for each antibody, rather the functional gene for each antibody results from a process of DNA rearrangement that takes place during B cell development in the bone marrow. Details on B cell development are considered in chapter 8.

In the bone marrow, *hematopoietic stem cells* produce immature pro-B cells. These *pro-B cells* have the genetic potential for making antibody that can bind to one of many different epitopes. However, as they mature within the bone marrow, each maturing B cell loses its "pluripotential" ability and develops into a mature B cell with a *single* antigenic specificity. Throughout the life of an individual, the stem cells continue to produce millions of B cells and thereby maintain our ability to secrete antibody to a vast array of antigens.

The details of the molecular mechanism responsible for the generation of antibody diversity are fairly complex (Figure 7.9). DNA segments containing coding for kappa and lambda L chains are located on human chromosomes 2 and 22, respectively, whereas DNA coding of the H chain is on chromosome 14. Three different sequences of DNA code for the L chain: the V (variable) segments which code for amino acids 1 to 95; the J (joining) segments that code for the remaining portion (thirteen amino acids) of the V region, and the C segment that codes for the constant region (~100 amino acids). In the human genome, there are forty different light chain V segments, five different J segments, but only one C segment. These coding regions are separated by noncoding regions of DNA (indicated in Figure 7.9 by placement of series of dots). As noted above, during B cell development in the bone marrow, recombination of the DNA coding for both the L and H chains occurs. In this process, one of the forty V segments is brought near one of the five J

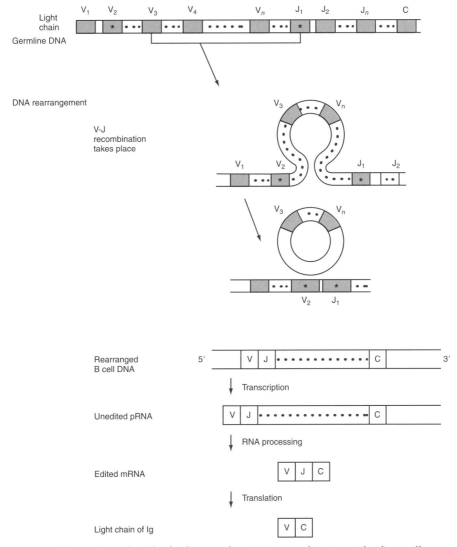

Figure 7.9. Generation of antibody diversity by DNA recombination. The figure illustrates the process by which germline DNA is rearranged and the heavy chain protein is produced during B cell development. One V segment (example, V_{2*}) recmobines with one J Segment (example J_1) to create the variable (V) region of the light chain.

segments, and the intervening DNA is enzymatically removed (Figure 7.9). The recombination process is essentially random, so that any one of the forty V segments may pair with any of the five J segments, resulting in ~200 different combinations of V and J. Once the newly- formed gene is produced, it is transcribed into RNA, noncoding RNA is excised by splicing, and a functional mRNA transcript is produced which is used for the synthesis of the L chain (Figure 7.9).

Within the same B cell, DNA recombination of the H chain V region loci also takes place. The H chain variable region is coded for by three different DNA segments, namely the Variable (V) which codes for amino acids 1 to 95, the Diversity (D) segments which code for one to fourteen different amino acids, and the Joining (J) segment which codes for the remainder of the H chain V region. In humans, there are an estimated fifty-one functional heavy chain V segments, twenty-seven D segments, and six J segments. Thus, by the random assortment of these segments, 8,262 different heavy chain VDJ combinations can be made. An especially high amount of diversity is found in the third CDR region of the H chain as both the D and J segments aid in coding for this area. Downstream from the V coding region are located DNA sequences which code for each of the H chain constant region isotypes (e.g., μ, δ, γ, α, and ε). Following recombination, a primary RNA transcript is made which contains information for the V region, the μ constant region and the δ constant region. The RNA transcript is produced, introns are excised, and RNA splicing takes place resulting in two mRNA transcripts. One codes for an IgM and one for an IgD molecule. This process explains how the same variable region can become associated with two different constant regions. Once the recombination process is complete, the B cell has committed itself to the production of a unique L and a unique H chain that pair to form an antibody molecule capable of interacting with a single epitope.

Since the L and H chain undergo DNA recombination independently, a single cell may produce one of 200 possible L chains and one of 8,262 possible H chains. As a result of random pairing of L and H chains, over 1.65 million antibodies with different antigenic-specificities can be produced. This result is obtained by multiplying the probability of the two independent events which gives the probability of any given event occurring simultaneously, thus $200 \times 8,262 = 1,652,400$. Although each B cell produces antibody of only one specificity, as many B cells exist, each of which has a different antibody determining gene produced by DNA recombination the number of possibilities is vast.

In addition to the antibody diversity resulting from "mixing and matching" of different DNA sequences, other modifications may occur during the recombination process. For example, during the rearrangement process when the DNA is cleaved and religated, two nucleotides from a codon of one V segment of DNA may be spliced next to one nucleotide of a codon from a J segment. As a result, an entirely new triplet may be produced and a different amino acid is incorporated into the chain. In addition, the enzyme *terminal deoxynucleotidyl transferase* (TdT) is able to add nucleotides randomly to the H chain between the time the DNA is broken at the V, D, and J segments, and the DNA is religated. This process also adds a significant amount of diversity to the recombinant CDR3 region. It is estimated that the human immune system can make over a billion different antibodies by randomly rearranging fewer than 200 segments of DNA. As a consequence, the immune system is able to respond to new pathogens it has never before encountered.

CHANGES IN THE AFFINITY AND CLASS OF ANTIBODIES DURING THE COURSE OF THE IMMUNE RESPONSE

Once mature B cells leave the bone marrow, they circulate in the blood and lymphatic system where they may encounter antigen. As noted previously, if a B cell comes in contact with a foreign antigen, i.e., molecule, it undergoes clonal expansion and some of the resulting daughter cells become plasma cells that secrete antibody. The first antibody they secrete is IgM (Figure 7.10). As the response progresses, more daughter cells are produced, resulting in production of a larger number of plasma cells, and greater amounts of antibody being produced. The newly produced B cells migrate into specialized areas in the lymph nodes and the spleen,

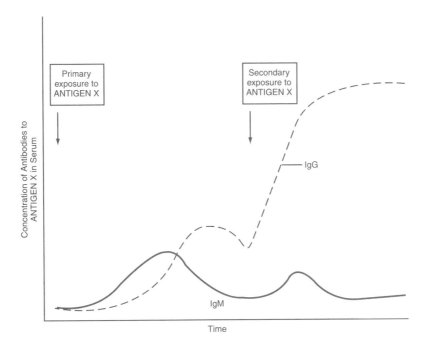

Figure 7.10.   Kinetics of a primary and a secondary antibody response to an antigen. The Y axis shows the amount of specific antibodies present in serum over time. At first, IgM antibodies are produced, but later, IgG (or possibly IgA) antibodies begin to appear. Following re-exposure to the same antigen, a rapid IgG response occurs because numerous memory B cells, which have already undergone isotype-switching, can be called rapidly into action.

called *germinal centers*, where two important events take place. First, in response to cues it receives, the B cell will undergo a process called *isotype-switching* and begins to secrete antibody other than IgM. For example, in response to a bacterial or viral infection the B cell may switch from IgM to IgG production while in response to a worm infection it may start producing IgE.

The second process that occurs within germinal centers is known as *somatic hypermutation*. The precise mechanism responsible for this is unclear, but one or more mutations may occur in the nucleotide sequences that code for the V region of the antibody molecule. As a result, daughter B cells are produced that express slightly different BCR. Since the mutations are random, some of the resulting B cells may have higher affinity receptors for the antigen, and some will have lower affinity receptors. As the immune response progresses and the amount of antigen decreases in the body, those B cells with higher affinity receptors out-compete those with lower affinity receptors. As a result, the overall affinity of the antibody produced during an immune response increases. Thus, during an immune response, IgM antibodies are replaced by either IgG, IgA, or IgE antibodies, and the affinity of these antibodies increases.

Once the antigen or infection producing the antigen is eliminated, many of the newly produced B cells will persist in an inactive state, and as a result, the person will retain a large number of B cells specific for the antigen. These cells are called *memory B cells*. When a person becomes infected again, a secondary response takes place. A large number of the retained memory B cells will respond. As a result of the presence of memory B cells, the secondary response is characterized by the rapid production of high affinity IgG, IgA, or IgE antibodies.

FUNCTIONS OF IMMUNOGLOBULIN CLASSES

A summary of the chemical and biological characteristics of human immuno-globulins is provided in Table 7.1. The five classes of immunoglobulins differ in molecular size, half-life in the plasma, carbohydrate content, and biologic activity. The serum levels of IgG, IgA, and IgM vary with several factors, one of which is age. The levels of these immunoglobulins are lowest soon after birth, peak during adolescence, and decline gradually with aging.

IgG is the most abundant of the immunoglobulins. As noted earlier, IgG (M.W. 150,000) is composed of two heavy (M.W. 50,000) and two light (M.W. 25,000) chains linked by disulfide bonds. Approximately 65 percent of IgG molecules in humans have kappa light chains, while 35 percent have lambda. IgG is found in high concentrations in serum, with levels of 6-18 mg/ml. About 40 percent of IgG is intravascular and 60% is in the interstitial fluid. Because of its ability to diffuse between intravascular and extravascular spaces, IgG is effective in neutralizing bacterial toxins in both blood and tissues and is active against infectious agents that are disseminated in the blood, principally the Gram-positive bacteria. It neu-tralizes viruses and enhances the phagocytosis of microorganisms. It is therefore an *opsonizing* antibody. It is synthesized during the latter part of the primary re-sponse and is the major antibody synthesized during the secondary immune re-sponse. The half-life of IgG varies inversely with its serum concentration and is about twenty-one days, the longest of all the immunoglobulins.

The differences in the four subclasses of IgG are related to differences in amino acid sequence. Subclass differences were originally demonstrated immunologically, demonstrating that each of the four subclasses has unique epitopes. The subclasses of IgG are present in different amounts, with IgG1 > IgG2 > IgG3 > IgG4. Besides being structurally different, the four subclasses of IgG also have different biologi-cal characteristics. For example, IgG3 has the greatest ability to activate comple-ment of any of the IgG subclasses, IgG1 has less, IgG2 even less, and IgG4 does not activate complement. Of the IgG classes, only IgG1 and IgG3 have the capacity to bind to surface receptors of macrophages and neutrophils. Organisms opsonized with IgG of these subclasses are thus readily phagocytized. All four subclasses of IgG are transported across the human placenta and provide passively transferred humoral immunity to the newborn.

IgM has a molecular weight of 900,000 and is a pentamer of five subunits in a circular configuration joined by disulfide bridges (Figure 7.4). An additional polypeptide chain, called the *J chain*, helps stabilize the molecule. The J chain (M.W. 15,000 daltons) is coded for by a non-Ig gene. IgM is the largest molecule of any antibody of the five classes; because of its size, it circulates primarily in the vascu-lar blood compartment. IgM is the first antibody to be made during a primary immune response. It is an efficient activator of the complement cascade, since only one bound IgM molecule is needed to lyse a cell. On the other hand, IgG requires two or more bound molecules to activate complement.

IgA is an important first line of defense. Its principal function is to protect mu-cous membranes from infection. It is synthesized by plasma cells in the submucosa of the respiratory, gastrointestinal and genitourinary tracts and in excretory glands and is found at high concentrations in the lymphoid tissues and in secretions such as saliva, sweat, tears, urine, nasal fluid and milk. IgA provides protection to the newborn. They obtain it by ingestion with the first milk or *colostrum*. IgA is the second most abundant Ig in serum.

IgA may occur as a monomer or as a polymer of two to five subunits. In serum, IgA exists primarily as a monomer (90 percent) with some polymeric forms, mostly dimers and trimers. Like IgM, the J (joining) chain helps bind the IgA subunits together. IgA present in extracellular secretions is referred to as *secretory IgA*. Secretory IgA is a dimer, consisting of two monomeric IgAs, a J chain and a nonimmuno-globulin glycoprotein called the *secretory component* (M.W. 85,000 daltons). After release from the plasma cell, IgA may bind to a poly-Ig receptor on epithelial cells. This binding process induces the transport of the IgA molecule through the endothelial cell by transcytosis. During the transport process, the poly-Ig receptor is cleaved and a portion of it, called the *secretory component* (SC), becomes bound to dimeric IgA (Figure 7.11). The SC is thought to make the IgA molecule resistant to attack by proteolytic enzymes.

In humans, IgE binds to basophils and their tissue counterparts, mast cells, and circulates in serum at very low levels. IgE has a role in many allergic disorders, such as bronchial asthma, hay fever, and anaphylaxis, which are probably extreme forms of basically protective inflammatory responses. Allergens stimulate IgE production particularly in areas such as the tonsils and Peyer's patches in the gastrointestinal tract. IgE attaches by its Fc portion to membrane receptors on mast cells and basophils, leaving the combining sites free to bind to antigen. When reexposure to the same allergen occurs, the allergen binds to the IgE on the cell and vasoactive mediators, such as histamine, are released. The clinical effects of the mediators include respiratory tract constriction, increased vascular permeability, and vasodilation resulting in difficulty in breathing, edema, and skin rashes. Another result of allergic reactions is the increase in production of secretions by cells on mucosal surfaces. IgE may also contribute to defense against parasitic worm infections.

IgD, like IgE, circulates in trace amounts in serum. It has a short half-life (2.8 days), possibly because of its susceptibility to proteolytic degradation. Its known function is to serve, along with IgM, as an antigen-binding receptor on the surface of B lymphocytes. IgD probably plays a critical role in differentiation of B cells and in the initiation of the immune response.

DETECTION OF ANTIBODIES: BASIC PRINCIPLES AND CONCEPTS
BEHIND SEROLOGICAL ASSAYS

When an individual or animal is immunized with a complex antigen, many different B cells respond, i.e, the response is *polyclonal*. As a result, antibodies will be produced that bind to different epitopes on the antigen, they will have different affinities, and be of different isotypes. Such anti-serum is commonly referred to as *polyclonal antiserum*.

In contrast to polyclonal antibodies produced by immunization, a large amount of antibodies with a single antigenic-specificity (i.e., monoclonal antibodies) can be produced by hybridomas. Kohler and Milstein developed the technique for "immortalizing" single antibody-secreting B cells. By fusing a pre-plasma cell (normal life span equals 4 days) with a tumor cell (life span, "forever"), the resulting hybridoma and its progeny will secrete antibody indefinitely. Since all of the antibody comes from the progeny of a single plasma cell (i.e, is monoclonal), all of the

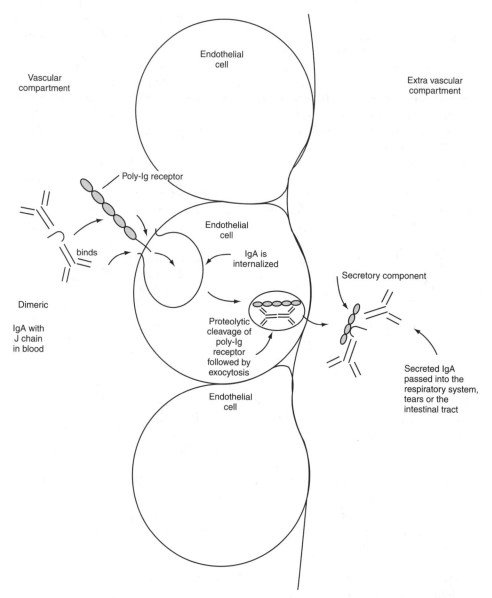

Figure 7.11. Transcytosis of dimeric IgA from the blood to secretions. Dimeric IgA circulating in the blood binds to the poly-Ig receptor on endothelial cells, where it is transported through the cell and released into the gut or respiratory tract. In the process, a piece of the poly-Ig receptor, called the secretory component binds to the dimer and helps protect the antibody from degradation.

antibody molecules produced by a single hybridoma have the same antigenic specificity, affinity and isotype. Although monoclonal antibodies are highly specific for a single epitope, they may have a low affinity, and have restricted biological functions. Thus, monoclonal antibodies cannot be used in all of the immunological assays described below. Monoclonal antibodies are currently being used in the development of diagnostic assays and immunotherapy. One strength of

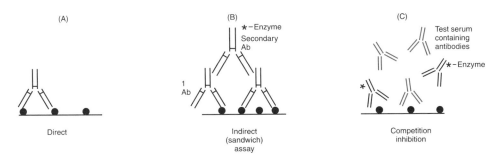

Figure 7.12.   Examples of direct, indirect and inhibition assays. Examples of a direct binding are shown in (A), and of indirect binding in (B). An inhibition assay is shown in (C).

hybridoma-derived antibodies is consistency, as large amounts of the same anti-body can be produced over a long period of time. In contrast, polyclonal antisera must be produced in individual animals and may differ from lot to lot.

Various methods have been used to detect the presence of antibody in serum, and these methods are referred to as *serological assays*. Serological assays can be divided into five different categories, based on the immunological principle they employ. In Table 7.2, the five basic types of serological test are listed along the top, namely, *precipitation, agglutination, complement-mediated cell lysis, direct binding*, and *biological function assays*, and their attributes are listed under each heading.

In some of these assays, the presence of antibody may be demonstrated by detect-ing the direct binding of the antibody to the antigen (Figure 7.12A). Such assays are known as *direct binding assays*. In other assays, a second antibody may be used to detect the presence of the antibody directly bound to the antigen. These are *indirect binding assays*. The antibody bound to the antigen is referred to as the *primary antibody*, and the antibody which binds to it is called the *secondary antibody*. The assay format shown in Figure 7.12B is called an *indirect, secondary*, or *sandwich assay*. Another assay approach is the *inhibition assay*. In this method, a solution known to contain a labeled antibody is mixed with the sample being tested (Figure 7.12C). If the sample contains antibody, it will compete with the labeled antibody for sites on the antigen and less labeled antibody will be bound. Direct, indirect, and inhibition methods can be used with any of the five basic categories listed across the top of Table 7.2.

Precipitation assays: In this assay, a solution containing a soluble antigen is com-bined with antibodies (Figure 7.13). The antibodies bind to, and cross-link, the an-tigen resulting in the formation of a large immune complex with a *lattice structure*, which precipitates from solution and settles to the bottom of the reaction tube. In order for a precipitation reaction to occur, the antigen must have multiple epitopes, and the antibody must be at least bivalent (i.e., Fab fragments cannot cross-link). As shown in the figure, if one keeps the amount of antigen constant and adds in-creasing amounts of antibody, there is a point where maximal precipitation occurs. This is known as the *zone of equivalence*, and occurs where antibody and antigen are present in approximately equal molar concentrations. Dilutions of the sample where precipitate is not formed because there is either too little or too much antibody are referred to as the *prozones*. Because maximal precipitation occurs when there are equal concentrations of antigen and antibody, the test was originally used as a semiquantitative assay to determine the amount of antibody present in serum.

Precipitation assays are commonly carried out today as *precipitation-in-gel assays*.

Table 7.2. Some aspects of serological tests.

| | Type of Test | | | | |
Attribute	Direct Binding	Precipitation	Agglutination	Complement-mediated Cell Lysis	Phagocytosis
Nature of the Antigen	any antigen	soluble antigen with 2 or more epitopes	solid antigen (particle with 2 or more epitopes	an intact cell	any substance
Nature of the Antibody	Fab, F(ab)'2, all classes of antibody	Bivalent antibody	Bivalent antibody	IgM >> IgG	IgG
Concentration		Equal molar amounts of antigen & antibody	Best at equal molar amounts of antibody & antigen; problem with prozone effect	IgM requires only 1 molecule per cell; usually 800-1,000 IgG/cell required	
Read out	usually biological assays, e.g. neutralization of virus	visible precipitate in a test tube or gel	agglutination of RBC or latex	cell death or release of intracellular components	Up-take phagocytes
Additional comments	often detected in an indirect or sandwich assay (see text)	best if multiple epitopes per antigen and polyclonal antibody			

Two examples are shown in Figure 7.14. A semisolid agar gel is poured, and holes are cut in the gel to produce wells. In Figure 7.14A, antibody was placed in one well and antigen in another. The two soluble molecules diffused through the agar, and a lattice structure was formed at the point where antigen and antibody were in approximately equivalent concentrations. This general format is known as a *double diffusion* or an *Ouchterlony* test, so named after the man who first described it. In the example shown in Figure 7.14B, antibody to human albumin was placed in the center well (well #1) and albumin isolated from two different humans was placed in wells 2 and 3. A continuous precipitin band was formed between the antibody and the two human albumin samples. This type of reaction is known as a *band of identity*, and shows that albumin isolated from the two humans is antigenically identical. Albumin isolated from chickens was placed in well 4. A precipitation band was formed that is continuous with the human precipitate, but there was also a small arc, or spur, seen. This is known as a *band of partial identity* and shows that albumin from humans and chickens share some, but not all, epitopes in common.

Immunoelectrophoresis is another type of a precipitation assay (Figure 7.15). In the example shown, an agar gel was prepared, serum from humans was added to the central well, and the sample was electrophoresed to separate the proteins. Then, two troughs were cut in the gel, and serum containing antibodies to human serum proteins was added to one trough, and antibody to human IgM was added to the other trough. Following incubation, a series of precipitin arcs formed. This proce-

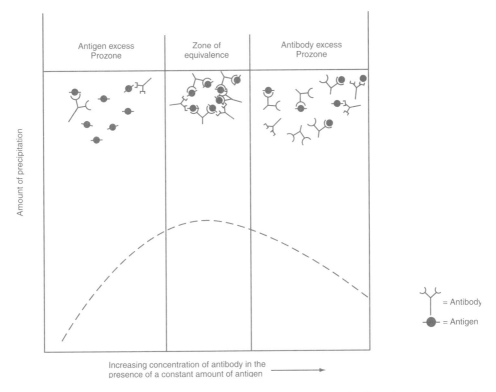

Figure 7.13.   In precipitation assays. Lattice formation is created when there are approximately equal molar concentrations of antigen and antibodies.

A. Ochterlongy or Double Diffusion
   The Principle

B. A Specific Example

Agar Gel

Ag → ← Ab → diffusion

A precipitate forms
when there are approximately
equal concentrations of
antigen and antibody

Well #1: antibodies to human albumin
Well #2 + #3: human albumin
Well #4: chicken albumin
Well #5: unrelated protein

Figure 7.14.   Two examples of precipitin-in-gel assays. (A) An example of a double diffusion or Ouchterlony assay. Antibodies are placed in one well and antigen in the other. As the two molecules diffuse, they meet and a precipitin band forms where there are equal amounts of antigen and antibody. (B) Antibody to human albumin was placed in well #1. Wells #2 and #3 contain albumin from two different humans, well #4 contains albumin from a chicken, and well #5 has an unrelated protein. A smooth, continuous band of identity is present between the two wells containing human albumin, whereas a band of partial identity is seen with chicken albumin. The results demonstrate that human and chicken albumin share some, but not all, epitopes in common.

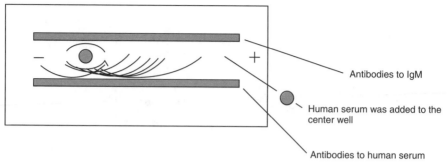

Figure 7.15. Immunoelectrophoresis. The presence of human IgM can be detected by comparing the position of the single band at the top of the slide with the complex band pattern of the whole serum sample.

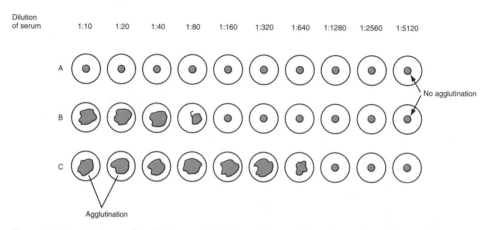

Figure 7.16. An example of direct and indirect hemagglutination assays. (A) Serial dilutions of normal serum which does not have antibodies to erythrocytes was added to the wells in row A. This is the negative control. (B) Serial dilutions of serum containing antibodies to erythrocytes were added to the wells in row B and direct agglutination occurred in the first 4 wells. Thus, the serum sample has titer of 1:80 by the direct dilution system. (C) Serial dilutions of the same serum containing antibodies to erythrocytes used in row B were added to the wells in row C and allowed to bind to the erythrocytes. Then, anti-antibodies were added, i.e., indirect agglutination was produced. A positive agglutination reaction was observed in the first 7 wells. This result shows that an indirect reaction is more sensitive than the direct reaction.

dure was used to determine the presence of IgM in the serum. Of course, there are numerous other applications for this general immunological method.

Agglutination assays: In an agglutination assay, the antigen is usually a cell (for example an erythrocyte) or an antigen coupled to a particle (i.e., latex). When the antigen is mixed with antibodies, the antibodies cross-link the particles, and a visible mass is seen with the naked eye. As with precipitation assays, the antibodies must be at least bivalent, and the antigen must contain multiple epitopes in order for cross-linking to occur. Again, the antibody and the antigen must be present in approximately equal molar concentrations for cross-linking to take place. A prozone effect also occurs in agglutination assays.

The classical example of an agglutination assay is the *direct hemagglutination assay* (Figure 7.16). In order to determine if a person has antibodies to antigens expressed on the surface of another person's erythrocytes, various dilutions of serum from the person are added to wells of a microtiter plate. Then, a suspension of the erythrocytes to be tested is added. If antibodies are present in sufficient concentration to cross-link the erythrocytes, the immune complex, which forms, precipitates as a fluffy layer on the bottom of the well. If antibodies are not present, the erythrocytes roll down the sides of the well, and a compact pellet of cells forms at the center of the well. In the example shown, a positive reaction is seen with serum diluted 1:20, 1:40 and 1:80, but not 1:160. The term *titer* is used to refer to the reciprocal of the highest dilution that gives a positive reaction. Thus, we would say that the serum used in the test had a titer of 1:80.

In the direct hemagglutination assay, anti-erythrocyte antibodies hold the complex together. In some cases, anti-erythrocyte antibodies may bind, but in amounts too low to hold the complex together. In this case, low levels of antibody may be detected using an *indirect agglutination assay*. After time has elapsed to allow the antibody present to bind to the erythrocytes, antibody to the anti-erythrocyte antibody is added and will cross-link the antibody on the erythrocyte and cause a precipitate to form. The indirect assay detects lower amounts of antibody than the direct assay. Thus, antibody titers in indirect hemagglutination assay (i.e., 1:640 in the example shown in Figure 7.16) will be higher than in corresponding direct assays (i.e., 1:80 in Figure 7.16).

Cell lysis using complement: In this assay, the antigen must be present on the surface of a cell. The antigen may be naturally present, e.g., carbohydrate A,B,O blood group antigens on erythrocytes, or the antigen may be covalently coupled to the surface of a cell. Antibody is added to the cell suspension, followed by the addition of complement. If antibody is present, it binds to complement and the complement produces a number of holes in the cell membrane. If erythrocytes are used, one can measure either the amount of hemoglobin released into the medium or a decrease in the number of unlysed erythrocytes remaining. If the cell is a leukocyte, one adds a dye, e.g., trypan blue, that cannot penetrate an intact cell membrane. If holes have been produced in the cell membrane, the dye will enter the cell and stain it. If antibody is not present, the cell membrane remains intact and the cell is colorless. Complement-mediated lysis assays can be conducted as either direct, indirect, or inhibition assays.

Binding assays: In this type of assay, antibodies bound directly to the antigen are detected by an antibody coupled to some type of label. This label may be either a radioisotope (i.e., ^{125}I), an enzyme (i.e., alkaline phosphatase), or a fluorochrome (i.e., fluorescein isothiocyanate or rhodamine). Assays using radiolabeled antibody are referred to as *radioimmunoassays* (RIA). The presence of antibody in a sample is detected by measuring the amount of radioactivity bound to the antigen using a scintillation or gamma counter. Assays in which enzymes are used are called enzyme-linked *immunosorbent assays* (ELISA or EIA). In this case, a substrate is added that changes color in samples where there is a positive reaction. When fluorochromes are used, the assays are referred to as *immunofluorescence assays* (IFA). If the antigen being studied is part of a cell or organism, then fluorescence is detected using a fluorescence microscopy. An example of a positive indirect IFA is shown in Figure 7.17. In RIA, ELISA, and IFA assays, various dilutions of sera are used so that antibody titers can be determined. These assays are very sensitive and detect nanogram or picogram amounts of antibody. Because of the sensitivity of these tests, serum can be diluted extensively and still give a positive reaction. It is not unusual for an indirect RIA or ELISA to have titers of 1:10,000 to >1:1,000,000. As with the

(A)

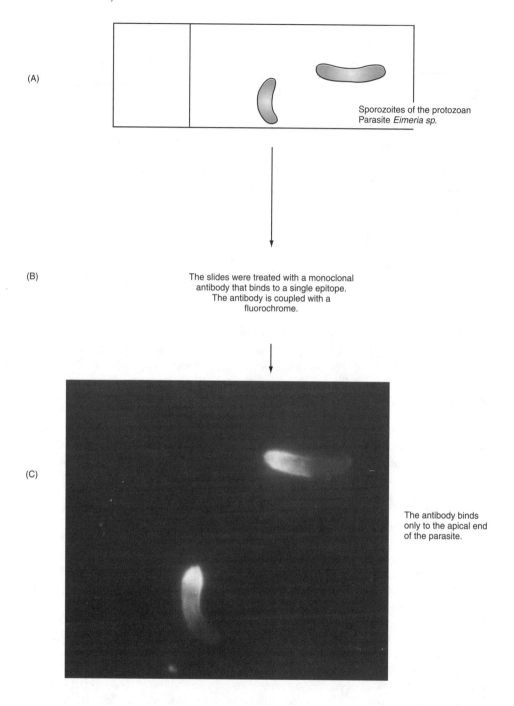

Sporozoites of the protozoan
Parasite *Eimeria sp.*

(B)

The slides were treated with a monoclonal
antibody that binds to a single epitope.
The antibody is coupled with a
fluorochrome.

(C)

The antibody binds
only to the apical end
of the parasite.

Figure 7.17. Binding assays: Results from a direct immunofluorescence assay. (A) Sporozoites of
the protozoan causing coccidiosis were fixed on a microscope slide. (B) they were treated with a
fluorescein isothiocyanate-labeled monoclonal antibody. (C) On examination with a microscope
using UV light, the monoclonal antibody was determined to bind to the apical end of the organism.

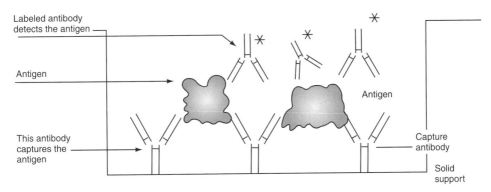

Figure 7.18. An example of an antigen-capture assay. An antibody is absorbed to a microtiter well, and then a sample which is suspected of containing the antigen is added. If the antigen is in the sample, it is captured by the antibody. After washing the well, a second antibody to the antigen which is labeled with an enzyme is added. Following the addition of a chromatographic substrate, the well will turn color in a positive reaction.

other assay approaches discussed above, RIA, ELISA, and IFA assays can be performed as inhibition assays, as well.

The majority of assays used today in hospitals and clinical laboratories for detecting the presence of antibodies to various pathogens are indirect RIAs, ELISAs, or IFA assays.

Biological assays: The presence of antibody can be detected using a variety of biological assay systems. In most cases, such tests utilize the basic principles described above. For example, antibody may bind to viruses and prevent them from entering cells. Such antibody is often called *neutralizing antibody*. In a viral neutralization assay, viruses are combined with dilutions of the serum being tested, and then the mixtures are added to a tissue culture flask containing a monolayer of cells. If antibodies are present, the virus will be neutralized; if antibodies are not present, the virus will invade the cells and cause cytopathic alterations of the cells that are then observed microscopically. A variety of inhibition of invasion or inhibition of growth assays are available for measuring antibody responses to different pathogens.

Antigen-detection methods: The above discussion focused on the detection of antibodies in serum or other body fluids. These assays can be modified to detect the presence of antigen. For example, RIA or ELISA are often formatted as *antigen capture assays* (Figure 7.18). In these assays, wells of a microtiter plate are coated with antibody (monoclonal antibodies are frequently used), and then a solution which may contain the antigen is added. If present, the antigen will be "captured" by the bound antibody. Unbound material is washed from the plate, and a second labeled-antibody which is specific for the antigen is added. The presence of the antigen is identified by detecting the binding of the secondary antibody. Today, this basic antigen-capture approach is being used in the development of simple, rapid assays for diagnosing a variety of infectious diseases.

Additional information on serological tests can be found in chapter 20.

SUMMARY

The goal of this chapter was to provide you with an appreciation of the importance of B cells and the antibodies they produce. A hallmark of the inducible immune system is specificity. During development of B cells in the bone marrow, a complex series of steps takes place whereby V(D)J segments of DNA are recombined to produce an almost infinite number of antibody H and L chains. The wide array of antibodies produced serve as receptors for antigen on the surface of B cells and as soluble molecules which are secreted into sera. Antibodies play an important role in the control of pathogens by enhancing phagocytosis, preventing spread from the site of infection, blocking key receptors needed by pathogens for entry into host cells and activation of the complement cascade. As an infection progresses, early IgM responses are replaced by IgG antibodies which are important in the control of pathogens in the blood or tissues, IgA which helps prevent the entry of organisms into the body, or IgE, which aids in elimination of parasitic worms or may cause allergies. Thus, in order to understand the inducible immune response, it is important to have a good appreciation of antibodies, including their structure and function.

In the latter part of this chapter, the subject of antibody detection was addressed. It was shown that antibodies can be detected by their ability to precipitate soluble antigens, agglutinate cells, activate complement-mediated cell lysis, and by binding directly to antigens. Antibodies can be detected directly, or by using secondary (indirect), or inhibitory immune interactions. Basic assays used to detect antibodies can be reformatted to detect antigens. It should be noted that a large number of commercial assays are currently available which are used routinely in both clinical and research settings. Some of these assays are described in more detail in chapter 20.

SUGGESTIONS FOR FURTHER READING

General Textbooks

1. Cox, F.E.G., J.P. Kreier, and D. Wakelin. "Immunology and Immunopathology of Human Parasitic Infections." Chapter 4 in *Topley and Wilson's Microbiology and Microbial Infections, Vol. 5: Parasitology*. 9th ed. London: Edward Arnold, 1998.
2. Janeway, C.A. Jr., P. Travers, M. Walport, and J.D. Capra. *Immunobiology: The Immune System in Health and Disease*. CB Current Biology Publications. New York: Garland Publishing, 1999.
3. Kuby, J. *Immunology*. 3d ed. New York: W.H. Freeman and Company, 1997.
4. Leffell, M.S., A.D. Donnenberg, and N.R. Rose. *Handbook of Human Immunology*. Boca Raton, FL: CRC Press, 1997.

Specific Review Articles on Molecular Biology of B Cells

1. Kelso, G. "V(D)H Hypermutation and Receptor Revision: Coloring Outside the Lines." *Current Opinions in Immunology* 11, no. 1 (1999):70-75.
2. Maizels, N. "Immunoglobulin Class Switch Recombination: Will Genetics Provide New Clues to Mechanisms?" *American Journal of Genetics* 64, no. 5 (1999):1270–1275.
3. Ross, D.A., M.R. Wilson, N.W. Miller, L.W. Clem, and G.W. Warr. "Evolutionary Variation of Immunoglobulin Mu Heavy Chain RNA Processing Pathways: Origins, Effects and Implications." *Immunological Reviews* 166 (1998):143–151.

Specific Antibody Function

1. Corthesy, B., and J.P. Kraehenbuhl. "Antibody-Mediated Protection of Mucosal Surfaces." *Current Topics in Microbial Immunology* 236 (1999):93–111.
2. Yssel, H., and colleagues. "The Role of IgE in Asthma." *Clinical and Experimental Allergy* 28, suppl. 5 (1998):104–109.

Reviews on Antibodies to Specific Pathogens & Their Roles in Pathology

1. Juompam, L., and colleagues. "Selective Alterations of the Antibody Response to HIV-1." *Applied Biochemistry and Biotechnology* 75, no. 1(1998):139–150.
2. Beck, J.M., and colleagues. "Lymphocytes in Host Defense Against *Pneumocystsis carinii*." *Seminars in Respiratory Infections* 13, no. 4(1998):330–338.
3. Paul, L.C. "Antibodies and Chronic Organ Graft Rejection." *Annuals of Transplantation* 2(1997):46–52.

QUESTIONS

1. Diagram a typical antibody molecule (i.e., IgG) and label the following parts: light chain, heavy chain, hinge, variable regions, Fc region.
2. How does the BCR differ from antibodies secreted by the same cell?
3. There are five major classes of immunoglobulin. Which immunoglobulin class is
   a. present in serum at the highest concentration?
   b. found only on the surface on B cells?
   c. the first antibody to be produced following a primary infection?
   d. present in high concentrations in the respiratory tract and gut?
   e. associated with allergies?
   f. able to cross the placenta and provide protection for neonates?
4. Why are there more antibodies produced following a secondary infection than during a primary infection?

ANSWERS

1. See Figure 7.3.
2. The BCR has a transmembrane domain that anchors it into the cell membrane. It is associated with several other proteins, called Igαβ. The constant region of the BCR is either mu or delta. On the other hand, secretory antibody does not have a transmembrane domain and the constant region may be either mu, gamma, epsilon or alpha.
3. a. IgG.
   b. IgD.
   c. IgM.
   d. IgA.
   e. IgE.
   f. IgG.
4. During the primary exposure to a pathogen, B cells with complementary receptors undergo clonal expansion and a large number of daughter cells are produced. Many of these become memory B cells. Thus, when a person is exposed to the pathogen again, there are large numbers of B cells available to respond. Thus, the response occurs much faster and large amounts of antibody are produced.

CHAPTER

8

INTRODUCTION
CELLS OF THE INDUCIBLE
    IMMUNE SYSTEM
    Lymphocytes
    B Lymphocytes
    T Lymphocytes
    Lymphocyte Antigen-Specific
        Receptors
    Gamma/Delta–Positive
        T Cells
THE IMMUNE SYSTEM
DEVELOPMENT OF THE
    IMMUNE SYSTEM
    Embryological Development
        of the Lymphoid Organs
        and Tissues
    Differentiation of Pluripoten-
        tial Hematopoietic Stem
        Cells
    Production of Antigen-
        Specific Receptors
    Antigen-Independent Differ-
        entiation of B Cells
    Antigen-Independent Differ-
        entiation of T Cells
ACTIVATION OF THE IM-
    MUNE SYSTEM BY
    ANTIGEN
    Initiation of a Primary Induc-
        ible Immune Response
    Antigen Processing and
        Presentation
    Interaction of Antigen-
        Presenting Cells (APC) and
        T Cells
    T Helper Cells Differentiate
        into either Th1 or Th2
        Cells
    Interaction of T Helper Cells
        and Macrophages
    Interaction of Th2 Cells and B
        Cells to Produce
        Antibodies
    Activation of Cytotoxic T
        Cells
SUMMARY
SUGGESTIONS FOR
    FURTHER READING
QUESTIONS
ANSWERS

The Inducible Defense System: The Induction and Development of the Inducible Defence

Michael A. Hickey and Diane Wallace Taylor

INTRODUCTION

As you learned in earlier chapters, the *inducible immune system* protects the host by recognizing and eliminating foreign antigens and pathogens. In addition, the inducible immune system recognizes abnormal self-proteins on the surface of cells, such as those that might be present on cancer cells, and eliminates them before they can grow. The cell type responsible for mediating the inducible immune response is the *lymphocyte*. Each lymphocyte has a unique antigen-specific receptor on its cell surface. When the cell comes in contact with the correct antigen, it undergoes proliferation and produces a number of daughter cells. Some of these cells play an active role in elimination of the disease-producing agent, whereas others become *memory* cells. Memory cells are very important if a person becomes reexposed to the same pathogen, in that they can rapidly respond and quickly eliminate the organism. Thus, the hallmark of the inducible immune system is said to be *"recognition, specificity, and immunologic memory."* This chapter will provide information on how lymphocytes recognize and respond to antigens, discuss factors that influence lymphocyte differentiation, and show how lymphocytes interact with each other to bring about immunity.

CELLS OF THE INDUCIBLE IMMUNE SYSTEM

Lymphocytes

Morphologically, the lymphocyte usually appears in the peripheral blood as a small, round uninucleate cell approximately 7 to 8 µm in diameter. The nucleus occupies the bulk of the cell, with a small amount of basic cytoplasm surrounding it (Figure 8.1). The lymphocyte that is commonly observed in blood films is in the resting stage

131

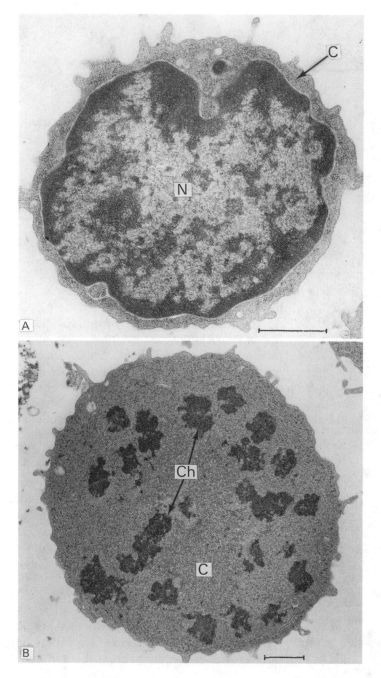

Figure 8.1.   Electron micrographs of lymphocytes: (A) A resting lymphocyte. The nucleus (N) occupies most of the cell. There is a thin rim of cytoplasm (C). This cell could be either a B or T cell. (B) Upon antigenic stimulation, cell division occurs and individual chromosomes (Ch) are observed. With further differentiation, B cells become plasma cells. (C) Typical mouse and (D) human plasma cells. The presences of a massive amount of endoplasmic reticulum (ER) in the cytoplasm of the lymphocyte is the distinguishing characteristic of the cells that are actively synthesizing and secreting antibody and cytokines, Bar represents 1 μm. (Photos courtesy of G.B. Chapman).

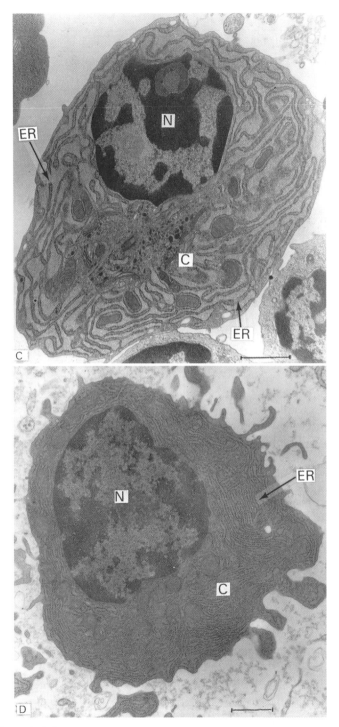

Figure 8.1. (*concluded*)

Table 8.1. Lymphocyte subsets.

Lymphocyte Subset	Function	Specific Surface Markers
B Cells	1) Antigen presenting cells. 2) Differentiate into plasma cells for antibody production.	sIgM, sIgD, Class II MHC
Plasma Cells	Antibody production.	sIg of antibody secreted, increased levels of Class II MHC
T Helper 1 Cells (Th1)	Activated cells secrete IL-2, IFNγ, and TNFβ, for the development of cellular immunity.	CD2, CD3, CD4, CD5, α/β TcR
T Helper 2 Cells (Th2)	Activated cells secrete IL-4, IL-5, IL-6 and IL-10, for the development of humoral immunity. B cell activation and differentiation.	CD2, CD3, CD4, CD5, α/β TcR
Cytotoxic T Cells (CTL)	Killing of foreign, cancerous, or virus infected cells.	CD2, CD3, CD8, CD5, α/β TcR
γ/δ T Cells	Unclear, but may be involved in defense along epithelium.	CD3, γ/δ TcRa

(G_0) of the cell cycle. The cytoplasm contains a few mitochondria, a small number of ribosomes, little or no endoplasmic reticulum, and an interphase nucleus. Upon activation by antigen, however, lymphocytes increase in size (≈ 12 μm) and differentiate into *lymphoblasts* (or *blasts*). Because lymphoblasts ultimately secrete products (for example, antibodies or cytokines) or transport intracellularly produced molecules to cell surfaces (for example, the interleukin-2 receptor), lymphoblasts have many of the morphologic characteristics of secretory cells. The Golgi apparatus becomes prominent and there are large amounts of rough endoplasmic reticulum and polyribosomes. Activated cells usually undergo cell division, during which chromosomes and spindle fibers are evident. Electron micrographs of resting, dividing, and activated lymphocytes with these attributes are shown in Figure 8.1.

Despite the fact that all lymphocytes look similar when examined by light or electron microscopy, lymphocytes can be divided into subsets that have a wide range of immunological functions. The major lymphocyte subsets are shown in Table 8.1. Lymphocytes express different proteins and glycoproteins on their surfaces. These proteins can be used to identify the different subsets and are commonly referred to as *surface markers* or *surface antigens*. An international system has been devised for "naming" cell surface markers which are commonly referred to as CD antigens. The immunologic importance of some of these surface markers has been established, but the functions of others are less clear. CD antigens expressed by different lymphocyte subsets are included in Table 8.1.

B Lymphocytes

As discussed in the previous chapter, the primary role of B lymphocytes is to produce antibodies. Antibody-producing lymphocytes were originally identified in the *Bursa of Fabricius* in chickens, and therefore called *bursa or B cells*. Further studies showed that they are also produced in the bone marrow of mammals. Thus, today they are referred to as bone-marrow derived or B cells. B cells may also serve

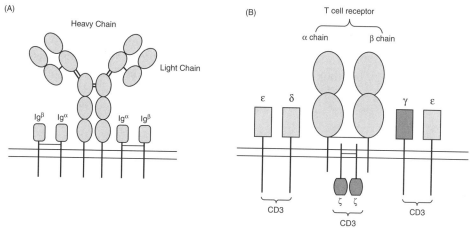

Figure 8.2. (A) B cell and T cell receptors. The B cell receptor is made up of a membrane bound IgM or IgD antibody molecule and a heterodimeric protein complex consisting of Igα and Igβ. Antigen binding by the Ig molecule causes the Igα-Igβ complex to transmit signal to the nucleus. (B) The T cell receptor is made up of the α and β chain which binds to MHC presented peptide antigens. The CD3 molecule is co-expressed with the T cell receptor and conducts transmembrane signals when the T cell receptor binds to processed antigen.

as antigen presenting cells (APC). Their role in antigen presentation is discussed later in this chapter.

T Lymphocytes

T cells have a variety of functions and can be divided into three functionally different subsets (Table 8.1). These include cytotoxic T cells, T helper 1 (Th1) cells that participate in inflammation, and T helper 2 (Th2) cells that provide help for antibody production. The primary role of cytotoxic T cells is to recognize foreign cells, (i.e., in skin grafts), tumors, and virus-infected cells and kill them. These cells express the surface marker CD8. Helper T cells express the surface marker CD4 and interact directly or produce soluble chemical signals called *cytokines*, which influence the activation and differentiation of other cells. *Th1 cells (T helper 1)* produce cytokines that activate cells involved in inflammation. For example, Th1 cells produce the cytokine *interferon-γ (IFN-γ)* which increases the ability of macrophages and neutrophils to kill invading pathogens. On the other hand, *Th2 cells (T helper 2)* interact with B cells to stimulate their activation and differentiation into *plasma cells* and are required for the production of antibodies.

Lymphocyte Antigen-Specific Receptors

Each B and T cell expresses an antigen-specific receptor on its surface that allows it to interact with a single epitope on an antigen. The receptor on B cells is called the *B cell receptor* (BcR). This receptor, which was discussed in the previous chapter, is made up of a membrane-bound antibody molecule which is associated with two transmembrane proteins, Igα and Igβ (Figure 8.2). The B cell receptor directly binds to epitopes expressed on antigens that can be made up of proteins, carbohydrates, lipids, as well as many organic compounds.

The antigen-specific receptor on T cells is called the *T cell receptor* (TcR) and is similar in structure to the receptor on B cells (Figure 8.2). It consists of the 40-50 kDa alpha chain which is joined to the 40-45 kDa beta chain. These two glycosylated protein chains are linked by a disulfide bond. Most T cells express alpha/beta TcR, which is highly specific for antigen. T cell receptors, however, cannot bind directly to intact antigen. They only bind to protein antigens, and these proteins must first be internalized by another cell, which digests the protein into peptides, and then presents the peptides on its cell surface. The process is known as *antigen processing and presentation* and the cells involved in this process are known as *antigen presenting cells (APC)*.

For both B and T cells, it is the unique *shape* to the binding site of the B cell receptor and the T cell receptor that creates "specificity." One question that originally bothered immunologists was how a person could produce millions of different lymphocyte receptors. We will return to this question later in the chapter

Gamma/Delta-Positive T Cells

A few T cells do not express the alpha/beta TcR, but rather express a TcR composed of a gamma and a delta chain. The α/β and the γ/δ TcR are structurally similar. T cells expressing the γ/δ TcR are found primarily along the epidermis and the lining of the small intestine. The exact function of γ/δ T cells is unclear. There is evidence that these T cells are involved in the early response to some infections that may enter the body through these surfaces. But it remains unclear if they recognize only processed protein antigens.

THE IMMUNE SYSTEM

A diagram of the major components of the immune system is shown in Figure 8.3A. Organs that provide mature lymphocytes—that is, the bone marrow and thymus—are termed *primary lymphoid organs*. Those that receive and maintain functional lymphocytes are called *secondary lymphoid organs*. Secondary lymphoid organs include lymph nodes, the spleen, Peyers patches (lymph nodes along the gut, also referred to as gut associated lymphoid tissue, or GALT), appendix, tonsils, and adenoids. Lymph nodes develop throughout the body and are concentrated in areas where pathogens are most likely to enter the body. They are especially concentrated in areas in the head around the mouth, and nose, and in the gut and limbs. The lymph nodes and spleen are connected by lymphatic channels (Figure 8.3A). The spleen, thymus, and bone marrow are connected to the rest of the immune system by the blood.

Lymphocytes within the immune system are not fixed within tissues but constantly migrate throughout the body during their lifetime in search of foreign material in a process called *lymphocyte trafficking*. Lymphocytes present in lymph nodes may leave them via the efferent lymphatics, circulate in the lymphatic vessels and lodge in other lymph nodes, or enter the blood via one of the two major lymphatic ducts (Figure 8.3A). In the blood, lymphocytes circulate through the spleen and peripheral circulation; then they ultimately enter venules from which they migrate back into the lymphatic system. Both T and B cells recirculate by this route.

Within the secondary lymphoid organs, lymphocytes are found in distinct areas such that they will be able to mount a maximal immune response. The architecture of a typical lymph node is shown in Figure 8.3B. A similar though more complex arrangement exists in the spleen. If an antigen enters the tissues, it will probably make its way into the lymphatics and enter the lymph nodes. If the antigen is in the blood, it will be "filtered-out" in the spleen. Within these organs, macrophages and

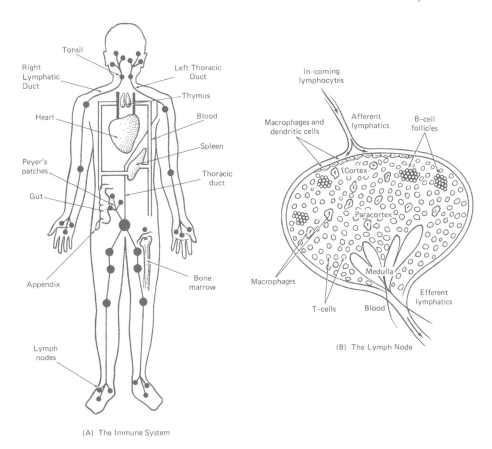

Figure 8.3.   The anatomy of the immune system: (A) The major components of the immune system of humans. The system consists of lymph nodes connected by lymph ducts; the Peyer's patches, which are masses of lymphocytes in the gut wall; the thymus, and the spleen. The other major component of the system, the bone marrow, which exists in bones throughout the body, is indicated by the drawing of a section of a femur. (B) The lymph node has a complex anatomy. Afferent lymph ducts bring lymph-containing antigens into the lymph nodes. In the outer region of the node, there are numerous macrophages and dendritic cells. Contact of antigen with these antigen-presenting cells initiates the immune response. As a result, B cell colonies (germinal centers) containing many plasma cells develop, and antibody is produced and released. The antibody leaves the node by the efferent lymphatic ducts that empty into the blood system. Lymphocytes also leave the node by the efferent duct to colonize other parts of the body.

other APC are strategically positioned so that they can capture foreign material by phagocytosis. Beneath this layer, T cells, macrophages, and dendritic cells are found in the paracortical region (Figure 8.3B). Within the *paracortex* are found discrete regions, called *follicles*, that contain B cells. Upon infection B cells divide within the follicle, the follicular region increases in diameter and may merge with an adjoining follicle. Regions containing rapidly dividing B cells are called *germinal centers*. During an infection, lymph nodes enlarge as a result of both B and T cell proliferation and increased immigration of lymphocytes into the organ. One sign of a localized immune response is an enlarged lymph node. Activated B and T cells will leave the lymph nodes and spleen, and disperse throughout the body.

DEVELOPMENT OF THE IMMUNE SYSTEM

Embryologic Development of the Lymphoid Organs and Tissues

The basic pattern of the immune system found in the adult animal is developed during embryogenesis. During the formation of the lymphoid organs, cells of endodermal and mesodermal origin form a loose matrix of connective tissue that becomes filled with developing lymphocytes. The cells in the matrix of the bone marrow and thymus not only provide structure for the organ but also provide factors required for stem cell and lymphocyte differentiation. We will first look briefly at the formation of the organs and then at the development of the cells within them.

All components of the human immune system begin formation during the first three months *in utero*. After about six weeks of development, the thymus, spleen, and bone marrow begin to form. In the formation of the thymus, endodermal and ectodermal tissue from the bronchial gill clefts grows inward, and two lobes of tissue are found on either side of the throat. These lobes migrate into the thoracic cavity, coalesce, and form a recognizable thymus by week ten. The development of the thymus is completed when the matrix becomes filled with developing lymphocytes of mesodermal origin that migrate from the yolk sac and bone marrow (described later). In bone marrow and spleen formation, mesodermal cells form a loose connective tissue network that becomes populated with developing lymphoid and stem cells.

The last portions of the immune system to form are the lymphatic channels (the lymphatic duct system) and lymph nodes. In humans, six lymphatic sacs of mesodermal tissue form. As the fetus develops, these elongate into channels. At about three months, masses of mesodermal cells form beside the channels, a connective tissue capsule forms around them, and they become vascularized. The newly developed lymph nodes sink into the channels and become populated with lymphocytes from the thymus and spleen. Lymph node development is completed within a short period of time after parturition.

During embryonic development, stem cells that give rise to lymphocytes can be identified in the yolk sac. The yolk sac is of endodermal origin (an outpocketing of the gut), but cells of mesodermal origin are thought to migrate there and develop into stem cells. In mammals, stem cells migrate from the yolk sac into the developing thymus and the fetal liver, and then from the fetal liver into the bone marrow. Following differentiation and development, lymphocytes leave the thymus as T cells and the bone marrow as B cells that migrate into the spleen. From the spleen, lymphocytes migrate to the developing lymph nodes and the blood. Immature pre-T-cells also emigrate from the bone marrow to the thymus, where they complete development. Self-renewing stem cells can be found in the bone marrow throughout the life of the animal.

Differentiation of Pluripotential Hematopoietic Stem Cells

Cells involved in both the innate and acquired immune systems, as well as platelets and erythrocytes, develop from a common stem cell, called the *pluripotential hematopoietic stem cell* (Figure 8.4). This stem cell, under the influence of many different cytokines, undergoes a complex sequence of differentiation steps during embryogenesis and throughout the life of adult animals (Figure 8.4). The exact sequence of events is uncertain, but it is known that the pluripotential hematopoietic stem cell first differentiates into a multipotential stem cell that gives rise to progenitor cells that are committed to develop into a specific cell type. Progenitor cells and their

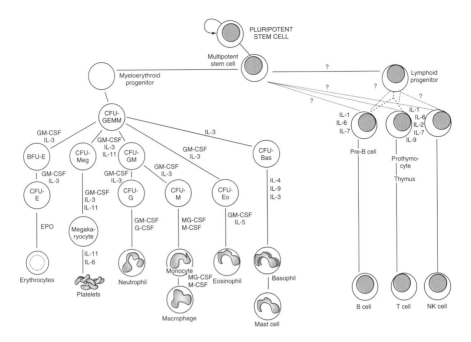

Figure 8.4. B cells and T cells as well as all other blood cells develop from the same hematopoietic stem cell. Differentiation of a stem cell into the different blood cells is mediated by the cytokine environment in the bone marrow.

progeny possess receptors for cytokines, which serve as growth and differentiation signals. Some of the cytokines known to be involved include interleukine (IL) IL-3, IL-7, and the *colony stimulating factors (CSF)*, which are produced by tissues in the bone marrow. Accordingly, these tissues have been referred to as the *hematopoietic-inducing microenvironment*. Under the influence of CSF, progenitor cells are induced to complete differentiation. Known progenitor cells include *granulocyte-macrophage-colony forming cells* (GM-CFC) that ultimately develop into macrophages and neutrophils; *eosinophil-colony forming cells* (EO-CFC) that become mature eosinophils; *megakaryocyte-colony forming cells* (MC-CFC) that become megakaryocytes and platelets; and *burst-forming unit erythrocytes* (BFU-E) that produce erythrocytes. The exact lineage that gives rise to mast cells and basophils is unclear.

The progenitor for lymphocytes has yet to be identified, but it also develops from the multipotential stem cell. It is currently unclear how B cells, T cells, and a lymphocyte-related cell—called a natural killer (NK) cell—differentiates from the stem cell. Several theories exist for the development of these cells, but a clear progression is as yet unresolved. Because mice and humans with severe combined immune deficiency (SCID) lack both B cells and T cells, it is believed that they may derive from a single progenitor (Figure 8.4). Although NK cells share many of the cell surface markers with T cells, they are likely to be of a different lineage, since the SCID defect prevents the formation of B and T cells without effecting NK cell development.

Production of Antigen-Specific Receptors

How do B and T cells produce antigen receptors that can recognize so many different antigens? This subject is treated in chapter 7 and is further developed next. The

Table 8.2. Minigene segments that make up mouse B and T cell receptors.

| | B cell receptor | | | T cell receptor | |
	heavy chain	light chains κ	λ	α chain	β chain
variable (V) segments	300-1000	300	2	100	25
diversity (D) segments	13	0	0	0 2	
joining (J) segments	4	4	3	50	12
combinations	VDJ	VJ		VJ,	VJ, VDJ, VDDJ

simplified answer is that lymphocytes possess a genetic mechanism of gene rearrangement that is not found in any other type of cell. By recombining a series of "mini-genes" or segments of DNA, they can generate millions of antigen-specific receptors. The mechanisms by which the process is realized is however not simple.

As B cells mature in the bone marrow and T cells mature in the thymus, genetic recombination takes place. B and T cells have a number of gene segments called *variable segments* (V) which code for about ninety-five amino acids; *diversity segments* (D) that code for one to fourteen amino acids; and *joining segments* (J) that code for the remainder of the variable region of the receptor (Table 8.2). There are many V, D and J genes segments that code for the heavy chain of antibody molecules and the gamma chain of the TcR. There are also numerous V and J segments that code for the light chain of antibodies and the alpha chain of the TcR. The approximate number of V,D,J segments is shown in Table 8.2.

The gene rearrangement process is similar in B and T cells. As shown in Figure 8.5, the first gene rearrangement that occurs randomly moves one D segment to join one of the J segments. This occurs first by a looping the DNA that brings the D and J regions into close proximity. Then the DNA between the D and J is cut out and the D and J segments are religated together. This process requires two enzymes called *RAG1* and *RAG2 (recombination-activating genes)*. Together RAG1 and RAG2 form a protein heterodimer which has a specific endonuclease activity. The interaction of the RAG1-RAG2 endonuclease with a *recombinational signal sequence (RSS)* catalyzes the breaking and joining of DNA needed for the DJ recombination. The intervening DNA forms a circle that is lost from the cells genome. During the cutting and splicing of the DNA, additional diversity is generated because DNA cutting and repair is not always precise. This imprecision leads to what as known as *junctional diversity*. To further increase the number of possible DNA sequences derived from the DJ rearrangement, nucleotides may be added to the ends of each newly cut DNA strand (Figure 8.5). This process is known as *N-nucleotide addition* and is mediated by the enzyme *terminal deoxynucleotidyl transferase (TdT)*. Then, the D segment is ligated directly to the J segment, but the rejoined DNA may have gaps in one or both chains of the DNA. These gaps are then filled with palindromeic nucleotides through a process called *P-nucleotide addition* (Figure 8.5). This completes the DJ recombination. The same steps occur to join a random V gene segment to the newly rearranged DJ segment.

Once the VDJ rearrangements are completed, the DNA is transcribed to produce the primary RNA transcript. Following splicing to remove the introns, the resulting VDJC mRNA is used to make one of the two receptor proteins. The other chain is produce by a similar process that requires only VJ recombination.

Although the antigen receptors for T cells and B cells are produced randomly by the combination of a limited number of DNA gene segments, they produce an ex-

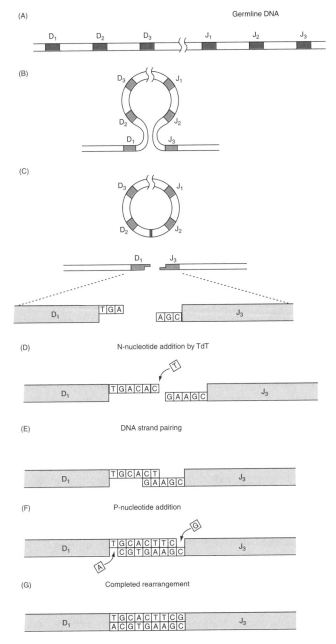

Figure 8.5. Antibody molecules and T cell receptors are formed through a process of DNA rearrangement. In this example, the D1 segment is being joined to the J3 segment. (A) The germline DNA (B) forms a loop bringing the D_1 and J_3 segments close together. (C) The DNA is cut by the RAG1-RAG2 complex. The DNA between the D_1 and J_3 segments forms a loop that is lost from the genome. The remaining DNA will be ligated connecting the D_1 segment to the J_3 segment. (D) While the D_1 and J_3 segments are being ligated random nucleotides are added to the ends of the DNA strands by terminal deoxynucleotidyl transferase (TdT), in a process known as N-nucleotide addition. (E) Pairing of the DNA strands and DNA ligation occurs. (F) The gaps in the DNA are filled with palindromic nucleotides (P-nucleotides) to complete the DNA ligation. (G) The final DNA strand has the D_1 minigene joined directly to the J_3 minigene.

tremely large number of possible antigen receptors. The *combinational diversity* produced through the random selection of V, D, and J segments, as well as junctional diversity caused by imprecise cutting of the DNA and the N and P nucleotide addition, dramatically increases the possible combinations. It is the combination of all of these random events that leads to the large number of different antigen receptors needed by the immune system to recognize all the possible pathogens to which the body is exposed.

Antigen-Independent Differentiation of B Cells

B cell development takes place in the bone marrow. As shown in Figure 8.6, the earliest B cell is called a *pro-B-cell*, and it does not yet express immunoglobulin either in the cytoplasm or on the cell surface. However, pro-B-cells do express some of the surface markers associated with B cells . Late pro-B-cells begin the process of gene rearrangement to produce the heavy chain of the IgM molecule. Once the IgM heavy chain is made, the cell becomes a *large pre-B-cell* and expresses immunoglobulin heavy chains in the cytoplasm. The heavy chain combines with a molecule known as the *surrogate light chain* that becomes expressed on the cell surface. Large pre-B-cells are able to replicate themselves in the bone marrow. This amplification step gives rise to clones that have the same heavy chain rearrangements. Once large pre-B-cells have undergone division, they become small pre-B-cells. At this stage, gene rearrangement takes place and a light chain molecule is produced that replaces the surrogate light chain. Now the B cells has a fully functional IgM molecule expressed on the surface. The expression of surface IgM is the defining event for the *immature B cell stage*. Immature B cells go through a selection process to eliminate self-reactive B cells before leaving the bone marrow. Mature B cells express all of the surface markers for B cells including IgM and IgD and are ready to interact with antigen as part of an immune response.

Antigen-Independent Differentiation of T cells

T cells, like B cells, begin their development in the bone marrow, however, they finish their development in the thymus. Cells destined to become T cells (*pro-T-cells*) leave the bone marrow and migrate through the blood to the cortex of the thymus. These cells lack many of the surface proteins normally found on mature T cells. The maturation of pro-T-cells into T cells can be followed by changes in surface protein expression (Figure 8.7). Upon arrival in the thymus, pro-T-cells begin to produce *CD2* (LFA-2) which will be expressed on the cell surface. The expression of CD2 marks the change from pro-thymocyte to *thymocyte*. The CD2+ thymocytes are often referred to as *double-negative thymocytes* because they lack both CD4 and CD8 cell surface proteins. The next change in the thymocyte occurs with the expression of the adhesion molecule CD44 and CD25. Gene rearrangement of the T cell receptor β chain begins in these cells (Figure 8.7), and the newly formed β chain is then expressed on the surface with a surrogate α chain which is known as the *pre-T cell β (pTα)*. The new β/pTα complex is found on the cell surface in association with CD3 which stabilizes the T cell receptor in the cell membrane and conducts the transmembrane signal upon T cell receptor binding. Along with the TcR/CD3 complex two other proteins, namely CD4 and CD8, appear at the cell surface. Because these thymocytes express both CD4 and CD8, they are now referred to as *double positive thymocytes*. Once the β chain is expressed, gene rearrangement for the β chain stops and gene rearrangement to produce the α chain

The **pro-B-cell** begins VDJ rearrangement of its heavy chain gene.

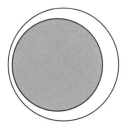

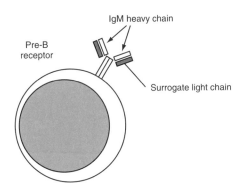

The **pre-B-cell** has completed VDJ rearrangement of the heavy chain. The IgM heavy chain is expressed on the cell surface with a surrogate light chain as a pre-B receptor.

An **immature B cell** has completed DNA rearrangement of both the light and heavy chain, and expresses the completed IgM molecule on the cell surface.

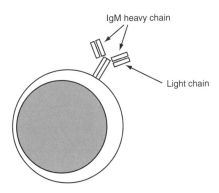

The **mature B cell** expresses both surface IgM and IgD.

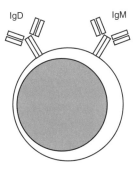

Figure 8.6.   Antigen-independent B cell development.

LIVERPOOL JOHN MOORES UNIVERSITY
LEARNING SERVICES

Pro-T-cells enter the thymus and differentiate into **thymocytes** and express the surface proteins CD2, CD44 and CD25. Thymocytes begin to undergo DNA rearrangement to produce the T cell receptor β chain.

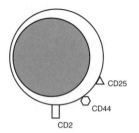

When the β chain rearrangement is complete it is paired with a surrogate α chain. This pro-T-cell receptor is expressed with CD3 on the cell surface. At this time CD44 and CD25 cease to be expressed and are replaced by CD4 and CD8 on the cell surface. These **double positive thymocytes** begin the DNA rearrangement of the α chain.

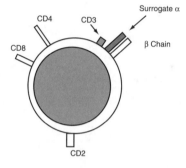

When the α chain is completed it replaces the surrogate α chain and the completed T cell receptor is expressed. This stage of the T cell undergoes positive and negative selection.

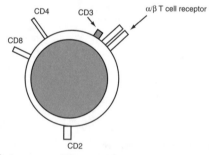

Thymocytes surviving the selection process will stop expressing either CD4$^+$ or CD8$^+$ to become **single positive thymocytes**. These single positive thymocytes leave the thymus as mature CD4$^+$ T helper cells or CD8$^+$ cytotoxic T cells.

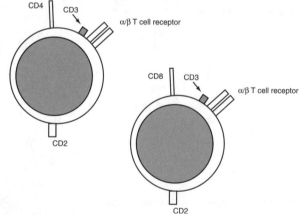

Figure 8.7. T cell development in the thymus.

begins. If the production of an α chain is successful, the resulting cell expresses the full complete α/β T cell receptor.

Because VDJ rearrangement is a random event, a large number of different TcR are formed, some of which may be able to interact with self proteins. Such anti-self-

LIVERPOOL JOHN MOORES UNIVERSITY

reactive T cells could induce an autoimmune response if they were allowed to mature and leave the thymus. Therefore, T cells with anti-self-receptors that recognize self-antigens in the thymus receive a signal that induces apoptosis (programmed cell death). This process is called *negative selection*. In addition, some of the TcR produced by random DNA recombination may not be functional in a particular individual. Therefore, a selection process takes place whereby useful TcR are *positively selected*. During positive and negative selection, the thymocytes stop producing either the CD4 or the CD8 protein to become *single positive* thymocytes. Thymocytes that survive both positive and negative selection have the ability to recognize foreign antigen expressed on self-cells. These now mature T cells express either CD4 or CD8 along with all the other T cell associated surface proteins including the T cell receptor and CD3. The mature T cells leave the thymus through the lymphatics or blood vessels and begin circulating throughout the body.

ACTIVATION OF THE IMMUNE SYSTEM BY ANTIGEN
Initiation of a Primary Inducible Immune Response
An inducible immune response may be induced whenever the body is invaded by a pathogen or a foreign substance is inadvertently introduced (i.e., through a cut or wound). Initially, cells in the noninducible (innate) immune system attempt to eliminate the foreign material. If they are successful, an inducible response does not occur. If, however, the pathogen is able to multiply rapidly, secrete toxic material, or if a large amount of foreign antigen is present, then the inducible response is needed.

Antigen Processing and Presentation
The first step in induction of an inducible immune response is the processing of antigen by antigen presenting cells (Figure 8.8). As discussed below, the major types of APC include macrophages, some types of dendritic cells, and B cells. Once an antigen is internalized by an APC, the contents of the phagocytic vesicle become acidified. This change in pH leads to the activation of proteases, which help fragment the antigen into peptides. Within the vesicle, some of the fragments become associated with Class II MHC molecules, whereas other fragments are completely degraded in the lysosomal vesicles. Following processing, endosomal vesicles return the antigenic peptide complexed to Class II molecules to the cell surface. As a result, a combination of the antigen segment bound to a Class II molecule is expressed on the antigen presenting cell surface. These processes are known as *antigen presentation*. In order for a protein fragment to be expressed, it must be of an appropriate size (thought to be eleven to twenty amino acids long) and of the correct shape, charge, and hydrophobicity to bind to the Class II molecules. Segments of antigens that can make successful interaction with Class II MHC molecules are generally termed *T cell epitopes* because they provide induction signals for T helper cells.

As you will recall from chapter 4, macrophages are able to internalize foreign antigen by phagocytosis or pinocytosis. Many cells of the macrophage lineage function as APC. These include *monocytes* in the blood, *histocytes* in the connective tissue, macrophages in the spleen, alveolar macrophages in the lungs, and *microglial cells* in the central nervous system.

The cells called Langerhan's cells are located in the skin. These are dendritic cells that arise from macrophases. Langerhan's cells are very efficient at phagocytosis and are able to process and express peptides on their surfaces. When these cells migrate to a lymph node, they differentiate into *interdigitating dendritic cells* (IDCs).

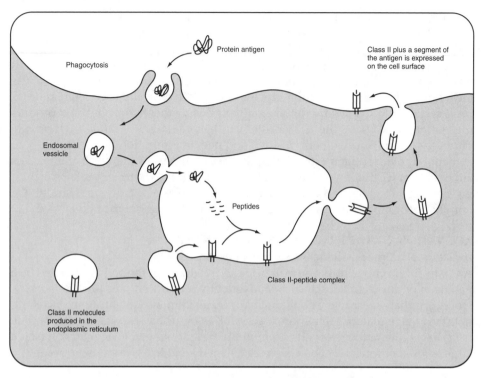

Figure 8.8. Phagocytized antigens are transported to the endosome where proteases break down the protein into peptides. Class II molecules made in the endoplasmic reticulum are transported to the endosome where they encounter and bind the peptides. The Class II-peptide complex is then transported to the cell surface where it can be recognized by CD4+ T helper cells.

Although IDCs are nonphagocytic, they express very large amounts of their previously collected antigens on their surfaces. As discussed below, the IDCs are very important in the activation of T cells during an immune response.

B cells may also function as APC. The BcR expressed on the surface allows B cells to bind antigen directly. This bound antigen is then internalized and processed in a manner similar to that of macrophages. Although B cells cannot phagocytose large particles, they are very efficient in capturing smaller soluble proteins in an antigen-specific fashion. Presenting these bound antigens to the T cells, not only activates the T cells, but also allows the activated T cell to ultimately activate the B cell to divide and produce antibodies.

Antigen processing is a key step in initiation of an inducible immune response. Many bacteria and larger particles are processed and presented by macrophages, whereas viruses invade and are presented by dendritic cells. B cells are most efficient in presenting soluble molecules, including many toxins. Thus, different APC participate in the response to different diseases-causing agents.

Interaction of Antigen-Presenting Cells (APC) and T Cells

The activation of T helper cells requires the interaction of the T cell with an APC. APC are not simply "holding" antigen to be recognized by the T cell, but are also active participants in the activation process. In order for the TcR to recognize a foreign peptide presented by the MHC Class II molecule, T cell and APC need to make direct cell to cell contact for an extended period of time. Accordingly, both the T cell and the APC have cell adhesion proteins on their surfaces that allow the cells to "stick" together for a short time. This interaction is illustrated in Figure 8.9A. If the T cell receptor does not recognize the peptide presented by the APC, the two cells disassociate. If the TcR recognizes the peptide, then the CD4 molecule binds to a site on the Class II molecule (Figure 8.9B). This interaction causes a structural change in the CD3 molecule, which transmits a signal through the membrane. This primary activation signal, or Signal #1, activates a number of biochemical pathways, including one which causes a structural change in the LFA-1 adhesion molecule. As a result, cell contact between the T cell and the APC increases, allowing the two cells to remain in contact for a longer period of time. In addition to Signal #1, the T cell needs a second signal (Signal #2) in order to undergo clonal expansion. Signal #2 is transmitted by the interaction of CD28 on the T cell with B7 on the APC (Figure 8.9C). CD28 is constitutively expressed on T cells, but B7 is not always present on APC's. To produce B7 on their surfaces and thus, to initiate an inducible immune response, APCs must respond to signals generated by carbohydrates for example, found in bacterial cell walls, cytokines such as *interferon-γ* (IFN-γ) produced by activated Th1 cells, or products of the complement cascade. The B7 molecule, so induced, provides Signal #2 for the activation of T helper cells.

After receiving Signal #1 and Signal #2, T helper cells begin to express a new protein called the *interleukin-2 receptor* (IL-2R or CD25) and then start secreting the cytokine IL-2. Secreted IL-2 binds to IL-2R on the same T cell, where it serves as a growth factor for cell proliferation (Figure 8.9D). Cytokines produced by a cell that bind to a receptor on the same cell are called *autocrine factors*. As a result of cell division, a large number of T cells all expressing the same TcR are produced. Some of the resulting daughter cells will secrete cytokines that activate other cells that participate in the immune response. The specific roles of these effector T cell are discussed below.

T Helper Cells Differentiate into either Th1 or Th2 Cells

Naive CD4+ T cells are referred to as Th0 cells. Based on the differentiation signals they receive, Th0 T helper cells will differentiate into either T helper 1 (Th1) or T helper 2 (Th2). A number of factors influence whether the cell becomes a Th1 or Th2 cell. For example, low quantities of soluble antigen tend to stimulate the production of Th2 cells, whereas large amounts of insoluble particulate antigen induce production of Th1 cells. In addition, APC have an effect on differentiation of Th0 cells. Antigens presented by macrophages tend to cause Th0 to differentiate into Th1 cells, whereas when presented by B cells, antigens tend to induce Th2 cells. As discussed below, cytokines also influence Th1/Th2 production. T helper 1 and 2 cells are referred to as *effector cells* because they have the ability to secrete cytokines that activate other cell types.

Th1 cells are defined by their production of the cytokine, interferon-γ (IFN-γ). They also produce GM-CSF, *tumor necrosis factor-α* (TNF-α), IL-2, and IL-3. IFN-γ activates macrophages, resulting in expression of B7, increased amounts of adhesion molecules, and of MHC Class II molecules. Therefore, activated macrophages become efficient APC. They also have an enhanced ability to kill pathogens either by phagocytosis or by the release of toxic products. IFN-α also suppresses differentiation of Th0 cells into Th2 cells. Differentiation of Th0 cells into Th1 cells results in the establishment of a predominantly cell-mediated immune response.

Th2 cells are primarily involved in the activation of B cells. They not only direct B cell growth and differentiation, but also are required for the production of anti-

148 • M.A. Hickey and D.W. Taylor

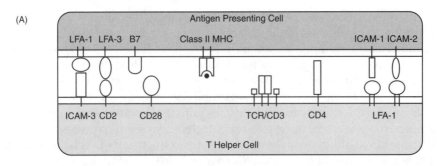

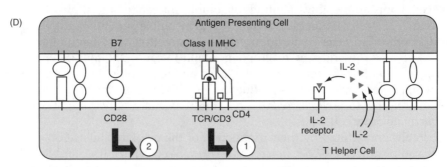

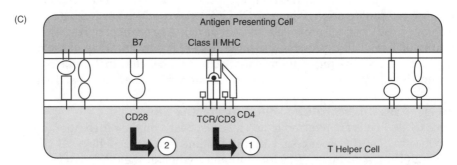

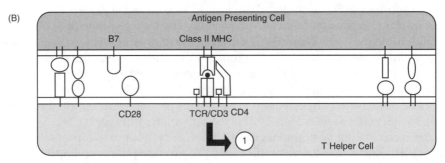

Figure 8.9. Activation of T cells involves intimate contact between an antigen presenting cell and the T cell. (A) Interaction between the APC and the T cells begins with the binding of cell adhesion proteins. (B) If the T cell receptor is able to recognize the antigen presented by the Class II molecule, then binding occurs. CD4 strengthens the Class II MHC-T cell receptor interaction by binding to the Class II molecule. This interaction gives the T cell its first activation signal. (C) Signal #2 is mediated by the binding of the antigen presenting cells B7 molecule with the CD28 on the T cell. These two signals activate the T cell. (D) The T cell will produce an IL-2 receptor which is expressed on the T cell surface. Then the cell secretes IL-2. Binding of the autocrine IL-2 to the IL-2 receptor causes the T cell to proliferate.

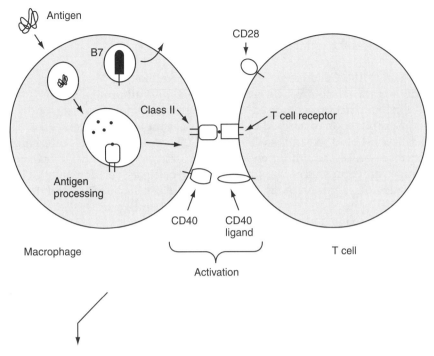

Activated Macrophage
1) Increased quantities of adhesion molecules.
2) Increased quantities of Class II MHC.
3) B7 expression.
4) Enhanced phagocytosis.
5) Release of reactive oxygen intermediates.

Figure 8.10.   Resting macrophages can be activated by activated T cells which express the surface protein CD40L. While the T cell receptor is bound to the Class II-peptide complex the CD40L can bind to CD40 on the macrophage. The interaction of CD40 with CD40L causes the activation of the macrophage.

body secreting plasma cells. Th2 cells are defined by their ability to secrete *interleukin-4* (IL-4) and *interleukin-10* (IL-10). They also produce other cytokines such as *interleukin-5* (IL-5) and *transforming growth factor-β* (TGF-β). IL-4 and IL-10 suppress Th0 differentiation into Th1 cells, thereby shifting the immune response toward the production of Th2 cells and ultimately induction of humoral immunity.

Once Th1 and Th2 cells have become activated and undergone clonal expansion, they begin to express a molecule known as the CD40 ligand (CD40L) on their surface. The presence of the CD40L on activated T helper cells is required for the activation of macrophages and B cells.

Interaction of T Helper Cells and Macrophages
As noted above, macrophages can be activated by contact with cytokine, bacterial compounds, and components of the complement cascade. They can also be activated by direct contact with activated T helper cells. In this interaction, the CD40L on the activated T helper cell binds to CD40 which is constitutively expressed on monocytes and macrophages (Figure 8.10). This interaction, plus a second signal activates macrophages. As noted above, activated macrophages are more efficient

in killing both intracellular pathogens (e.g., the bacteria that cause tuberculosis and leprosy) and extracellar bacteria than are resting macrophages. Thus, the Th1 cell greatly enhances the cellular immune response.

Interaction of Th2 Cells and B Cells to Produce Antibodies

In order for a B cell to produce antibodies to almost all protein antigens, a direct B cell:T cell interaction is required. Such antigens are known as T-dependent antigens. The production of antibodies by B cells is a multistep process. First, the BcR on B cells must bind the antigen (Figure 8.11). Then, the antigen is internalized by endocytosis, processed within endosomal vessels, and the peptide fragments of the antigen are expressed on the surface of the B cell in association with MHC Class II molecules. Once this happens, the TcR on the Th2 cells interacts with this newly created T cell epitope and makes direct contact with the B cell. This combined interaction provides Signal #1 to the B cell.

Like T cells, B cells require two signals in order to become activated. Signal #2 is the combination of CD40, which is naturally expressed on B cells, with the CD40L, which is only expressed on activated T helper cells. Together, Signal #1 and Signal #2 activate B cells and allow them to receive growth and differentiation signals provided by soluble cytokines. Factors that are important in B cell clonal expansion include IL-4, IL-5, and IL-6, which are secreted by Th2 cells. Thus following activation, B cells divide and produce a large number of daughter cells. Some of these daughters will differentiate into plasma cells and secrete IgM antibodies. Some may become memory B cells. A few daughter cells, however, will migrate into B cell follicles in lymph nodes or the spleen (Figure 8.2B). There they continue to divide and the follicle increases in size to create a germinal center. Within the germinal centers, B cells receive additional signals from Th2 cells. Some of the B cells are induced to undergo isotype-switching and start secreting IgG, IgA, or IgE antibodies. While in the germinal centers, B cells also receive signals that induce the region of their DNA that codes for the variable region of the BcR to undergo somatic hypermutation. As a result, B cells are able to secrete antibodies with slightly higher or lower affinity for the antigen. Within the germinal centers, B cells with higher affinity BcR are selected for. Thus, with time, the overall affinity of the antibodies produced increases as the infection progresses (see Figure 7.10). Th2 cells are thought to play an important role in induction of both isotype-switching and somatic hypermutation.

Activation of Cytotoxic T Cells

Cytotoxic T cells are able to recognize and directly kill cancerous and virus-infected cells. Since cytotoxic T cells have the ability to kill, their function must be highly regulated so that they kill only "the bad" cells and not normal, healthy neighboring cells. Cytotoxic T cells do not interact directly with viruses, rather they only kill cells that are infected with virus. Since viruses live in the cytoplasm of the cell, viruses cannot be detected by cytotoxic T cells unless some of the viral proteins are transported to the cell surface. Likewise, tumor cells often produce abnormal self-proteins, and these too must be presented on the cell surface to be recognized. Host cells have the ability to process intracellular proteins, including tumor and viral antigens, into peptides that are then presented on the cell surface in association with Class I molecules (Figure 8.12). As a result, intracellular viruses "blow their cover," and infected cells can be killed by cytotoxic T cells.

All nucleated cells in the body have the ability to process intercellular proteins

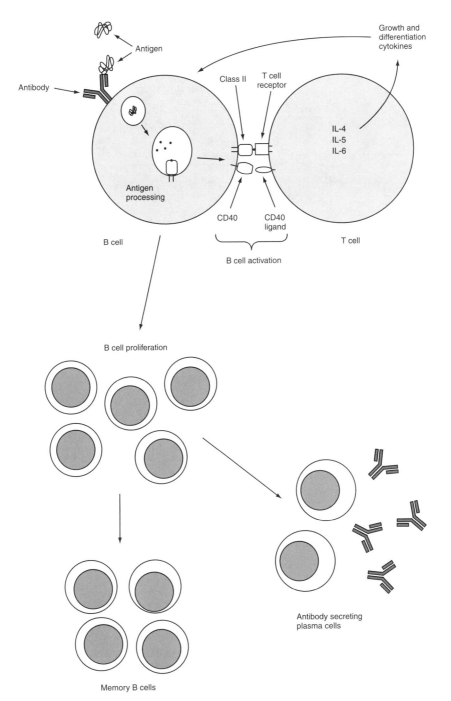

Figure 8.11.   B cells internalize antigen bound by the surface immunoglobulin receptor. The antigen is then processed and presented on a Class II molecule. The recognition of the Class II molecule by the T helper cell allows the T cells CD40L to bind the CD40 on the B cell. The CD40-CD40L interaction activates the B cell. Once the B cell is activated, cytokines which are released by the T helper cell act as growth and differentiation factors for the B cell. The B cell will then undergo proliferation and produce many daughter cells. Some of these daughter cells return to the resting stage and become memory cells. Others differentiate into antibody secreting plasma cells.

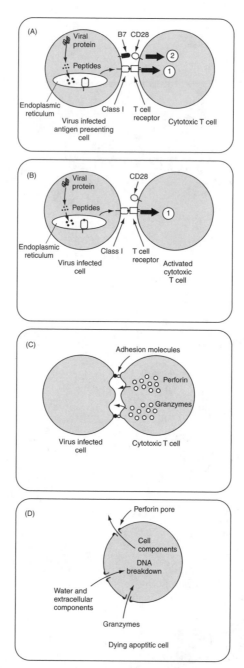

Figure 8.12. (A) Viral proteins produced in the cytoplasm are broken down into peptides. These are transported into the endoplasmic reticulum to be bound by the Class I molecules, and then they are transported to the cell surface. Cytotoxic T cells need two activation signals. These are the interaction of the T cell receptor with the Class I molecule and the interaction of B7 on an antigen presenting cell with CD28 on the T cell. (B) Once the cytotoxic T cell is activated, only T cell receptor-Class I interaction is required for the release of the cytotoxic compounds (C). (D) Perforin released by the T cell inserts into the membrane and polymerizes to produce a pore in the cell membrane. This allows cellular components to leak out of the cell and lets water leak into the cell. Granzymes, also released by the T cell, enter the cell through the perforin pores and mediate DNA breakdown and apoptosis.

into peptides and present them on the cell surface (Figure 8.12). That is, specialized APC are required to process extracellular pathogens (i.e., pathogens that live outside of cells), whereas, intracellular viruses, parasites, and proteins in abnormal tumor cells can be directly processed and presented by the infected cell. In this process, a small amount of protein present in the cytoplasm of the cell is broken down into peptides by a complex of enzymes known as the *proteosome*. Then, a combination of two proteins, *TAP1 and TAP2*, transport the peptides made by the proteosome from the cytoplasm into the endoplasmic reticulum. The Class I molecule is made up of two proteins, the Class I protein and an accessory molecule called β-2 *microglobulin*. The Class I molecule and the β-2 microglobulin are made in the endoplasmic reticulum and are able to capture the peptide. This trimolecular complex is then transported from the endoplasmic reticulum to the Golgi and finally to the cell surface.

Cytotoxic T cells have the same requirement for activation as T helper cells. Signal #1 is provided by the binding of the T cell receptor to the Class I molecule containing the foreign peptide followed by Signal #2, which is produced by the binding of B7 to the T cells CD28. B7 is found only on activated macrophages, activated B cells, and dendritic cells (Figure 8.12). Thus, one of these B7-bearing cells must be involved in the initial activation of cytotoxic T cells. This process usually takes place in a lymph node or in the spleen. Once the cytotoxic T cell is activated, it undergoes clonal expansion and develops into an *armed effector cell*. Effector cytotoxic T cells are then armed for killing infected cells or tumor cells, and circulate through the body in search of abnormal cells.

If they find them, i.e, if the TcR on the cytotoxic T cell binds specifically to the peptide being presented by the Class I molecule, they are able to directly kill the cell. Cytotoxic T cells kill their target cell by making direct membrane to membrane contact with them (Figure 8.12). Then, within the zone of contact, they release molecules called *perforin* which polymerize to form a hollow ring or pore in the membrane of the target cell. The cytotoxic T cells then release several serine proteases, called *granzymes*, directly into the abnormal cell. These proteases break down the DNA in the cell, which causes the cell to die through a process called *apoptosis*. The DNA in the nucleus is broken down and the cell eventually breaks up into vesicles which are phagocytosed by macrophages. Thus, virus-infected cells are killed before the viruses can complete their replication and tumor cells are killed before they divide. Because cytotoxic T cells make direct, intimate contact with the target cells and directly release perforin and granzymes into them, only abnormal cells and not innocent by standard cells are killed.

Cytotoxic T cells also produce interferon-γ, a powerful activator of macrophages, which heightens the immune response by providing more activated B7-bearing APC as well as by increasing the ability of the macrophages to eliminate apoptotic cells.

SUMMARY

The inducible immune response plays a critical role in protecting the body from viruses, bacteria, parasites, and toxic substances. Once a foreign substance enters the body and reaches high enough levels, an inducible immune response begins. The initial response requires antigen-presenting cells and T cells. Pathogens that enter through the skin will come in contact with the interstitial fluid and drain into a nearby lymph node. If the pathogen or foreign substance is in the blood, it will enter the spleen. As shown in Figure 8.3B, the outer regions of these secondary lymphoid organs contain a large number of macrophages, dendritic cells, and some B cells which serve as APC. Here, bacteria and parasites can be phagocytosed by macrophages, viruses may infect dendritic cells, and soluble molecules may be internalized by B cells. Some foreign proteins will be processed into peptides within endosomes and presented on their cell surfaces by Class II molecules. Now Th0 cells with appropriate TcRs can recognize the antigen, undergo clonal expansion, and differentiate into either Th1 or Th2 helper T cells. The overall dynamics of the infection, including amount of antigen, type of antigen-presenting cell, and cytokine environment, help determine if a Th1 or Th2 cell response is produced. If Th1 T cells are produced in the lymph node or spleen, they migrate to the place in the body where the pathogen is located, e.g., the skin, and mediate their effector function. As shown in Figure 8.10, T helper cells make direct contact with macrophages and secrete cytokines such as IFN-γ, that activate macrophages. Activated macrophages develop an increased efficiency in antigen presentation and are able to release cytotoxic factors, such as reactive oxygen intermediates and nitric oxide, which leads to killing of the pathogen. Thus, Th1 cells enhance general inflammatory responses which are mediated by macrophages, neutrophils and other cell types.

On the other hand, if Th2 cells are produced, they remain in the lymph node or spleen and interact with B cells. As shown in Figure 8.11, Th2-cell provides activation signals and cytokines that induce B cells to develop into antibody-producing plasma cells. Antibodies circulate in the blood and lymphatic fluid in search of antigen. When antibodies bind to microorganisms, they induce several effector functions. Antibodies may agglutinate the pathogens and prevent them from spreading, or block key receptors preventing their entry into host cells. Antibodies can also activate the complement cascade, which lyses the organism. The coating of the microbe makes it easier for macrophages and other phagocytic cells to destroy the microbe. If the pathogen is a virus or a foreign cell (e.g., tissue graft), cytotoxic T cells will be activated to become armed effector cells which kill the cells infected with the virus or the foreign cells. The inducible immune response may continue to develop and function in a highly coordinated fashion until the pathogen is eliminated.

As a result of the primary inducible immune response, a large number of memory lymphocytes, including Th1, Th2, cytotoxic and B cells, are produced. These cells are now responsible for recognizing and responding to the pathogen should the host become reinfected. Thus, the inducible immune response plays a major role both in dealing with microorganisms and preventing infectious diseases.

SUGGESTION FOR FURTHER READING

1. Janeway, C.A. Jr., P. Travers, M. Walport, and J.D. Capra *Immunobiology: The Immune System in Health and Disease*. CB Current Biology Publications. New York: Garland Publishing, 1999.
2. Kuby, J. *Immunology*. 3d ed. New York: W.H. Freeman and Company, 1997.
3. Lai, L., N. Alaverdi, L. Maltias, and H.C. Morse 3rd. "Mouse Cell Surface Antigens: Nomenclature and Immunophenotyping." *Journal of Immunology* 160, no. 8 (April 15, 1998):3861–3868.
4. Berke, G. "Killing Mechanisms of Cytotoxic Lymphocytes." *Current Opinion in Hematology* 4, no. 1 (Jan 1997):32–40.
5. "Clinical Use of B- and T-Cell Gene Rearrangement Analysis in Hematopoietic Disorders." *Clinics in Laboratory Medicine* 16, no. 1 (March 1996):1–21.
6. Haynes, B.F., and L.P. Hale. "The Human Thymus. A Chimeric Organ Comprised of Central and Peripheral Lymphoid Components." *Immunologic Research* 18, no. 3 (1998):175–192.

7. Dudler, J., and A.K. So. "T Cells and Related Cytokines." *Current Opinion in Rheumatology* 10, no. 3 (May 1998):207–211.
8. Lappin, M.B., I. Kimber, and M. Norval. "The Role of Dendritic Cells in Cutaneous Immunity." *Archives in Dermatological Research* 288, no. 3 (March 1996):109–121.

QUESTIONS

1 Since both B and T cells are morphologically identical by light and electron microscopy, how do immunologists tell them apart?

2 In what discrete region of the lymph node do B cells primarily reside? In what region of the lymph node do rapidly dividing B cells reside?

3 If all the cells of the blood are derived from the pluripotential hematopoietic stem cell what causes some stem cells to become B cells and others to become macrophages?

4 How does the enzyme terminal deoxynucleotidyl transferase (TdT) contribute to the diversity of the B and T cell receptors?

5 From a limited number of DNA gene segments, an extremely large number of possible antigen receptors exist for both T and B cell receptors. What processes contribute to this great abundance of possible receptors?

6 T cells need two transmembrane signals in order to become activated. Where do these signals come from?

7 Cytotoxic T cells require two signals (the first resulting from TcR interaction with a Class I + peptide and the second from CD28 interaction with B7) for activation. Since *non*-APC do not express B7, how do they kill virus- infected cells that are not APC?

8 When a cytotoxic T cell binds to and recognizes a virus-infected cell, what mechanism does it use to kill the virus-infected cell?

9 The Th0 cell becomes either a Th1 or a Th2 cell. What factors determine the outcome of Th0 differentiation?

10 T helper cells recognize antigens presented by the Class II MHC molecule and cytotoxic T cells recognize antigens presented by Class I antigens. How are the antigens presented by Class I and Class II molecules different?

ANSWERS

1 B cells and T cells have different proteins on their surfaces. For example, B cells have surface Ig molecules which are not found on T cells and T cells have the T cell receptor which is not found on the B cell.

2 B cells group together along the paracortex of the lymph node in follicles. When the B cells respond to antigen and begin to divide rapidly the follicles become germinal centers.

3 Cytokines within the bone marrow regulate the differentiation of the pluripotential hematopoietic stem cell. Interleukines such as IL-3 and IL-7 and colony stimulating factors together regulate stem cell development.

4 TdT adds random nucleotides to the ends of the V, D, and J DNA segments during gene rearrangement. This adds small fragments of DNA between each minigene; DNA that was not encoded by the genome.

5 Combinational diversity is caused by the random selection of V, D, and J segments. Imprecise cutting of the DNA leads to junctional diversity. Finally, the addition of N and P nucleotides dramatically increases the number of possible receptors.

6 Signal one is produced by CD3 when the TcR binds to the peptide -MHC Class II

complex. The second signal is the binding of B7 on the antigen presenting cell to the T cells CD28 protein. To induce a cytotoxic T cell, viruses must infect a cell type that is capable of expressing B7. The inducing cells, the interstitual dendridic cells (IDC) are highly susceptible to viral infections, are located in strategic locations in the lymph node and express large amounts of Class I + viral peptide as well as B7. The cytotoxic T cells become activated by recognizing the viral peptides expressed by the Class I MHC on these cells. Once activated the cytotoxic T cell becomes an effector cell and circulates through the body. As an effector cell, it only needs the TcR binding to the Class I molecule-peptide complex to initiate killing.

7 The cytotoxic T cell makes direct contact with the virus-infected cells, the members of the two cells make a junction, and the cytotoxic T cells release perforin and granzymes onto the infected cell.

8 A number of factors influence the differentiation of Th0 into Th1 or Th2 cells including the nature of the pathogen, the amount of antigen, its type of antigen-presenting cell, and the initial types of cytokines produced.

9 Antigens found *outside* of cells, are internalized by antigen-presenting cells by phagocytosis or receptor-mediated endocytosis, enzymatically degraded into peptides within endosomes, and then returned to the cell surface where they are presented by Class II molecules. Antigens produced *inside* of cells (for example viral antigens) are enzymatically digested into peptides in the cytoplasm, transported into the endoplasmic reticulum by TAP-1 and TAP-2 where they bind to Class I molecules, and then they are presented on the surface of the cell.

CHAPTER 9

INTRODUCTION
ANTIBODY-MEDIATED
   EFFECTOR MECHANISMS
   Antibody-Mediated
      Phagocytosis
   Inactivation of Toxins by
      Antibody
   Prevention of Microbe
      Attachment to Host Cells
   Bacteriolysis
   Agglutination
COMPLEMENT-MEDIATED
   EFFECTOR MECHANISMS
   Introduction
   Antibody-Dependent
      Activation of
      Complement: The
      Classical Complement
      Pathway
   The Alternative Pathway of
      Complement Activation
   Biological Activities of
      Complement
      Components
   Regulation of Complement
      Activity
CELL-MEDIATED EFFECTOR
   MECHANISMS
   Introduction
   Macrophage Activation and
      the Elimination of Intra-
      cellular Parasites
   Delayed-Type Hyper-
      sensitivity
   Macrophage Activation and
      Microbiocidal Activity
   Tumoricidal Activity
   Natural Killer Cells
   Antibody-Dependent Cell
      Cytotoxicity (ADCC)
   Cytolytic T Lymphocytes
   The Biological Significance
      of MHC Restriction of
      CTLs
SUMMARY
SUGGESTIONS FOR
   FURTHER READING
QUESTIONS
ANSWERS

Specific Host Restance: The Effector Mechanisms

Ralph A. Sorensen

INTRODUCTION

In the complex interplay of host and parasite, the induction of immunity to specific nonself antigens is a favorable outcome for the host. Inducible immunity against an infectious agent persists after recovery from an infection because of changes in the lymphocyte (both B and T) populations brought about by contact with these antigens. These changes not only aid in the control of the primary infection but also permit the rapid mobilization of a secondary immune response for the elimination of the pathogens or other noxious agents on subsequent exposure.

The secretion of antibody and the binding of a T cell receptor to a processed antigen are necessary but not sufficient to destroy the invading organism. A variety of *effector mechanisms* has evolved to accomplish this task after specific recognition of the foreign antigen has occurred.

The many effector mechanisms of specific immunity arose during evolution in response to the complex mechanisms that pathogens developed to colonize their hosts, just as the efficiency of these invasive mechanisms evolved in response to the host's immune effector mechanisms. Selective pressures come to bear on both the host and the parasite. If the host on which parasites feed is consumed rapidly in the process, neither the host nor the parasite have much opportunity to pass on their genes to their heirs. It is usually better for both if the parasite works out a living arrangement that does not destroy its home. The host must keep the parasite in check to preserve its own life, and the microbe does its best to counter the defenses thrown at it by the threatened host. Around and around it goes, a virtual arms race until an uneasy truce is reached.

157

We call the defenses of the host which enforce this truce the immune system. We call violations of the truce infectious disease.

Most of the effector mechanisms to be described arose from simpler constitutive mechanisms used by organisms without inducible immunity. Phagocytosis is one example of such a mechanism. An existing mechanism that is utilized in a newly developed system is called a *preadaptation*. These preexisting defense mechanisms were integrated into the inducible system when it evolved and, in the process, their efficacy was increased dramatically. These effector mechanisms are, therefore, part of both the constitutive and inducible host defense systems

Microbial pathogens have many molecular components of which the proteins and polysaccharides are particularly immunogenic. Of all the immune reactions specific for parasite proteins and polysaccharides that develop during infection, those which are specific for *virulence factors* are most vital for protection of the host. Virulence factors can be as diverse as a secreted toxin, a polysaccharide capsule that prevents phagocytosis, or a receptor on a microorganism that mediates its attachment to a host cell. Humoral and cell-mediated immunity are both generated in response to all infections; however, the magnitude of each and their relative importance in the immune protection developed in any particular infection varies with the nature of the infection and the types of virulence factors present.

In this chapter we will describe several of the specific immune effector mechanisms that are responsible for host defense against infection with pathogenic bacteria, viruses, protozoa, and worms. Effector mechanisms mediated directly by antibody will be described first, followed by effector mechanisms mediated by antibody indirectly through the activation of the complement and phagocytic systems. The specific cell-mediated immune responses will be described subsequently. The number and variety of these mechanisms speak both to the complexity of infectious processes and to the plasticity of host responses. Mutation and gene recombination provide the variability upon which natural selection works to yield the remarkable world we see around us of which the immune system is but a small part.

ANTIBODY-MEDIATED EFFECTOR MECHANISMS
Antibody-Mediated Phagocytosis

The binding of an antibody molecule to a parasite, in and of itself, does little damage to the parasite. Clumping may inhibit dispersal and bound antibody may block receptors important in the entry into host cells, but, perhaps more importantly, bound antibody can prepare the parasite for destruction by ingestion by several types of phagocytic cells. This process of preparing the parasite for ingestion is called *opsonization*. The word *opsonin* is from the Greek for "to prepare to eat." Antibody of the IgG class is the most efficient opsonin of all the opsonic antibodies. There are numerous receptors for the Fc portion of IgG on all phagocytic cells. The two most important types of phagocytic cells are neutrophils and macrophages, with the latter possessing three different classes of Fc receptors, one of which has a very high affinity for IgG. These Fc receptors help the phagocyte bind to the antibody-coated parasite much more tightly. The receptors for the Fc portion of antibody and the receptors for complement products (such as $\overline{C3b}$) function similarly on macrophages and neutrophils.

The binding of antibody-coated microbes to phagocytes by the Fc receptors generates an intracellular signal which activates the phagocytes. To be fully-activated, macrophages require an additional costimulatory signal from interferon-γ (IFN-γ) and, once activated, are known as activated or *angry macrophages*. Activated phagocytes increase the energy-dependent movement of their membranes causing them to engulf the bound particle. When the process is complete, the particle is encased within an endocytic vesicle, the *phagosome*. Lysosomes, membrane bound organelles filled with hydrolytic enzymes, merge with the phagosome to form a *secondary lysosome* or *phagolysosome*. Proton pumps acidify the phagolysosome and more than forty different acid hydrolases attack all of the different macromolecules that comprise the microbe. The monomers resulting from this digestion of the microbe then diffuse through the phagolysosome membrane into the cytoplasm of the host cell.

In the case of parasites that are too large to be taken up by phagocytosis, worms for example, the phagocytes, after attaching to the worm, may secrete the contents of their lysosomes into the space between the worm and the attached macrophage, thus destroying the parasite without ingesting it. In the case of a worm infestation, eosinophils are more likely to assume the defensive role. For this reason, when an elevated eosinophil count is detected in a differential white cell count of a sick individual, a worm infection is suspected.

Killing of the pathogen in the phagolysosome is assisted by the oxygen-dependent release of several toxic substances, including hydrogen peroxide (H_2O_2) and superoxide anion (O_2^-). This accounts for the sudden increase in oxygen consumption associated with phagocyte activation, the well-studied but misnamed "respiratory burst." Since H_2O_2 and O_2^- are toxic to the host's tissues as well as those of the parasite, enzymes such as superoxide dismutase (which converts O_2^- to H_2O_2) and catalase (which converts H_2O_2 to water) are also released into the cytoplasm of the macrophage and into the intercellular spaces in order to limit potential damage to the host.

The efficiency of antibody-mediated phagocytosis is much greater than the efficiency of clearance by constitutive mechanisms. Antibody-mediated clearance is enhanced further if $\overline{C3b}$ is also deposited on the surface of the parasite since $\overline{C3b}$ receptors as well as Fc receptors are then involved in attachment. The rapid clearance by phagocytosis brought about by the inducible response is often the difference between life and death in a host infected with a rapidly reproducing microbe.

Antibodies important in the protection of the host are usually directed against external structures on the microbes. Such antibodies may be specific for polysaccharide microbial capsules, the lipoteichoic acids of Gram-positive bacterial cell walls, or bacterial fimbriae. The IgG antibody response to the M protein-lipoteichoic acid complex on the surfaces of group A beta hemolytic streptococci has been extensively studied. Antibody of this specificity inhibits the streptococcus from binding the host's fibrinogen. A fibrinogen coat can prevent phagocytosis by veiling the parasite in a covering of host material. The serum titer of anti-M protein antibody correlates well with resistance to infection by these bacteria.

Another antibody response to a surface component of a microbe that has been well studied is that to the capsule of pneumococcus. The uptake of pneumococci only occurs in the presence of antibody to the microbe's capsule. In its absence the microbes are not phagocytized and reproduce unimpeded. As a result the host may die of severe pneumonia. This system, by the way, was historically important as it led Avery, McLeod, and McCarty in 1945 to discover that the material capable of transforming a bacterium into one capable of making this capsule was DNA. This was the first identification of DNA as the genetic material in bacteria.

Inactivation of Toxins by Antibody

Microbial toxins are of two types, *exotoxins* and *endotoxins*. As their names suggest, exotoxins are secreted by the microbe, and endotoxins are not secreted but, instead, are released when the microbe dies. They differ in chemical nature, as well, and the host deals with them in distinct ways. Exotoxins are proteins secreted by only a few of the many bacterial pathogens, but they may be extremely potent virulence factors for the microbes that secrete them. Some exotoxins produce disease when they are ingested with food or water. In such cases there may be no microbial infection or growth in the poisoned individual. Botulism and staphylococcal food poisoning are examples of such exotoxin poisoning. Production of food poisoning in the absence of infection is clearly of no use to the microbe. It is possible that such toxins perform functions important to the microbe which are still unknown and it is only chance that makes them toxic.

The roles of many exotoxins in the pathogenesis of disease are clear. The toxins secreted by the clostridia causing gas gangrene, for example, kill the host's tissue, thus making food available for the infecting bacterium. Many toxins secreted by streptococci and staphylococci kill or impair the functions of leukocytes, thereby preventing phagocytosis of the microbes. Coagulase causes deposition of fibrin on the staphylococci that produce it, providing an antigenic disguise for the microbe. Regardless of the function of the toxin in the microbe's ecology, its inactivation is clearly important to the host.

Exotoxins are very immunogenic. Inactivation is a result of the binding of induced antibody to sites on the molecule that are responsible for the toxic effects. In most cases antibody can block intoxication if it is available before the toxin binds to its target, but it cannot reverse damage already done. This is the case with tetanus antitoxin. It must be given prophylactically and is of little use for treatment after infection. If antitoxin is given, it is given just after injury before infection can develop. Prophylactic immunization with *toxoid*, a detoxified but still immunogenic toxin, permits a rapid secondary antibody response by the host after infection. This antibody neutralizes the toxin, thus blocking intoxication.

The toxin-antibody complexes formed are removed by the macrophages and neutrophils (Figure 9.1). Because the bound Fc receptors and the precipitated immune complexes are a much larger target than the toxin molecules themselves, phagocytosis of the exotoxin and destruction by lysosomal enzymes in the immune individual is very efficient. In the absence of antitoxin, the phagocytic cells may be destroyed by the action of the exotoxins.

Antibodies formed in response to immunization with a toxoid are important in the development of immunity to diseases caused by a variety of exotoxin producing microbes. Some examples of such diseases are gas gangrene caused by *Clostridium perfringens*, diphtheria caused by *Corynebacterium diphtheriae*, tetanus caused by *Clostridium tetanus*, and botulism caused by *Clostridium botulinum*.

Endotoxins are lipopolysaccharides that are a part of the cell walls of Gram-negative enterobacteria. They are not secreted but are released when the bacteria die and disintegrate. Endotoxin does induce antibody production, but the antibodies are not specific for the endotoxin. This is because lipopolysaccharide is capable of inducing the expansion of numerous B cell clones without acting through the surface immunoglobulins and without calling upon antigen-specific helper T cells. LPS thus acts as a T cell independent antigen. It is as if lipopolysaccharide is the calling card of the enterobacteria and the response of the host to its presence is rapid and severe. A severe inflammatory response induced by endotoxin can lead to anaphylactic shock and the death of the host. Endotoxin is also an efficient acti-

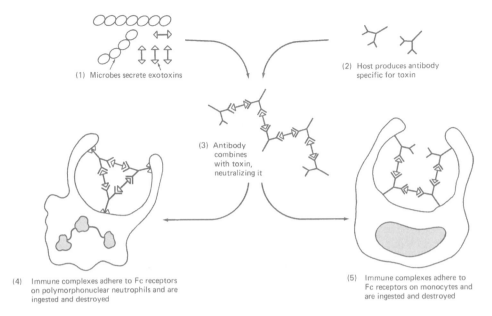

(1) Microbes secrete exotoxins

(2) Host produces antibody
specific for toxin

(3) Antibody
combines
with toxin,
neutralizing it

(4) Immune complexes adhere to Fc receptors
on polymorphonuclear neutrophils and are
ingested and destroyed

(5) Immune complexes adhere to
Fc receptors on monocytes and
are ingested and destroyed

Figure 9.1.   Microbial exotoxins (1) are rendered innocuous through neutralization by specific
IgG antitoxins (2). After combination with antibody, the immune complexes (3) are ingested and
degraded by phagocytic cells of the polymorphonuclear (neutrophilic) (4) and monocytic (5) classes.

vator of complement through the alternative complement pathway. It is primarily
the complement system that protects the host from the effects of endotoxin. When
complement is activated through binding to endotoxin it induces phagocytosis of
the endotoxin through C3b receptors. The phagocytes then reduce the ingested
endotoxin to nontoxic fragments.

Prevention of Microbes Attachment to Host Cells

Intracellular parasites, such as viruses, some bacteria, and some protozoa enter
their host cells through attachment to specific receptors on the host cell surface.
The attachment of antibody by itself does not kill the parasite. Instead, antibodies
of the IgG, IgM, and secretory IgA classes directed against the surface molecules of
an intracellular parasite may prevent attachment to and infection of the host cell.
The IgG antiviral antibody in the blood, for example, is responsible for the lifelong
immunity to polio. The polio virus normally infects intestinal lining cells where it
causes little damage. When, however, the virus binds to and infects neurological
cells of the host it causes paralysis. The antibodies produced upon immunization
specifically block this binding.

Many bacteria use fimbriae, short hairlike projections, to adhere to mucosal surfaces of the respiratory tract, the urogenital tract, and gut. Secretory or dimeric IgA
directed against fimbrial antigens can inhibit the colonization of mucosal surfaces
in these areas. For example, antibody to capsules and fimbriae of pseudomonads
inhibits infection of the trachea and lungs. Antibody to some intracellular protozoan parasites can prevent their attachment and entry into their host cells. To some
degree antibody-mediated inhibition of attachment to the red blood cell of the protozoan that causes malaria contributes to antimalarial immunity.

Table 9.1. List of the antimicrobial actions of antibodies.

1. Opsonization for phagocytosis
2. Inducing complement activation and enhancing phagocytosis
3. Prevention of attachment to host cells
4. Prevention of penetration of host cells
5. Neutralization of toxins
6. Inhibition of motility of parasites
7. Agglutination of parasites
8. Inhibition of microbial growth and metabolism

Bacteriolysis

Antibody alone does not bring about the osmotic lysis of bacteria. When antibody binds to the surfaces of parasites, however, the immune complexes that are formed will bind and activate complement. It is the products released by the activated complement that lyse the bacteria. Gram-negative bacilli are particularly susceptible to complement-mediated lysis. Antibodies of the IgA, IgM, and IgG classes activate complement. In addition to blocking microbial attachment to mucosal surfaces, secretory IgA also functions by activating complement. Bacteriolysis probably occurs rarely *in vivo* since complement components generated early in the reaction provide such potent opsonins that microbes are likely to undergo phagocytosis before they can be lysed.

Agglutination

Microbes are agglutinated just as molecules are precipitated by antibody cross-linking to form large immune complexes. Although the agglutination of parasites by antibody does not kill them outright, agglutination leads to a decrease in their infectiousness and their eventual destruction. The number of infectious units available for dissemination through the host is decreased by agglutination. Agglutinated microorganisms are also much easier to ingest by phagocytic cells than are single cells. Clumps of parasites are readily filtered from the blood by phagocytic cells in the spleen and lungs. Antibodies to the flagella of motile bacteria form clumps in which their movement, and thus their spread, is inhibited. Agglutinating antibodies to *Mycoplasma* may inhibit growth by blocking receptors on the bacteria necessary for the uptake of nutrients. In general, however, antibody-mediated agglutination alone is not a major impediment for microbial growth. Table 9.1 summarizes the major antimicrobial actions of specific antibodies.

COMPLEMENT-MEDIATED EFFECTOR MECHANISMS
Introduction

As described in chapter 4, there are two pathways for activation of the complement system, the classical and the alternative pathways (Figure 9.2). The term "classical" is derived from the fact that this pathway was discovered earlier than the alternative pathway. The significant difference between the two pathways is the nature of the substances that trigger them. In the classical pathway, complement is activated by immune complexes (soluble antigens agglutinated by IgG or IgM), microbes coated with IgG, by C-reactive protein, and some viruses. In contrast, alternative pathway activation occurs following contact with the polysaccharide-bearing surfaces of a variety of microorganisms and by lipopolysaccharide from Gram-negative bacteria. Alternative pathway activation does not employ antibody. The terminal sequence of the reactions that leads to the formation of a membrane attack complex is identical in both pathways. It is thought that the alternative pathway arose earlier in evolution since it provides an anti-

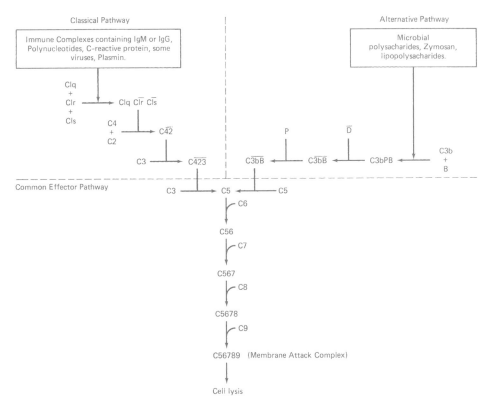

Figure 9.2.   The reaction sequences of the complement components in the classical and alternative pathways. Activating substances for each pathway are shown in the boxes. Lines over the complement proteins (e.g., $\overline{\text{C1s}}$) indicate enzymatic activity. The two pathways differ not only in the nature of the initiating step, but also in the subsequent amplification reactions leading to cleavage of C5. The pathways share the same effector mechanisms, including the membrane attack complexes.

microbial defense in the absence of a specific immune response. As such, the term "alternative" is somewhat of a misnomer. The classical pathway of complement activation was probably superimposed on the alternative pathway of activation with the result that the functions of the complement system were coordinated with the actions of the antibody system.

The complement components, designated by a capital C, are all proteins. They comprise ten percent of total human serum protein. Each component is identified by a numbered suffix, C1, C2, etc., that reflects the order in which they were originally purified rather than the order in which they react. Additional serum proteins called factors B, D, and P (properdin) are also involved in complement activation. The complement components circulate in the blood in inactive form. During the activation process, they may change in conformation, undergo proteolytic cleavage, or aggregate into multisubunit proteins. By convention, when a complement protein is split in two, the fragments are designated by a lower case a (for the smaller piece) and b (for the larger piece). The activation mechanisms can generate a protein with an enzymatic site or a binding site not exposed on the inactive component. The sites generated enable each component to react with the next component in the cascade. Activated complement proteins have biological activities that play a variety of roles in eliminating the invading microbe. In the classical pathway, fac-

Table 9.2. Biological activities of complement components

Component	Activity
$\overline{C4a}$	Anaphylatoxin, histamine release
$\overline{C3a}$	Anaphylatoxin, weak chemotactic factor
$\overline{C5a}$	Anaphylatoxin, strong chemotactic factor
$\overline{C3b}$ (membrane)	Immune adherence, opsonization
$\overline{C4b}$ (membrane)	Immune adherence, opsonization
$\overline{C5b}$ (membrane)	Initiates formation of membrane attack complex
$\overline{C8C9n}$ (membrane)	Membrane disruption

tors B and D and properdin (P) amplify reactions after they have been initiated. For this reason, the classical pathway is sometimes known as the *properdin pathway*.

Antibody-Dependent Activation of Complement: The Classical Complement Pathway
The principal triggers for the classical complement pathway are soluble antigen-antibody complexes (called *immune complexes*) and antibody bound to the surfaces of target cells. When antibody molecules are bound, complement proteins are also bound, and the reaction cascade is set in motion. This initial process is referred to as *complement fixation*, a name that makes reference to the surface location of the complement. The end game in this activation is the osmotic lysis of the cell. Although lysis of an infected host cell or of a parasitic microorganism is of obvious benefit to the host, other less obvious benefits occur as a result of complement activation. Some of the most important contributions to host defense that result from complement activation result from the biologic activities of the fragments cleaved from complement proteins at various points in the complement cascade. The fragments are either released into the general circulation or act at the cell surface (Table 9.2).

The first step in activation of complement by the classical pathway is binding of C1 Fc receptors to two or more IgG antibody molecules. The proximity of IgG molecules in soluble immune complexes or attached to the surfaces of target cells brings two IgG molecules close enough together to bind two of the C1 Fc receptors (Figure 9.3A). Pentameric IgM antibodies bound to antigens on the surface of a target cell undergo a conformational change, exposing their several Fc receptors.

C1 consists of three parts: C1q, C1r, and C1s. There is only one C1q in each C1 molecule, but there are two each of C1r and C1s. The C1q part is composed of six subunits with the extended ends tied together in a "stalk" and six globular "heads," the Fc receptors that bind to constant regions of the antibody molecules (Figure 9.3B). The binding of C1q to the antibody molecules triggers an internal rearrangement in one of the C1r molecules to expose its active site. The activated $\overline{C1r}$ then cleaves the $\overline{C1s}$ molecule, exposing its active site. Active $\overline{C1s}$ is a serine protease.

The second step in the cascade is the enzymatic cleavage of C4 and C2 by the active C1s serine protease since a single serine protease is able to catalyze the proteolysis of many C4 and C2 molecules, the small initial reaction is quickly amplified. Each serine protease may cleave approximately two hundred C4 molecules into $\overline{C4a}$ and $\overline{C4b}$ fragments. $\overline{C4b}$, the larger of the two fragments, binds to the cell membranes of any cell near the activating immune complex (Figure 9.4). The C2 molecule is also cleaved by the serine protease into a large fragment ($\overline{C2b}$) which binds to the membrane bound $\overline{C4b}$ forming a $\overline{C4b2b}$ complex. The unbound smaller fragments from the cleavage of C4 and C2 ($\overline{C4a}$ and $\overline{C2a}$) diffuse from the area where they were produced into the fluid phase of the blood. These soluble fragments are pharmacologically active and enhance the inflammatory reaction that develops at the site. In turn, the $\overline{C4b2b}$ complex cleaves the C3 and is therefore

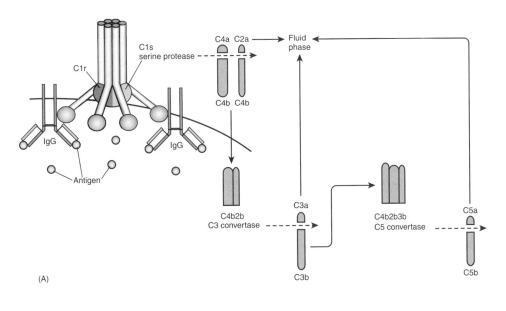

(A)

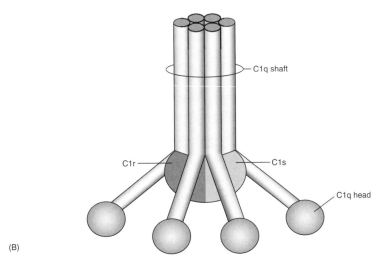

(B)

Figure 9.3. (A) The initial reactions of the classical complement pathway occur on membranes or on immune complexes. The first reaction is the recognition of bound IgG (or IgM) antibody by the C1q subunit. Self-activation by rearrangement and cleavage within C1 generates a C1s serine protease that cleaves both C4 and C2. The membrane-bound $\overline{C4b2b}$ serves first as a C3 convertase and then as a C5 convertase following attachment of $\overline{C3b}$ to $\overline{C4b2b}$. The smaller complement fragments in the "fluid phase" have potent inflammatory activities. (B) C1q is a hexameric protein with extended portions of the six subunits joined together in a "stalk" and six globular "bulbs" that bind to the constant region of IgG and IgM antibodies.

given the name *C3 convertase*. $\overline{C3a}$ and $\overline{C3b}$ are the fragments produced. The larger fragment, $\overline{C3b}$, binds to the $\overline{C4b2b}$ complex to form a $\overline{C4b2b3b}$ aggregate that now possesses a new enzymatic site specific for C5. Cleavage of C5 by this *C5 convertase* is the last enzymatic step in the pathway. Each molecule of C5 convertase may split fifty to one hundred C5 molecules. The small fragments resulting from complement activation, $\overline{C3a}$ and $\overline{C5a}$, diffuse away from their sites of production. The $\overline{C5b}$

fragment is hydrophobic and binds to the lipid bilayer of cells near its site of production.

The $\overline{C5b}$ fragment on the membranes of cells serves as the initiating point for the assembly of the remaining complement components, C6 through C9, into a structure termed the *membrane attack complex* (MAC). The assembly of the complex occurs in several steps. The $\overline{C5b}$ fragments bind C6, C7, and C8. C7 and C8 undergo conformational changes exposing hydrophobic regions that embed into the cell membrane. The $\overline{C5b678}$ complex serves as a nucleation point that brings about the polymerization of up to sixteen C9 molecules. The polymerized C9 molecules form a cylindrical tubule that inserts into the cell membrane making a hole. This transmembrane channel permits water and ions to flow into the cell. As a consequence the cell swells and bursts. Before bursting, the proton gradient used by a bacterium to generate ATP is also destroyed. Nucleated cells often simply lose their cytoplasm through the pores rather than swelling and bursting (Figure 9.4).

While the entire process is very complex in its details, the basic principles are few: in the classical pathway complement fixation is triggered by antibody binding to antigen; complement proteins are activated by proteolysis; some fragments become active proteases, furthering and amplifying the entire process, and others become soluble molecules that play other roles in the immune response. The final step is the production of a macromolecular complex that forms a hole in the membrane and destroys the microbe.

The membrane attack complex usually enters the membranes of cells to which antibody is bound. A few of these complexes, however, may detach from the antibody-coated cell on which they formed and deposit on adjacent cells, resulting in the loss of healthy host cells in the vicinity. When this occurs it is referred to as a *bystander* effect of complement activation.

The Alternative Pathway of Complement Activation

The alternative pathway also results in the deposition of $\overline{C5b}$ on microbial surfaces, but by a different pathway. The alternate route of complement activation is a mechanism for generating complement components with inflammatory activity and for assembling the $\overline{C5C9}$ lytic complex in the absence of antibody.

Activation of complement by the alternative pathway begins in the plasma. A small amount of C3 hydrolyzes spontaneously ("tickover") to form $\overline{C3a}$ and $\overline{C3b}$. The $\overline{C3b}$ binds to the surfaces of cells, including those of the host. The lipopolysaccharide of Gram-negative bacteria and the carbohydrates of yeast cell walls, however, provide particularly hospitable sites for the stable deposition of $\overline{C3b}$. Bound $\overline{C3b}$ associates with Factor B, an inactive protease in the plasma, to form a complex, $\overline{C3bB}$. After deposition on the microbe, the Factor B in the complex is cleaved by the action of Factor D. The products of this reaction are $\overline{Ba}$, which diffuses away, and $\overline{C3bBb}$. $\overline{C3bBb}$ is a C3 convertase. When it is stabilized by the binding of properdin (P) molecules, it cleaves many C3 molecules, amplifying the deposition of $\overline{C3b}$ on the cell surface. The stabilized large complex of $\overline{C3b\text{-}Bb\text{-}C3b(n)\text{-}P(n)}$ eventually undergoes a conformational change to expose another enzymatic site on $\overline{Bb}$ which is a C5 convertase. When C5 is cleaved and $\overline{C5b}$ is deposited on the cell surface, the assembly of the membrane attack complex follows.

The classical and alternative pathways are functionally intertwined by their common C3 and C5 convertases. Therefore, the activation of one pathway can amplify the activity of the other through the generation of $\overline{C3b}$ and $\overline{C5b}$.

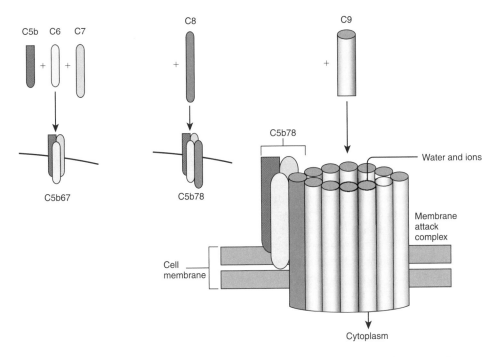

Figure 9.4. Outline of the assembly of complement proteins into a membrane attack complex. The deposition of $\overline{C5b}$ on a membrane site as a trimolecular complex of $\overline{C5b67}$ allows the binding of C8 to the site. C8 initiates the formation of a transmembrane tubule due to the polymerization of ten to sixteen C9 molecules. This "membrane attack complex" allows the free passage of water into the cell resulting in the cell's lysis.

Biological Activities of Complement Components

Complement activation induces inflammation, attracts leukocytes from the circulation to the site of inflammation, facilitates phagocytosis of parasites, facilitates clearing of dangerous immune complexes from the circulation, and produces membrane attack complexes. All of these processes are mediated by complement components (Table 9.2). $\overline{C3a}$, $\overline{C4a}$, and $\overline{C5a}$ stimulate inflammation and are called *anaphylatoxins*. Anaphylatoxins trigger the release of histamine from platelets, mast cells, and basophils. Histamine causes vasodilation, increases capillary permeability, and constriction of bronchial smooth muscle. These changes in the capillaries cause edema, the accumulation of plasma in the inflamed site. The plasma contains additional antibodies and complement thereby accelerating the elimination of the pathogens.

Chemotactic factors are substances that attract leukocytes. Under their influence polymorphonuclear leukocytes are induced to adhere to vascular endothelial cells, pass through the spaces between the endothelial cells of the capillaries (extravasation), and move into the inflamed site by moving up the concentration gradient of the factor. The presence of additional leukocytes increases the likelihood of phagocytosis of any parasites present. $\overline{C3a}$ and $\overline{C5b67}$ are weakly chemotactic; $\overline{C5a}$ is strongly chemotactic.

Immune adherence brings about the strong attachment of phagocytic leukocytes to parasites. The complement components responsible for immune adherence are

LIVERPOOL
JOHN MOORES UNIVERSITY
AVRIL ROBARTS LRC
TEL. 0151 231 4022

$\overline{C4b}$ and $\overline{C3b}$ which serve as powerful opsonins. As opsonins, these components are also important for the solubilization and clearance of immune complexes. $\overline{C4b}$ and $\overline{C3b}$ also bind to receptors on erythrocytes. The erythrocytes are then cleaned of their attached immune complexes by macrophages in the spleen and liver. Failure to remove these immune complexes can result in their deposition in the kidney glomeruli, a pathological condition in many autoimmune diseases.

Regulation of Complement Activity

Since the activation of complement by invading parasites generates potent products which may cause injury to host cells in the neighborhood, the activation of the complement cascade must be closely regulated to prevent unnecessary damage to the host. Moreover, the complement proteins as noted previously spontaneously activate to a small degree, a process called "tickover" that is fundamental in the activation of the alternative pathway. The primary safeguard protecting the host is the very short half-life of activated complement. For example, the binding site on $\overline{C3b}$ undergoes very rapid spontaneous hydrolysis unless it is bound to a cell.

Other regulatory mechanisms include serum or cell-surface proteins of the host. The enzymatic step mediated by C1 is inhibited by a normal serum protein, C1-inhibitor, that binds $\overline{C1r-C1s}$ and causes it to dissociate from $\overline{C1q}$, thereby limiting the activation of C2 and C4 and the formation of C3 covertase. C3 convertase can also be inactivated by a serum protein called C4 binding protein or a cell-surface protein called decay-accelerating factor (DAF). The key step in both the classical and alternative pathways is the deposition of $\overline{C3b}$ on cells. Factor I in normal serum is a $\overline{C3b}$-inactivator that degrades $\overline{C3b}$ and $\overline{C4b}$ unless they are bound to a cell surface. Another normal serum protein, Factor H, enhances the inhibitory action of Factor I. Protectin is a protein on host cell surfaces that prevents the formation of membrane attack complexes.

The factors that stimulate or inhibit complement activation are in exquisite balance. In the absence of parasites or other foreign antigens, complement activation is extremely-limited and such slight activation as does occur (the "tickover" described above) yields activated products which, in the absence of alternative activating factors, are quickly inhibited. Even in the presence of parasites and other foreign antigens activation is controlled so that it occurs only in the immediate vicinity of the initiating factor. Such control is vital to prevent the occurrence of an uncontrollable chain reaction that would destroy the host as well as the parasite.

CELL-MEDIATED EFFECTOR MECHANISMS

Introduction

Cell-mediated immunity is a major factor controlling the growth of bacteria, protozoa, and viruses in a host cell. The mycobacteria, which are responsible for the human diseases of tuberculosis and leprosy, grow inside the phagosomes of the macrophages that ingest them. By preventing lysosome fusion and the acidification of the phagosome, they create a niche for themselves that is protected from antibody and cytotoxic T cells. The response to this type of infection is *activation* of the infected macrophage which gives the activated macrophage a heightened ability to kill the parasites they have ingested. Helper T cells play an important role in this activation process. Viruses replicating inside cells of the host are destroyed by killing of the infected host cell by *cytolytic T lymphocytes* (CTLs). Parasitic worms dwelling in the tissues of the host may also be killed by CTLs.

All of the effector responses of cell-mediated immunity require activation by T cells[1]. This means that with the elimination of T cells, the cell-mediated protective response is eliminated. There are two basic classes of T cells that can be distinguished by CD (short for *cluster of differentiation*) marker proteins on their surface. CD4+ cells include the inflammatory T cells (T_H1) and the helper T cells (T_H2). CD8+ cells are the cytotoxic T cells. Because of the affinity of the CD4 protein for the human immunodeficiency virus (HIV), it is this class of T cells that is destroyed in people with AIDS. The severe immunodeficiency that results is the direct consequence of the destruction of CD4+ cells.

Macrophage Activation and the Elimination of Intracellular Parasites
The distinctive characteristic of cell-mediated immunity is that it can be transferred from an immunized animal to a naive recipient by the adoptive transfer of T lymphocytes. The role of macrophage activation in resistance to parasites developing inside macrophages was first shown by George MacKaness and his colleagues. In the early 1960s they clearly demonstrated that T cells from mice that had been immunized with attenuated *Listeria monocytogenes* (a parasite which grows inside macrophage phagosomes) when transferred to nonimmune mice, conferred resistance to *Listeria* infection (Figure 9.5). Neither immune serum nor macrophages could transfer this immunity. A surprising outcome of this study was the observation that with the transfer of resistance to *L. monocytogenes*, resistance to unrelated intracellular pathogens also developed in the T cell recipients. This relatively nonspecific resistance was probably a result of a generalized T cell mediated activation of macrophages throughout the body of the recipient of the transplanted T cells.

Delayed-Type Hypersensitivity
Macrophage activation is part of a well-studied phenomenon known as *delayed-type hypersensitivity* (DTH). The skin reaction which develops following tuberculin injection, originally described by Robert Koch in 1882 (chapter 5), is a prime example of DTH. This skin reaction is a visible manifestation of events that may occur in any tissue where tubercle bacilli are present. The events which occur at the site of tuberculin injection in a tuberculin-sensitive individual are the same as those which occur in appropriately-sensitized individuals when tissue-dwelling worms or intracellular protozoa, bacteria, or viruses release antigen at their sites of growth. Despite the name hypersensitivity, the reaction is normally beneficial to the host and detrimental to the parasite. If, however, it becomes excessive, tissue damage can occur. The granulomatous skin lesions in leprosy and the lung abscesses seen in tuberculosis are examples of such pathological tissue damage.

DTH requires an initial sensitization phase in which inflammatory T cells undergo clonal expansion. These cells were originally named T_{DTH} cells, but the current term is *inflammatory T cells* or T_H1 *cells*, a subset of CD4+ cells. T_H1 cells are only sensitized by antigen if antigen fragments are presented to them on the surface of an antigen-presenting cell in association with a Class II MHC protein. Not only do macrophages or other antigen presenting cells present processed antigen to the T_H1 cells, but they also secrete the cytokine interleukin-1 (IL-1). Interleukin-1 stimu-

---

1 Apparent exceptions to this rule are those portions of the immune response mediated by natural killer lymphocytes (NK cells). These cells, however, appear not to be thymic lymphocytes but cells of a separate lineage.

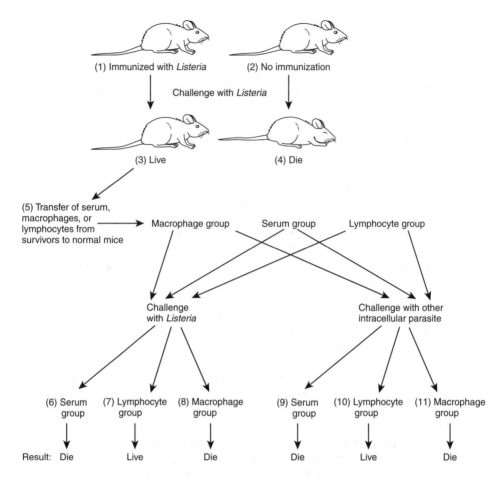

Figure 9.5.   The mechanism of immunity in *Listeria monocytogenes* in mice. Nonimmunized mice (2) die upon challenge with *Listeria* (4). Mice immunized with *Listeria* (1) survive the *Listeria* challenge (3) and display heightened resistance. The nature of the immune effector mechanisms is revealed by the transfer experiments (5). Mice that receive immune lymphocytes (7, 10) but not immune serum or macrophages (6, 8, 9, 11) resist challenge with *Listeria* and with unrelated intracellular parasites. Thus, the triggering of the immune response is antigen specific, but the antimicrobial activity generated is nonspecific.

lates the clonal expansion of T_H1 cells by stimulating the production of new surface receptors on the T_H1 cells. These new receptors allow the cells to respond to interleukin-2 (T cell growth factor) and divide. IL-2 is secreted by the T_H1 cells themselves, making IL-2 an *autocrine* hormone (Figure 9.6).

Following sensitization, the clonal expansion which occurs results in a large population of T_H1 lymphocytes that respond aggressively on reexposure to the antigen. This *effector phase* is focused back upon the macrophage, which, once activated, destroys its internal parasites and stimulates a localized inflammatory response. The initial sensitization provides enough of the appropriate T_H1 lymphocytes to mount a delayed hypersensitivity response at any site where antigen is deposited.

The hallmark of the delayed type reaction is a massive infiltration of lymphocytes and macrophages into the site where the antigen occurs. Only 0.1 percent of the T cells in a sensitized host respond *in vitro* to the antigen used to sensitize the host

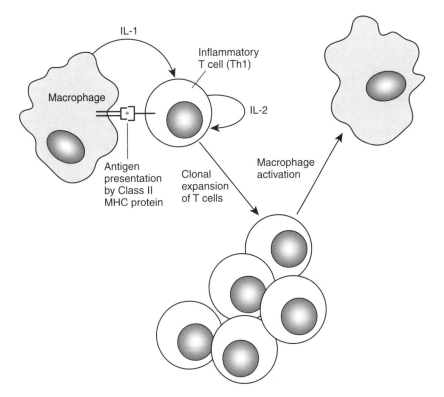

Figure 9.6. Mechanism for the sensitization of T cells by macrophages in a DTH reaction. Antigen in association with a Class II MHC protein is presented to an inflammatory (T_H1) T cell. In response to this stimulation and to IL-1 produced by the antigen-presenting macrophage, the T cell secretes autocrine IL-2 and undergoes clonal expansion. These sensitized T cells activate macrophages.

and only 5 percent of the lymphocytes at the site of a delayed type reaction in an animal sensitized by passive transfer are lymphocytes which were transferred. The sensitized T_H1 cells must therefore recruit a large number of unsensitized lymphocytes and macrophages to the site by the secretion of a variety of chemotactic cytokines. Circulating monocytes and lymphocytes attach to and pass through the endothelial lining of the capillaries and enter the infected tissues. These infiltrating cells continue the process of T_H1 clonal expansion and macrophage activation (Figure 9.7). This effector response peaks at about forty-eight hours after exposure to antigen. For this reason, the reaction is called *delayed-type* (as opposed to *immediate*) hypersensitivity.

Macrophage Activation and Microbiocidal Activity
The activation of infected macrophages by T_H1 cells is the central event in the DTH response. Macrophage activation at the site of a delayed-type reaction can be reduced to a series of events which take place over a few hours (Figure 9.8). Monocytes are stimulated by T_H1 cell cytokines to leave the blood and accumulate in the inflamed area. These newly arrived monocytes are potentially responsive macrophages. They are first *primed* and then *activated* by the action of the antigen-specific T_H1 cells that were produced at the infection site by clonal expansion. An antigen-

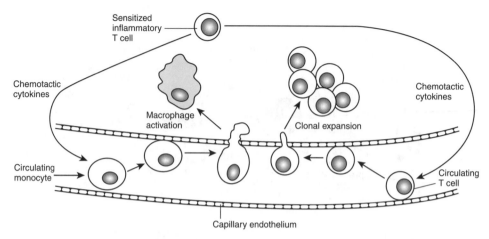

Figure 9.7.   The role of initially sensitized inflammatory cells in recruiting additional cells from the circulation in a DTH reaction. Circulating unsensitized T cells and monocytes are stimulated by chemotactic cytokines to attach and pass through the capillary epithelium into the infected tissue. In the tissues, these cells undergo clonal expansion and activation (shown in Figures 9.7 and 9.9).

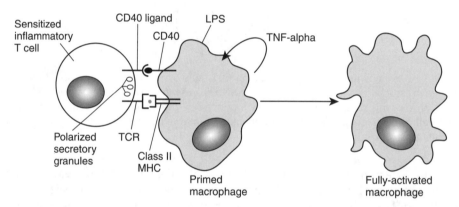

Figure 9.8. The sequence of events involved in the activation of macrophages. Responsive macrophages differentiate into primed macrophages when stimulated by antigen-specific sensitized inflammatory T cells. T cells recognize specific antigen displayed by the macrophage in association with its Class II MHC. Priming of the macrophage occurs when the CD40 ligand on the T cell binds the CD40 on the macrophage. Activation of the macrophage occurs when γ-interferon (γ-IFN) is released from secretory granules. TNF-α also plays an autocrine role in activating the macrophage.

specific sensitized inflammatory (T_H1) T cell binds to the infected macrophage by recognizing antigen fragments presented by the macrophage in association with its class II MHC proteins. These T_H1 cells also express a surface protein, *CD40-ligand*, on their surface that interacts with a CD40 protein on the macrophage. Interaction between the CD40-ligand and CD40 primes the macrophage. Priming can also be accomplished by very small amounts of bacterial lipopolysaccharide (LPS). Activation is accomplished by the secretion of interferon-γ (IFN-γ, originally known as macrophage activating factor) by the T_H1 cell. The IFN-γ secretory granules

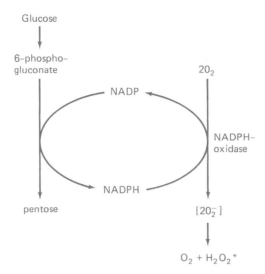

Glucose

6-phospho-
gluconate

$2O_2$

NADP

NADPH-
oxidase

NADPH

pentose

$[2O_2^-]$

$O_2 + H_2O_2$*

Figure 9.9. Some mechanisms used by phagocytes in production of the "respiratory" burst. The degradation of glucose is linked through by NADP-NADPH cycle to the activation of oxygen. The active oxygen products, O_2^- and H_2O_2, are antimicrobial because of their strong oxidizing capabilities.

become localized at the site of macrophage attachment and the release of IFN-γ is therefore site specific so that bystander damage is limited. Both the CD40-ligand and IFN-γ are synthesized *de novo* when the T_H1 cell binds to its target macrophage. This process takes several hours. The macrophage is also involved in its own activation through the secretion of tumor-necrosis factor (TNF-α). The TNF-α binds to receptors on the macrophage itself, serving as an autocrine hormone.

T_H1 cells produce a variety of other cell surface proteins and secreted cytokines that play important roles in the inflammatory response. *Fas ligand* and *TNF-β* can kill chronically infected macrophages, releasing the infecting microbes for destruction by other activated macrophages. IL-3 and *granulocyte-monocyte colony-stimulating factor* (GM-CSF) stimulate the bone marrow to produce more monocytes. IL-2 continues T_H1 cell proliferation.

During macrophage activation arachidonic acid metabolism is enhanced. This results in greatly increased secretion of prostaglandins and leukotrienes. These products mediate inflammation. Activated macrophages also have an increased capacity for oxidative metabolism. The metabolic burst of activated macrophages following phagocytosis is twenty to fifty times that of resting macrophages. The metabolic burst is carried out by a NADPH-dependent oxidase enzyme complex that resides in the macrophage membrane (Figure 9.9). These enzymes generate superoxide (O_2^-) ion which is rapidly dismutated to H_2O_2 and hydroxyl radicals (OH-). These potent oxidizing agents are effective mediators of host defense. All of the effector mechanisms used by macrophages in the inducible immune response were developed as parts of the constitutive resistance system. The inducible response, however, amplifies their effects.

Activated macrophages are also able to kill pathogens in their vicinity. Activated macrophages destroy the extracellular protozoan[2] *Pneumocystis carinii* in this way.

---

2 or fungus, depending on the taxonomist to whom you speak.

Infection by *Pneumocystis carinii* is very common in HIV-infected individuals in the U.S., and such infection is therefore considered to be suggestive of AIDS, the disease brought about by the HIV-induced deficiency of CD4+ T cells.

Tumoricidal Activity

Activated macrophages also have tumoricidal activity. The fact that the activated macrophages have an enhanced capacity to destroy not only the microbe that brought about their activation but other cells as well is the basis of the use of BCG (Bacillus Calmette-Guerin, an attenuated *Mycobacterium bovis* preparation) as a therapeutic agent for treatment of solid tumors. The BCG is injected into the tumor mass. The monocytes that concentrate at the site differentiate into macrophages which upon activation destroy tumor cells. Despite the initial promise of this innovative therapy, the clinical results have not been very promising.

Natural Killer Cells

Natural killer (NK) cells are a distinct class of lymphocytes that do not fit into either the T cell or B cell categories. Because they lack surface immunoglobulins, TCRs, and other distinctive markers of the T or B cells, they are also referred to as *null cells*. NK cells possess large cytoplasmic granules that resemble those of the granular leukocytes. Because of this attribute, another name given to the natural killer cell is *large granular lymphocyte*. NK cells comprise five to ten percent of the circulating lymphocyte population in humans.

Natural killer cells kill a variety of pathological cells including host cells that have been infected with viruses, cells in allografts, and some cancer cells, especially leukemic cells. They are also capable of destroying some fungi and protozoa. Natural killer cells kill without prior sensitization. Thus, natural killer cell activity may be considered a component of constitutive immunity. Natural killer cells also have receptors for the Fc portion of IgG and can therefore be mobilized as effector cells by antibody through the antibody-dependent cell-mediated cytotoxicity (ADCC) mechanism. In this latter respect they may be considered effectors for the inducible immune system.

Natural killer cells lyse a wide range of target cells with no apparent restriction by the major histocompatibility complex. They are, therefore, distinct from cytotoxic T lymphocytes. Natural killer cells increase in number when exposed to IFN-α, IFN-β, and IL-12, cytokines that are released by virally-infected cells (Figure 9.10A). In this capacity NK cells function to hold the line against a viral infection until a specific immune response can be mobilized.

The mechanisms whereby natural killer cells function are quite similar to those used by cytotoxic T cells (see below). Both types of cells release cytotoxic chemicals from cytoplasmic vacuoles. An important difference is that NK cells do not need to be primed. Their granules are always present which means they can be mobilized rapidly. There is no type of self-restriction since NK cells are able to kill just as efficiently if they are transferred to a host of a different genotype.

Since NK cells seem to show no specific binding to their targets (at least none by conventional mechanisms) it has long been a mystery how they kill infected or transformed cells and not normal cells. Various models have been proposed to explain their specificity. One model invokes two receptors. First the NK cells bind to a cell through a receptor specific for surface glycoprotein and prepare to kill. The killing signal is overridden by binding of a second receptor to Class I MHC pro-

(A)

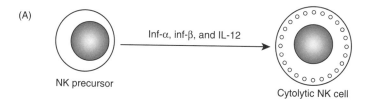

(B)

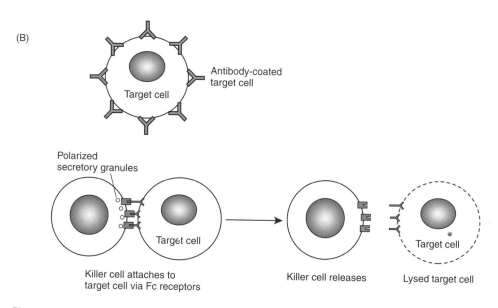

Figure 9.10. (A) Natural killer cell precursors differentiate into strongly cytolytic NK cells through the effects of the cytokines INF-α, INF-β, and IL-12 released by virally infected cells. (B) Antibody-dependent cell-mediated cytotoxicity (ADCC) is mediated by secreted IgG antibody molecules which bind to the target cell. Cytolytic cells, including NK cells, macrophages, neutrophils, and eosinophils, bind to the target cell via membrane-bound Fc receptors. Killing involves the release of secretory granules in the direction of the target. Having killed, the cytotoxic cells release and prepare to kill again.

teins. Since virally infected and transformed cells down-regulate MHC Class I expression, they may be killed while normal cells with a normal level of MHC Class I expression avoid being killed.

Antibody-Dependent Cell Cytotoxicity (ADCC)

Antibody-dependent cell cytotoxicity is an effector mechanism that depends on the joint activity of leukocytes of various types (NK cells, monocytes and macrophages, neutrophils, and eosinophils) and antibody. The killer cells themselves are not capable of killing specifically: the reaction is made specific by the antibody. The antibody involved is of the IgG type. To bring about cytolysis, the killer cells must be bound to antibody on the target cell by their Fc receptors (Figure 9.10B). Antibody-dependent cell cytotoxicity may be an important part of the host defense against a variety of parasites, including worms, fungi, and protozoa.

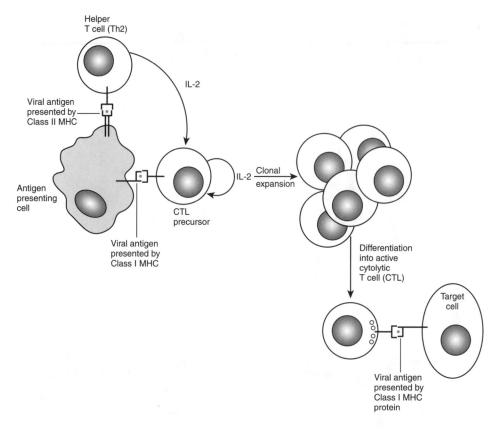

Figure 9.11.   The cellular events controlling the proliferation and differentiation of cytotoxic T lymphocytes (CTLs). An antigen presenting cell presents a viral (or other internal parasite) antigen, in association with a Class I MHC protein, to a CTL precursor cell. The CTL precursor responds by secreting the cytokine IL-2 to which it responds. In many cases, IL-2 may also be provided by a helper T cell which responds to the same antigen presented by a Class II MHC protein. The IL-2 stimulates the cell to proliferate and differentiate into an active CTL. The active CTL binds to target cells that display the same antigen in association with a Class I MHC.

Cytolytic T Lymphocytes

Cytolytic T lymphocytes (CTLs) are lymphocytes programmed to destroy target cells in an antigen-specific fashion. They are T cells identified by the CD8 protein on their surface and are therefore referred to as CD8+. They have been extensively studied because they are the cells primarily responsible for graft rejection (chapter 11). CTLs are also capable of recognizing virus and other parasite-produced proteins present on the surfaces of host cells in association with Class I MHC molecules (Figure 9.11). Despite the damage to the host which may result from the destruction of infected host cells, the recognition and destruction of viruses and other intracellular parasites by the destruction of infected host cells is the only way the host can rid itself of such infections.

Prior to infection, CTLs exist as precursor cells, incapable of killing until they are activated. The formation of competent CTLs requires that they receive an antigen-specific Class I MHC-restricted activation signal. The precursor CTLs express IL-2 receptors on their surface and proliferate in response to IL-2 stimulation. The IL-2 is produced by the CTL precursor cell itself and by helper T cells that have recognized the antigen presented by a Class II MHC. After proliferation, they differentiate into competent CTLs replete with cytoplasmic vesicles filled with cytotoxins.

For cytotoxic lymphocytes to kill, contact with the target cell is required. In the case of virally infected cells, specific CTLs bind to target cells by recognizing viral antigen in association with Class I MHC proteins in the infected cells' membranes. The attached CTL releases the contents of its lytic vesicles into the target cell. After this "kiss of death," the CTL can release the cell and move off to kill again.

The contents of the lytic vesicles of CTLs include a group of serine proteases, known collectively as *granzymes*, and TNF-â, also known as *lymphotoxin*. Both of these molecules trigger the target cell to commit suicide, a process known as *apoptosis*. TNF-â binds to a receptor on the target cell surface, triggering an internal signaling cascade, whereas granzymes enter the cells through pores made by a membrane attack complex called *perforin*. Perforin is similar in structure and function to the complement protein C9. Apoptosis is a programmed cell death involving a very characteristic fragmentation of the chromatin, vesiculation of the cytoplasm, shrinkage of the cell, and disruption of the cell membrane. It was originally thought that the action of the perforin was to cause osmotic lysis and death of the cell, but this is likely to be an *in vitro* artifact.

CTLs also secrete a number of cytokines that participate in the immune response. Principle among these cytokines is IL-2 which interferes with viral replication, increases Class I MHC expression on target cells, and stimulates macrophage chemotaxis and activation.

The Biological Significance of MHC Restriction of CTLs

The single most important mechanism among the many mechanisms governing the sensitization and effector activities of T cells is that which limits antigen recognition to antigens presented in association with membrane proteins coded for by the MHC complex. Major histocompatibility restriction of antigen recognition by cells of the inducible immune response is a complicated mechanism which at first glance defies our understanding. But since it has evolved, it is a good bet that it serves a vital function. It cannot have evolved to prevent the acceptance of foreign tissue grafts, but rather must have arisen as part of the mechanism required to prevent colonization of the host's tissues by parasites. Since antigen presenting cells display parasite components on their surfaces, it would not be in the interest of a host to use its cytolytic mechanisms to destroy these cells. By restricting killing to cells with foreign antigen on Class I MHC, the disaster that would be caused by the death of Class II bearing antigen presenting cells is avoided.

Self-recognition is also required to permit differentiation from nonself. If all members of a species were identical in self components, some parasite could potentially develop an outer coat similar to that of the host's self and thus escape detection in all members of the species. Given the extreme polymorphism of the MHC proteins in a population, each member of the species is distinct in its self-markers. This means that no parasite can develop a pattern to deceive *all* members of the species. The diversity of self-types is increased by the recombination and reassortment of genes during gamete formation and fertilization. This system precludes any parasite becoming self to all members of the species. The systems of self-recognition and MHC restriction are thus systems which permit parasite recognition in the face of individuality.

SUMMARY

The purpose of the inducible immune response is to eliminate or control the growth of pathogens that threaten the survival of the host. To this end, a variety of effector mechanisms have evolved which destroy or reduce the growth and spread of infecting parasites. There are two basic arms of the immune response: humoral and cell mediated. The humoral arm produces antibody molecules specific to the antigens of the parasite. When these antibodies bind, they do not kill or damage the microbe directly. Instead, they call upon several nonspecific defense mechanisms of the host. Antibody serves as a powerful opsonin, giving a target to phagocytes which bind the antibody through its Fc portion. Antibody can also bind to and block the active sites of microbial exotoxins, prevent the binding of the microbe to host cells by blocking receptors on the microbe's surface, or agglutinate the microbes, further facilitating phagocytosis and also impeding the spread of the parasite.

Many of the effects of antibody are mediated by a group of blood serum proteins called collectively complement. The binding of antibody to a microbial surface will cause the deposition and serial activation of complement proteins. Complement binding facilitates phagocytosis among its many actions. The ultimate effect of these activated proteins is, however, inflammation at the site of the infection and osmotic lysis of the infecting pathogen.

The cell-mediated arm of the immune system does not employ antibodies to kill parasites, but, instead, it uses at least two types of lymphocytes. One type, the inflammatory T lymphocytes (T_H1 cells), undergo clonal expansion in response to the infection, release inflammatory cytokines, and activate macrophages that have microbes growing inside their phagosomes. An activated macrophage will respond by killing the microbe and releasing additional inflammatory cytokines. This type of response is referred to as delayed type hypersensitivity since the process takes time to develop. Uncontrolled, DTH can do severe damage to the host.

A second class of T lymphocytes, the cytotoxic T lymphocytes (CTLs), differentiate into cells capable of outright killing of virally infected host cells, some invading parasites, foreign tissue grafts, and some tumor cells. The killing is accomplished by the release of granules onto the surface of the target cell. These trigger the suicide of the cell, a process called apoptosis. Killing of cells can also be accomplished by nonspecific natural killer cells or by many other types of cells that bind to cells coated by antibody.

The effect of all of these mechanisms is to maintain the health of the host in a world of potentially hostile pathogens. The purpose of MHC restriction of these actions seems to be to prevent the accidental killing of T helper cells and to prevent parasites from mimicking their host as a means of successful infection.

SUGGESTIONS FOR FURTHER READING

1. Berke. G. "Functions and Mechanisms of Lysis Induced by Cytotoxic T lymphocytes and Natural Killer Cells." Chapter 27 in *Fundamental Immunology*. 2d ed. Edited by W.E. Paul. New York: Raven Press, 1989.
2. Carroll, M.C. "The Role of Complement and Complement Receptors in Induction and Regulation of Immunity." *Ann. Rev. Immunol.* 16 (1998):545–568.
3. Clark, W.F., "Cell-Mediated Cytotoxity." Chapter 14 in *The Experimental Foundations of Modern Immunology*. New York: John Wiley and Sons, 1989.

4. Eichenfeld, L.F., and R.B. Johnson Jr. "The Complement System." Chapter 13 in *Immunology and Inflammation: Basic Mechanisms and Clinical Consequences.* L.H. Sigal, and Y. Ron. New York: McGraw-Hill, Inc., 1994.
5. Janeway, C.A., and P. Travers. "T-cell Mediated Immunity." Chapter 7 in *Immunobiology: The Immune System in Health and Disease.* 3d ed. New York: Garland Publishing, Inc., 1997.
6. Klein, M.R., S.H. van der Burg, O. Pontesilli, and F. Miedema. "Cytotoxic T lymphocytes in HIV-1 infection: a killing paradox? *Immunology Today* 19, no. 7 (1998):317–324.
7. Kuby, J. "Immune Effector Mechanisms." Part III in *Immunology.* 3d ed. New York: W.H. Freeman and Company.
8. Lanier, L.L. "NK Cell Receptors." *Ann. Rev. Immunol.* 16 (1998):359–393.
9. Meltzer, M.S. and C.A. Nacy. "Delayed-Type Hypersensitivity and the Induction of Activated, Cytotoxic Macrophages." Chapter 28 in *Fundamental Immunology.* 2d ed. Edited by W.E. Paul. New York: Raven Press, 1989.
10. Mosser, D.M. and A. Brittingham. "Leishmania, Macrophages and Complement: A Tale of Subversion and Exploitation. *Parasitology* 115 Suppl:S9-S23, 1997.
11. Verret, C.R. "Specific and Non-Specific Cell-Mediated Cytotoxicity." Chapter 8 in *Immunology and Inflammation: Basic Mechanisms and Clinical Consequences.* Edited by L.H. Sigal, and Y. Ron. New York: McGraw-Hill, Inc., 1994.

QUESTIONS

1. How does antibody increase the efficiency of phagocytosis?
2. How do antibodies directly interfere with the process of infection?
3. What is the most important difference between the classical and the alternative pathways of complement activation?
4. How does a very small amount of complement fixation lead to a very large effector response?
5. How have parasites developed a niche inside phagocytic cells?
6. Why is delayed-type hypersensitivity delayed?
7. Compare the ways CTLs and NK cells kill their targets.
8. What are some ideas as to why killing by CTLs is MHC restricted?

ANSWERS

1. Antibody that is produced as part of a humoral response will coat the cell surface of pathogens that induced the response. Since many phagocytic cells have receptors on their surface that can recognize the Fc portion of the antibody, they can bind to the pathogen much more tightly and increase the efficiency of phagocytosis.
2. Pathogens that infect the host by entering the host cells (intracellular microbes and viruses) gain entry by binding to receptors on the surface of the host cells. Antibodies directed against these receptor ligands on the parasite can therefore physically block infection. Antibodies can also block the active sites on exotoxins. To the extent that exotoxins aid the infectious process by, for example, mobilizing food for the pathogen, infection may be limited, antibody blocking of exotoxin action.
3. The alternate pathway is commonly activated by bacterial surface components and not by antibody. As such, it is not nearly as specific as the classical pathway. Because of its relatively nonspecific nature, the alternative pathway is likely to be the primitive pathway from which the classical pathway evolved.

4. Complement is activated by a cascade of reactions in which many of the steps are enzymatic. Since a single enzyme molecule can catalyze a large number of reactions rapidly, the activation process is greatly amplified as it progresses.

5. When a microbe is endocytosed by a phagocyte, it is encased inside a membrane-bound phagosome. Normally, it would be destroyed by hydrolytic enzymes from lysosomes that fuse with the phagosome. Some parasites have evolved means to prevent lysosome fusion as well as the acidification of the phagosome, thereby creating a niche inside the cell.

6. DTH is due to the inflammatory activities of activated macrophages. A macrophage is activated by the MHC-restricted binding of an inflammatory T cell to an infected macrophage. The bound T cell releases the inflammatory cytokine IFN-γ and binds its CD-40 ligand to the CD-40 protein on the macrophage. Both IFN-γ and CD-40 ligand must be synthesized by the T cell after it binds. This takes time.

7. The most fundamental difference is that CTLs killing is antigen-specific and MHC-restricted. Natural killer cells bind target cells without such a restriction. The limited specificity of natural killer cells seems to be due to the down-regulation of MHC Class I receptors on the target cells which are recognized by the NK cell. But this binding is not antigen-specific.

8. Since there are two types of MHC proteins, Class I and Class II, and only the Class I proteins are involved in CTL killing, the killing of Class II restricted T helper cells is avoided. More importantly, MHC Class I proteins are highly polymorphic in the host cell population. This means that no parasite can successfully infect all members of a population by mimicking a single MHC specificity.

CHAPTER **10**

INTRODUCTION
AUTOIMMUNE DISEASES
  Breakdown of Self-
    Tolerance
  Pathogenesis
THE HYPERSENSITIVITIES
  Type I Hypersensitivity
  Type II Hypersensitivity
  Type III Hypersensitivity
  Type IV Hypersensitivity
SUMMARY
SUGGESTIONS FOR
  FURTHER READING
QUESTIONS
ANSWERS

Immunologically Mediated Diseases and Allergic Reactions

Kim A. Campbell and Caroline C. Whitacre

INTRODUCTION

The immune system is critical for maintenance of health, and its purpose is to protect the host. Through the complex interaction of lymphocytes, macrophages, cytokines, antibodies, complement, and other biochemical factors, the immune system performs such functions as eradicating infectious agents or generating protective antibodies following vaccination. Immune responses are all regulated by an exquisite system of checks and balances. In some cases immunoregulatory mechanisms fail, and inappropriate reactions are generated in response to innocuous foreign agents, as in **allergy**, or in response to self-antigens, leading to **autoimmune disease**. The immunological mechanisms that mediate allergic and autoimmune responses are identical to the responses to infectious agents, only the antigens are different. In this chapter, we will discuss the deleterious effects of "inappropriate" responses to self-constituents and overactive immune responses to environmental antigens.

AUTOIMMUNE DISEASES

In the early 1900s, Paul Ehrlich introduced the term *horror autotoxicus* to describe the inability of the immune system to react against self-constituents. Parallel to this concept is the notion that immune responses of sufficient strength and duration generated against self-constituents would result in harmful autoimmune diseases. In the years since the introduction of the *horror autotoxicus* concept, abnormal autoimmune responses have been recognized to be the primary cause of, or a secondary contributor to, several human diseases.

Breakdown of Self-Tolerance

The central role of the immune system is to discriminate

Table 10.1. Autoimmune diseases.

Organ-specific Pathology

Autoimmune Disease	Autoantigen	Hypersensitivity Reaction
Graves' Disease	Thyroid-stimulating hormone receptor	Type II
Multiple Sclerosis	Myelin antigens in CNS	Type IV
Autoimmune Hemolytic Anemia	Blood group antigens	Type II
Type I Insulin-Dependent Diabetes	Pancreatic islet cells	Type IV
Hashimoto's Thyroiditis	Thyroglobulin	Type II
Pernicious Anemia	Cofactor for the intestinal absorption of vitamin B_{12}	Type II
Addison's Disease	Adrenal cortical enzymes	Type II
Myasthenia Gravis	Acetylcholine receptor	Type II

Non-organ-specific or Systemic Pathology

Autoimmune Disease	Autoantigen	Hypersensitivity Reaction
Goodpasture's Syndrome	Non-collagenous domain of Type IV collagen in basement membranes	Type II
Rheumatoid Arthritis	Gamma globulin	Type IV
Systemic Lupus Erythematosus	DNA, histones, ribonuclear proteins	Type III

self from nonself. Competent lymphocytes must recognize and respond to foreign antigens, yet remain nonresponsive to self-antigens. In order to avoid autoreactivity, the immune system functions within the confines of **self-tolerance**, which is defined simply as the unresponsiveness of the immune system to a self-antigen. Tolerance mechanisms actively prevent the maturation and expansion of potentially self-reactive lymphocytes to maintain a self-tolerant repertoire of mature immune cells, as discussed in chapter 8. Self-tolerance mechanisms include (1) the deletion of all self-reactive lymphocytes during their maturation, (2) the preferential inactivation of helper T cells specific for self-antigens, and (3) the suppression of self-reactive T cells by regulatory cells. How then is it possible that autoimmune responses are generated in light of the fact that control mechanisms are working to prevent such occurrences? Autoimmune responses result from a breakdown of immunological tolerance. There may be an abnormal selection of self-reactive lymphocytes or an inappropriate stimulation of normally nonresponsive or anergic T cells. A breakdown in tolerance may also occur as a result of inhibiting suppressive surveillance mechanisms, or there may be a release of antigens that are normally inaccessible to immune recognition. A number of factors may be responsible for breaking self-tolerance, including genetic predispositions, infections, or immunological anomalies.

Pathogenesis
Autoimmune disease affects one to two percent of the United States population. The pathogenesis of most autoimmune diseases involves one or more of the mechanisms that mediate hypersensitivity reactions. Table 10.1 lists some of the more common autoimmune diseases, the self-antigen recognized by the immune system, and the type of immunopathogenic mechanism operating in each disease. There

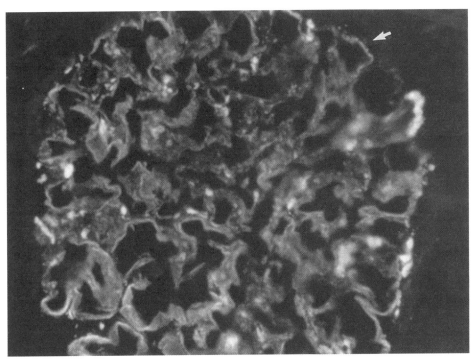

Figure 10.1. A micrograph of a section of kidney from an individual with lupus, demonstrating the presence of immunoglobulin in the glomerular capillary loops. The section was stained with fluorescent labeled antiglobulin. Arrow indicates an individual capillary loop, demonstrating granular immunofluorescence.

are at least two broad categories of autoimmune diseases based on type of lesions observed. *Organ-specific* autoimmune diseases demonstrate a restricted tissue specificity, whereas *organ-nonspecific or systemic* autoimmune diseases affect multiple tissues due to their specificity for an antigen that is widely disseminated in the body. An example of an organ specific autoimmune disease is **Hashimoto's thyroiditis**, which is a chronic condition marked by hypoactivity of the thyroid gland. Both antibodies directed against thyroglobulin and cytotoxic T cells mediate the progressive destruction of thyroid follicular cells, which eventually prevents the production of thyroid hormone. In contrast to the localized effects of Hashimoto's thyroiditis, nonorgan specific or systemic autoimmune diseases manifest clinical symptoms in many organ systems, including the skin, joints, kidney, and muscle. An example of a systemic autoimmune disease is **systemic lupus erythematosus**, referred to as SLE or lupus. SLE occurs most frequently in females (9:1 female-to-male ratio), usually between the ages of twenty and fifty years. Symptoms include fever, extreme fatigue, weight loss, skin rashes, sensitivity to sunlight, central nervous system signs, and arthritis in several joints. In these patients, autoantibodies are produced against DNA (both single-stranded and double-stranded), ribonuclear proteins, and histones. Immune complexes of DNA and autoantibodies are deposited in the skin, joints, muscle, and glomeruli of the kidney which produces a Type III hypersensitivity reaction. The deposition of immune complexes in the kidney is most damaging and can result in life-threatening glomerulonephritis. Figure 10.1 shows a section of kidney with the immune complexes that have been deposited in the glomeruli visualized by immunofluorescence. The mechanism thought to be responsible for causing the pathology observed in SLE and other immune complex diseases will be discussed in the section entitled "Type III Hypersensitivity."

One of the most common autoimmune diseases is **rheumatoid arthritis**, which affects approximately 2 million Americans, the significant majority of which are female. Unlike osteoarthritis, which develops in aging adults, rheumatoid arthritis typically strikes people between the ages of twenty-five to fifty years, but this disease can occur in young children, including infants. Clinically, rheumatoid arthritis is characterized by painful inflammation of the joints and synovium. Individuals with rheumatoid arthritis have serum IgM or IgG autoantibodies that react to the Fc portion of their own IgG, such autoantibodies are referred to as *rheumatoid factors*, and their presence is diagnostic for the disease. Immune complexes of IgG and autoantibodies accumulate in the joints and blood vessels and mediate a Type IV hypersensitivity reaction that leads to the joint inflammation and vasculitis characteristic of this disease.

The vast majority of the autoimmune diseases listed in Table 10.1 are thought to be due to humoral immunity and autoantibody formation; however, there are autoimmune diseases in which cell-mediated immunity is the primary mediator. For example, **multiple sclerosis** is due to a cellular immune response to myelin in the central nervous system. Lesions in the brain and spinal cord of MS patients have been shown to contain lymphocytes and macrophages, which mediate demyelination of the myelin sheath. As a result of these lesions, MS patients, who are generally adults between the age of twenty and forty years, suffer vision and motor abnormalities.

THE HYPERSENSITIVITIES

As previously mentioned, the immune system is essential for curing disease, but it can also be the cause of numerous clinical disorders. The hypersensitivities are inappropriate or excessive immune responses that produce tissue injury upon secondary or subsequent contact with an agent that is not intrinsically harmful. Examples of hypersensitivity reactions include allergy to ragweed pollen, a transfusion reaction following transfer of mismatched blood, the skin reaction following contact with poison ivy, and the severe glomerulonephritis that occurs following injection of antiserum obtained from another species of animal. Similar to any immune response, hypersensitivities display specificity and memory. In the 1950s, Gell and Coombs proposed a classification scheme to delineate the four types of hypersensitivities based upon the immunological mechanism involved (Table 10.2).

Type I Hypersensitivity

Type I hypersensitivity, also known as *immediate hypersensitivity*, is defined as an allergic reaction that occurs within minutes following exposure to antigen. In 1921, Prausnitz and Küstner described a phenomenon that provided insight into the mechanism of allergic reactions and provided the basis for the skin puncture test used in clinics to correlate symptoms with specific allergens. Küstner was allergic to fish, but no antibodies directed against fish antigens could be detected in his serum. Prausnitz injected a small amount of Küstner's serum into his own skin, the next day he injected a fish extract into the same site and a rapid reaction occurred. A sharply delineated, soft swelling (the "wheal") quickly appeared at the site of injection, and the skin surrounding the wheal became reddened (the "flare" or ery-

Table 10.2. The four types of hypersensitivity.

Gell & Coombs Classification		Mechanism	*Example*
Type I	Immediate Hypersensitivity	Release of allergic mediators from IgE-sensitized mast cells upon reexposure to antigen	Hay fever drug allergies
Type II	Antibody-mediated Cytotoxicity	Antibodies directed against antigens on the surface of cells mediate cytotoxic reactions	Hemolytic disease of the newborn
Type III	Immune-complex Hypersensitivity	Antigen-antibody complexes deposited in tissue activate the complement pathway and cause inflammation and tissue damage	Serum sickness
Type IV	Cell-mediated Hypersensitivity	Secondary contact with an antigen induces T lymphocytes to secrete cytokines which recruit macrophages to the site	Contact dermatitis

thema). Prausnitz and Küstner postulated that an 'atopic reagin' was present in the serum of atopic individuals. Half a century later, Ishizaka and colleagues described the atopic reagin as IgE, a new class of immunoglobulin present in the serum at very low concentrations. The wheal and flare reaction demonstrated that the skin is a suitable site for examination of antibody-mediated allergies. In order to identify an offending antigen in patients with allergies, a panel of suspected antigens, called allergens (extracts of ragweed or grass pollen, animal dander, etc.), are injected into the skin, and the injection sites are scored for any wheal and flare responses.

Allergic rhinitis (hay fever) is the most common type of immediate hypersensitivity reaction. Hay fever affects between ten to twenty percent of the U.S. population. Hay fever is a misnomer because hay does not cause the problem nor is there any fever associated with the symptomatology. The symptoms of hay fever that occur following exposure to ragweed pollen or other allergens include sneezing, itchy nose, watery eyes, headache, congestion, and sinusitis. Seasonal allergic rhinitis occurs between the months of June and September when concentrations of windborne fungus and pollen from grass, trees, and weeds are greatest. The culprits of perennial rhinitis can include pet hair, dust mites, mold spores, and cockroaches. Bronchial asthma, eczema, urticaria (hives), and food allergies are less common than hay fever but are additional examples of immediate hypersensitivity reactions to environmental allergens.

The immunological mechanism of an immediate hypersensitivity reaction involving both IgE and mast cells is shown in Figure 10.2. Once an allergen comes in contact with an individual's mucosal surface, it is phagocytosed by antigen-presenting cells (macrophages, dendritic cells) which process and present that antigen to T_H2 cells which then secrete cytokines such as IL-4 and IL-13. These cytokines induce IgE production by B lymphocytes. IgE then binds to mast cells via high affinity FcεRI receptors which specifically interact with the Fc region of IgE antibodies. The interaction of IgE with the mast cell surface is a relatively stable one, since mast cells have been shown to retain IgE molecules on their surface for up to twelve weeks. Upon reexposure to the sensitizing antigen, the surface bound IgE reacts with it and as a result FcεRI receptors become cross-linked, which activates the mast cell through a series of biochemical events, one of which is an increase in

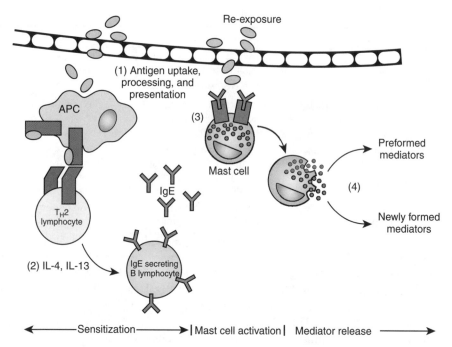

Figure 10.2. *Type I Hypersensitivity.* Sensitization of mast cells begins with primary exposure to an allergen that enters the skin or mucosal surface. Antigen-presenting cells engulf the allergen then process and present it to T helper cells (1). T_H2 cells secrete IL-4 and IL-13 which induce B cells to produce allergen-specific IgE (2). IgE molecules bind to FcεRI receptors on the surface of mast cells (3). Upon reexposure to the allergen, IgE and therefore FcεRI receptors are cross-linked, initiating mast cell activation and inducing (4) degranulation and release of preformed and newly synthesized mediators of inflammation.

intracellular calcium. Preformed mediators (histamine and proteases) and newly formed mediators (leukotrienes and prostaglandins) are subsequently released by the mast cell. Cytokines, such as TNFα and IL-4, are also released from mast cells to amplify the inflammatory response. Within two to four hours after the initiation of an immediate hypersensitivity response, a late phase reaction can occur. The late phase reaction arises after the wheal and flare have diminished and at the site of inflammation there is an accumulation of eosinophils. The late phase component of immediate hypersensitivity reactions is IgE-dependent and cannot be inhibited by antihistamines.

Mast Cells and Basophils
Mast cells are derived from bone marrow progenitor cells. Two types of mast cells have been described based on their tissue distribution, staining characteristics, and the proteases they contain. The two types of mast cells are also functionally different in their response to drugs that stimulate degranulation or that inhibit histamine release. **Connective tissue mast cells** are found around blood vessels in most tissues, and **mucosal mast cells** are found predominantly in the mucosa of the gut and lung (Figure 10.3). Mucosal mast cells contain relatively little histamine, and chondroitin sulfate is the predominant proteoglycan present in their granules. Connective tissue mast cells predominantly contain the proteoglycan heparin in their

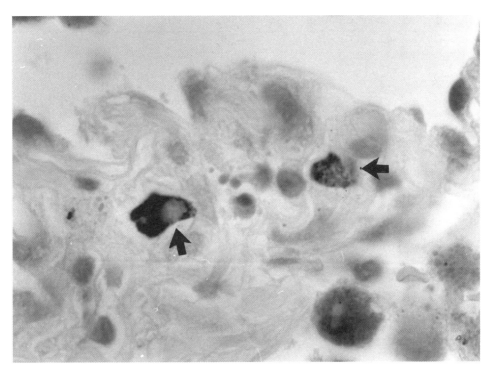

Figure 10.3. Photomicrograph of mucosal cells from the lung alveolar septa stained with methylene blue. Note the intensely staining granules within these mast cells. Arrows indicate mast cells in the tissue. (Oil immersion view.)

granules, and they produce large quantities of histamine. Experiments in mice suggest that mast cell phenotypes can be interchanged depending on the micro-environment. Thus, the type of mast cell and its chemical mediators can vary depending on its anatomic location.

Basophils are similar to mast cells, but they are found mostly in the bloodstream. They are derived from the bone marrow and can synthesize many of the same mediators as mast cells. Both mast cells and basophils bind IgE on their surface via Fcε receptors, and both cell types degranulate when their Fcε receptors are cross-linked. Basophils are terminally differentiated, circulating granulocytes that can infiltrate tissues through the action of their adhesion molecules. Basophils are distinct from mast cells because they are derived from a separate lineage, mature in the bone marrow, and circulate upon maturity. In contrast to basophils, mature mast cells do not normally circulate but mature within the vascularized tissues where they reside.

IgE-Mediated Activation of Mast Cells and Basophils
Mast cells and basophils are activated by antigen-bridged IgE molecules bound to FcεRI molecules on their surface. The biochemical events that occur following receptor cross-linking and which result in mast cell degranulation are not completely understood or have only been partially elucidated. However, it is clear that several intracellular signal transduction pathways are activated. While FcεRI subunits lack any known enzymatic activity, this receptor associates with protein tyrosine kinases, and protein tyrosine phosphorylation is essential for FcεRI-

Table 10.3. Mediators of immediate hypersensitivity reactions.

Preformed Mediators (stored in cytoplasmic granules)

Examples	Biological Effects
Histamine	Vasodilation; contraction of smooth muscle in bronchial and gastrointestinal tract
Heparin	Anticoagulant; modulation of proteases; inhibition of complement
Neutral proteases	
Tryptase	Tissue destruction
Chymase	Digestion of basement membranes

Newly Generated Mast Cell Mediators

Examples	Biological Effects
Prostaglandin D_2	Bronchoconstriction; peripheral vasodilation; inhibition of platelet aggregation; neutrophil chemoattractant
Leukotrienes C_4, D_4, E_4	Potent bronchoconstriction; increase vascular permeability
Platetlet Activating Factor (PAF)	Aggregation of platelets; chemotaxis and degranulation in eosinophils and neutrophils; increase vascular permeability; bronchoconstriction

Cytokines

Examples	Biological Effects
TNFα, IL-1, IL-4, IL-5, IL-6 and IL-3	Modulation of IgE synthesis; recruitment of inflammatory cells; leukocyte adhesion

mediated degranulation. Tyrosine phosphorylation of phospholipase C induces the breakdown of membrane phosphatidylinositol 4,5-bisphosphate, resulting in the formation of 1,2-diacylglycerol (DAG) and inositol 1,4,5-triphosphate (IP_3). IP_3 and DAG serve as second messenger molecules, which release cytoplasmic calcium from internal stores and activate protein kinase C, respectively. Activation of PKC and a rise in Ca^{2+} concentration leads to maximal mast cell secretory activity; however, IP_3 alone does not account for the elevation of intracellular calcium. It has recently been shown that FcεRI activates a sphingosine kinase pathway to mobilize calcium. Many of the regulatory functions of calcium are mediated through the Ca^{2+}-binding protein calmodulin. Ca^{2+}-calmodulin complexes are involved in the disassembly of the cytoskeleton, which allows granules to fuse with the plasma membrane and release their preformed mediators into the extracellular environment. In addition, Ca^{2+}-calmodulin complexes mediate activation of phospholipase A_2, which is important for generation of arachidonic acid, an important intermediate in lipid (prostaglandin and leukotriene) biosynthesis. Lastly, crosslinking FcεRI activates the adenylate cyclase pathway, which results in the conversion of ATP to cAMP and subsequent activation of protein kinase A. Both cAMP and protein kinase A may also be involved in the regulation of degranulation processes.

Preformed and Newly Formed Mediators
Because mast cells are heterogeneous, the same mediators are not released by all mast cells once degranulation occurs. However, the mediators synthesized by most mast cells and basophils can be divided into three general types: 1) preformed mediators that are packaged into granules, 2) newly formed mediators (membrane-derived lipids), and 3) cytokines. Examples of these types of mediators are outlined in Table 10.3. Preformed mediators are low molecular weight compounds that struc-

turally contain an amine group and functionally exhibit vasoactive properties. This group includes histamine, proteases, heparin, eosinophil chemotactic factor, and neutrophil chemotactic factor. These substances are stored in the cytoplasm within granules and can be released immediately upon degranulation. These mediators have a variety of biological effects. For example, histamine, which is the major pre-formed mediator present in the human mast cell, causes contraction of smooth muscle in the bronchioles, vascular dilation with accompanying increases in vascular permeability, and increases in nasal secretions. Histamine also produces the wheal and flare response. Histamine binds to specific receptors on different target cells and initiates intracellular biochemical events that invoke different results depending on the target cell type. Such effects are usually evident within one to two minutes after exposure of an allergic individual to the inciting antigen. Proteases such as tryptase and chymase may increase vascular permeability by digesting the blood vessel basement membrane. Heparin may complex with the proteases within the granule and may decrease their deleterious effects once the granules are released into the extracellular space. Finally, chemotactic factors for eosinophils and neutrophils are present in the granules and account for the influx of these cells into areas of mast cell degranulation.

The second class of mediators released by activated mast cells are the newly formed mediators. Generation of lipid mediators begins with the activation of the enzyme phospholipase A_2, which catalyzes the release of arachidonic acid from the membrane phospholipids. Arachidonic acid is then sequentially metabolized by the enzymes in one of two separate pathways: **the cyclooxygenase pathway** that produces the prostaglandins or **the 5-lipoxygenase pathway** that forms the leukotrienes. During allergic reactions, prostaglandin D_2 induces vasodilation and bronchoconstriction. The leukotrienes C_4, D_4, and E_4, previously referred to as slow-reacting substance of anaphylaxis, mediate prolonged bronchoconstriction, vasopermeability, and mucus secretion. Another derivative of phospholipid is platelet activating factor, which aggregates platelets, leading to microthrombi. Platelet activating factor also causes severe bronchoconstriction, increases vasopermeability, and augments chemotaxis of neutrophils. Whereas mast cells have been shown to produce prostaglandin D_2, the leukotrienes, and PAF, basophils apparently synthesize only the leukotrienes (See chapter 4).

Mast cells have recently been shown to synthesize and secrete cytokines. Cytokines are a diverse group of glycoproteins secreted by a variety of cells, and they modulate immune responses through their ability to alter the function of responsive target cells. TNFα, IL-1, IL-3, IL-4, IL-5, IL-6, IL-8, and chemokines, which are involved in the migration of leukocytes to a site of inflammation, are among the cytokine mediators produced by mast cells. Cytokine-dependent processes in allergic inflammation include upregulation of IgE synthesis and recruitment of eosinophils, macrophages, and T cells to the inflamed area. In addition, cytokines enhance leukocyte expression of adhesion molecules, such as E-selectin , vascular cell adhesion molecule-1 (VCAM-1), and intercellular adhesion molecule-1 (ICAM-1) on vascular endothelial cells. The function of these cytokines is particularly important during the late phase reaction of Type I hypersensitivity.

Immunotherapy for Allergies
Allergies to certain foods, dust, or animal dander can be controlled by avoidance of the allergen. However, ubiquitous allergens such as ragweed, grasses, or certain

tree pollens are difficult to avoid. Many allergy patients undergo **allergen immunotherapy,** which is a technique that involves subcutaneous injection of increasing doses of an allergen over a period of weeks or months in hopes of reducing allergen-specific IgE levels. Allergen immunotherapy has proven successful for treatment of allergic asthma and rhinitis, but the mechanism by which this treatment improves clinical symptoms is not entirely clear. Following repeated injections of allergen, there is an increase in antigen-specific IgG antibodies, which are postulated to function by neutralizing antigen, by blocking the interaction of antigen and IgE, and by negatively regulating IgE production through antibody feedback mechanisms. Desensitization through continued allergen injection could also downregulate IgE production by shifting the predominance of antigen-specific T_H2 T lymphocytes to T_H1 cells or by inducing specific T cell tolerance.

New immunotherapeutic treatments for allergies are currently in the initial stages of evaluation. Peptide immunotherapy involves the injection of allergen peptides that maintain T cell reactivity but possess reduced IgE-binding. Some patients allergic to cats showed marked improvement when immunized with an immunodominant peptide derived from a cat dander protein. Treatment with anti-IgE antibodies has also been shown to be effective in decreasing serum IgE levels and in blocking IgE-mediated allergic symptoms in humans.

Pharmacologic Interventions in the Treatment of Allergies
Current therapies for allergy attempt to prevent the release of inflammatory mediators from mast cells or to interfere with the actions of such mediators. For example, **antihistamines** are administered to antagonize the binding of histamine to its receptors and to counteract the effects of histamine. Antihistamines inhibit the wheal and flare response, but they do not block constriction of smooth muscle. **Sodium cromolyn** benefits patients with allergic disorders, such as asthma, and is thought to inhibit inflammatory cell activation and mediator release. **Epinephrine** and **theophylline** also inhibit mast cell activation. In addition, these drugs counteract the effect of leukotrienes on smooth muscle by acting as bronchodilators. Prevention of bronchoconstriction is currently being attempted by administration of drugs that inhibit leukotriene synthesis and antagonize leukotriene receptors. **Corticosteroids** are the most potent anti-inflammatory drugs available. Corticosteroids not only diminish inflammatory cell activation and function, they also block the transcription of cytokine genes, including those for TNF and IL-4 production. Corticosteroids can be detrimental to health and produce undesirable effects, so they must be used with great care.

Type II Hypersensitivity
Type II hypersensitivity (also referred to as *cytotoxic hypersensitivity*) is mediated by IgG or IgM antibodies that bind specifically to cell surface or extracellular matrix constituents. Antibodies bound to cell surface constituents can bind and activate complement. Complement participates in Type II hypersensitivity reactions by acting as an opsonin or by directly lysing the antibody-coated cells. Examples of Type II hypersensitivity reactions include incompatible blood transfusions, hemolytic disease of the newborn, and autoimmune hemolytic anemia. The transfusion of incompatible blood results in antibody and complement-mediated destruction of the transfused erythrocytes. Patients with autoimmune hemolytic anemia produce antibody directed against their own red blood cells. In some cases, antibodies are directed against drugs (penicillin, quinine, and sulphonamides) or drug metabolites

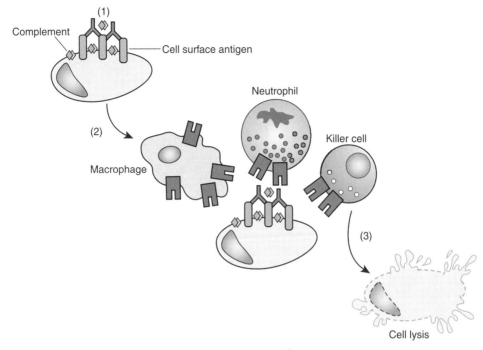

Figure 10.4. *Type II Hypersensitivity.* (1) IgG or IgM antibodies bind to cell surface constituents. Complement then binds to the antibodies and becomes activated. (2) Complement activation results in recruitment of cytotoxic cells such as macrophages, neutrophils, or killer cells. These effector cells bind to the target cell via Fc and/or complement receptors and (3) attempt to destroy the cell through lysis or phagocytosis.

that are bound to the erythrocyte or platelet surface. Immune complexes consisting of drug and antibody can also be adsorbed onto the RBC surface.

The critical event in any Type II hypersensitivity reaction is the binding of IgG or IgM antibodies to cell surface antigens (Figure 10.4). Events occurring after the antibody initially binds to the target cell depend on the class or subclass of antibody and the nature of the cell involved. If the antibody is IgM, IgG_1, IgG_2, or IgG_3, then the $\overline{C1q}$ component of complement binds to the Fc region and becomes activated. This initiates activation of the classical complement pathway and terminates with the formation of the $\overline{C5b6789}$ membrane attack complex in the lipid bilayer leading to osmotic lysis of the affected cell (see chapter 9). Induction of the classical complement pathway also generates $\overline{C3b}$, which can covalently bind to the membrane of target cells. $\overline{C3b}$ serves as an opsonin, since neutrophils and macrophages have CR1 receptors which specifically bind $\overline{C3b}$. As a result, effector cells phagocytize the entire cell-antibody-$\overline{C3b}$ complex and destroy it.

A well-known example of a disease mediated by Type II hypersensitivity reactions is erythroblastosis fetalis, also known as **hemolytic disease of the newborn** (Figure 10.5). This condition affects infants born to mothers who do not express the Rhesus (Rh) blood group antigen. The erythrocytes of these babies are Rh^+ because of paternal Rh^+ genes. An Rh^- mother carrying an Rh^+ fetus becomes sensitized to Rh^+ erythrocytes during gestation and the delivery process. During subsequent pregnancies, maternal IgG specific for fetal erythrocytes crosses the placenta and mediates red cell destruction, which can lead to death of the fetus. Prevention of

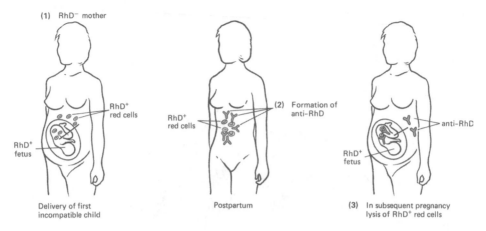

(1) RhD⁻ mother

RhD⁺ red cells

RhD⁺ fetus

Delivery of first incompatible child

RhD⁺ red cells

(2) Formation of anti-RhD

Postpartum

(3) In subsequent pregnancy lysis of RhD⁺ red cells

anti-RhD

RhD⁺ fetus

Figure 10.5. Immunologic events occurring in erythroblastosis fetalis. An RhD⁻ mother carrying an RhD⁺ fetus is exposed to fetal red blood cells carrying the RhD antigen during delivery of the baby (1). During the postpartum period, the mother forms antibodies directed against the RhD antigen (2). In subsequent pregnancies where the fetus is RhD⁺, maternal antibodies (containing anti-RhD antibodies) cross the placenta and can cause red cell destruction (3). Erythroblastosis fetalis can be prevented by giving the mother an injection of antibody directed against the RhD antigen upon birth of the fetus, thus eliminating the fetal cells from the maternal circulation before antibody can be formed.

erythroblastosis fetalis involves immunologic intervention once an incompatibility between mother and father at the Rh locus is detected. Immediately after each birth, an Rh⁻ mother is injected with preformed anti-RhD-antibodies, which bind to fetal Rh⁺ cells and prevents the maternal immune system from recognizing the fetal erythrocytes.

There are additional antibody-mediated diseases in which autoantibodies to cellular and tissue antigens produce immunopathological damage through Type II hypersensitivity mechanisms. For example, patients with **Goodpasture's syndrome** produce IgG antibodies specific for a domain of type IV collagen in glomerular basement membranes. Clinically, patients with Goodpasture's syndrome develop nephritis that is sometimes associated with lung hemorrhages as a result of the local activation of complement and neutrophils in the renal glomeruli and pulmonary alveoli. **Myasthenia gravis** is an example of a disease in which antibody inhibits the function of particular cells. Patients with myasthenia gravis produce antibodies to acetylcholine receptors on the surface of muscle cells. The binding of antibody to acetylcholine receptors interferes with neuromuscular transmission by downmodulating the number of receptors responsive to acetylcholine. Progressive muscle weakness results from a failure of muscle cells to respond to nerve impulses. While autoantibodies are associated with certain immunologic diseases, the question remains as to whether the antibodies are the cause or the result of tissue and cellular damage.

Type III Hypersensitivity

Type III hypersensitivity, also known as *immune-complex disease*, is triggered by the deposition of immune complexes in tissue (Figure 10.6). Each time an antibody binds its antigen, immune complexes are formed, but they are usually removed

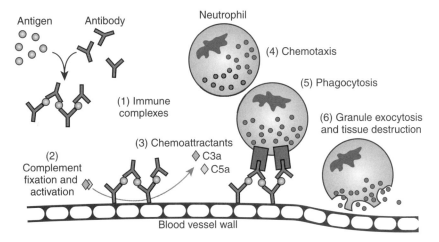

Figure 10.6. *Type III Hypersensitivity.* Immune complexes (1), formed when antigen and antibody molecules combine, deposit on tissues, where they fix complement (2). Activation of complement results in the release of complement split products $\overline{C3a}$ and $\overline{C5a}$ (3). The $\overline{C5a}$ is chemotactic (4) for neutrophils which attempt to phagocytose (5) the complexes. Exocytosis of granules (6) and release of enzymes causes damage to endothelial cells and the underlying basement membrane, whether in the kidney, lung, or blood vessel walls.

without incident by the reticuloendothelial system (mononuclear phagocytes in the liver, spleen, and lungs). However, immune complexes that persist in the circulation can be deposited in arteries, renal glomeruli, or joint synovia where complement and inflammatory cells are activated and cause tissue damage. This effect was discovered when patients became ill after being passively immunized with horse derived antiserum for diphtheria or tetanus infections. The horse antiserum was given to save the patient's life; however, it often produced a syndrome characterized by fever, hives, arthritis, and proteinuria. This syndrome was later referred to as **serum sickness**. The immunopathology associated with serum sickness was studied experimentally in animals. Rabbits injected with a foreign antigen, in this case bovine serum albumin (or BSA), produced anti-BSA antibodies, which complexed with BSA to accelerate clearance of the antigen from the blood. During this process, large immune complexes became deposited in various tissues, where they fixed and activated complement. As discussed previously, the activation of the classical complement pathway not only induces recruitment of inflammatory cells, such as neutrophils, but complement activation also results in the production of **anaphylatoxins** $\overline{C3a}$ and $\overline{C5a}$ (Figure 10.6). These products elicit the release of vasoactive amines, including histamine, which increase local vascular permeability. In addition, $\overline{C5a}$ is chemotactic for polymorphonuclear neutrophils (PMNs), basophils, and eosinophils. PMNs attempt to bind and phagocytize immune complexes through their Fc and $\overline{C3b}$ receptors; however, they are unable to accomplish this feat due to the fact that the immune complexes are bound to vessel walls. As a result, the neutrophils exocytose the enzymatic contents (lysosomal enzymes) of their granules onto the vessel endothelium, causing local tissue damage. The hallmarks of Type III hypersensitivity are necrosis and neutrophil infiltration. An example of immune complex mediated vasculitis is the **Arthus reaction**, which is a characteristic skin lesion induced by the subcutaneous injection of antigen into a

Table 10.4.   Factors that influence the deposition of immune complexes.

1) The **size** of the circulating immune complexes

2) The **ability of the host to clear immune complexes** from the circulation. Patients with deficiencies in their complement system cannot properly solubilize or clear immune complexes. The rate of clearance is also dependent on the efficiency of the mononuclear phagocyte system.

3) **Biochemical properties** of the antigen and antibody, such as immunoglobulin isotype, molecular charge, antibody valence, and the avidity of the interaction between antibody and antigen.

4) **Anatomic** and **hemodynamic factors**

hyperimmune animal. The resulting inflammation and tissue injury peaks four to eight hours after initiation of the reaction; therefore, the Arthus reaction develops more slowly than immediate hypersensitivity but more rapidly than delayed-type hypersensitivity. An example of an immune complex-mediated disease is **systemic lupus erythematosis (SLE)** in which immune complexes formed between DNA and anti-DNA antibody are deposited in the glomeruli of the kidneys and at other sites where they cause nephritis, arthritis, and vasculitis.

There is some evidence that individuals who develop Type III hypersensitivity have a defect in the macrophage mediated clearance of immune complexes. There are a number of factors that determine the extent of immune complex deposition (Table 10.4). First, the size of immune complexes in part determines their persistence in the blood. Very small complexes are not deposited, whereas large immune complexes are removed quickly by mononuclear phagocytes because larger antigen-antibody complexes bind and activate complement more efficiently. Small and medium-sized immune complexes are more likely deposited. Secondly, the deposition of immune complexes in tissue appears to be triggered by an increase in local vascular permeability. For example, complement split products as well as mediators released by mast cells, basophils, and platelets, participate in the release of vasoactive amines. When this release occurs within a blood vessel, these mediators cause retraction of endothelial cells, exposure of the underlying basement membrane, and increased blood flow and capillary permeability. The plasma containing the complexes passes into the tissues where they are deposited. Third, immune complex deposition is observed in certain locations within the body more often than in others. For instance, sites of biological filtration such as the renal glomerulus or choroid plexus are particularly susceptible to immune complex-mediated damage. At these sites, fluids in the blood pass through filtering membranes, and the complexes are often retained on the filtering surfaces. Sites of high blood pressure and turbulence, such as the glomerular capillaries, are also susceptible to immune complex deposition, since the turbulence may bring the small complexes together and result in their aggregation and deposition.

Type IV Hypersensitivity
Type IV hypersensitivity is also known as *delayed hypersensitivity* since the obvious signs of these reactions are observed twenty-four hours or more after contact with the antigen. In contrast to the first three types of hypersensitivity, which are antibody-mediated, type IV hypersensitivity reactions are cell-mediated immune responses involving T lymphocytes and activated macrophages (Figure 10.7). The most commonly recognized form of delayed hypersensitivity is **allergic contact**

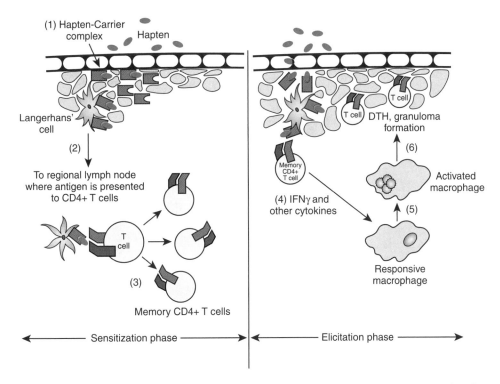

Figure 10.7. *Type IV Hypersensitivity.* During the sensitization phase, hapten molecules complex with carrier proteins in the skin (1). Hapten-carrier complexes are picked up by Langerhans' cells, which then migrate to the regional lymph nodes and present antigen to $CD4^+$ T cells (2). Hapten-specific, memory T cells are generated (3). Reexposure to the specific antigen initiates release of IFNγ and other cytokines from the memory T cells (4). These cytokines drive the activation of resting macrophages (5). Activated macrophages participate in the cell-mediated reactions such as delayed type hypersensitivity and granuloma formation (6).

dermatitits, best exemplified by the acute eczema that develops following exposure to poison ivy. Other common allergens that induce allergic contact dermatitis include rubber, nickel, fragrances, cosmetics, and topical antibiotics. The contact dermatitis that may develop following exposure of a sensitized individual to bath soap is a typical form of DTH (Figure 10.8). More severe forms of DTH reactions have been observed in certain disease states such as leprosy or tuberculosis, where the antigen is persistent and cannot easily be eliminated by macrophages.

The mechanisms responsible for delayed type hypersensitivity reactions are quite different from the antibody-mediated hypersensitivities discussed previously. A person must first become sensitized to an allergen for a DTH response to occur. Generally, the agents that incite delayed-type hypersensitivity are usually very small, low molecular weight, but highly reactive haptens, which are not immunogenic by themselves. The sensitization phase of DTH begins when haptens penetrate the skin and complex with a carrier (Figure 10.7). When coupled to a carrier protein in the skin, the complexes can elicit a cell mediated immune response. Langerhans' cells located in the epidermis (basal cell region) process and present the antigens on their surface in the context of MHC Class II molecules. The Langerhans' cells migrate from the skin to regional lymph nodes where they interact with $CD4^+$ Th

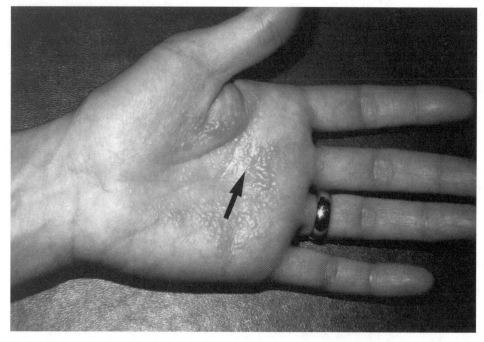

Figure 10.8.   Photograph of a hand affected by allergic contact dermatitis (arrow) following exposure to bath soap. Low molecular weight chemicals contained in the soap bind to skin proteins, and the combination produces a hapten-carrier conjugate that is immunogenic. This reaction is T cell-mediated, and histologically, both macrophages and lymphocytes are seen infiltrating the underlying tissue.

cells which recognize the antigen/MHC via the T cell receptor complex. Both the T cells and the Langerhans' cells become activated. The Langerhans' cells secrete IL-1, which stimulates T cells to secrete IL-2. IL-2 mediates the expansion of T cells capable of recognizing the hapten. The antigen-specific T cells circulate through the vasculature and come to rest in the skin.

Upon reexposure to the allergen, the Langerhans' cells again process and present the antigen to the primed T cells, which initiate the elicitation phase of DTH in the skin. Activated, memory T cells release a number of soluble mediators termed cytokines. In particular, interferon gamma (IFNγ) activates macrophages and enhances their ability to eliminate the antigen. IFNγ increases phagocytosis, antigen presenting efficiency, and microbicidal activity. Because it is a potent macrophage activating cytokine, IFNγ is the most potent mediator of DTH reactions. IFNγ also increases the expression of adhesion molecules on endothelial cells and potentiates the release of proinflammatory cytokines and chemokines. This complex cascade of events results in the recruitment and activation of many T cells and macrophages in the local inflammatory site. Upon gross examination of the DTH reaction site, the area is erythematous and "indurated" or hard to the touch. Resolution of DTH reactions occurs after forty-eight to seventy-two hours, and the mechanism of suppression involves secretion of prostaglandin E_2 and downregulatory cytokines, such as TGFβ and IL-10. Both TGFβ and PGE_2 have inhibitory effects on IL-1 and IL-2 synthesis; whereas, IL-10 downregulates Class II molecules and inhibits antigen-specific proliferation of IFNγ-secreting T cells.

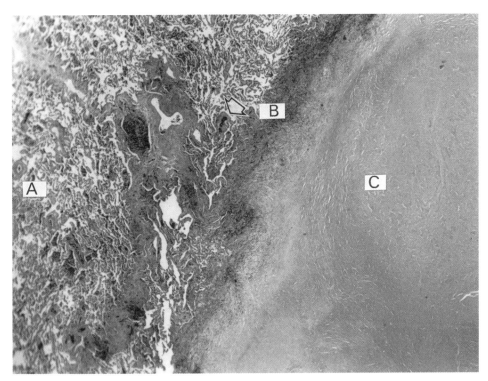

Figure 10.9. Photomicrograph of a tissue section containing a granulomatous reaction in the lung of an individual with tuberculosis. Note lung tissue (A), zone of inflammation with lymphocytes and macrophages (B), and remains of dead tissue (C). The lesion (C) is an example of caseous necrosis. Arrow indicates a multinucleated giant cell (low power view).

From a clinical standpoint, the most significant of the DTH reactions is the **granulomatous** inflammation (Figure 10.9) that develops following infection with microbes such as *Mycobacterium tuberculosis, Mycobacterium leprae,* or *Schistosoma.* These pathogens persist because macrophage microbicidal mechanisms fail to effectively eliminate them from host tissues. Granulomatous inflammation results from an attempt by the host to localize and prevent the spread of the invading microorganisms. Granuloma formation involves macrophages and epithelioid cells. Contained within the granuloma core may be **giant cells**, which are formed by the fusion of multiple epithelioid cells or macrophages. Giant cells are visible as large cells with many nuclei located around their outer edge. Epithelioid cells and giant cells are believed to be derived from macrophages and represent a terminal stage of differentiation. Surrounding the granuloma core is an area of actively proliferating lymphocytes, and there may be an area of fibrosis (scarring) due to the body's healing response to tissue injury. The end result is a palpable, granular mass of inflammatory tissue, the center of which contains dead tissue (referred to as *caseous necrosis*) due to the frustrated actions of T cells and macrophages.

SUMMARY

In this chapter, we have discussed various ways in which the immune system can mediate pathological damage to the host. For example, the immune system may react against self-antigens, such as DNA in the case of lupus, or against thyroid antigens in the case of thyroiditis. The end result may be systemic autoimmune disease in the former case, or organ-specific disease in the latter case. Systemic and organ-specific autoimmune diseases may also be classified according to the mechanism responsible for their immunopathology. Type I hypersensitivity, exemplified by hay fever, is due to the formation of excessive amounts of IgE antibodies specific for an allergen. These antibodies are capable of binding to FcεRI molecules on the surface of mast cells and basophils. Binding of antigen to IgE cross-links FcεRI molecules, and the mediators contained within mast cell cytoplasmic granules are then released, causing tissue damage. Type II hypersensitivity, as illustrated by transfusion reactions, is caused by IgG or IgM antibody directed against a cell surface antigen. Binding of antibody to the cell is accompanied by fixation of complement and destruction of the cell to which the antibody is bound. Type III hypersensitivity, exemplified by systemic lupus erythematosus, is due to immune complex deposition in tissues. Fixation of complement by the immune complexes causes the release of complement split products, which are chemotactic for neutrophils and also cause basophil degranulation. The contents of neutrophil and basophil granules may directly damage host tissue. Lastly, there is Type IV hypersensitivity, which mediates poison ivy, tuberculosis, and leprosy. This type of hypersensitivity is caused by T cell and macrophage activation in response to a skin-sensitizing compound or a persistent infection. Although there are four discrete types of hypersensitivity reactions, it is important to remember that any combination of these reactions may occur simultaneously in a given individual.

SUGGESTIONS FOR FURTHER READING

1. Baker, J.R. "Primer on Allergic and Immunologic Diseases." *Journal of the American Medical Association* 278, no. 22 (1977):1799-2034.
2. Middleton, E., C.E. Reed, E.F. Ellis, N.F. Adkinson, J.W. Yunginger, and W.W. Busse. *Allergy, Principles & Practice.* St. Louis: Mosby-Year Book, 1998 .
3. Roitt, I., J. Brostoff, and D.K. Male. *Immunology.* New York: C.V. Mosby, 1998
4. Abbas, A.K., A.H. Lichtman, and J.S. Pober. *Cellular and Molecular Immunology.* Philadelphia: W.B. Saunders, 1994

QUESTIONS

1. Discuss the various immunological failures that may lead to the development of autoimmune diseases.
2. List the distinguishing characteristics of connective tissue and mucosal mast cells.
3. Describe the differences between Type I vs. Type IV hypersensitivities. Give an example of a disease whose pathology is mediated by each of these reactions.
4. Describe the conditions that lead to granuloma formation and list the histological features of a granuloma.

ANSWERS

1. Autoimmune diseases result from a breakdown of immunological self-tolerance. Failure to maintain self-tolerance may occur if immunological surveillance mechanisms are inhibited or if there are faulty selection processes occurring in the thymus or bone marrow during lymphocyte development. Likewise, tolerance can be reversed if self-antigens normally sequestered in immunologically privileged sites

somehow become readily available to interact with and be recognized by immune cells.

2. Mast cells can be differentiated based on their anatomical location and cytoplasmic granule content. Connective tissue mast cells are often found adjacent to blood vessels in most tissues; their granules contain high levels of histamine; and heparin is the major proteoglycan present in their granules. Mucosal mast cells, on the other hand, are found mostly in the gut and lung; their granules contain lower levels of histamine than connective tissue mast cells; and chondroitin sulfate is the predominant proteoglycan in their granules.

3. Both immediate and delayed-type hypersensitivity reactions require prior sensitization to an antigen; however, the symptomatology and effector mechanisms that mediate each of these reactions are quite different. Type I reactions are rapid, producing a wheal and flare reaction within minutes after exposure to an allergen. Type I hypersensitivity reactions involve IgE and mast cell mediators. Hay fever and hives are classic examples of immediate hypersensitivity. In contrast, Type IV reactions produce an indurated lesion within twenty-four to forty-eight hours after antigen exposure. Antibody is not involved in Type IV hypersensitivity reactions. The cellular constituents of Type IV hypersensitivity are T cells and macrophages. Rheumatoid arthritis and multiple sclerosis are two autoimmune diseases whose pathologies involve Type IV reactions. Tuberculosis and leprosy are two chronic, infectious diseases in which Type IV granulomatous hypersensitivity is apparent.

4. Granuloma formation is consistently associated with infections involving *Mycobacterium tuberculosis* and *Mycobacterium leprae*, intracellular parasites which persist in macrophages because microbicidal mechanisms fail. Essentially, the immune system tries to localize the infection by building a wall around the site of infection. As a result, there is formation of a granulomatous lesion, which upon histological examination is shown to contain macrophages or giant cells, epithelioid cells, T lymphocytes, and fibrosis.

CHAPTER **11**

THE PHENOMENON OF
  REJECTION
TYPES OF GRAFTS
FORMS OF GRAFT RE-
  JECTION
  Hyperacute Rejection
  Acute Rejection
  Chronic Rejection
HISTOCOMPATIBILITY
  ANTIGENS
IMMUNOLOGIC MECH-
  ANISMS OF ALLOGRAFT
  REJECTION
T CELL ALLORECOGNITION
  PATHWAYS
T LYMPHOCYTE ACTIVA-
  TION
CYTOKINES
CYTOKINE PROMOTER
  REGION POLYMORPHISM
MIXED LYMPHOCYTE
  CULTURES
GENERATION AND DETEC-
  TION OF CYTOTOXIC T
  LYMPHOCYTES
CLINICAL STRATEGIES FOR
  AVOIDANCE OF GRAFT
  REJECTION
  Tissue Matching
  Immunosuppression
SPECIAL CONSIDERATIONS:
  RETRANSPLANTS
SPECIAL CONSIDERATIONS:
  TRANSPLANTATION OF
  SPECIFIC TISSUES
SUMMARY
SUGGESTIONS FOR
  FURTHER READING
QUESTIONS
ANSWERS

The Host Response to Grafts and Transplantation Immunology

Armead H. Johnson

THE PHENOMENON OF REJECTION

Early attempts at tissue transplantation revealed the existence of strong, immunologic responses that destroy transplanted tissues. These responses effectively eliminate the possibility of tissue transplantation into immunologically competent recipients in the absence of tissue matching or immunosuppression. Since the practice of tissue transplantation is a product of twentieth century medicine, it is difficult to explain the evolutionary significance of an immunologic process designed to prevent tissue exchange, and thus frustrate transplant surgeons. In fact, graft rejection is caused by immunologic mechanisms that are regularly employed to assure survival of the individual by controlling infection. The rejection of foreign tissues is therefore the result of strongly selected and highly conserved immunologic mechanisms, the functions of which are the identification and elimination of "nonself" or foreign, be that infectious agents or transplantated foreign tissue.

In general, the vertebrate immune system is capable of mounting a rapid, efficient response to foreign material which invades its body. Frequently invasion by microorganisms follows trauma to tissue or destruction of tissue, and tissue damage may be one of the initial factors alerting the immune system to infection. Tissue damage activates the bradykinin, clotting, fibrinolytic, and complement systems, and thus initiates inflammation in the damaged site. If the invaders are capable of rapid reproduction, then the immune system must rapidly mobilize its responses to contain the invader before it can become widely disseminated. The immune system cannot know the nature of the foreign material it might encounter at the site of invasion, and thus, it cannot selectively mobilize factors specific for any particular infectious agent, but rather must concentrate all of its defense mechanisms at the site of injury. This may explain why a variety of defensive cells accumulate at sites of tissue injury. Presumably, these cells are called to the site as part of the localized inflammatory response by general chemotactic mechanisms. If no microorganisms are encountered, the tissue damage is repaired and the inflammatory response wanes. However, if microorganisms are encountered, additional immune mechanisms are triggered that direct development of an inducible immune response. If a tissue graft is present instead of a microorganism at the site of injury, the response is the same. An immune response is mounted against the transplanted tissue. Rejection of the foreign tissue is accompanied by a prominent inflammatory response and considerable infiltration of the grafted tissue by cells. In the absence of treatment to induce immunosuppression, the destruction of grafted tissue is, however, usually efficient and relentless.

TYPES OF GRAFTS

Most of the grafts that are transplanted are *allografts*, or grafts between individuals of the same species. Such individuals are not genetically identical unless they are identical twins. *Allografts* can come from twins, parents, relatives, or unrelated individuals. Transplantation of grafts between identical siblings, or between mice of the same strain, are termed *syngeneic*. Not many humans needing grafts are lucky enough to have an identical twin to supply grafts. Such grafts, when available, are not recognized as foreign by the host because they are the same as self, i.e, not foreign. The term *autograft* means that the grafted tissue is from the same individual, such as skin transplanted from one part of the body to cover a part that has been damaged by a burn. Finally, the term *xenograft* refers to grafts between individuals of different species. Successful xenografting is a desirable goal since there are not enough human organs to be transplanted into all of the individuals that need an organ graft. Miniature pigs, because they are of a similar size with a similar circulation to that of humans, have been farmed to use as organ donors for humans. Recently, ethical review boards have blocked transplantation of organs between animals and humans because of the possibility of transmission of animal retro viruses to humans. An example of such a transfer is the human immunodeficiency virus that causes AIDS. AIDS is believed to have been transferred from chimpanzees, in whom it does not cause disease, to humans, in whom it does.

FORMS OF GRAFT REJECTION

The most practical definition of graft rejection derives from its most obvious clinical manifestation, loss of graft function. Functional impairment is the result of progressive destruction of the graft, most of which is due to immunological rejection. Currently, there are at least three recognized forms of graft rejection by the immune system that can be distinguished on the basis of rate, immunologic characteristics, and degree of susceptibility to immunosuppressive strategies. These are hyperacute rejection, acute rejection, and chronic rejection.

Hyperacute Rejection

This form of rejection occurs in recipients of vascularized grafts that have graft-reactive antibodies circulating in their blood prior to transplantation. These recipients have been sensitized to tissue antigens previously by blood transfusions, previous allografts or pregnancy where the tissues of the fetus, containing histocompatibility

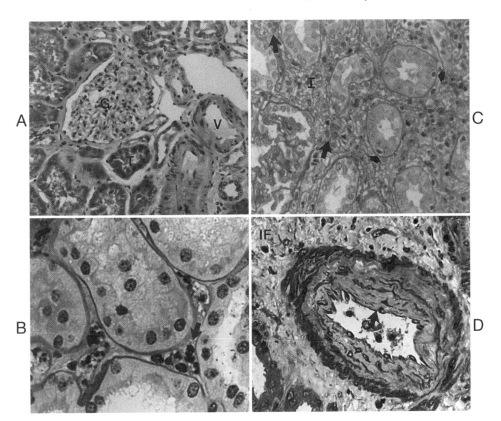

Figure 11.1. (A) Photomicrograph of a normal kidney. Glomerulus (G), tubule (T), vessel (V) (Hematoxylin and Eosin, original magnification 40x). (B) Renal allograft undergoing hyperacute rejection. The peritubular capillaries are filled with neutrophils (arrows). (Periodic acid schiff, original magnification 160x.) (C) Renal allograft undergoing acute cellular rejection. The interstitium (I) is expanded by edema and a mononuclear cell infiltrate (arrows). Mononuclear cells focally invade the tubules (arrowheads). (Periodic acid schiff, original magnification 100x.) (D) Renal allograft undergoing chronic rejection. An artery shows fibrointimal hyperplasia (arrows) and there is interstitial fibrosis (IF). (Gomori's trichrome, original magnification 100x.)

antigens from the father, are in essence an allograft. It can occur within minutes to hours of graft revascularization. Immunologically, hyperacute rejection is characterized by deposition in the graft of antibody and complement on the capillary walls, aggregation of platelets in the capillary lumens, and lining of the capillaries with polymorphonuclear leukocytes (Figure 11.1). The clotting cascade is initiated. As a result of these reactions, the capillaries and arterioles in the graft rapidly become blocked. The clots in the vasculature of the graft stop blood flow to the graft. Tissue necrosis ensues and the graft dies. There is no known medical procedure that can stop the process of hyperacute rejection. Thus, testing for donor-specific, preformed antibodies in the recipient is a vital part of a pretransplant work-up, and their detection is a serious contraindication for transplantation of that organ into that recipient.

Acute Rejection
Acute rejection is the first phase of rejection which occurs within a few weeks or months of graft implantation. This form of rejection occurs in graft recipients that

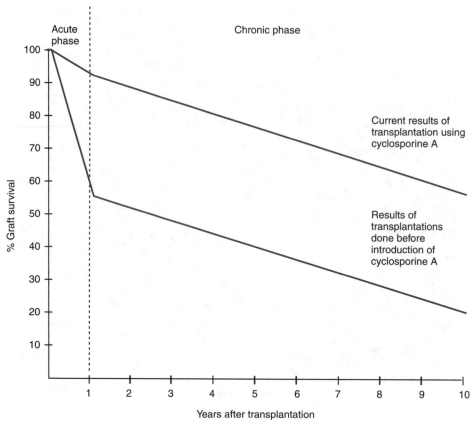

Figure 11.2. Two phases of rejection, acute and chronic. Improvements in medical procedures have reduced the rate of graft loss during the acute phase, but the rate of graft loss in the chronic phase has not improved.

possess mature, graft-reactive T lymphocytes and is characterized by infiltration of the graft tissue with these lymphocytes. The first change is accumulation of small lymphocytes on the capillary and venule walls. The lymphocytes pass through the vascular endothelium and infiltrate the grafted tissue. With the passage of time the infiltration becomes intense and diffuse. This response is self-sustaining and has been called a vicious cycle caused by the local release of cytokines, which up-regulate expression of MHC molecules, which activate more cytokine release, and so on. The infiltrating cells cause the progressive disruption of the capillaries and venules. Fluids accumulate in the tissues, and eventually the blood flow to the grafted tissue is interrupted. With the failure of the blood supply, the graft dies. A renal allograft undergoing acute cellular rejection is shown in Figure 11.1C.

Acute cell mediated rejection, unlike the other forms of rejection, can be controlled by appropriate medical treatment. Because of the armamentarium of immuno-suppressive drugs available to treat acute rejection episodes, most transplant centers lose very few grafts to acute rejection. Figure 11.2 shows two phases of rejection, acute and chronic. The rate of graft loss during the acute phase has improved, mainly because of the use of Cyclosporine A (discussed later.)

Acute rejection is the best understood of the three forms of rejection. There is considerable evidence that acute allograft rejection is carried out primarily by

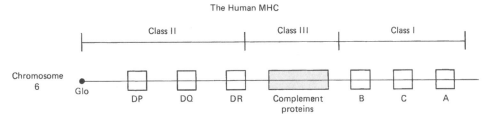

The Human MHC

Figure 11.3.   Strong human histocompatibility genes of the major histocompatibility complex (MHC) that are responsible for vigorous rejection responses are encoded on chromosome 6. At the gene loci e.g., DP, DQ, DR, B, C, and A, many alleles are available that are reassorted during sexual reproduction yielding many unique and therefore histoincompatible individuals. These genes, of course, have important functions in the immunological response quite apart from their role in tissue rejection. These are described in chapter 8.

T lymphocytes. First, mice that are made deficient in T lymphocytes by neonatal thymectomy, and the so-called "nude" mice that are genetically incapable of making T lymphocytes, fail to reject allografts. In contrast, a deficiency in B lymphocytes does not interfere with allograft rejection. This does not mean that B cells and antibodies are not involved in acute rejection. Rather, their involvement must be dependent on T lymphocytes. Second, it has been shown that T lymphocytes obtained by thoracic duct cannulation of dogs bearing allografts, but not autografts, have the ability to destroy cells derived from the donors of their grafts. This destruction is rapid, efficient, and specific for the graft. The cells which mediate this destruction are the cytolytic T lymphocytes. Since these lymphocytes destroy graft cells *in vitro*, it has been hypothesized that they destroy grafts *in vivo* also.

Chronic Rejection
Chronic rejection occurs in graft recipients whose grafts survive past the period of acute rejection. It usually occurs some months after graft implantation. This is clearly a second phase of graft rejection. When chronic rejection occurs, there is a gradual deterioration of the graft. Manifestations associated with chronic rejection are similar to arteriosclerosis. Severe narrowing of the arteries in the grafted tissues occurs. Endothelial cells respond to the immunological attack by producing TGF-β, which causes fibrosis and, with platelet-derived growth factor, proliferation of smooth muscle cells. The narrowing of the arteries results from deposition of antibody and complement, and the formation of platelet and fibrin aggregates on the vessel walls. These deposits become covered with endothelium and are incorporated into the intima. The arterial narrowing causes reduction in blood flow, resulting in ischemia and progressive fibrosis. It is hypothesized that early, intense acute rejection episodes may be responsible for the development of graft vessel sclerosis and chronic rejection. A renal allograft undergoing chronic rejection is shown in Figure 11.1D.

The immunosuppressive regimes in use to prevent acute rejection have little or no effect on chronic rejection. Currently, there are no satisfactory methods available to control chronic rejection. Because of this, the gradual rate of graft loss due to chronic rejection has not changed over the years. This is illustrated in Figure 11.2.

HISTOCOMPATIBILITY ANTIGENS
The tissue or histocompatibility antigens which cause vigorous rejection responses and are the primary obstacle to transplantation are encoded within the *Major Histocompatibility Complex*, or MHC (Figure 11.3). In the human, the MHC encodes the

so-called *HLA* or *Human Leukocyte Antigens*, while in the mouse it encodes a similar set of molecules called *H-2* or *Histocompatibility-Locus 2* antigens. All vertebrates studied to date possess a major histocompatibility complex. In the mouse, the MHC is found on chromosome 17 while in the human, it is found on chromosome 6. There are also weaker histocompatibility antigens that cause milder rejection responses. In both species, the weaker histocompatibility antigens are encoded at many different chromosomal sites and are collectively called minor histocompatibility antigens.

Although first identified by transplantation reactions, the MHC antigens are now known to play key roles in an immune response. In both humans and mice, the MHC genes are organized into regions encoding three classes of molecules: Class I, Class II, and Class III (Figure 11.3). Class I and Class II molecules are the molecules which influence the response to transplanted tissues and are expressed as heterodimers on the cell surface. The various gene products encoded by the Class I and Class II genes are structurally and functionally homologous. The Class I molecules in the human are HLA-A, -B, and -C and H-2 K, D, and L in the mouse. The Class II molecules are HLA-DR, -DQ, and -DP in the human and I-A and I-E in the mouse. Class III genes encode different products including soluble complement components, steroid 21-hydroxylase enzymes, tumor necrosis factors (TNF), and heat shock proteins, which will not be discussed further in this section. There are still other genes within the MHC, including nonclassical Class I molecules, Class I and Class II pseudogenes, genes for chaparoning peptide loading (DM, DO), genes for the proteosome components (LMP), and the peptide transporters (TAP). Many of the molecules encoded by these genes also play roles in the immune response but are not considered histocompatibility antigens and will not be discussed in this chapter.

The Class I molecules are heterodimers composed of a 44 kDa glycoprotein heavy chain, encoded within the MHC, which is noncovalently associated with a 12 kDa protein, called beta-2 microglobulin encoded on another chromosome. The MHC encoded heavy chain spans the cell membrane and is oriented with its amino terminus to the outside of the cell. Class I molecules are encoded in the human MHC by three separate genes. Thus, cells from a given individual can display up to six different Class I molecules, one product encoded by each of three loci on two chromosomes (Table 11.1). An individual inherits three of these genes from each of his parents.

The Class II molecules are heterodimers composed of two noncovalently associated transmembrane glycoporteins, an α-chain (33–35 kDa) and a β-chain (26–28 kDa). Both α and β chains are encoded within the MHC. Both polypeptides have intracellular, transmembrane and extracellular domains, and like Class I, the amino terminus is oriented to the outside of the cell. Class II molecules are encoded in the human MHC by at least three different loci. There are either one or two HLA-DR molecules expressed depending on the haplotype as well as one HLA-DQ and one HLA-DP molecule. Hence, cells from a given individual can display up to six or eight different Class II proteins depending on the haplotypes inherited. Again, three or four of these proteins are encoded by genes which are inherited by the individual from each of his parents.

MHC antigens are inherited *en bloc* by offspring. As shown in Figure 11.4, each parent has a pair of homologous chromosomes, each encoding an HLA haplotype. Haplotype refers to the set of MHC genes, one from each locus, encoded on one of the homologous chromosomes. The offspring inherit one haplotype from each parent. Therefore, children inherit one of four possible combinations. The genes are closely linked on the chromosome and crossing over occurs infre-

Table 11.1. MHC-encoded proteins.

	Class I	Class II
Molecular weight	44,000 daltons	26,000-28,000 daltons 33,000-35,000 daltons
β2-microglobulin	+	–
human chromosonal loci	HLA-A HLA-B HLA-C	HLA-DR HLA-DQ HLA-DP
function	target structure for CTL and allo-antibody	induction of cytokine secretion
distribution	most nucleated cells	highly selective distribution

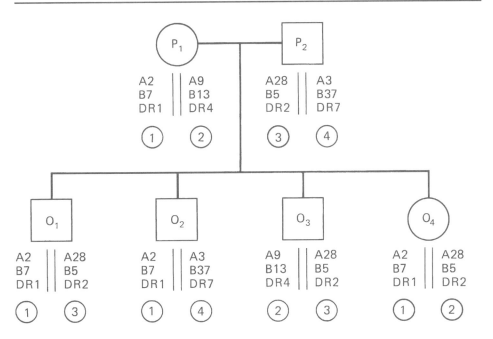

Figure 11.4. The reassortment of some of the histocompatibility genes. Each parent (P_1, P_2) has unique alleles at the various sites. The offspring (O_1, O_2, O_3, and O_4) have different combinations of the genes than their parents, a result of segregation of chromosomes during gamete formation and occasionally a recombination event during fertilization. Note: Not all HLA loci are shown in the figure.

quently (~1 percent). Crossing over occurs when genetic material is exchanged between chromosomes during meiosis.

One striking characteristic of the Class I and Class II genes is their high degree of polymorphism. Each of the Class I and Class II genes has multiple alternate forms (or alleles) within the population. The number of alleles identified currently for HLA-A, -B, and -DR is more than 150 at each locus. As each individual has genetic information for only two alleles at each locus, products encoded by all other alleles at that locus are "foreign" to that individual. The alleles inherited by an individual determine the histocompatibility molecules that they express (i.e., HLA or tissue type). The differences in amino acid sequence encoded by the different alleles form antigenic determinants that are recognized by the immune system by both antibody and cell mediated mechanisms. It is clear from experimental and clinical evidence that both *in vivo* and *in vitro* immune responses are strongest when there are incompatibilities for all Class I and Class II alloantigens. Thus, to decrease the immunological assault elicited by a foreign allograft, both the patient (recipient) and the donor graft are HLA typed and, when possible, the organ is transplanted to the recipient with the fewest HLA allelic differences or incompatibilities. Because the density of HLA molecules expressed on the cell surface of different organs varies considerably, the necessity for matching also differs among the different transplanted organs. For kidney transplantation, matching for HLA is not absolutely necessary, although, matching is beneficial for long-term engraftment (> five to ten years). Matching for liver transplantation is not required, partly because of the low level of expression of MHC antigens on the surface of hepatic cells. However, the story is very different for bone marrow transplantation. Some degree of matching is required. The best results are obtained from HLA-A, -C, -B,- DR, -DQ matched marrow transplants. However, matching for HLA-DR appears to be the most critical and some mismatches at HLA-A and -B can be tolerated.

The minor histocompatibility antigens have been difficult to identify and to devise tests to detect. Minor histocompatibility antigens are peptide fragments from a polymorphic protein by which the donor and the recipient differ. They are primarily presented by Class I molecules to CD8 T cells although minor antigens, presented by Class II to CD4 T cells, have been identified. Because minor histocompatibility antigens are recognized by cytotoxic T cells from individuals who have received an allograft, reagents to detect these antigens (i.e., cytotoxic T cells) frequently are individual specific and of limited accessability for reagents. Generation *in vitro* is difficult. The precursor T cell frequency is the same as that for nominal antigens, which is much lower than the precursor frequency of T cells which recognize MHC antigens. Although eliciting weaker immune responses, in the absence of immunosuppression, even minor histocompatibility antigens can induce allograft rejection, and multiple minor histocompatibility antigen incompatibilities can cause major barriers to transplantation. One minor histocompatibility antigen, the Y antigen, is known to be a "major" minor histocompatibility antigen, and when possible, female recipients are not given marrow transplantations from male donors.

IMMUNOLOGIC MECHANISMS OF ALLOGRAFT REJECTION

Allograft rejection *in vivo* is an extremely complex event which, although dependent on T lymphocytes, is not exclusively a T lymphocyte phenomenon. There is evidence for the participation of virtually every major immune effector mechanism in graft rejection. But, in general, rejection can be classified into (1) cell-mediated killing, (2) antibody-mediated damage and (3) inflammatory damage (Figure 11.5). Antibody specific for the histocompatibility antigens accumulates on a graft. Antibody can mediate destruction by activating the complement cascade and by focusing the mechanism of antibody-dependent cellular cytotoxicity. A large fraction of the cells that infiltrate allografts are macrophages, and activated macrophages are mediators of antibody-dependent cellular cytotoxicity. Some cytokines can directly cause nonspecific tissue destruction. For example, tumor necrosis factor from activated macrophages also destroys cells and is a major mediator of chronic rejection.

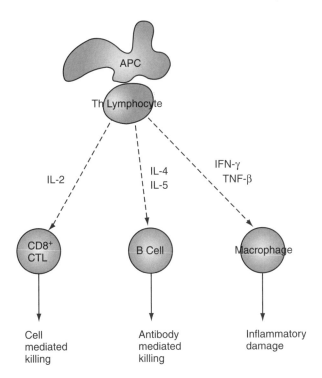

Figure 11.5. Graft rejection is by (1) cell mediated killing, (2) antibody mediated mechanisms, and (3) inflammatory mechanisms.

During rejection, the graft is thus subject to a variety of destructive mechanisms, all regulated by the cytokines.

The activation of naive allospecific T cells by the recognition of foreign tissue antigens in the grafted tissue is central to the rejection process. These T cells produce cytokines, which are required for the activation of effector mechanisms which inflict tissue damage within the graft such as that brought about by cytotoxic T lymphocytes, macrophages, antibodies, and inflammatory responses. Each of these mechanisms may play a greater or lesser role in the rejection process depending on several factors, such as the tissue transplanted, the histocompatibility match, and the immunosuppressive agents administrated.

T CELL ALLORECOGNITION PATHWAYS

The job of T cells is to survey the surface of antigen presenting cells in order to detect any foreign invaders. T cells accomplish this via their antigen specific receptors, i.e., the T cell receptor (TCR). The TCR has many similarities with the other antigen specific receptor, immunoglobulin [covered in chapters 7 (Ig) and 8(TCR)]. T cells circulate through lymphoid organs surveying the antigenic fragments presented by MHC molecules on the surfaces of antigen presenting cells. Self-antigens are ignored; however, when a T lymphocyte encounters a MHC—foreign peptide complex for which it has specificity, the affinity of interaction triggers a series of events which result in activation of the T cell and the initiation of an immune response.

The allograft reaction is unusual because it involves two different sets of APC,

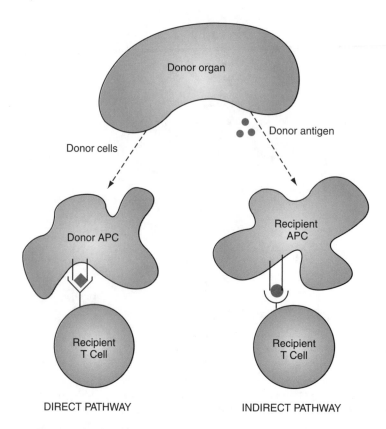

Figure 11.6.   Direct and Indirect activation of recipient T cells. The Direct pathway of recognition is the recognition of the MHC/peptide complex present on donor APC, whereas the Indirect pathway of recognition is the recognition of self MHC plus peptides of donor origin presented by self APC.

those of the donor as well as those of the recipient. Having two recognition pathways is a fundamental feature of allograft rejection that distinguishes it from other types of immune responses. These two pathways are called the *Direct* and the *Indirect* pathway (Figure 11.6). Direct recognition is the stimulation of recipient T cells by the MHC/peptide complex present on donor lymphocytes. Indirect recognition is the stimulation of recipient T cells by self-APC which present peptides of donor origin. Peptides of MHC antigens are better at stimulating an indirect response than are peptides from other antigens, which is not surprising, since they are the major histocompatibility antigens. Therefore, the majority of mature alloreactive effector T cells have specificity for MHC antigens.

Until recently, direct recognition of alloantigens was thought to be the main pathway for graft rejection responses. However, recent studies comparing the strength of both direct and indirect responses manifested following graft rejection suggest that the indirect response plays the predominant role in graft rejection, at least of solid organ grafts. If, indeed, indirect recognition is the predominant recognition pathway, the way that one thinks about MHC matching for graft survival will need to change since peptide fragments of MHC molecules and not the MHC molecule itself would be the stimulus. Studies in MHC matching are underway to determine whether a reduction in the number of foreign peptides mismatched will better re-

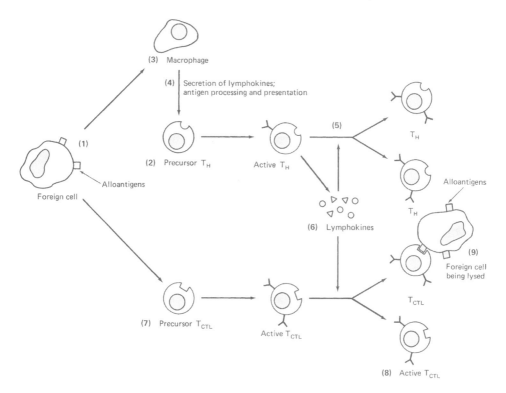

Figure 11.7. The indirect pathway activation of T lymphocytes by alloantigens on foreign cells is by processes similar to activation by other antigens. The alloantigens (1) on the foreign cell are processed and presented to helper T lymphocytes (T$_H$) (2) by macrophages (3) and the macrophages are induced to secrete lymphokines (4). These processes cause helper T lymphocyte clones (CD44) of appropriate types to expand (5) and provide help (6) to appropriate precursor lytic (T$_C$) (7) lymphocytes (CD84). These lytic lymphocytes become activated and reproduce, yielding large numbers of active cytolytic lymphocytes (8) capable of lysing any foreign cells (9) bearing the alloantigen that induced the process.

duce graft rejection than a reduction in the number of intact MHC molecules mismatched.

T LYMPHOCYTE ACTIVATION

When a naive lymphocyte encounters a relevant MHC-peptide complex, ligation of the TCR induces a conformational change in an adhesion molecule, LFA-1, greatly increasing its affinity for its ligand (Figure 11.7). T cells receiving this signal cease to migrate. Progression toward an alloreactive effector cell does not proceed unless the T cell receives a costimulatory signal, delivered by the same cell that delivers the signal through the TCR. The best characterized costimulatory signal is that delivered by ligation of the B7 molecule (CD80 and CD86) on the APC and the CD28 molecule of the T cell. If signal one (i.e. TCR/MHC-peptide ligation) is received without receiving a costimulatory signal, the T cell becomes nonresponsive or anergic. The lymphocyte which receives a costimulatory signal expresses active receptors for interleukin-2, the cytokine that triggers lymphocyte proliferation and differentiation, begins to produce interleukin-2, and expresses the CD40 ligand. Animal experiments show that long-term graft acceptance, with minimal or no immunosuppression, can be induced by blocking the costimulatory signal(s) and the activation molecule CD40. This tolerance or anergy is very desirable because it is antigen specific. Unfortunately, while highly desirable, this state of anergy cannot yet be accomplished routinely and therefore is not yet used in clinical settings.

If growth and differentiation factors are available, the partially activated lymphocyte continues to differentiate, acquiring full cytolytic capability or helper T cell function. CD8+ cytolytic T cells are activated by Class I-peptide complexes, whereas CD4+ helper T cells are activated by Class II-peptide complexes. Cytotoxic T cells require help from activated T helper cells to become mature "killers" and fully active. The above mechanism assures that specific clones, which are selected by antigen for activation and expansion, are activated and expanded while clones not reactive with the available antigen remain inactive.

CYTOKINES

Cytokine production is a capacity of most types of T lymphocytes, not just helper lymphocytes. The primary function of T lymphocytes may be, in fact, to produce cytokines, and thus regulate and coordinate the behavior of the cells involved in immune responses. The cytokines are the hormones of the immune system. As such, they operate like other peptide hormones affecting many cell types that display the appropriate receptors.

Progeny of a single helper lymphocyte can produce a variety of cytokines that collectively influence macrophages, B lymphocytes, other T lymphocytes, and lymphoid cell progenitors. There are two types of T-helper lymphocytes, Th1 and Th2. Th1-type helper lymphocytes produce proinflammatory cytokines such as interferon-γ, which causes natural killer cell and macrophage activation and interleukin-2, which causes T lymphocyte proliferation. Th2-type helper lymphocytes produce anti-inflammatory cytokines such as interleukin-4, which promotes activation and growth of B cells, and interleukin-10, which inhibits Th1 cells. This list of cytokines and their activities is far from inclusive.

The level and types of cytokines that a recipient produces are important to the survival of the graft. One type of T-helper cell can become predominant over the other and over the immune response to a particular antigen because of the immunoregulatory ability of certain cytokines. Interferon-γ (a Th1 cytokine) suppresses the activation of Th2 lymphocytes, whereas interleukin-10 (a Th2 cytokine) suppresses the activation of Th1 lymphocytes. When this happens the response is said to have become polarized toward a cellular or a humoral response. Th1-like cytokines activate cell-mediated mechanisms of acute rejection. In contrast, Th2-like cytokines are involved in the activation and proliferation of B lymphocytes, thereby promoting humoral mechanisms of rejection. Th2 cells also produce transforming growth factor β (TGF-β) and granulocyte-macrophage colony-stimulating growth factor, cytokines that are involved in the activation of T-suppressor cells. Therefore, a Th2 response favors the establishment of anergy or tolerance. However, one of these same cytokines, TGF-β, may contribute to the pathology of chronic rejection.

CYTOKINE PROMOTER REGION POLYMORPHISM

The activation of cytokine genes is dependent on the binding of protein transcription factors to the DNA directly upstream from the cytokine gene, the promoter region. Genetic polymorphisms have been identified in the promoter regions which influence the expression of cytokine genes by controlling the strength of binding of certain transcription factors. This difference in binding predisposes an individual to higher or lower production of a given cytokine. Although the cytokine itself is the same, the amount produced can differ from four- to fifty-fold.

These promoter region polymorphisms, because they polarize responses toward cell-mediated or antibody-mediated responses, may influence allograft rejection. Thus, an individual who has a genetically encoded tendency to make higher levels of interleukin-10 and lower levels of interferon-γ has a tendency to polarize toward antibody mediated responses. Studies have shown that transplant receipts with the genetic profile for high interferon-γ/low interleukin-10 production have significantly more frequent and more severe acute rejection episodes. In contrast, individuals with the genetic profile for low interferon-γ/high interleukin-10 production have significantly longer graft survival with fewer acute rejection episodes. Some transplant surgeons are now beginning to use cytokine promoter region allele typing to tailor immunosuppressive drug therapy for a specific recipient. Cytokine promoter region alleles also may influence chronic rejection. Individuals who have a high TGF-β production phenotype have more severe chronic rejection in a recent study. As mentioned earlier, TGF-β is a potent smooth muscle mitogen and probably accounts for some of the smooth muscle cell proliferation in the intima of vessels in the graft that occurs during chronic rejection. TGF-β is also involved in the fibrosis seen in the lesions.

MIXED LYMPHOCYTE CULTURES

The mixed lymphocyte culture has been used as an *in vitro* model of the allograft reaction, but it is now thought to represent primarily the direct recognition pathway. Still, it is used by a number of laboratories to determine tissue compatibility for bone marrow transplantation. When lymphocytes from two different individuals are mixed in tissue culture, the cells of each will stimulate the lymphocytes of the other to form blasts and divide. To differentiate between the ability of a lymphocyte to respond and stimulate, a one-way MLC is used, in which the stimulating cells are treated with either mitomycin-C or x-irradiation. Proliferation in the mixed lymphocyte reaction is controlled by the Class II antigens. T cell proliferation is detected by analysis of incorporation of tritiated thymidine (Figure 11.8). Tritiated thymidine is a radioactive DNA precursor that is incorporated into DNA by dividing cells. In the MLC, the lymphocytes identify each other as "nonself" or foreign through recognition of the cell surface histocompatibility antigens, e.g., HLA in man.

GENERATION AND DETECTION OF CYTOTOXIC T LYMPHOCYTES

Cytolytic T lymphocytes are generated *in vitro* in mixed lymphocyte cultures. Like the graft-reactive lymphocytes from the thoracic ducts of grafted animals, the cytotoxic lymphocytes that develop in mixed lymphocyte cultures can only lyse cells that display the alloantigens present on the stimulator cells. These cytotoxic lymphocytes are thus alloantigen specific. When a lymphocyte population is cultured with foreign cells, only a fraction of the lymphocytes in the population develop cytolytic activity, specifically, those lymphocytes with antigen receptors that can recognize the foreign histocompatibility antigens. The other lymphocytes are not stimulated and do not become lytic cells.

It requires five to seven days for cytotoxic lymphocytes to develop in mixed

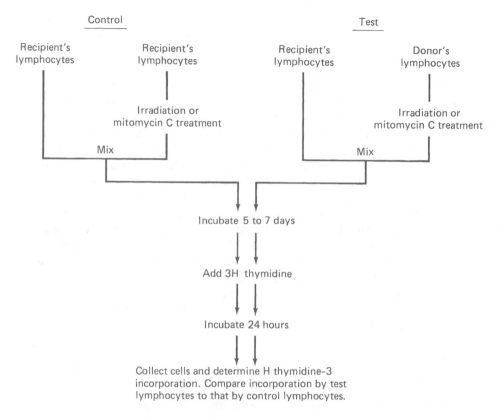

Figure 11.8. The procedure for determining the degree to which a graft recipient will be activated by alloantigens in a donors' lymphocytes. The donors' lymphocytes are treated by irradiation or with mitomycin C to prevent them from dividing. This treatment does not affect their ability to stimulate cell division of the recipient's lymphocytes. After mixing, the culture is incubated for five to seven days, then tritiated (^{3}H) thymidine is added; after twenty-four hours additional incubation, the degree of incorporation of label is determined. A compatible control using the recipient's lymphocytes is also run. A stimulation index (incorporation by test system divided by incorporation in control) indicates degree of compatibility.

lymphocyte cultures. The presence of cytotoxic lymphocytes is assessed by determining the ability of the lymphocytes to lyse cells that have been radiolabeled with ^{51}Chromium (Figure 11.9). The cells which may be destroyed are called target cells. ^{51}Chromium binds to proteins of the target cell cytoplasm. If the cell is lysed, the cytoplasm leaks out and the label with it. The amount of radioactivity released from the target cells is an index of the amount of lysis that occurred in the target cell population. This method of detecting target cell destruction by cytotoxic lymphocytes is called the Chromium-51 release assay.

CLINICAL STRATEGIES FOR AVOIDANCE OF GRAFT REJECTION
Treatments designed to prevent rejection of grafts must take into account the fact that rejection can occur by at least three dissimilar mechanisms. To avoid hyperacute rejection, potential graft recipients are tested; those who have antibodies reactive with the donor lymphocytes are not transplanted. Hyperacute rejection mediated by antibodies may be partially controlled by plasmapheresis, a process that selec-

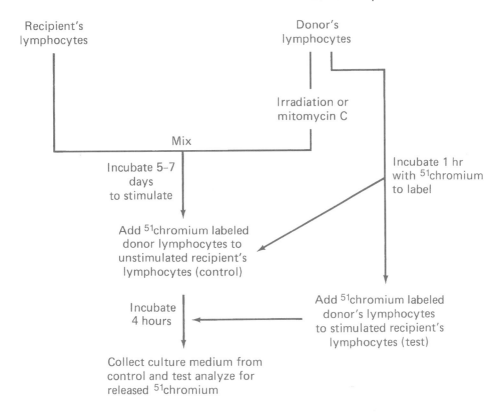

Figure 11.9.   The degree to which cytolytic lymphocytes are generated in a mixed lymphocyte culture can be determined by the chromium-51 release assay. The donor's lymphocytes are labeled with ^{51}Cr, a label which binds to the proteins in the cytoplasm and is released along with the cytoplasm during cell lysis. The donor's lymphocytes are mixed with the recipient's lymphocytes and the cultures are incubated by five to seven days to permit generation of cytotoxic lymphocytes. Then fresh ^{51}Cr labeled donor's lymphocytes are added to the culture. After four hours the amount of radioactivity in the culture medium is measured. A cytotoxicity index is constructed by dividing the amount of radioactivity released in the test system by the amount released by labeled donor lymphocytes mixed with unstimulated recipients' lymphocytes. The larger the value of the index, the greater the incompatibility; an index of one indicates complete compatibility.

tively removes antibodies. There are two primary strategies used to avoid acute allograft rejection: these are tissue matching and selective immunosuppression. Chronic rejection is initiated by cellular, antibody, and viral attack of graft endothelium. Current immunosuppressive drugs have no effect on chronic rejection.

Tissue Matching
Lymphocyte Cross-match. One of the major contraindications for transplanting a given graft into a specific recipient is the presence of antibodies in the recipient which react with the HLA molecules of the donor. Therefore, candidates for transplants are routinely screened for the presence of graft-reactive antibodies. These antibodies can develop after an earlier transplantation, after blood transfusion, or after pregnancy. Serum samples from transplant candidates are tested for their ability to mediate complement-dependent lysis of lymphocytes obtained from the blood of

the tissue donor. This test is the T cell cross-match. Transplant candidates with no detectable donor-reactive antibodies have little risk of hyperacute rejection.

Blood Group Matching. ABO blood group antigens are important histocompatibility antigens as blood group antigens are present on vascular endothelium as well as on erythrocytes. Because of this, a primary criterion for transplantation is ABO blood group compatibility between a transplant candidate and the tissue donor. Hyperacute rejection can occur when the graft donor and recipient are of different ABO blood groups.

"Tissue Typing" or "Histocompatibility Typing." To avoid acute rejection, attempts are made to match the histocompatibility proteins of the graft candidate with those of the tissue donor. In tissue matching, primary attention is given to the major histocompatibility molecules with little effort being expended on attempts to match minor histocompatibility antigens. "Tissue typing" or "histocompatibility typing" is the procedure used to determine the HLA alleles of donor and recipient. DNA-based typing procedures are rapidly replacing serological methods. The DNA-based typing procedures use the Polymerase Chain Reaction (PCR) to generate billions of copies of the HLA alleles. These PCR products are then characterized by one of two methods. Probably the most frequently used method is Sequence Specific Polymorphism (SSP), in which the specificity of the test is in the primers, and the product or absence of a product is visualized on a gel. The other method is Sequence Specific Oligonucleotide Probe (SSOP) typing where the specificity of the test is in the oligonucleotide probes that are used to characterize the PCR product. Basically, a given gene is amplified using PCR and the product blotted onto membranes. These membranes are then probed with sequence specific oligonucleotide probes. Unique patterns of binding of the oligonucleotide probes characterize each allele. Serological typing is still used to a limited extent, particularly for Class I typing. In this procedure, blood lymphocytes from donor and recipient are tested to determine if they can be lysed by antibodies and complement. A panel of antibodies, each antibody of which reacts with known HLA antigens, is used in this test. The antibodies are usually obtained from the sera of multiparous women. These sera contain high titers of complement-fixing antibodies specific for the major histocompatibility antigens of their children. The specificities of the antibodies in the sera are determined before it is used as a "typing serum."

It is most often not possible to find a donor/recipient combination that is completely matched for all MHC-encoded molecules. Some matches are more important than others. For example, matching of HLA-DR is more important than matching of HLA-B, which is more important than matching of HLA-A, which is more important than matching of HLA-C.

Immunosuppression

Long-term graft survival in transplant recipients is largely a result of increased sophistication in the use of immunosuppressive agents. There are transplant centers that have not had an acute rejection episode in several years. Without immunosuppression, few, if any, allografts would survive. The importance of immunosuppression in graft acceptance is made apparent by the fact that with treatment with immunosuppressive drugs, such as Cyclosporine A, it is possible to perform transplants without regard for HLA matching. However, HLA matched transplants do have better long-term survival rates.

A wide variety of immunosuppressive drugs and treatments have been evaluated in clinical transplantation studies. Many procedures like high energy irradiation, which destroys all dividing cells, or thoracic duct drainage, which removes graft reactive T cells, are either too destructive or too complicated to be practical. Many drugs, like cyclophosphamide, are similar to irradiation in that the negative effects of the treatment exceed the benefits. These treatments are often so immunosuppressive that they leave the patient too susceptible to infection and cancer. Immunosuppressive drugs that improve graft acceptance with minimal undesirable side effects that are in general use today are azathioprine, prednisone, anti-TCR monoclonal antibodies, antilymphocyte globulin, Cyclosporine A, and FK506. The various immunosuppressants operate by different mechanisms. In fact, therapeutic strategies use combinations of these drugs in controlling acute graft rejection.

Azathioprine is an analogue of 6-mercaptopurine. This drug competes for enzymes necessary for production of nucleic acids, and thus impairs synthesis of DNA and RNA. For this reason, rapidly dividing cells are most sensitive to azathioprine. Presumably, this drug is immunosuppressive because it interferes with the synthesis of cytokines and with expansion of alloreactive lymphocytes. Undesirable side effects of this drug include leukopenia, anemia, bone marrow depression, and hair loss.

Corticosteroids such as prednisone have wide-ranging physiologic effects, including immunosuppression. Prednisone, or more properly its active metabolite, prednisolone, interferes both with cytokine production by helper T lymphocytes and with lymphocyte accumulation at a graft site. Prednisone is capable of reversing ongoing graft rejection. Undesirable side effects include avascular necrosis of bone, peptic ulceration, impairment of wound healing, and cataract formation.

Antilymphocyte globulin is a purified preparation of antibodies raised to lymphocytes. These antibodies interfere with immune responses by causing lymphocytes to be destroyed by complement-mediated lysis or by phagocytes of the reticuloendothelial system. Patients will become sensitized to these antibodies, since being made in horses, they are foreign proteins. Patients quickly generate neutralizing antibodies, making therapy with antilymphocyte globulin or monoclonal antibodies ineffective.

Cyclosporine A and FK506 are fungal metabolites. These two drugs have a relatively selective effect on helper T lymphocytes. They block T cell proliferation by reducing the expression of several cytokine genes, those which rely on activation of the gene by a particular transcription factor. Included in this group of cytokines are interleukin-2, interleukin-4, and tumor neucrosis factor-α. Both Th1 and Th2 helper T cells are affected, and thus, both cellular and humoral immune responses are reduced. However, Cyclosporine A and FK506 interfere only with acute rejection responses and are not effective at all for treatment of chronic rejection. A disadvantage of these two drugs is that they do not stop immune responses once they have begun. Cyclosporine A also has a number of undesirable side effects, including toxic effects on the kidneys and liver. FK506 has fewer side effects, but those it has are similar to those listed above for Cyclosporine A. Both drugs, because they cannot be synthetically made, are very expensive.

Acceptance of allografts is facilitated by donor-specific blood transfusions (DST). This procedure is only practical when tissues from a living donor are to be transplanted. Three transfusions of 200 cc of donor blood are given to the transplant candidate at biweekly intervals prior to transplantation. These transfusions can cause sensitization of the transplant candidate to histocompatibility antigens of the donor. The incidence of sensitization can be reduced by treating the transplant candidate with azathioprine during the three-week period when the transfusions are being given. When the transfusion process is complete, the recipient is tested for the presence of antibodies reactive with donor lymphocytes. If no antibodies are present, the candidate is transplanted with the donor tissue.

The effect of this procedure is to minimize the immune reactivity of the recipient to the donor's alloantigens. Reduced donor-reactivity makes immunosuppression easier and post-transplant clinical complications less frequent and more manageable. The reasons why this procedure works are unclear. It has been suggested that the transfusions stimulate production of a population of suppressive T cells, which, in turn, dampen immune responses to donor alloantigens after transplantation. It has also been suggested that the transfusions stimulate the production of antibodies which recognize the alloantigen binding structures on alloantibodies and on T lymphocytes. These anti-idiotypic antibodies would be circulating by the time of transplantation and would interfere with the ability of the immune system to respond to the alloantigens of the graft.

SPECIAL CONSIDERATIONS: RETRANSPLANTS

The immunologic events associated with retransplantation are not the same as events associated with primary transplantation. The most obvious difference is the accelerated rate and increased intensity with which graft rejection proceeds, even with immunosuppressant treatments that are highly effective against primary rejection. Lymphocytes from unsuccessfully transplanted individuals will proliferate and generate cytolytic activity in culture much more rapidly than naive lymphocytes. This second set response, like all secondary immunologic responses, is the result of the presence of large numbers of graft-reactive lymphocytes available to the immune system upon secondary contact with the alloantigens. The minor histocompatibility antigens, which are numerous but appear to contribute relatively little to primary acute rejection responses following the stimulation of the first encounter, may also make a significant contribution to the immune response to the secondary transplant. Retransplant patients also frequently have high levels of alloantibodies which react with a large percentage of HLA antigens. Thus, finding a donor for whom a given recipient has a negative cross-match is much more difficult compared to a primary transplant patient.

The various immunosuppressive drugs are less effective at interfering with rejection of second transplants. The net effect is that retransplants are rejected more often and more rapidly than primary transplants.

SPECIAL CONSIDERATIONS: TRANSPLANTATION OF SPECIFIC TISSUES

Most of the information available on allograft rejection is derived from studies of the most commonly transplanted organ, the kidney. Other organs and tissues behave differently.

Some tissues, such as corneas, are poorly vascularized, and have little contact with the immune system; also there are few technical complications with corneal transplants. For these reasons, corneal transplants are highly successful.

The most serious impediment to liver transplantation is the technical complexity of the surgical procedure, rather than control of subsequent rejection. Indeed, livers are not easily rejected. The large liver mass may overwhelm or absorb the immune responses directed at it. Nonetheless, liver transplant recipients must be immunosuppressed if rejection is to be avoided.

Transplantation of the pancreas has not been particularly successful. The major impediment to transplantation of the pancreas is the surgical procedure. For anatomic reasons, the pancreas must be transplanted with a segment of the donor gut. Infection of the immunosuppressed transplant recipient with microorganisms of the gut occurs frequently.

Heart transplantation is complicated by several factors. Hearts must be obtained from donors who have just died, and the organ must be rapidly transferred from donor to recipient. Heart transplant candidates are usually in poor health, and in addition, it is unusually difficult to diagnose rejection before it becomes uncontrollable. The relative technical ease and the efficiency of the immunosuppressive strategies now available have however made cardiac transplantation a widely accepted procedure.

Skin transplantation is one of the least successful tissue transplant procedures. The reasons for this are unclear. The graft procedure is not technically demanding, and autografts, are usually retained. The failure of foreign skin grafts to be accepted may result from the existence of an usually potent, skin-specific immune response or a unique system of histocompatibility antigens. The need for rapid vascularization of skin and the effect of immunosuppressants on the process of vascularization may also limit skin graft survival.

Bone marrow transplantation, which has enormous clinical potential, is still under development and has been increasingly successful. Bone marrow transplantation is most successful when the donor and recipient are completely histocompatible. Bone marrow transplantation is an immunologically unique procedure, and has a variety of correspondingly unique complications. For this technically simple transplant procedure, bone marrow is aspirated by needle from the pelvis or sternum of the graft donor, and transfused into a recipient that has been made immunodeficient by lethal irradiation or chemical preconditioning. Complications arise when immunocompetent lymphoid cells in the donor bone marrow recognize the foreign histocompatibility antigens of the immunocompromised recipient and initiate a rejection response, resulting in a potentially fatal attack on the host by the graft (graft-versus-host disease). Bone marrow recipients are also often severely immunocompromised and are thus susceptible to opportunistic pathogens.

SUMMARY

When a foreign tissue or organ is transplanted into a histoincompatible recipient, a number of immunologic events occurs. There are inflammatory responses in the tissues damaged by the surgical procedure, and there is damage caused by the handling of the graft. This inflammatory response causes the damaged tissues to be infiltrated by a variety of inflammatory cells, including macrophages and T lymphocytes.

At the same time, foreign cells and proteins escape from the transplanted tissues and are trapped by the lymph nodes along the lymph ducts draining the area. In the lymph nodes, T cells respond to the foreign histocompatibility antigens and expand into populations of graft-reactive T lymphocytes. These graft-reactive lymphocytes, which can secrete cytokines and mediate cytolysis, leave the lymph nodes and travel through the blood to the graft site where they enhance the local inflammatory response and participate in tissue destruction.

The activated T lymphocytes which accumulate at the graft site participate in graft destruction by lysing graft cells. They, and other graft-reactive T lymphocytes, secrete cytokines which potentiate immunologic events at the graft site. Some cytokines increase graft antigenicity by increasing the expression of MHC-encoded proteins. Other cytokines directly kill graft tissues. Still others mobilize and orchestrate the graft-reactive immune responses of antibodies and macrophages.

There are a variety of ways for immunosuppressants to interfere with graft rejection. Many immunosuppressants destroy dividing cells, preventing formation of clones of lymphocytes capable of rejecting the graft. Other immunosuppressants interfere with the basic signalling systems used by lymphocytes to potentiate immune responses at a graft site. In addition to these effects, some immunosuppressants interfere with the mechanisms by which lymphocytes are accumulated at the graft site. If immunosuppressants are used effectively, most primary acute allograft rejection can be avoided. However, new immunosuppressive strategies need to be developed which are effective against chronic graft rejection, and against acute graft rejection in retransplanted patients. In general, much has been learned about the phenomenon of graft rejection and therapeutic strategies have been developed to control it to some degree. Nevertheless, there is still much to be learned about the immunology of transplantation.

SUGGESTIONS FOR FURTHER READING

1. Calne, R. "The Development of Immunosuppression in Organ Transplantation." In *Progress in Transplantation*, vol. 1. Edited by P. Morris and N. Tilney, 1–10., New York: Churchill Livingstone, 1984.
2. Dinarello, C., and J. Mier. "Lymphokines." *New England Journal of Medicine* 315 (1987):94–945.
3. Flavell, R., H. Allen, L. Burkly, D. Sherman, G. Waneck, and G. Widera. "Molecular Biology of the H-2 Histocompatibility Complex." *Science* 233 (1986):437–443.
4. Halloran, P., A. Wadgmar, and P. Autenreid. "The Regulation of Expression of Major Histocompatibility Complex Products." *Transplant* 41 (1986):413–420.
5. Henkart, P. "Mechanism of Lymphocyte-Mediated Cytotoxicity." *Ann. Rev. Immunol.* 3 (1985):31–58.
6. Kirkpatrick, C. "Transplantation Immunology." *Journal of the American Medical Association* 258 (1987):2993–3000.
7. Mason, D. "Effector Mechanisms of Allograft Rejection." *Ann. Rev. Immunol.* 4 (1986):119–145.
8. Mickey, M. "HLA Effects." In *Clinical Transplants*. Edited by P. Terasaki, 303–316. Los Angeles: UCLA Tissue Typing Laboratory, 1987.
9. Steinmuller, D. "Tissue Specific and Tissue Restricted Histocompatibility Antigens." *Immunology Today* 5 (1984):234–240.
10. Tilney, N., J. Kupiec-Weglinski, C. Heidecke, P. Leary, and T. Strom. "Mechanisms of Rejection and Prolongation of Vascularized Organ Allografts." *Immunol. Rev.* 77 (1983):185–216.
11. Weiss, A., J. Imboden, K. Hardy, B. Manger, C. Terhorst, and J. Stobo, "The Role of the T3/Antigen Receptor Complex in T Cell Activation." *Ann. Rev. Immunol.* 4 (1986):593–619.

QUESTIONS

1. Name the types of grafts.
2. What are the forms of allograft rejection and how are they mediated?
3. Describe the major histocompatibility complex.
4. What are the differences that characterize Class I and Class II molecules?
5. How many HLA molecules does an individual express?
6. How are HLA antigens inherited?
7. What are minor histocompatibility antigens?
8. What is the feature of allograft recognition that distinguishes it from T cell recognition of nominal antigen? Describe the differences.
9. What mechanism determines whether a T cell becomes activated or tolerized?
10. How do T helper subtypes, Th1, and Th2, influence graft survival?
11. How do cytokine promoter region genes affect graft survival?
12. List the clinical strategies for avoidance of graft rejection.
13. What is the mode of action of Cyclosporin A and FK506? Do they act on all types of rejection?
14. Why are retransplants less successful than first transplants?

ANSWERS

1. (A) Allograft, (B) autograft, (C) xenograft.
2. (A) Hyperacute rejection-mediated by preformed antibodies in the recipient which react with the cells of the donor graft. (B) Acute rejection-mediated primarily by T lymphocytes. (C) Chronic rejection-mediated by antibody which causes endothelial cells to produce TGF-β and platelet-derived growth factor causing fibrosis and proliferation of smooth muscle cells with subsequent narrowing of arteries.
3. The Major Histocompatibility Complex consists of a group of genes which encode for cell surface molecules that are involved in the initiation of an immune response. These molecules are very polymorphic and represent the tissue antigens against which the majority of an alloresponse is directed.
4. Class I molecules - Class I molecules are transmembrane heterodimers consisting of a 44 kDa lycoprotein heavy chain which is encoded within the MHC, and a non-covalently associated 12 kDa protein, β2 microglobulin which is encoded on another chromosome. There are three different loci, HLA-A, -B, and -C, each with many different alleles.
   Class II molecules - Class II molecules are transmembrane heterodimers consisting of an α-chain (33-35 kDa) and a β-chain (26-28 kDa). Both α and β chains are encoded within the MHC. There are three types of Class II molecules, HLA-DR, -DQ, and -DP.
5. An individual expresses six Class I molecules, three from each homologous chromosome (2, HLA-A, 2, HLA-B, and 2 HLA-C) and between six and eight Class II molecules depending on the haplotypes inherited (2-4 HLA-DR, 2 HLA-DQ, 2 HLA-DP).
6. HLA antigens are inherited *en bloc* in a Mendelian fashion. One chromosome is inherited from each parent. Thus, children inherit one of four possible combinations.
7. Minor histocompatibility antigens are peptide fragments from a polymorphic protein by which the donor and the recipient differ.
8. The allograft reaction involves two different sets of APC, those of the donor as well

as those of the recipient. The two pathways are called the *Direct* and the *Indirect* pathways. Direct recognition is the stimulation of recipient T cells by the MHC-peptide complex present on donor cells. Indirect recognition is the stimulation of recipient T cells by self APC which present peptides of donor origin.

9. A lymphocyte which receives signal one (TCR ligation) without receiving a costimulatory signal becomes tolerized. If the T cell instead receives a costimulatory signal, it becomes activated.

10. Th1 type T lymphocytes produce inflammatory cytokines such as interferon-γ and interleukin-2 which causes T lymphocyte proliferation thus, promoting cellular immune reactions. Cell-mediated reactions promote allograft rejection. Th2 type T lymphocytes produce anti-inflammatory cytokines such as interleukin-10 and cytokines that are believed to be involved in the activation of T suppressor cells. Thus, Th2 like responses favor the establishment of anergy or tolerance.

11. Cytokine promoter region polymorphisms influence the level of expression of cytokine gene products by controlling the strength of binding of certain transcription factors. An individual who has a genetically encoded tendency to make lower levels of the Th2 cytokine IL-10 and a higher level of the Th1 cytokine interferon-γ has a tendency to polarize toward cell-mediated responses and more severe graft rejection.

12. (A) Lymphocyte cross-match to detect the presence of antibodies in the recipient which react with the HLA antigens of the donor and thus, prevent hyperacute rejection. (B) Blood group matching. (C) Tissue Typing or Histocompatibility Typing. (D) Immunosuppression.

13. These two drugs have a relatively selective effect on helper T lymphocytes, blocking T cell proliferation by reducing the expression of several cytokine genes. Both Th1 and Th2 helper T cells are affected. These drugs act only on acute rejection.

14. Retransplant patients have been previously sensitized, thus, they have an accelerated rate and increased intensity with which graft rejection proceeds. Cycloporine A and FK506 are not as effective because they do not stop responses once they have begun.

CHAPTER

12

INTRODUCTION
EXPERIMENTAL TUMOR
  IMMUNOLOGY
  Oncogenic RNA Viruses
    and Oncogenes
  Oncogenic DNA Viruses
  Chemically-Induced
    Tumors and Spontan-
    eous Tumors
  Immuno Surveillance
  Escape of Tumor Cells
    from Immune Responses
IMMUNITY TO VIRUS-
  INDUCED NEOPLASIA
  Marek's Disease
  Immune Respones to
    Marek's Disease Virus
  Feline Leukemia
  Immunity to Feline
    Leukemia
  Vaccines
HEPATOCELLULAR
  CARCINOMA
CONCLUSIONS FROM
  IMMUNIZATION
  STUDIES AGAINST
  VIRAL-INDUCED
  NEOPLASIA
IMMUNOLOGICAL
  APPROACHES FOR THE
  CONTROL OF TUMORS
PROSPECTS FOR IMMUN-
  OLOGICAL CONTROL
  OF NEOPLASIA
SUMMARY
SUGGESTIONS FOR
  FURTHER READING
QUESTIONS
ANSWERS

The Immunological System and Neoplasia

K.A. Schat

INTRODUCTION

All cells of multicellular organisms except the germ line cells have a defined life span, and their cell cycle is tightly regulated by interconnected pathways. A balance between cell division and programmed cell death or **apoptosis** is essential to maintain stability within multicellular organisms. The proportion of cells undergoing division versus apoptosis is high during embryonal development and remains high for certain cells (e.g., hemapoietic stem cells). In most tissues cell division slows down after embryonal development has been completed, but the balance can be changed in favor of increased replication when tissues need to regenerate. Two important mechanisms play a role in controlling the cell cycle. **Proto-oncogenes** are positive regulators driving cells out of the G_0 phase into cell division and thus proliferation. Proto-oncogenes are often switched off after homeostasis has been reached. Negative regulators or **tumor suppressor genes** inhibit cell division and thus proliferation. Cells unable to complete the cell cycle will enter apoptosis, which is the default pathway. Tumors (from *tumere*, meaning "to swell") can develop when cells proliferate in an uncontrolled manner or when cells are prevented from entering the apoptotic pathway, while normal cell division continues. Tumors may regress or progress depending on a complex set of factors.

The immune system is only one of the factors determining if a tumor will progress or regress. Cell-mediated immune responses are an important part of the defense against cells expressing foreign antigens on their surfaces after infection with intracellular pathogens such as viruses, protozoa, and certain bacteria. These cells can be lysed by antigen-specific **cytotoxic T lymphocytes** (CTL) if the antigenic epitopes are presented by self major histocompatability complex (MHC) Class I antigens or by **natural killer** (NK) cells if the MHC Class I antigens are down-regulated, absent, or changed. Tumor cells expressing **tumor-specific antigens** (TSA) or **tumor-associated antigens** (TAA) can be eliminated by CTL, NK cells, or other cells. For example, antibody-dependent killer cells can lyse tumor cells if specific antibodies to surface antigens to TSA or TAA are present. In the next section, some of the experimental work supporting the elimination of tumor cells by different immune responses will be discussed.

Immunization against tumors has been a popular idea since the end of the nine-teenth and extending well into the twentieth century. The belief was held that if one could immunize an individual against pathogens foreign to the host, it must also be possible to immunize against a tumor, which is also foreign to the host. As early as 1895, two French scientists inoculated a donkey and two dogs with cells from a human osteosarcoma and tested the sera from these animals in human pa-tients with the same type of tumors. The treatment resulted in some improvement in some of the patients, but unfortunately the patients did not recover. Although these experiments seem naive in light of our current understanding of the immune system, it has to be noted that more than 100 years later we have still not succeeded in developing an immunological approach to combat tumors in man. However, as will be discussed in the last section of this chapter, considerable progress toward this goal has been made using the techniques of molecular biology to alter immu-nological responses to tumor cells.

Other investigators at the end of the nineteenth century made the discovery that certain mammalian tumors could be transplanted from one animal to another. Some of the animals which received tumor fragments either failed to develop a tumor, or showed spontaneous regression of the tumor after it had grown for a period of time. It was not until Little and Tyzzer established the basic principles of tissue transplantation genetics that it was realized that the immunological responses re-ported from studies with random-bred animals were directed primarily against normal transplantation antigens present both in the tumors and normal tissues. After this time it was realized that only studies with homozygous inbred strains of animals, which share the same major histocompatibility antigens, could distinguish between antigenic differences in tumor and normal host tissues. The development of inbred strains of mice including nude and **scid** (severe combined immunodefi-ciency) mice and, more recently "knock-out" mice in which specific genes have been inactivated, has been essential for our current understanding of antitumor immunity.

The development of tumors is a complex process in which different immune responses may play a role. In this chapter we will examine briefly how tumors arise (etiology) and how tumor cells may be eliminated by the immune system or, alter-nately, why these cells escape immune surveillance. In addition, three examples of virus-induced tumors for which vaccines exist will be discussed and future devel-opments will be outlined.

EXPERIMENTAL TUMOR IMMUNOLOGY

Tumors develop as a result of changes in the DNA of cells. These changes are caused by spontaneous mutations and by chemical or physical treatments. In addition, infection with certain viruses can also lead to tumor development (Table 12.1). The etiology of a given tumor is important for the understanding of the development or

Table 12.1. Virus families associated with naturally occurring tumors.

Virus Family	Virus subfamily or genus	Virus genome	Examples of naturally occurring tumors
Retroviridae	Oncovirinae	RNA	Feline leukemia Avian leukosis Human T cell leukemia
Herpesviridae	Alphaherpesvirinae Gammaherpesvirinae	DNA DNA	Marek's disease in chickens Burkitt lymphoma and nasopharyngeal carcinoma in humans
Hepadnaviridae	Hepatitis-B virus and Hepatitis-B like viruses	DNA	Livercarcinoma in man and woodchucks
Papovaviridae	Papillomavirina	DNA	Papillomas in man and many mammalian species

lack of development of immune responses to that tumor. For example, the tumor may lack neo-antigens if the tumor develops as the consequence of one or more point mutations of **proto-oncogenes** (see below) or tumor suppressor genes. In that case the resulting mutated protein may no longer function in the proper fashion, but the change of one or a few amino acids in the mutated protein may not lead to the expression of an epitope that is recognized as nonself. Both chemically- and virally-induced tumors have contributed to the understanding of tumor immunology and examples of each group will be discussed in more detail.

Oncogenic RNA Viruses and Oncogenes
As early as 1911, Peyton Rous, who received the Nobel prize for this work almost sixty years later, demonstrated that a filterable agent could cause sarcomas when inoculated into chickens. It was later shown that this filterable agent, now known as Rous sarcoma virus, belongs to the subfamily of oncovirinae of the family Retroviridae. These viruses are unique because their RNA is transcribed backwards (*retro* means "backward") into DNA through an RNA-dependent-DNA polymerase or reverse transcriptase. It was later shown that the Hepadnaviridae (Table 12.1) also contain genes coding for a reverse transcriptase. The family of Retroviridae contains three subfamilies: the oncovirinae, which can cause tumors; the lentivirinae, which includes human immunodeficiency virus (HIV) causing AIDS; and spumavirinae. Retroviruses are found in many vertebrate species and can induce several types of tumors, some of which are important causes of neoplasia in domesticated animals (e.g., feline leukemia virus in cats).

The basic structure and the genomic map of retroviruses are depicted in Figure 12.1. Purified viruses contain a limited number of viral proteins. Two glycoproteins are expressed on the cell surface and are important for the attachment of the virus to the cells: a transmembrane protein or spike protein to which the second glycoprotein or "knob" is attached. These proteins are identified as glycoprotein (gp) 15 and gp 70, respectively in feline leukemia virus (FeLV), the number indicating the molecular mass in kilodaltons. In addition, the virion contains the reverse transcriptase and four structural proteins: p27 (capsid protein), p15 (matrix protein), p10 (nucleocapsid protein), and p12 (inner coat protein). After virus enters the cells, the RNA is reverse transcribed into DNA, which is incorporated into the cellular genome. The incorporated DNA will persist in these cells. This group of retroviruses does not transform

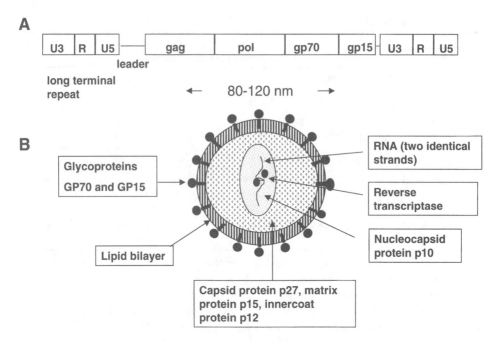

Figure 12.1. Genome and structure of feline leukemia virus (FLV), a member of the oncovirinae subfamily of the family of Retroviridae. (A) The double-stranded DNA form of the genome after reverse transcription. The long terminal repeat consists of the unique 3' end of the RNA genome, a repeat region and the unique 5' end of the genome. Gag codes for the structural proteins, pol codes for the reverse transcriptase, and env for the two glycoproteins. (B) Schematic structure of the FLV particle. Note that the glycoproteins are inserted in the lipid bilayer and are accessible to virus neutralizing antibodies.

cells *in vitro* and tumors develop only after a prolonged incubation time in hosts. Some retroviruses, however, transform cells easily *in vitro*, and tumors develop rapidly *in vivo*. These acutely transforming viruses have captured a proto-oncogene (see below) from the cellular genome replacing part of the viral genome or adding it after the *env* gene. The captured proto-oncogene has become a viral oncogene or *v-onc*. The long terminal repeat or LTR (see Figure 12.1) is a strong promoter that can overexpress the *v-onc* gene leading to the development of tumor cells.

In addition to the horizontally transmitted or **exogenous** retroviruses, most vertebrates contain complete or incomplete endogenous retroviruses in their germ line. Based on this observation and the finding that some retroviruses were able to rapidly transform cells *in vitro*, Huebner and Todaro of the National Cancer Institute proposed the oncogene hypothesis in 1969 to explain the induction of cancers by agents such as viruses, chemicals, and radiation. They postulated that endogenous retroviruses contained "oncogenes" which were normally repressed but could be activated by physical or chemical carcinogens or other factors leading to the development of cancer. This hypothesis led to important studies showing that oncogenes are indeed found in many cells. It was shown however through very elegant studies that cellular oncogenes were normally present in the cellular genome and were not introduced as a consequence of a virus infection. In contrast, viruses containing oncogenes had obtained these oncogenes from the cellular genome (see the previous section). In order to distinguish viral from cell oncogene types, distinct names were required. The cellular oncogenes were therefore called proto-oncogenes (*proto*: Gr., first) or *c-onc*, and the viral oncogenes are now known as *v-onc*. Since then a long list of *c-onc* genes have been cloned and sequenced. It is clear that *c-onc* genes have important roles in cellular pathways leading to cell division. Many *c-onc* genes are active during embryonal development and cell differentiation. Mutations or inappropriate activation of *c-onc* genes by carcinogens can cause abnormal cell division leading to cancer induction. As mentioned before, retroviruses integrate in the cellular genome and it has been shown that the LTR (Figure 12.1) of the integrated retrovirus is a powerful transactivator. If the retrovirus integrates near a *c-onc* gene such as *c-myc*, the LTR can transactivate the expression of c-myc or other onc genes causing abnormal production of proteins that are able to stimulate cell division.

Oncogenic DNA Viruses

Several DNA viruses can transform cells *in vitro* or after inoculation of experimental animals. For example, polyoma virus, belonging to the family Papovaviridae, is capable of transforming cells *in vitro* as well as inducing tumors after inoculation of newborn mice and hamsters. One of the polyoma viruses, simian virus (SV)40, attracted the attention of tumor virologists when it was learned that a large number of humans were vaccinated with polio vaccine prepared in cell cultures contaminated with SV40. Fortunately, there is no evidence that SV40 causes cancer in humans. The mechanism of transformation by SV40 has been well studied. Cells can only be transformed by SV40 if the cells are nonpermissive for virus replication but allow early gene products to be made. One of these gene products called "middle T antigen" acts as a receptor for a growth factor, which causes constitutive activation of the cell cycle. The importance of polyoma viruses for tumor immunology was the finding that these tumors express virally induced tumor-specific antigens—a fact which was used in early studies on tumor rejection. Based on our current knowledge of the transformation process by polyoma viruses, it is clear that these immune responses are probably directed toward the "T antigen" family.

More relevant for tumor immunology are the DNA viruses causing cancer after natural infection of vertebrates, including humans (Table 12.1). Although the three groups of viruses (herpesvirus, hepatitis B virus, and papillomavirus) are very different from a virologist's point of view, a common denominator has emerged as far as the transformation process is concerned. Epstein-Barr virus, causing nasopharyngeal carcinomas and Burkitt's lymphomas in humans, produces several proteins in tumor cells that can 1) inhibit apoptosis, 2) stimulate division of B cells by activation of growth factor receptors, 3) activate cytokine-cytokine receptor pathways resembling antigen stimulation, and 4) activate probably the proto-oncogene *c-myc*. These virus-derived proteins provide potential target antigens for immune responses. Papilloma viruses transform cells *in vivo* by activation of receptors for growth factors such as platelet-derived growth factor and by inactivation of the tumor suppressor gene p53. As with tumor induction by SV40, after infection with papillomaviruses, tumor induction can only occur if virus replication does not occur and only early proteins (E5, E6, and E7) are made. Transformation of hepatocytes by hepatitis B virus is poorly understood. Viral DNA is frequently integrated in clonally expanded tumor cells, but virus proteins are seldom detected. It has been suggested that *c-myc* can be activated in *cis* by integrated viral DNA. Another hypothesis states that one of the viral proteins inflicts cell damage leading to frequent cell divisions and thus an increased risk for mutations leading to the development of hepatocellular carcinomas.

It is clear that oncogenic DNA viruses of the different families use different viral pathways to activate cell division. However, the actual mechanism of transformation is remarkably similar in that growth factors coded for by proto-oncogenes or receptors for growth factors are improperly activated. This has important consequences for immunological approaches to prevent or perhaps treat these tumors. The targets for immune intervention are viral proteins if they are expressed in the tumor cells, while prevention of infection by conventional vaccination may offer another approach as will be discussed in the section on Marek's disease.

Chemically-Induced Tumors and Spontaneous Tumors

Tumors can also arise after chemical (for example, 3-methyl-cholanthrene) or physical (for example, irradiation, ultraviolet light) treatment. These treatments can cause changes in the DNA of proto-oncogenes coding for growth factors, genes coding for growth factor receptors, proteins that activate these receptors, or transcription factors stimulating transcription of one or more of these genes. Normally, tumor suppressor genes will induce apoptosis in cells with abnormal DNA if the DNA cannot be repaired in order to prevent neoplastic transformation. "Spontaneous" tumors are therefore often characterized by multiple mutations in the DNA. The immune response will not be able to detect tumor cells which lack epitope changes in the mutated proteins. This is because these proteins were recognized during the education of the thymus-derived lymphocytes as self, thus eliminating that population of T cells from the T cell repertoire during the education process in the thymus. Sometimes, however, the mutations result in the production of neo-antigens which are also called **tumor-specific antigens** or **TSA**. An example of this possibility was provided early during the studies on tumor immunology when inbred mice were used for studies on immune responses to 3-methyl-cholanthrene-induced tumors. For example, when 3-methyl-cholanthrene-induced tumor cells were injected into the C3H strain of mice, the tumor cells grew and then regressed after a period of time. When these same mice were injected for a second time with the same tumor cells, either no growth, or temporary growth followed by rapid regression of the tumors occurred suggesting an immune response. All nonimmunized control mice rejected the tumor cells only after the cells grew for a period of time (Figure 12.2). These findings were not fully accepted because it was believed that the 3-methyl-cholanthrene tumor cells had mutated during passage in the mice, which resulted in diminished growth potential *in vivo* rather than rejection by immune responses. However, it was finally accepted that the tumor cells expressed antigens not present in normal mice and furthermore, that each 3-methyl-cholanthrene-induced tumor was immunologically distinct. Others showed that allogeneic inhibition, which is based on differences between donor and recipient mice, played no role in establishing immunity to tumor challenge in mice injected with irradiated methyl-cholanthrene-induced autochthonous tumor cells. Thus, it was established that these chemically induced tumors contained new or neoantigens on the cell surface that were responsible for immunity to the tumors.

Immuno Surveillance

In the previous section, the basic concepts regarding tumor cell development were discussed. In this section, the importance of the immune system for the elimination of these cells will be discussed. The notion that the immune system is able to recog-

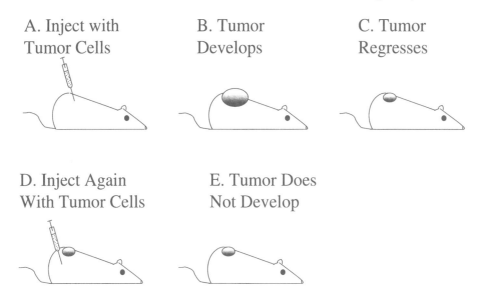

A. Inject with Tumor Cells

B. Tumor Develops

C. Tumor Regresses

D. Inject Again With Tumor Cells

E. Tumor Does Not Develop

Figure 12.2.   Rejection of 3-methyl-cholanthrene-induced tumors in "immunized" C3H mice. Mice rejecting the tumor cells after the primary inoculation are resistant to tumor development after a second injection.

nize and destroy continuously arising tumor cells was first proposed by Ehrlich and later eloquently formulated by Burnet (1970) as follows: *"The 'thymus-dependent' immune system arose from the evolutionary need to counter the development of malignant disease. Wandering cells ancestral to lymphocytes developed the capacity to recognize anomaly ('not-self') on another cell surface and to react destructively on such recognition."* As soon as this immunosurveillance hypothesis was formulated, it was questioned by several investigators because many observations failed to support this hypothesis. For example, nude or athymic mice and rats, as well as mice and rats thymectomized at birth, do not have an increased susceptibility to chemically induced or "spontaneous" tumors, although they tend to develop tumors of the lymphoreticular system more frequently than intact mice.

Although the immune surveillance theory has been rejected to a large degree, experimental studies have shown that specific anti-tumor responses can be induced. Moreover, these anti-tumor responses are directed against tumor-specific antigens (TSAs) as shown in Figure 12.2. In reality, the use of immunological approaches to eliminate tumor cells has been remarkably unsuccessful. In the next section, the reasons why tumor cells escape destruction by immune responses will be briefly discussed.

ESCAPE OF TUMOR CELLS FROM IMMUNE RESPONSES

There are many reasons why tumor cells escape specific responses by T cells. This is somewhat surprising because several types of tumors give rise to tumor-specific lymphocytes that often infiltrate into tumors. These tumor-infiltrating lymphocytes (TIL) can be cultivated *in vitro* and are able to kill tumor cells in *in vitro* assays. However, these cells are often inactive *in situ* (see next page).

An obvious explanation for the escape from immune responses is that tumors arising from mutations may lack epitope changes in the mutated proteins, which was

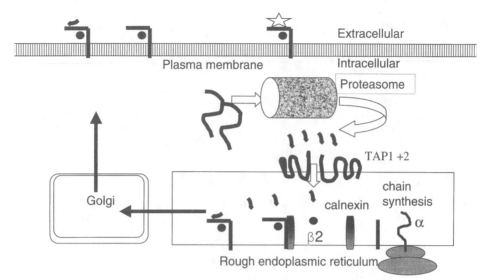

Figure 12.3. Interference of tumors with antigen processing and presentation of nonapeptides by the major histocompatibility complex I antigens (MHC-I). Proteins are processed in the proteasome to nonapeptides and transported into the rough endoplasmic reticulum by the transporter of antigens, the proteins (TAP)1 and 2. The MHC-I is formed from the α-chain, the β2-microglobulin, and calnexin. The nonapeptides bind to and stabilize MHC-I, the complex is transported through the Golgi apparatus to the membrane. Tumor cells may have changes interfering with (1) transport of nonapeptides by TAP1+2, (2) mutations in the β2-microglobulin leading to instable MHC-I, (3) lack of recognizable epitopes, (4) decreased expression of MHC-I.

discussed in the previous section. However, tumor cells expressing altered proteins or TSAs also often escape destruction by antigen-specific cytotoxic T cells (CTL) or natural killer cells (NK cells). The escape from CTL can be caused by additional mutations in the tumor cells leading to variants that no longer present recognizable epitopes. Another mechanism interfering with recognition by CTL is decreased MHC Class I antigen expression. Researchers have found that human melanomacarcinomas, highly malignant and often fatal tumors if not removed early by surgery, frequently exhibit a decreased expression of MHC Class I proteins. This decrease is apparently caused by mutations in the first exon of the β2-microglobulin, leading to translational defects as well as additional changes affecting the expression of MHC Class I antigens (Figure 12.3). The transport of peptides by the TAP-1 and -2 proteins into the **endoplasmic reticulum** (ER) can also be affected in tumor cells similarly to cells infected with certain viruses (e.g., herpesvirus simplex).

The absence of MHC Class I antigens on tumor cells should in theory allow NK cells to eliminate these cells, but some tumors are able to prevent NK cell-induced lysis. NK cells receive an inhibitory signal if they recognize self-MHC Class I antigens. Some tumor cells may synthesize molecules resembling classical MHC molecules that are able to interact with the receptor for the inhibitory signal thus preventing the activation of the lytic signals.

A second mechanism used by tumor cells to escape destruction by CTL and NK cells is the production of immunosuppressive products. For example, cytokines that interfere with the development of CTL (e.g., IL-10 and TGF-β) or with NK cell activation. Antigen-specific CTL lyse target cells by the induction of apoptosis through either the perforin-granzyme pathway or activation of **Fas** (also known as

CD95) expressed on tumor cells. The latter, a member of the TNF receptor family, is activated by the ligand **FasL** or **CD95L**, which is expressed on CTL. The interaction between CD95L and CD95 initiates a signaling cascade resulting in activation of a protease named **FLICE** for **Fas-associated death-domain-Like IL-1β-Converting Enzyme** and ultimately cell death by apoptosis. Tumor cells can counter the apoptotic pathway by producing specific anti-apoptotic proteins. A family of inhibitors, called **FLIPs** for **FLICE inhibitory proteins**, has been found which can be made in tumor cells thus preventing CTL-induced apoptosis. Interestingly, CD95L is expressed in colon carcinoma cell lines and melanoma cell lines. This finding suggests that in colon cancer and melanomas direct pathways exist whereby cancer cells expressing CD95L cause immunosuppression by the induction of apoptosis in CTLs expressing CD95.

It was mentioned before that tumor-infiltrating lymphocytes or TILs are often inactive *in situ*. Ellem et al. (1998) advanced the hypothesis that this state of anergy may actually be the result of two sets of interactions. First, TILs infiltrating into metastatic tumors are primed after the encounter with the primary tumor or after vaccination with autologous tumor cells. The lack of antigenic stimulation of the TILs in the metastatic tumor (for example by a decrease in MHC Class I antigens on the tumor cells or elimination of the autologous tumor cells used as a vaccine) results in a decrease of cytokine production, especially IL-2, causing a decrease in anti-apoptotic proteins and consequently an increase in apoptosis of TILs. Stromal factors produced by the connective tissue in the tumor mass, however, actually prevent apoptosis of the activated TILs which have infiltrated into the metastatic tumor. The result is that the TILs become quiescent *in situ*, but can be activated in the presence of IL-2, which is exactly the approach used to demonstrate *in vitro* activity.

Another reason why tumors are not eliminated by primed tumor-antigen reactive CTL is that the small blood vessels growing into the tumor lack the homing signals for CTLs preventing exvasation from the small blood vessels into the tumor mass. The processes involved in exvasation of lymphocytes are still poorly understood, but it has become clear that many of the integrins needed for this process are not expressed in the microvasculature of tumors. The consequence is that even if tumor-antigen specific CTLs are generated, they may not be able to leave the blood vessels and destroy the tumor cells.

In conclusion, immunotherapy for the control of tumors has been a disappointing road to travel, although not without hope for future success. In the final section of this chapter, new immunologically based approaches for the control of tumors will be discussed.

IMMUNITY TO VIRUS-INDUCED NEOPLASIA

In the previous section, we discussed the fact that certain viruses can cause cancer in the appropriate hosts. Vaccines are routinely used to protect chickens against Marek's disease, a lymphoma caused by a herpesvirus, cats against neoplasia induced by feline leukemia virus, a retrovirus, and humans against hepatocelular carcinomas as a sequella of infection with HBV. In this section, the immunological basis for vaccine-induced protection will be discussed.

Marek's Disease

Marek's disease is a lymphomatous disease of chickens which is found in all poultry-producing countries. The disease is characterized by tumors in visceral organs, musculature, nerves and around the feather follicle epithelium in the skin. The tumor cells are mostly CD4+ T cells, but other nontransformed lymphocytes are often present in the tumors. In addition to tumors, infection can also cause a loss of myelin around the nerves, loss of lymphocytes in the thymus and bursa of Fabricius causing **immunosuppression**, and under certain conditions, atherosclerosis. Damage to the bursa of Fabricius results in decreased antibody responses, because this organ is the source of B lymphocytes in chickens and other bird species. In 1970 different vaccines were introduced in the U.S., U.K., and the Netherlands thus providing protection against a virus-induced neoplastic disease for the first time.

Pathogenesis of Marek's Disease
Marek's disease virus (MDV) belongs to the group of alphaherpesviridae, a classification based on its genomic organization, although it was originally classified as a gammaherpesvirus similar to Epstein-Barr virus based on its infectivity for and transformation of lymphocytes. Marek's disease virus strains are divided into three serologically distinct groups. All oncogenic strains belong to serotype 1, while serotype 2 contains naturally occurring, nononcogenic chicken strains. A related, nononcogenic group of strains isolated from turkeys (HVT or herpesvirus of turkeys) forms serotype 3. Marek's disease virus is unusual because it is strictly cell-associated in most cells in infected chickens with the exception of cells of the feather follicle epithelium where cell-free, infectious virus is produced. In most other virus infections virus is released from all infected cells and thus can infect other cells or be neutralized by virus-neutralizing (VN) antibodies.

The pathogenesis of Marek's disease (MD) is of interest from an immunological point of view because it is a good example of how a virus can subvert host immune responses for its own purposes (Figure 12.4). The initial replication of MDV occurs in B lymphocytes resulting in a lytic infection. As a consequence viral antigens are presented to CD4+ T helper cells, which become activated as a part of the immune response. Unfortunately it is not yet possible to differentiate between Th1 and Th2 cells in chickens. Activated, but not resting T cells, are susceptible to infection with MDV and the infection switches from B to T cells, in which MDV establishes a latent infection. Some of the virus-positive lymphocytes locate in the feather follicle epithelium, where infectious virus is formed and shed into the environment with feathers and dander. Depending on a number of variables the latently infected T cells can become transformed by a still unknown mechanism. The virus probably integrates into the DNA of the tumor cells, although it is also possible that it remains in the nucleus as episomal DNA. Complete virus can be rescued from the tumor cells *in vitro* by cocultivation with permissive cell cultures. If latently infected lymphocytes are removed from the host and cultured *in vitro*, synthesis of viral antigens and DNA occurs. The addition of recombinant chicken interferon (IFN)α or IFNγ to these lymphocyte cultures will significantly reduce the synthesis of viral proteins suggesting that the host immune response plays a role in the maintenance of latency.

Resistance to Marek's Disease
All chickens are susceptible to infection resulting in latent infections, but not all chickens develop tumors (Figure 12.5). The development of tumors depends on the combination of oncogenicity of the infecting virus strain, the genetic background of the chicken, vaccine status, and environmental factors such as age of infection

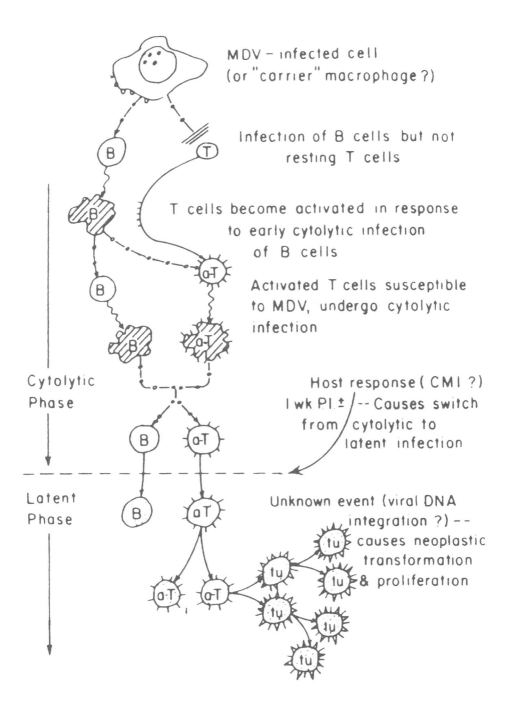

MDV – infected cell
(or "carrier" macrophage?)

Infection of B cells but not
resting T cells

T cells become activated in response
to early cytolytic infection
of B cells

Activated T cells susceptible
to MDV, undergo cytolytic
infection

Cytolytic
Phase

Host response (CMI?)
I wk P.I. ± /-- Causes switch
from / cytolytic to
latent infection

Latent
Phase

Unknown event (viral DNA
integration?) --
causes neoplastic
transformation
& proliferation

Figure 12.4.   Pathogenesis of Marek's disease. Virus infection results in a lytic infection of B lymphocytes. T cells responding to viral antigens become susceptible to infection and can undergo a lytic infection cycle or become latently infected. Latently infected T cells can become tumor cells. In: Calnek, B.W. Proceedings of the International Symposium on Marek's Disease (Calnek, B.W., and J.L. Spencer, eds), pp: 374–390, 1984. Reproduced with permission from the American Association of Avian Pathologists, Kennett Square, PA.

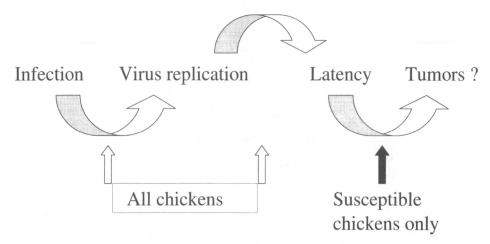

Figure 12.5. Induction of tumors by Marek's disease virus as an example of herpesvirus-induced tumors. Virus infects the host and replicates followed by latency. During latency only very few virus genes are transcribed. Depending on a number of factors, transformation may occur resulting in the formation of tumors.

with MDV, stress, and infection with other pathogens (Figure 12.6). A major part of the genetic resistance is linked to the expression of certain MHC Class I antigens. The basis for the MHC-based resistance is still unknown but it is probably related to T-cell-mediated immune responses (see below). Although birds of all ages are susceptible to tumor development, young chicks are in general more susceptible because they are still immunologically immature and therefore less able to control virus replication. Maternal antibodies, which are IgG or IgY in chickens, derived from the yolk provide limited protection during the first three weeks.

Immune Responses to Marek's Disease Virus
Immunity to MD has been divided into antiviral and antitumor immune responses although the presence of tumor-specific, nonvirus coded antigens on tumor cells has not been demonstrated. In contrast, viral proteins can be expressed on tumor cells and immune responses to these antigens are similar to antiviral responses. Both innate and acquired immune responses are involved in MD immunity.

Innate Immunity
Infection of chickens with MDV strains of all serotypes will activate natural killer (NK) cells as early as three days postinfection. The actual role of NK cells in MD immunity has not been elucidated, but it is probably directed toward the elimination of virus-infected lymphocytes. MD tumor cell lines are resistant to lysis by chicken large granular lymphocytes (which are cells with NK cell activity) suggesting that NK cells do not play a role in eliminating MD tumor cells. Suppressor macrophages also reduce virus replication in part by limiting T cell proliferation. It is also likely that macrophages restrict virus replication by the induction of nitric oxide (NO) and cytokines.

Inducible Immunity.
Antigen-specific cytotoxic T cells (CTL) have been demonstrated in infected and vaccinated chickens starting at six to seven days postinfection. These T cells express CD3, CD8, and TCRαβ1, but not CD4 and represent classical CTL. Chickens

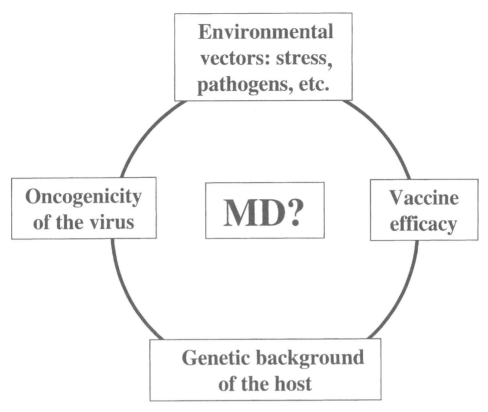

Figure 12.6. Interactions between the oncogenicity or virulence of Marek's disease virus and the genetic resistance or susceptibility of the host determine the outcome of infection. Vaccination status and environmental factors (e.g., age of exposure, stress induced by other pathogens, heat stress, etc.) are major factors influencing the outcome of infection.

have three T cell receptors, TCRαβ1, TCRαβ2, and TCRγδ, in contrast to only two, TCRαβ and TCRγδ, in mammals. These CTLs recognize different viral proteins and the generation of CTLs against ICP4, an immediate early viral protein, may be linked to MHC Class I associated resistance.

Viral neutralizing (VN) antibodies can be demonstrated starting at six days post-infection. At least some of the VN antibodies are directed against glycoprotein B, but it is likely that antibodies are also present against other glycoproteins. The importance of VN antibodies is limited in MD because the virus is strictly cell-associated. As a consequence, cell-free virus is only accessible to neutralization during the first phase of infection prior to initiation of replication in lymphocytes. However, antibodies can lyse infected cells by antibody-dependent cell-mediated cytotoxicity (ADDC) or complement activation.

Vaccination against Marek's Disease
Vaccines are prepared from attenuated oncogenic (serotype 1), serotype 2, and serotype 3 strains or a mixture of two or three serotypes. The use of these polyvalent vaccines became necessary when more virulent, oncogenic strains of MDV emerged during the late 70s. The vaccines are given to all chicks at one day of age or at seventeen to eighteen days of embryonation. Challenge with virulent virus occurs

as soon as the chicks are placed in the houses. Protection is directed against viral replication resulting in a decreased level of infected lymphocytes and the absence of virus-induced immunosuppression. These factors, in turn, reduce the risk that lymphocytes become transformed and form tumors. The mechanism of vaccine-induced protection has not been fully established, but NK cells are activated shortly after vaccination and antigen-specific CTL are generated. Although killed vaccines protect to some degree, live vaccines are used because they induce antigen-specific CTL, which are essential for optimal protection. The generation of antigen-specific CTL depends on *de novo* production of viral proteins, which are ultimately presented as nonapeptides by MHC Class I antigens (see chapter 8 for details). Infection with live vaccines follows the same basic pattern as infection with all herpesviruses resulting in the establishment of latency. Whenever immune responses to the vaccine virus decrease, virus will be reactivated resulting in replication followed by enhanced immunity.

Feline Leukemia

Feline leukemia is a complex disease caused by a horizontally transmitted exogenous retrovirus. One of the common consequences of infection with feline leukemia virus (FeLV) is immunosuppression due mostly to lymphopenia as a result of a reduction in T lymphocytes. The immunosuppression was originally linked to survival of tumor cells rather than to a disease entity in its own right. The discovery of a human immunodeficiency virus (HIV), a retrovirus, as the etiological agent of the acquired immunodeficiency syndrome (AIDS) and the subsequent finding of additional retroviruses linked to immunodeficiencies in other mammalian species including cats stimulated reexamination of retroviral diseases in animals. The isolation of a feline immunodeficiency virus (FIV) was important because it not only provided a model for AIDS research, but because it complicated the clinical picture of the disease syndrome linked to FeLV infection. Furthermore feline leukemia is the first mammalian cancer for which vaccines have been developed and which are marketed by commercial companies in many countries of the world.

Pathogenesis of Feline Leukemia

Feline leukemia virus (FeLV) was first described by Jarrett and his colleagues. Exogenous FeLVs associated with chronic infection are divided into subgroups A, B, and C. In addition, defective viruses containing cellular *onc* genes and endogenous viruses or sequences have been described. FeLV-A is present in all infected cats and is the only FeLV transmitted through saliva in the natural infection cycle. Subgroup B virus is always found in the presence of FeLV-A and results from a recombination of subgroup A virus with endogenous sequences coding for the viral glycoprotein. Subgroup C virus develops from subgroup A by point mutations in the *env* gene (Figure 12.7). The recombinations and mutations occur in approximately fifty percent and two percent of infected cats, respectively, but after these changes occur the new subgroup viruses are not transmitted horizontally.

The pathogenesis of feline leukemia is complex and not yet fully understood. Contact with infectious saliva results in infection in approximately seventy percent of the cats, it is not clear why the remaining thirty percent of nonimmune cats are resistant to infection. In susceptible cats, virus replicates first in lymphocytes, but many of these cats develop antibodies and become virus-free and immune soon after infection. Infection spreads to the bone marrow in cats that fail to develop an early antibody response, a spread resulting in persistent infection. A high percentage of these

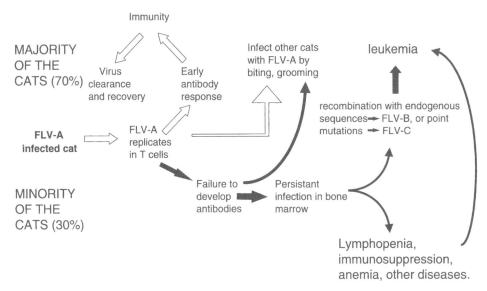

Figure 12.7. Pathogenesis of infection with feline leukemia virus A. In most infected cats (open arrows), virus replicates in T cells, cats develop antibodies and clear the infection. Transmission of the virus to other cats occurs through biting and grooming. In a minority of the cats (closed arrows), antibodies do not develop, persistent infection develops in the bone marrow, virus recombines or mutates to develop FeLV-B or -C, and tumors develop.

cats develop immunosuppression, anemia, lymphosarcomas, and other diseases (Figure 12.7). The lymphosarcomas often develop after cellular oncogenes are activated by the virus LTR or after recombination of these sequences with FeLV subgroup A viruses.

Resistance to Feline Leukemia
Two types of resistance have been recognized: (1) resistance to infection and (2) the ability to develop antibodies leading to viral clearance. Resistance to infection is likely caused by the absence of viral receptors for the glycoprotein on the virus envelope. The second type of resistance is clearly related to the ability to develop a vigorous humoral immune response, which is lacking in cats with a persistent infection.

Immunity to Feline Leukemia
It was mentioned in the previous section that the rapid production of antibodies is one of the deciding factors for the outcome of infection. These antibodies are directed against gp70 of subgroup A virus. In the past it had been proposed that immunity to feline leukemia was associated with antibody responses against **FOCMA** (**F**eline **O**ncornavirus-associated **C**ell **M**embrane **A**ntigen). However, it has recently been shown that FOCMA is actually the transmembrane p15E coded for by the *env* gene of subgroup C FeLV. This protein also has immunosuppressive properties and has been implicated in the pathogenesis of the disease. Antibodies against other viral proteins (e.g., proteins coded for by *gag*, see Figure 12.1) are often present in persistently infected cats. These antibodies do not neutralize the virus and can be detrimental by causing immune complex glomerulonephritis especially if the levels of circulating viral antigens are high.

Cell-mediated immune responses are also believed to be important in protective immunity, but the exact role of CTLs has not been established. Cats with depressed macrophage responses are more susceptible to virus infection, but it is not clear if this is the consequence of inadequate antigen presentation or cytokine dysfunctions.

Vaccines
Several vaccines against feline leukemia consisting of different preparations of FeLV-infected, inactivated cells are currently on the market. Some of the vaccines are FOCMA positive, while others are negative. The key to protection is the presence in the vaccines of gp70 of subgroup A FeLV and the subsequent development of neutralizing antibodies against this glycoprotein. Vaccination with recombinant gp70 of subgroup A has been shown to be equally effective as the inactivated whole virus vaccines.

During the last few years an increase in the incidence of soft-tissue sarcomas has been associated with vaccinations of cats against rabies virus. The vaccines are often given with adjuvants. However, an association between these sarcomas and the presence of FeLV or the use of FeLV vaccines has not been reported. Examination of these sarcomas for the presence of gp70 of FeLV by immunohistochemistry or the LTR of FeLV by polymerase chain reaction assays have been negative.

HEPATOCELLULAR CARCINOMA
Hepatocellular carcinoma (HCC) is a common tumor in humans especially in regions of Southeast Asia and subSaharan Africa causing more than 1 million deaths annually. HCC is most commonly associated with chronic hepatitis B virus (HBV) infections and subsequent liver cirrhosis. Worldwide an estimated 300 million people are carriers of HBV, but the prevalence of infection varies with the geographical region. Southeast Asia and subSaharan Africa have a high incidence (ten to twenty percent) of carriers, while West Europe and North America have a low incidence (one-tenth to two percent). The major mode of HBV transmission is perinatal in the high incidence areas which occurs probably through direct contact between the carrier mother and the infant. Infection at an early age prolongs replication and incomplete clearance of HBV from the liver and blood leading to low-level replication of HBV after the initial replication . Vaccines against HBV infection were introduced in 1982. Vaccination of populations at high risk have led to a sharp decline in chronic HBV infections and in Taiwan also in a marked reduction in the incidence of HCC. Infection with other viruses such as hepatitis C virus, alcoholism, or other factors leading to liver cirrhosis may also result in HCC.

Pathogenesis of Hepatocellular Carcinoma
Replication of HBV results in the formation of a major surface protein called S (approximately ninety percent of the total amount), and two minor (L and M) surface proteins. The S protein, or **HBsAg**, can form subviral particles which are exocytosed from the hepatocytes and enter into the blood stream. HbsAG is also a major component of infectious virus particles, thus the development of virus-neutralizing (VN) antibodies against HbsAg is critical for the clearance of HBV (Figure 12.8A). Infection of infants, young children between one and five years of age, or immunocompromised adults is characterized by a lack of antibody response to HbsAg and prolonged presence of HBV in the circulation. Approximately ninety percent of infants infected before one year of age develop chronic infections often without developing acute hepatitis or cirrhosis. The chronic infection can be divided into three phases. During the first phase, the majority of these children will remain positive for HbsAg over the next twenty to thirty years with a high risk of infecting their children at an early age. During the second phase virus clearance starts to occur often accompanied by lysis

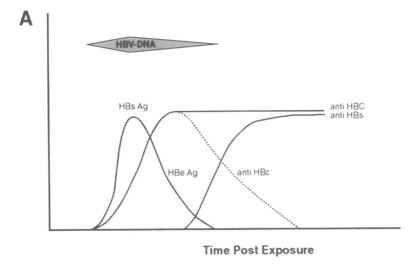

Time Post Exposure

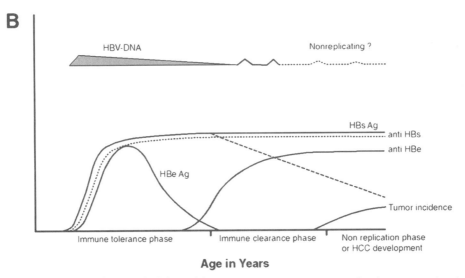

Age in Years

Figure 12.8.   (A) Infection of adults with hepatitis B virus: virus DNA can be demonstrated in the blood during the replication phase and HBsAg is present in the blood. Immunity (anti HBC) develops consisting of a IgM response (broken line) and IgG response (solid line) as well as an IgG response against HBs, both IgG responses remain present for life. (B) Infection of newborn babies causes a prolonged virus replication, as demonstrated by the detection of HBV DNA in the blood. The virus may be cleared during the immune clearance phase. HBsAg is continuously produced even in the presence of an antibody response to HBsAg, but levels will become low or absent if the immune clearance phase results in the nonreplicative phase of infection. Early core proteins (HBeAg) are produced, and antibodies against this protein develop. If immune clearance does not occur, the risk of developing hepatocellular carcinomas is high. (Adapted from Schiff's Diseases of the Liver, with permission from Lippincott-Raven, Philadelphia, PA).

of infected hepatocytes probably as the consequence of immune-mediated lysis of these cells. Finally, replication of HBV may cease during the third phase although some of these patients may remain positive for HbsAg. The consequences of the chronic infection range from none, with the development of asymptomatic, appar-

LIVERPOOL JOHN MOORES UNIVERSITY
LEARNING SERVICES

ently cured patients to the development of cirrhosis and HCC (Figure 12.8B). The actual mechanism(s) by which HCC develops in the latter group have not been fully elucidated. Integration of HBV DNA in the DNA of hepatocytes has been demonstrated in the presence as well as the absence of cirrhosis. Although integration of HBV DNA has been found near cellular oncogenes (e.g., *c-myc*) or tumor suppressor genes, it can also be found in many other locations on the chromosomes. Recently it has been suggested that one of the HBV proteins, **HBx**, may play a role in regulating viral and cellular genes. HBx may bind to the tumor suppressor gene p53 thus leading to a decrease in cell death. In addition, continuous low-level damage to hepatocytes and subsequent repair may lead to increased changes in mutations involved in the regulation of the cell cycle. Once HCC develops the tumor progresses and the survival rate is poor.

Resistance to Hepatitis B Virus Infection and Hepatocellular Carcinoma.
Obviously, prevention of infection by HBV is important for the prevention of HCC. Once infection has been established, patients can be treated with **interferon-α (IFN-α)**, but this approach has yielded disappointing results in infected infants. The use of antiviral drugs may provide another approach and several drugs have been evaluated in clinical trials. However, the development of effective vaccines may reduce the need to use drugs in infants and young children.

Immunity to Hepatitis B Virus
Infection of immunocompetent individuals with HBV results in the production of a polymerase, envelope surface proteins S, L, and M, nucleocapsid protein or hepatitis B core antigen (HBcAg), precore antigen and its secretory products HBeAg, and HBx. Only antibodies against HBsAg are protective and in most patients these antibodies persist for life. Anti-HBc-IgM can be detected early in the infection before HBsAg or anti-HBs are present. The presence of HBeAg is associated with chronic infection and its has been suggested that this protein may interfere with the development of immune responses. The appearance of anti-HBe is associated with the second phase of chronic infection and disappearance of infectious virus.

The importance of cell-mediated immune responses in clearance of HBV is not fully understood. It has been suggested that cytotoxic T cells (CTL) may cure cells infected with HBV through the production and targeted delivery of interferon-γ. These HBV-specific CTL do not use the perforin or FAS pathways to kill virus-infected hepatocytes.

Vaccination against Hepatitis B Virus
The first vaccine was developed and marketed in 1982 using HBsAg as the immunogen. The HBsAg was derived from blood plasma obtained from infected individuals. Since 1986 recombinant vaccines have been introduced, in which HBsAg is produced by *Saccharomyces cerevisiae* (also known as baker's yeast) containing the gene for HBsAg. Thus far this is the only example of a recombinant vaccine commercially available for use in humans. Currently over eighty countries have implemented vaccination programs resulting not only in protection in vaccinated children but also in reducing the overall rate of infection in nonvaccinated groups. If the mother is HBsAg positive, the vaccine needs to be given within twelve hours of birth in combination with high-titered HBV-specific immunoglobulin to achieve protection. The protection given by the vaccine is based on the development of antibodies against HBsAg. The antibodies neutral-

ize HBV particles. The vaccine is similar to other inactivated antiviral vaccines. The vaccine-induced protection against HCC is solely based on protection against virus infection.

CONCLUSIONS FROM IMMUNIZATION STUDIES AGAINST VIRAL-INDUCED NEOPLASIA

Marek's disease and feline leukemia vaccines have often been described as examples of antitumor vaccines. However, in both instances the vaccine-induced immunity is directed against viral components, and these immune responses are fundamentally identical to other antiviral immune responses. Immune responses against non-virus-coded tumor-specific antigens (TSA) have not yet been demonstrated in naturally infected or vaccinated chickens with Marek's disease nor in cats with feline leukemia. In contrast it has never been suggested that the vaccine against HBV is an antitumor vaccine. The reduction in HCC in high risk countries, e.g., Taiwan, is a desirable secondary effect of successful implementation of HBV vaccine programs.

IMMUNOLOGICAL APPROACHES FOR THE CONTROL OF TUMORS

Predictions by immunologists that new advances in tumor immunology would lead to significant improvements in the struggle against cancer in the near future have invariably been followed by disappointing results. It is therefore dangerous to once more predict a successful role for immunological-based therapies, but some strategies have emerged during the last few years that may actually provide some degree of effectiveness. These strategies may become important in those cases of human cancers where chemical or radiation therapies with or without surgery are not effective. In order to be successful the strategy has (a) to overcome the lack of recognition of the tumor cells by the immune system, and (b) to increase the immunogenicity of TSAs. Upregulation of MHC Class I expression on tumor cells has been achieved in experimental tumors by vaccination with engineered tumor cells expressing cytokines such as Il-2, Il-4 and IFN-γ. Another promising approach is to transfect tumor cells lacking MHC Class I expression with the appropriate MHC Class I gene. These tumor cells can be injected into the tumor, where they can be recognized by tumor infiltrating lymphoccytes (TIL) that have been activated by *in vitro* stimulation. The consequence of this recognition is that cytokines are produced by the activated TIL recruiting other cells such as granulocytes. It has been proposed that a complex and only partially understood series of interactions between T lymphocytes, granulocytes, and cytokines may be involved in rejection and elimination of tumor cells.

In the case of human melanocarcinomas, a series of antigens like MAGE, BAGE, and MART-1 have been identified on the tumor cells. These antigens may also be expressed on normal melanoma cells (e.g., MART-1) or on normal testis (MAGE, BAGE and others). These antigens can be recognized when presented by MHC Class I proteins and the actual epitopes have been identified for these TSAs. Cell lines established from melanomas can be used to stimulate and expand *in vitro* CD8+ TILs obtained from patients with melanocarcinomas. In a limited number of clinical trials patients with melanocarcinomas went into remission after treatment with autologous *in vitro* activated TILs.

A more complex but potentially rewarding technique is the possibility of engineering tumor-specific killer cells. Chen and colleagues (1997) developed a killer lymphocyte that recognized an antigen overexpressed on a number of human cancers and which delivered a potent toxin to the tumor cells. They cloned the heavy and light chain genes of the monoclonal antibody for this antigen in frame with the genes for a potent toxin. This construct was transfected into lymphokine activated killer cells. Inoculation of these cells into nude mice grafted with tumors led to clearance of the tumor. Although this approach has yet to be proven to work in humans in actual clinical trails, it may become feasible to develop such cells especially since a number of TSA have been identified.

PROSPECTS FOR IMMUNOLOGICAL CONTROL OF NEOPLASIA

During the last ten years, tremendous progress has been made in the understanding of the molecular changes leading to the development of tumors and the ways in which tumor cells can prevent their elimination by immune responses. Less progress has been made in using this knowledge to treat cancer by immunotherapy. The two viral-induced cancers for which vaccines are available (Marek's disease and feline leukemia) are not really good models for studies leading to the development of future cancer vaccines, because in both cases the relevant immune responses are antiviral and do not differ fundamentally from vaccine-induced immune responses against nononcogenic virus infections. Although tumor immunology has not lived up to its early expectations, the combination of molecular technology and increased understanding of the complex interactions involved in tumor rejection may still lead to a bright future for immunotherapy to combat cancer in humans and other animals.

SUMMARY

Tumors develop as the consequence of changes in cellular genes controlling the cell cycle (proto-oncogenes become cellular oncogenes or *c-onc*) or after infection with viruses that activate *c-onc* genes or contain *v-onc* genes. Immune responses against these altered or viral genes may develop if the protein is recognized as foreign, but tumors have developed several mechanisms interfering with immunity. Marek's disease herpesvirus (MDV) and feline leukemia virus (FLV) (a retrovirus) can cause tumors in chickens and cats, respectively. Vaccines exist to protect chickens and cats against tumor development as a consequence of MDV or FLV infection. However, both vaccines induce antiviral immune responses rather than antitumor immune responses. Hepatitis B virus (HBV) causes liver infection in humans and can cause hepatocellular carcinomas especially if the infection becomes chronic. Vaccines against the surface antigen of HBV (HBsAg) protect against virus infection and indirectly against hepatocellular carcinomas. Recently, several tumor specific antigens have been defined in human melanomas. Knowledge gained from the study of such antigens may lead to effective methods for using immune responses to combat cancer.

SUGGESTIONS FOR FURTHER READING:

Papers of historical interest on immune surveillance:
1. Burnet, F.M. "A Certain Symmetry: Histocompatibility Antigens Compared with Immunocyte Receptors." *Nature* 226 (1970):123–126.
2. Möller G., and E. Möller, eds. "Experiments and the Concept of Immunological Surveillance." *Transplantations Reviews* 28 (1976):3–96.

Current Reviews on Ways that Tumor Cells Escape Immune Recognition and Future Developments

1. Ellem, K.A.O., C.W. Schmidt, C.-L. Li, I. Misko, A. Kelso, G. Sing, G. Macdonald, and M.G.E. O'Rourke. "The Labyrinthine Ways of Cancer Immunotherapy —T Cell, Tumor Cell Encounter: 'How Do I Lose Thee? Let Me Count the Ways.'" *Advances in Cancer Research* 75 (1998):203–249.
2. Chen, S-Y., A-G. Yang, J-D. Chen, T. Kute, C.R. King, J. Colliers, Y. Cong, C. Yao, and X.F. Huang. "Potent Antitumour Activity of a New Class of Tumour-Specific Killer Cells." *Nature* 385 (1997):78–80.
3. Several papers in *Immunology Today* volumes 18 and 19 (1997, 1998). This is a good journal to read to keep informed on new developments.

Marek's Disease

1. Schat, K.A. "Immunity to Marek's Disease, Lymphoid Leukosis and Reticuloendotheliosis." In *Poultry Immunology*. Edited by T.F. Davison, T.R. Morris, and L.N. Payne, 209–234. Abingdon, UK: Carfax Publishing Company, 1996.
2. Calnek, B.W., and R.L. Witter. "Marek's disease." In *Diseases of Poultry*. Edited by B.W. Calnek, H.J. Barnes, C.W. Beard, L.R. McDougald, and Y.M. Saif, 367–413. Ames, IA: Iowa State University Press, 1997. (Textbook article on all aspects of Marek's disease)

Feline Leukemia

1. Sparkes, A.H. "Feline Leukemia Virus: A Review of Immunity and Vaccination." *J. Small Animal Practice* 38 (1997):187–194. (Specific for the immunity to feline leukemia).
2. Hardy, W.D. Jr. "Feline Oncoretroviruses." In *The Retroviridae*, vol 2. Edited by J.A. Levy, 109–180. New York: Plenum Press, 1993. (Textbook article on all aspects of feline leukemia)

Hepatitis B Virus and Hepatocellular Carcinoma

1. *Diseases of the Liver*. 8th ed. Edited by E. R. Schiff, M. F. Sorrell, and W. C. Maddrey. Philadelphia/New York: Lippincott-Raven, 1998.

The following chapters in Schiff's *Diseases of the Liver* are recommended:
a. Doo, E.C., and T.J. Liang. "The Hepatitis Viruses." Vol. I, 725–744.
b. Chan, H.L., M.G. Ghany, and A.S.F. Lok. "Hepatitis B.: Vol I, 757–792.
c. Koff, R.S. "Hepatitis Vaccines." Vol I, 897–905.
d. Di Bisceglie, A.M. "Malignant Neoplasms of the Liver." Vol II, 1281–1304.

QUESTIONS

1. What are proto-oncogenes, cellular oncogenes and viral oncogenes?
2. Do tumors always develop as a consequence of uncontrolled cell division?
3. Name a virus group and an example of a RNA virus that can transform cells. Briefly describe two mechanisms by which this virus transforms cells.
4. Name three DNA virus families that can cause tumors.
5. Describe how these viruses can transform cells into tumor cells.
6. How do chemically induced tumors and spontaneous tumors develop?
7. Are the changes in tumor cell genomes always detectable by the immune system?
8. What is the immunosurveillance hypothesis and who formulated the hypothesis?
9. How do tumor cells escape detection by the immune system?

10. Does infection with Marek's disease virus always result in the formation of tumors? Explain your answer.
11. Why are virus-neutralizing antibodies not very important in Marek's disease?
12. Describe how Marek's disease vaccines protect. Is the protection directed against viral or tumor antigens?
13. What are the groups of feline leukemia virus and what are the differences between the groups?
14. What happens normally when a cat becomes infected with FeLV-A?
15. When do cats develop sarcomas or other diseases associated with infection with FeLV?
16. What is the major immune response in cats infected with feline leukemia virus and how has this been used in vaccines?
17. Is there formation of neutralizing antibodies against FeLV-B?
18. Do FeLV or MDV infect humans?
19. What happens when an adult becomes infected with hepatitis B virus?
20. What happens when babies get infected with hepatitis B virus?
21. What is novel about the HBV vaccines?

ANSWERS

1. A. A proto-oncogene is a positive regulator for the cell cycle, thus activation of a proto-oncogene results in the cell leaving G_0 and entering the cell cycle.
B. A cellular oncogene is a proto-oncogene that has been mutated and is switched on permanently leading to uncontrolled cell division.
C. A viral oncogene is part of a proto-oncogene that has been incorporated in a virus and is altered such that it is permanently switched on driving infected cells to uncontrolled cell division.
2. No, inhibition of apoptosis or programmed cell death can also lead to the development of tumors even if the cell division remains normal. This is because the cells remain alive much longer while dividing at the normal level leading to an increase in absolute cell numbers.
3. Retroviruses and more specifically members of the subfamily of retrovirinae (e.g., feline leukemia virus). These viruses transform cells by insertion of their genome into the cellular genome after reverse transcription into DNA. These viruses transform cells by a) insertion next to or close to a cellular proto-oncogene resulting in enhanced transcription and translation of that gene or b) by containing a viral oncogene that is inserted into to cellular genome.
4. Herpesviridae, Hepadnaviruses, Papovaviridae.
5. The DNA viruses can transform cells by activating receptors for growth factors, inhibition of apoptosis, activation of c-myc, or activation of cytokine- cytokine receptor pathways by methods resembling antigen stimulation. The latter is especially important in the development of lymphomas. A general condition for transformation by DNA viruses is that the lytic viral replication is prevented.
6. Point mutations in proto-oncogenes or tumor supressor genes may lead to uncontrolled cellular division. Chemicals or physical factors (e.g., ultraviolet light) may induce these point mutations in the DNA.
7. No, only if the changes cause the expression of proteins that are normally not expressed and for which tolerance has not developed (e.g., MARGE in melano-

mas) or if the point mutations cause changes in epitopes presented to the immune system that are no longer recognized as self.

8. The hypothesis was formulated by F.M. Burnet. It states that ancestral lymphocytes developed the capacity to eliminate cells expressing not-self antigens (e.g., tumor cells).

9. Tumor cells have developed mechanisms interfering with antigen presentation (e.g., transport of nonapeptided by the TAP 1+2 proteins, changes in the β2 microglobulin leading to instable MHC complexes and lowered MHC Class I expression). A second mechanism at evasion is production of immunosuppressive products or by interference with the Fas-induced apoptotic pathway. A third mechanism is alteration in cytokine production resulting in mutations in genes programming their production. The tumor-infiltrating lymphocytes which lack ability to undergo antigenic stimulation and effector cells which either undergo apoptosis or become quiescent in vivo. A fourth mechanism is prevention of CTLs leaving the blood vessels growing into tumors due to a lack of homing signals in these vessels.

10. No, there are many factors that can influence the outcome of infection such as the virulence of the infecting virus, the age at infection, the genetic resistance or susceptibility of the chicken, infection with other immunosuppressive viruses and the degree of stress at the time of infection.

11. Marek's disease virus has a strictly cell-associated replication cycle and usually spreads from cell to cell directly. The exception is in the case of infection of the feather follicle epithelium (the parts of the skin where the feathers are inserted) where cell-free virus is produced. Antibodies can therefore only neutralize the virus before it enters B and T lymphocytes.

12. Vaccination activates natural killer cells early after infection which is followed by the generation of antigen-specific cytotoxic T cells. Virus-neutralizing antibodies are also made, but these are only important early in infection or when vaccinated chickens become infected with MDV. Vaccinated birds that are challenged have a significantly lower level of virus replication suggesting that the vaccine-induced immune responses are mostly antiviral in nature.

13. a) FeLV-A, B and C.
    b) FeLV-A spreads horizontally, FeLV-B develops by recombination of FeLV-A with endogenous sequences coding for viral glycoprotein, and FeLV-C develops by point mutations.

14. The cat develops neutralizing antibodies, becomes immune and clears the infection.

15. When a chronic infection develops and the virus replicates in the bone marrow. Recombinations or mutations then occur and these recombined or mutated viruses can activate cellular proto-oncogenes which act as c-onc genes thus driving cells into reproduction.

16. The major response is the development of neutralizing antibodies against glyco-protein (gp)70 of FeLV-A. Recombinant vaccines expressing this glycoprotein protect cats against leukemia and other diseases associated with this infection.

17. No, the glycoprotein in FeLV-B is derived from an endogenous gene and this is not recognized by the immune system as foreign.

18. No, both viruses need species specific receptors to enter cells for replication. These receptors are not present in humans. These viruses do not constitute a human health risk.

19. Hepatitis develops, antibodies against the hepatitis surface antigen (HBsAg) develop and may clear virus infection.
20. They are not able to clear the virus, they continue to have HBsAg in their blood as a result in chronic virus replication. After twenty to thirty years some individuals clear the infection but a small group will not clear the virus and develop hepato-cellular carcinomas.
21. The new vaccines against HBV are the first vaccines for human use that are made by recombinant technology. The gene for HBsAg has been inserted in to yeast and the expressed protein is used to vaccinate inducing a virus-neutralizing immune response against HBV.

INTRODUCTION
IMMUNITY IN
  INVERTEBRATES
  Introduction
  Phagocytosis
  The Prophenoloxidase
    System
  Humoral Immunity
  Cell-Mediated Immunity
IMMUNITY IN FISH
  Introduction
  Inflammation
  Lymphoid Organs
  Lymphocytes
  Antigen Receptors
  Immunoglobulins
  Immunoglobulin Gene
    Arrangement
  Complement
  Antibody Responses
  T Cell Responses
IMMUNITY IN AMPHIBIANS
  Introduction
  Lymphoid Organs
  Lymphocytes
  Immunoglobulins
  Immune Responses
  T Cell Responses
IMMUNITY IN REPTILES
  Introduction
  Lymphoid Organs
  Immunoglobulins
  Immune Responses
  T Cell Responses
IMMUNITY IN BIRDS (AND
  DINOSAURS)
  Introduction
  Lymphoid Organs
  Lymphocytes
  Immunoglobulins
  Immune Responses
  T Cell Responses
IMMUNITY IN MAMMALS
  Introduction
  Monotremes and Marsupials
  Some Differences Between
    Humans and Common
    Domestic Mammals
  Absorption of Colostrum
SUMMARY
SUGGESTIONS FOR
  FURTHER READING
QUESTIONS
ANSWERS

Comparative Immunology

Ian Tizard

INTRODUCTION

All living organisms, regardless of their complexity or evolutionary history are potential targets for pathogenic microorganisms. They must therefore be able to exclude invaders that might cause disease or death. Although the defense mechanisms employed by invertebrates and vertebrates have a superficial similarity, they usually have a different evolutionary origin. Thus, the defenses of invertebrates are considered to be functional analogs of vertebrate immune mechanisms insofar as they have similar effects but are of different origin. In contrast, the various vertebrate immune systems are usually homologous, not only having similar functions, but also having the same origins. Figure 13.1 provides a phylogenic tree of animal life on earth. The points of separation of the various forms are indicated and its perusal will permit the reader to obtain a rough grasp of the relationships among the various groups discussed in the remainder of this chapter.

IMMUNITY IN INVERTEBRATES

Introduction

Invertebrates may be divided into two major groups based on the presence or absence of a body cavity (coelom), (1) the acoelomates, including the sponges and coelenterates (jellyfish and sea anemones) and (2) the coelomates. The coelomates themselves are divided into two subgroups, the protostomes which subgroup includes the annelids, mollusks, and arthropods, and the deuterostomes which subgroup includes the echinoderms, protochordates, and chordates. It is from deuterostome-like ancestors that the vertebrates evolved.

Invertebrates protect themselves against invasion by processes of phagocytosis, humoral immunity, and cell-mediated immunity as well as by physical barriers. For

247

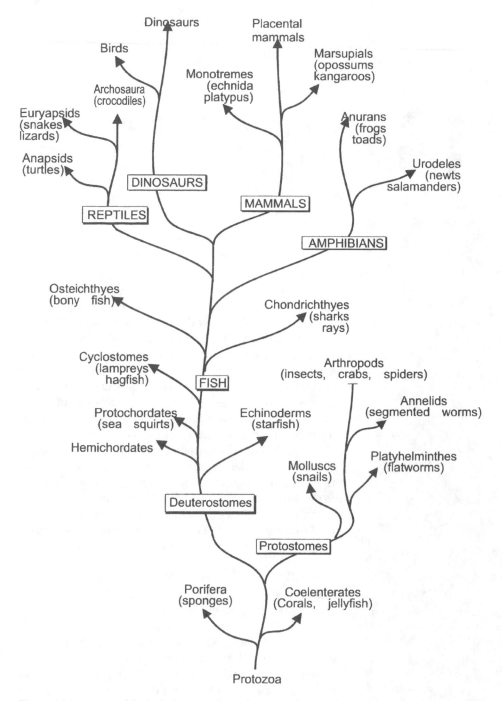

Figure 13.1. A simplified phylogeny of vertebrates and invertebrates.

example, arthropods have tough exoskeletons made of chitin that can protect them against all types of attackers. The horseshoe crab (*Limulus polyphemus*) not only has a hard exoskeleton but can also protect itself against bacterial endotoxins by secreting a specialized glycoprotein through pores in the carapace. On contact with bacterial endotoxins, this glycoprotein coagulates, sealing the pores and immobilizing any invading bacteria. Other invertebrates such as the coelenterates, annelids, mollusca, and echinoderms may secrete masses of sticky antibacterial mucus when attacked thereby immobilizing potential invaders.

Phagocytosis

In 1884, Eli Mechnikoff discovered phagocytosis while examining starfish larvae. He showed that mobile cells attacked rose thorns introduced into the coelom of these larvae. Several different types of phagocytic cell are recognized in invertebrates; the most important are blood leukocytes (hemocytes) and body cavity cells (coelomocytes). These cells act like mammalian phagocytes and undergo chemotaxis, adherence, ingestion, and digestion. They contain proteases and may produce reactive oxygen radicals. Some phagocytic cells may be hemostatic and can aggregate in and plug wounds. In cases where these cells are unable to control invaders by phagocytosis, granulomas may form.

The Prophenoloxidase System

Arthropods possess a family of enzymes that when activated, can generate a cascade of proteases leading to the production of phenol oxidase. They are activated by the interaction of bacteria, and fungi with hemocytes. Phenoloxidase is an enzyme that binds to foreign surfaces. It acts on tyrosine and dopamine to generate melanin around sites where immune defense reactions occur. In addition phenoloxidase enhances phagocytosis, plasma coagulation, and killing of bacteria and fungi.

Humoral Immunity

Soluble protective factors have been detected in the body fluids of both acoelomates and coelomates. When sea anemones are injected with bovine serum albumin (BSA), they produce a protein in tissue fluid that can bind to the BSA. This protein binds more strongly to BSA than it does to human serum albumin, suggesting some specificity of the reaction. Certain snails can produce proteins that bind and immobilize invading schistosome miracidia (larval forms of schistosome parasites). These proteins appear to be specific for the schistosome.

If insects are injected with heat-killed bacteria, proteins appear in their hemolymph that can prevent bacterial growth or cause bacterial lysis. For example, following infection of tomato hornworms, their hemocytes and hemolymph plasma enzymes degrade bacterial cell walls releasing peptidoglycans. These peptidoglycans in turn elicit increased synthesis of antibacterial proteins which accumulate in the hemolymph. In some insects toxins induce proteins that mimic antibody molecules. Among the proteins induced in this way is lysozyme. These antibacterial proteins appear about two hours after exposure to the bacteria and reach peak levels at twenty-four hours. In some insects, the activity is short-lived and disappears by four days; in others, it may last for several months. Passive immunity can be conferred on recipient insects by transfer of hemolymph from immune insects. Little is known about the mechanisms involved in the production of these antibacterial proteins.

Natural agglutinins are found in the coelomic fluid of coelenterates and annelids and in the hemolymph of arthropods and mollusks. These agglutinins are carbohydrate binding proteins (i.e., lectins). Most invertebrates make multiple lectins that recognize different carbohydrates. Horseshoe crab agglutinin binds N-acetyl-D-glucosamine, while scorpion and lobster agglutinins bind sialic acid and its derivatives. When these lectins bind carbohydrates on the surface of invading microorganisms, they may act as opsonins.

Echinoderms such as the starfish, *Asterias rubens*, possess an "axial organ." This organ contains cells that can bind antigens, respond to mitogens, and secrete lymphokine-like and antibody-like proteins. These proteins are pentamers of 120 kDa whose production involves cooperation between two different cell populations. If starfish are injected with the hapten trinitrophenol (TNP) attached to a carrier protein, the proteins produced by the axial organ will bind and lyse TNP-coated red blood cells in the presence of mammalian complement.

In some protostomes, proteins that resemble the terminal components of the complement pathway have been found in hemolymph. For example, the horseshoe crab and sipunculid worms have a lytic activity in their hemolymph that is inducible after treatment with cobra venom factor (a protease that activates C3). The coelomic fluid of earthworms can lyse vertebrate erythrocytes and digest some vertebrate serum proteins.

Cell-Mediated Immunity

Analogs of cell-mediated immunity are identifiable in simple organisms such as the sponges. Cell-mediated graft rejection is seen in sponges, coelenterates, annelids, and echinoderms. For example, sponges show allogeneic incompatibility. When two identical sponge colonies are placed side by side and made to grow in contact with each other, no reaction occurs. If, however, sponges from two different colonies are made to grow in contact, local destruction of the sponge tissue occurs along the area of contact as each sponge attempts to destroy the other. Allograft reactions have not been demonstrated among mollusks although these protostomia can reject xenografts. Annelids such as earthworms can reject both allografts and xenografts. The rejection of xenografts (grafts from other species of earthworms) takes about twenty days. Lymphocyte-like and phagocytic cells invade the graft. The grafted tissue turns white, swells, becomes edematous, and eventually dies. If the recipient worms are grafted with a second piece of skin from the same donor, the second graft is rejected faster than the first. This ability to reject second grafts rapidly may be adoptively transferred by coelomocytes from sensitized animals.

Echinoderms and tunicates are also able to reject allografts. Certain colonial tunicates have an analog of a histocompatibility locus that determines whether a new individual can be accepted into a parabiotic colony. (A parabiotic colony is one in which all the individuals are linked and so share vascular and nutrient functions.) Urochordates reject allografts by the actions of lymphocyte-like cells. First-set allografts are rejected in about forty days. Second-set allografts are rejected in twenty days. Specific memory lasts for at least fifty days after the first graft is rejected.

Many invertebrates possess either genes or proteins that are related to those found in vertebrates. Thus tunicates possess a protein related to mammalian CD5 as well as proteins coded by genes related to the J segments of mammalian immunoglobulin heavy chains. CD90, a molecule associated with vertebrate T cells, has been identified in squid, oysters, and locusts, as well as in tunicates. Tunicate CD90 shows close homology to the μ chains of fish immunoglobulin. β2-microglobulin, the β chain of MHC Class I molecules has been identified in the leukocytes of earthworms and in cultured *Drosophila* cells. IL-1α, IL-1β, and TNF-like activity have been identified in echinoderms and annelids as well as in urochordates.

IMMUNITY IN FISH

Introduction

The animals called fish include three very different classes of vertebrates. They include the Agnatha, jawless fish such as the lampreys, and the hagfish. A more developed class is the Chondrichthyes. These are fish with cartilaginous skeletons and include the elasmobranchs such as the skates, rays, and sharks. The most complex are the bony fish of the class Osteicthyes. These include the overwhelming majority of modern fish, the teleosts. Significant differences exist between the immune systems of each of these three classes.

Inflammation

Fish can mount acute inflammatory reactions involving granulocytes, macrophages, and lymphocytes. Granulocytes enter the inflammatory site first, and this is followed by a later wave of macrophages and possibly lymphocytes. The granulocytes are attracted by microbial products and leukotrienes. Fish have macrophages in many tissues, especially in the mesentery, the spleen, the kidney, and the heart. They are highly phagocytic and closely resemble mammalian macrophages although they may lack Fc and C3 receptors. Fish neutrophils are phagocytic, and their numbers increase in response to infection. They possess most of the enzymes of mammalian neutrophils. However the phagocytic activity of fish neutrophils varies between species and it has been suggested that in some fish, neutrophils may carry out their bactericidal function extracellularly rather than intracellularly.

The release of free oxygen radicals from neutrophils during inflammation may cause severe tissue damage. Fish lipids are highly polyunsaturated as an adaptation to low temperatures. These polyunsaturated fats are highly susceptible to oxidation and fish must therefore have mechanisms to prevent lipid oxidation. Melanin-containing cells serve this function. They are found in the lymphoid tissues of most bony fish, as well as in inflammatory lesions. Because melanin can quench free oxidizing radicals, it has been suggested that these cells protect tissues against free radicals produced by phagocytic cells.

Lymphoid Organs

Cartilaginous and bony fish have three major lymphoid organs. These are a head kidney, a thymus, and a spleen. Fish lack bone marrow. The development of a bone marrow depends upon the presence of suitable bones, and fish do not have suitable bones. These bones did not appear until vertebrates became adapted to a terrestrial existence, and therefore, fish do not have a bone marrow. There is no detectable thymus in cyclostomes. A thymus does, however, appear in cartilaginous and bony fish. It is found just above the pharynx. In immature fish small pores lead from the pharynx to the thymus suggesting that it may be exposed directly to antigens in the water. Thymectomy in fish can prolong allograft survival and reduces antibody responses. Antibodies and antigen-binding cells can be detected in the fish thymus. The thymus involutes in aged fish and in response to hormones or season.

Like the thymus, the spleen first appears in cartilaginous and bony fish and is absent from cyclostomes. Its overall structure and location are similar to that in mammals. The fish kidney, unlike that in mammals is divided into two sections. The posterior kidney (opisthnephros) is an excretory organ with the same function as the mammalian kidney. In contrast, the head kidney (pronephros) is a lymphoid organ containing antibody-forming cells and phagocytes. Its function is analogous to mammalian bone marrow and lymph nodes.

Lymphocytes
The cyclostome hagfish has two blood leukocyte populations. One is monocyte-like and the other is lymphocyte-like. These lymphocytes originate from the pronephros and about seventy percent of them have surface antigen-binding molecules. Plasma cells have not been observed in cyclostomes but cartilaginous and bony fish possess both lymphocytes and plasma cells. Immunoglobulin-positive lymphocytes can be found in the thymus, kidney, spleen, and blood, and they are assumed to be B cells. Fish lymphocytes can respond to bacterial lipopolysaccharide and PPD tuberculin. Lymphocytes from the pronephros respond only to LPS while thymocytes will not respond to either. T cells can be detected in fish by using antiserum directed against the fish homolog of CD90. These fish T lymphocytes also respond to phytohemagglutinin and concanavalin A. Fish T cells can perform a helper function and stimulate B cells to provoke antibody formation. NK cells have been described in bony fish.

Antigen Receptors
The immune system depends upon possession of three key antigen receptor systems, the T cell antigen receptor (TCR), the B cell antigen receptor (BCR), and the major histocompatibility complex (MHC). Both the TCR and BCR require the rearrangement of gene segments in order to form functional receptors. Thus for a vertebrate to possess an immune system equivalent to that seen in mammals the minimal requirements are possession of these three antigen receptors, and the ability to rearrange receptor genes. The least developed vertebrates that possess all three components are the cartilaginous fish.

Immunoglobulins
The cyclostomes make antigen-binding molecules that are induced by injection of bacteria. These proteins bind to streptococci and enhance phagocytosis of yeast by leukocytes. However, their amino acid sequences more closely resemble those of the complement components such as C3 than those of antibody molecules. It is probable that these molecules are part of a nonclonal complement-related humoral defense system.

IgM is the only immunoglobulin universally found in vertebrates, and it is therefore believed to be the ancestral immunoglobulin molecule. In fact, bony and cartilaginous fish produce primarily IgM. Cartilaginous fish usually have serum IgM in pentameric and monomeric forms while bony fish have tetrameric and monomeric forms of IgM. Recently several new immunoglobulin isotypes have been identified in elasmobranchs. These include IgW in the sandbar shark and IgR in the skate. The heavy chain of IgW contains six C_H domains, two more than IgM. Sequence analysis suggests that IgW may be an evolutionary precursor of IgD or IgA. IgR on the other hand has only two C_H domains.

The blood vessel walls of fish are permeable to immunoglobulins. As a result, antibodies are found in tissue fluids, in plasma, lymph, and skin mucus. In blood they constitute about forty to fifty percent of the total serum proteins. IgM is also found in the skin-covering mucus of bony fish. It appears to be locally synthesized. Fish antibody in the presence of normal serum as a source of complement is capable of lysing target cells. Likewise, fish antibodies can cause agglutination. There is no evidence that fish antibodies can function as opsonins nor have Fc receptors been detected on fish phagocytes.

Immunoglobulin Gene Arrangement

The way in which immunoglobulin molecules are coded for by light and heavy chain genes and the structures of the V, J, and C gene segments are conserved throughout the vertebrates. Nevertheless there are major differences among species in the organization of these immunoglobulin gene segments. For example, sharks and other elasmobranchs have clustered immunoglobulin genes where one V, D, J segment is linked to its own constant segment thus;

-VDJC–VDJC–VDJC–VDJC–VDJC–

There are more than 500 of these VDJC clusters and each cluster is about 16 kilobases in size. This arrangement is different from that in teleost fish which have a mammalian type of arrangement with multiple Vh genes arranged thus;

-V-V-V-V-V-V-V-V-D-D-J-J-J-J-C–

The low molecular weight immunoglobulin of lungfish, amphibians, reptiles, and birds is called immunoglobulin Y. Like the immunoglobulins of mammals, IgY consists of two heavy and two light chains. The heavy chains, called upsilon (υ) chains, usually consist of one variable and four constant domains and the complete molecule has a molecular weight of about 180 kDa. However, a truncated isoform that has only two constant domains is also found. This isoform has a molecular weight of about 120 kDa. Some other vertebrates such as ducks and geese, turtles and the lungfish have both full-sized and truncated IgY. Others such as chickens have only full-sized molecules while some turtles produce only truncated molecules. The truncated isoform of IgY is produced as a result of an alternative splicing of heavy chain mRNA. Its correct name is therefore IgY(ΔFc). Because this molecule lacks a Fc region, it lacks the capacity to initiate the usual immunoglobulin effector functions such as complement activation and FcR binding. Its function is unclear. Similar truncated immunoglobulins have also been found to occur in some fish [IgM(ΔFc)], some turtles and in the quokka (*Setonix brachyurus*), a marsupial.

Complement

Cyclostomes have a complement system that consists only of the alternate pathway. Thus lamprey C3 genes retain features of the common ancestor of mammalian C3 and C4 and the lamprey factor B gene resembles the common ancestor of factor B and C2. The lamprey complement system promotes phagocytosis rather than lysis. Cartilaginous and bony fish possess complement acting by both classical and alternate pathways and contains components similar to the mammalian components C1, C3, and C5. Fish complement generates a membrane attack complex similar to that formed in mammals. However, it works at a lower temperature, generally around 25°C.

Antibody Responses

Soluble antigens are usually poorly immunogenic in fish, while particulate antigens such as bacteria or foreign erythrocytes are highly immunogenic. In bony fish, IgM antibodies are produced in response to particulate antigens, while IgG or IgY antibodies are associated with the response to soluble antigens. Many cartilaginous fish show seasonal effects on antibody production, in that under constant conditions of light and temperature immune responses are poorer in winter than in summer.

Fish respond to antigens faster and with a greater immune response at higher temperatures. At low temperatures, the lag period may be long, or there may be a complete absence of an immune response. Only certain phases of the antibody response are temperature dependent. Thus, secondary immune responses may be elicited at low temperature, provided primary immunization is carried out at a high temperature. There is some evidence that the cells that are sensitive to temperature in fish are helper T cells and that the poor response of chilled fish to antigens is due to a loss of T cell membrane fluidity and reactivity to interleukins. Acclimatization to low temperatures can also occur. For example, goldfish that are acclimatized at a low temperature may be able to produce a similar number of antibody-forming cells to that of those that have remained at a warmer temperature. The nature of the antigen is also critical in that certain T cell dependent mitogens are ineffective at low temperatures, again implying that the target cell is a helper T cell.

T Cell Responses

Fish TCR genes are organized in multiple -VDC- clusters in the same pattern as shark immunoglobulin genes. The MHC Class I and II genes evolved before the emergence of cartilaginous fish. The basic structure of each MHC molecule has been conserved as has the organization of the Class I and Class II genes.

Hagfish kept under good conditions in a warm environment can reject skin allografts. First-set grafts take about seventy-two days at 18°C to be rejected; second-set grafts are rejected in about twenty-eight days. This suggests that immunologic memory has developed. Lampreys also reject skin allografts slowly, and their lymphocytes will divide in the presence of cells from a second lamprey and phytohemagglutinin. Elasmobranchs reject scale allografts slowly as do lampreys but bony fish reject them rapidly. Repeated grafting leads to accelerated graft rejection. The rejected allografts are infiltrated by lymphocytes and show destruction of blood vessels and pigment cells. As in all ectotherms, graft rejection is slower at lower temperatures.

IMMUNITY IN AMPHIBIANS

Introduction

There are two major orders of amphibians: the Urodeles, which include the long bodied, tailed amphibians such as the salamanders and the newts; and the Anurans, a more advanced order that includes the frogs and toads. Analysis of the amphibian immune response is further complicated by the fact that many undergo significant metamorphosis from an aquatic form (tadpole) to an amphibious adult form.

Lymphoid Organs

Amphibians have a variety of lymphoid tissues, some of which differ significantly from those in fish. Thus some Urodeles may have a small amount of lymphoid tissue within their long bones. They possess a thymus that arises from the pharyngeal pouches. It develops slowly, only appearing at the seventh week of life. Thymectomy delays or blocks rejection of skin allografts. This thymus is not divided into cortex and medulla. The thymus of anurans also arises from the pharyngeal pouches and involutes by about one year of age. In contrast to the urodele thymus, the anuran thymus has an outer cortex and central medulla. The cortex is full of proliferating lymphocytes. The medulla contains fewer lymphocytes, but thymic corpuscles are present. Larval thymectomy in the toad (an anuran) reduces the response to foreign red blood cells, but the response to bacterial lipopolysaccharide is unaffected, suggesting this is a T-independent response. Thymectomy also slows but does not completely prevent allograft rejection in toads. A limited degree of T cell function develops several months after larval thymectomy suggesting that extrathymic T cell development may occur in these animals.

The kidney retains its lymphopoietic function in amphibians. Stem cells arise from the intertubular areas of the kidney in both urodeles and anurans. The spleen of urodeles is not clearly divided into red and white pulp, but the spleen of anuran amphibians is. Thus in frogs and toads, the red pulp and the periarteriolar white pulp are separated by boundary layer cells. Lymph nodes are absent in urodeles, but structures that resemble lymph nodes are seen in some anurans. These proto-lymph nodes consist of a mass of lymphocytes surrounding blood sinusoids, and they filter blood rather than lymph.

Larval amphibians such as the bullfrog tadpole have special lymphoid organs in their branchial region called ventral cavity bodies. Sinusoids in the organ are lined with macrophages which effectively remove particulate antigen from the blood. Removal of these organs makes tadpoles incapable of making antibodies to soluble antigen. They disappear at metamorphosis.

Lymphocytes are found in large numbers in the subcapsular region of the liver in fish, amphibians, and reptiles. These lymphocyte accumulations occur close to blood sinuses and may have a lymphopoietic function.

Lymphocytes
Both adult and larval amphibians have circulating lymphocytes. Although some investigators have suggested that these lymphocytes arise in the thymus, it is more likely that they originate in the ventral cavity bodies or the liver. The thymic lymphocytes and about eighty percent of circulating lymphocytes carry surface IgM. Frogs possess NK-like and T-cytotoxic-like cells.

Immunoglobulins
Anuran amphibians can have two or three distinct immunoglobulin classes. They have an IgM that consists of either pentamers or hexamers (in *Xenopus*) and one or two low molecular weight molecules. They have an IgY with a 66 kDa υ heavy chain and/or a IgX with a 64 kDa χ heavy chain. Xenopus immunoglobulins also contain two types of light chain perhaps equivalent to mammalian κ and λ chains. Anuran amphibians possess secretory immunoglobulins in bile and the intestine (but not in skin mucus). These consist of IgM and IgY but not IgA. In the axolotl (*Ambystoma mexicanum*) IgY is a secretory immunoglobulin found in close association with secretory component-like molecules. This is different from what occurs in Xenopus where IgY behaves like avian IgY or mammalian IgG. Amphibian antibody diversity is generated in a fashion similar to that of mammals.

Immune Responses

Urodeles produce a monomeric IgM and can mount a good but slow antibody response against particulate antigens. They do not respond to soluble protein antigens such as serum albumin or ferritin.

Anurans such as frogs given particulate antigens such as bacteria or foreign erythrocytes will produce only IgM. In contrast, injection of bacteriophages or soluble proteins induces both IgM and IgY. Soluble antigens and bacteriophage can induce the production of both IgY and IgM in adult toads. The IgY takes up to a month to appear, and its level is very low. Anuran larvae will only make IgM antibodies unless challenged repeatedly in which case low levels of IgY are produced. Amphibians do not mount a secondary immune response to erythrocytes and bacteria, but memory does occur in response to the antigens that stimulate an IgY response. Studies on immunologic memory are complicated by the fact that antigen may persist in the circulation for several months following injection.

Both urodeles and anurans possess a complement system similar to mammals but one that is more effective at 16°C.

T Cell Responses

It takes about twenty-eight to forty-two days for a skin allograft to be rejected by urodele amphibians. The allograft looks healthy for about three weeks, and it is then slowly rejected. Destruction of the pigment cells makes destruction of the graft readily visible since it turns white. Second-set rejection takes about eight to twenty days in the newt, and the alloimmune memory lasts at least ninety days. Anurans, in contrast, show a fairly rapid allograft rejection. A first-set reaction takes about fourteen days at 25°C. The graft shows capillary dilatation, lymphocyte infiltration, and disintegration of pigment cells. Second-set allografts do not even become vascularized and are destroyed within a few days. If graft recipients are kept in the cold, a skin allograft may take as long as 200 days to be rejected.

During amphibian metamorphosis from larval stage to adult, there is a temporary immunosuppression as shown by a slowing in allograft rejection. Some allografts may even be tolerated at this time. As tadpoles change into frogs or toads, the thymus shrinks, and there is a drop in the numbers of immunoglobulin positive lymphocytes and a drop in antibody levels.

Toad lymphocytes respond to phytohemagglutinin and respond in the mixed lymphocyte reaction. The intensity of this reaction depends upon the degree of incompatibility between the cell populations.

Xenopus has a well-characterized MHC with Class I, II and III regions called XLA. The Class II region contains genes for both α and β chains. About twenty Class I and thirty Class II alleles are believed to exist. The Class III region contains a gene for C4. It is possible that Xenopus may also possess Class IV products related to those seen in birds. It is interesting to note that while MHC Class II molecules are expressed early in larval development on B cells and tadpole epithelia, MHC Class I molecules are not expressed on the surface of cells prior to larval metamorphosis.

IMMUNITY IN REPTILES

Introduction

Three subclasses of reptiles currently exist: the Anapsids which contains the turtles; the Lepidosaurs which includes the lizards and snakes; and the Archosaurs which includes the crocodiles and alligators.

Lymphoid Organs
Structures that closely resemble lymph nodes are seen for the first time in reptiles. They have a simple structure consisting of a lymphoid parenchyma with phagocytes and intervening sinusoids. A fully functional bone marrow is present in reptiles. The reptilian thymus is structurally similar to that seen in other classes of vertebrates. Age involution of the reptile thymus has been reported as well as a seasonal involution—the thymus shrinks in winter and enlarges in summer. The reptilian spleen usually shows a clear separation between red and white pulps. Primitive lymph nodules surrounding the aorta, vena cava, and the jugular veins are seen in some reptiles. Lymphocytes and plasma cells are found in nodules in the intestinal wall of all the more developed vertebrates. Some turtles and snakes (but not alligators) have lymphoid aggregations (the cloacal complex) that project into the cloacal lumen. These aggregates are larger in adults than in young turtles and are therefore not primary lymphoid organs and cannot be regarded as a primitive bursa. A few lymphocytes are found in the kidney of reptiles.

Immunoglobulins
The reptiles that have been studied possess both IgM and IgY. The IgM of turtles is comparable to mammalian IgM in size, chain structure and carbohydrate content. The IgY is found in both the full-sized and truncated isoforms, but some turtles may have only the truncated isoform.

Immune Responses
Turtles and lizards immunized with bovine serum albumin, pig serum, or red blood cells can mount both primary and secondary antibody responses. The antibody produced in the primary response is IgM; the antibody produced in the secondary response is IgY. All reptile antibody responses appear to be T-dependent. Secondary responses and IgY antibody production do not occur in response to certain bacterial antigens such as *Salmonella adelaide*, *Brucella abortus*, or *S. typhimurium*.

T Cell Responses
As in other ectotherms, the rate of allograft rejection in reptiles is very temperature dependent. Turtles, snakes, and lizards reject allogeneic skin grafts in about forty days at 25°C. The antigen-recognition step is less temperature-dependent than the rejection process. Graft-versus-host disease can be induced by injection of cells from their parents into newborn turtles and can lead to death. The severity of the disease depends upon the genetic disparity between the turtles. Mortality, however, is greater at 30°C than at 20°C. Other evidence of cell-mediated immune responses such as mixed lymphocyte reactions and delayed hypersensitivity reactions have been demonstrated in reptiles.

Reptiles, being ectotherms, are unable to change their body temperature by physiologic mechanisms. As a result, they will not develop a fever if maintained in a constant temperature environment. If maintained in an environment with cool and warm areas, they will cycle between these areas and maintain their body temperature within well-defined limits. It has been observed that normal iguanas (*Dipsosaurus dorsalis*) maintain their temperature between 37° and 41°C. However iguanas infected with *Aeromonas hydrophila* modify their behavior, so that they spend more time in the warm environment. As a result, their temperatures cycle between 40° and 43°C. Once the bacterial infection is cured, the iguanas resume their normal behavior. Thus the iguanas effectively induce a fever by their behavior.

IMMUNITY IN BIRDS (AND DINOSAURS)
Introduction
The dinosaurs, although related to the reptile Archosaurs, were sufficiently different from true reptiles to be placed in a class of their own, the Dinosaura. Although the great majority of dinosaurs disappeared 65 million years ago at the end of the cretaceous period, their modern descendants are probably the birds, the members of the class Aves. Unlike the reptiles, birds are, and dinosaurs probably were, endothermic (warm blooded). As a result of this, birds share with mammals all the benefits that come from greatly increased physiological and biochemical efficiency. The thymus in birds and in primitive mammals is essentially similar to that seen in most mammals. Germinal centers cannot be found in fish, amphibian, and reptile spleens. In contrast, the germinal centers of birds are large and well defined.

Lymphoid Organs
Although birds are commonly considered not to possess lymph nodes, they do possess structures that can be considered to be their functional equivalent. These avian lymph nodes consist of a central sinus that is the main lumen of a lymphatic vessel. It is surrounded by a sheath of lymphoid tissue that contains germinal centers. Avian lymph nodes have no external capsule.

Birds are also characterized by possessing a bursa of Fabricius. The bursa of Fabricius is a lymphoid organ found only in birds. It is a round sac located just above the cloaca. Like the thymus, the bursa reaches its greatest size in the chick about one to two weeks after hatching and then gradually shrinks. Like the thymus, the bursa consists of lymphocytes embedded in epithelial tissue. This epithelial tissue lines a hollow sac connected to the cloaca by a duct. Inside the sac, folds of epithelium extend into the lumen, and scattered through the folds are lymphoid follicles containing lymphocytes, plasma cells, macrophages, and epithelial cells.

Bursectomized birds produce very little antibody and in them antibody-producing plasma cells disappear. They still possess circulating lymphocytes however, and can reject foreign skin grafts. Thus bursectomy has little effect on the cell-mediated immune response. Bursectomized birds are more susceptible than normal to leptospirosis and salmonellosis but not to bacteria against which cell-mediated immunity is important, such as *Mycobacterium avium*. These results have been interpreted to suggest that the bursa is a primary lymphoid organ that functions as a maturation and differentiation site for B cells. Its follicles contain more than ninety percent B cells. Indeed, the bursa acts like the thymus insofar as its B cells are proliferating rapidly with more than five percent of bursal lymphocytes dividing per hour. However up to ninety-nine percent of B cells produced here die rapidly through apoptosis. This apoptosis is probably a reflection of negative selection of self-reactive B cells. Several different hormones have been extracted from the bursa. The most important of these is bursin; a tripeptide (lys-his-glycylamide) that activates B cells but not T cells.

Lymphocytes
Birds possess lymphocytes that originate in the yoke sac and migrate either to the bursa or to the thymus. Immature lymphocytes that enter the thymus mature under the influence of hormones from thymic epithelial cells, and cells with recognizable T cell markers emigrate from the thymus. In avian blood, T cells constitute between sixty and seventy percent of the total lymphocyte population.

Immature lymphocytes that enter the bursa emigrate as immunoglobulin positive B cells.

Immunoglobulins

The predominant serum immunoglobulin in birds is IgY. Some investigators have reported the existence of three subclasses, termed IgY1, IgY2, and IgY3, although this has not been completely substantiated. As relatively advanced birds, chickens possess only the full-sized isoform of IgY. The somewhat less developed ducks and geese possess both the full-sized and truncated isoforms. Chicken IgM is formed predominantly during the primary immune response. Chickens also possess polymeric IgA in secretions.

Birds generate antibody diversity in a manner that is quite distinct from that seen in mammals. The germ line contributes little to diversity since there is only one V gene and one J gene segment for both light and heavy chains. Only D gene segments exist as a cluster of sixteen gene segments. Immunoglobulin diversity is generated by somatic mutation involving gene conversion. For example, birds have a large number of pseudogenes that serve as sequence donors to diversify the initial light chain V genes by gene conversion. The gene conversion process also affects the D region since all the pseudogenes consist of fused VD segments. During recombination of the V and J segments, single bases are added to each segment (N-region addition) and joining occurs at random. Chicken immunoglobulins are further diversified by somatic point mutations and imprecise V-J joining. The frequency of somatic mutations is the same as in the mouse.

Rearrangement of immunoglobulin genes in birds is not an ongoing process as in mammals. The B cell progenitors rearrange their immunoglobulin genes as a single wave between ten and fifteen days of embryogenesis at a period when there is clonal expansion of B cells in the Bursa of Fabricius. The total number of possible rearrangements is thus limited to the number of B cell precursors that colonize the bursa. The chicken can generate about 10^6 different immunoglobulin molecules. This is approximately one order of magnitude less than that of the mouse.

Immune Responses

Birds produce primary and secondary responses in a manner similar to mammals. The predominance of IgM production in the primary immune response and of IgY in the secondary response is less marked than in mammals.

T Cell Responses

Chickens have T cells that can respond to the mitogens phytohemagglutinin and concanavalin A. Avian T cells can participate in delayed hypersensitivity reactions, graft-versus-host disease, and allograft rejection. Avian homologs of mammalian γ/δ TCR(TCR-1) and α/β TCR (TCR-2 and TCR-3) have been identified. TCR-2 and TCR-3 are subsets of α/β TCRs that use distinctly different Vβ gene segments. TCR-2 cells undergo V-DJ joining by gene deletion while TCR-3 cells undergo V-DJ joining by chromosome inversion.

Birds reject skin allografts in seven to fourteen days. There is massive infiltration of the grafted tissue with lymphocytes. These cells are believed to be T cells, since neonatal thymectomy results in a loss of ability to reject allografts.

If chicken T cells are dropped onto the chorioallantoic membrane of thirteen- to fourteen-day-old chick embryos, the cells will attack the chick tissues. This will result in pock formation on the membrane and splenic enlargement. The grafted cells attack the hematopoietic cells of the recipient. A few days after hatching, chicks become resistant to this form of graft-versus-host attack.

IMMUNITY IN MAMMALS
Introduction
The mammals consist of three orders: the Monotremes or egg laying mammals such as the platypus and the echidna; the Marsupals, or pouched mammals such as the opossum and the kangaroos; and the Eutherians, or placental mammals. Immunity in placental mammals is the subject of much of this text and therefore, will not be discussed at any length in this chapter. It should be pointed out however that mammals, unlike the other classes of vertebrates face an immunological dilemma. They carry their young within the uterus for a long period of time. The fetal mammal is in very close association with its mother where it effectively acts as an allograft. Thus mammals are faced with the necessity of not permitting immunological rejection of the fetus. This requires complex immunological control systems that will permit survival of the fetal allograft.

Monotremes and Marsupials
Monotremes such as the platypus and echidna are egg-laying mammals that do not have to concern themselves about immunological rejection of the fetus. They have an immune system that is similar to other mammals and make IgG rather than IgY. Their lymphoid organs show some structural differences from those in more evolved mammals. Thus, they have lymph nodes that consist of several lymphoid nodules, each containing a germinal center, suspended by its blood vessels within the lumen of a lymphatic plexus. Thus, each nodule is bathed in lymph. There is usually just one germinal center per nodule.

Marsupials are characterized by having very short gestation periods, and their premature young migrate from the uterus to the pouch where they develop attached to the mammary gland. This may well be a device to remove the fetus from the uterus before it can be immunologically rejected. Marsupials can synthesize IgA and IgE as well. Like other mammals, marsupials produce predominantly IgM in the primary immune response and IgG in secondary immune responses. The marsupial opossum (*Didelphis*) resembles more primitive vertebrates in that it responds well to particulate antigens such as bacteria, but poorly to soluble antigens.

Some Differences Between Humans and Common Domestic Mammals
Although the immune systems of the placental mammals are very similar, they also show significant differences between species. Some of the more interesting differences are described below.

Pig Lymph Nodes
Domestic pigs have lymph nodes with a very different structure than other mammals. Their nodes are orientated so that the cortex is located toward the center of the node while their medulla is at the periphery. Each node is served by afferent lymphatics that penetrate to the central cortex. Thus afferent lymph is carried deep into the node. Outside the cortex is a paracortex and a medulla. Lymph passes from the cortex at the center of the node to the medulla at the periphery before leaving through the efferent vessels. Thus the pig, and related mammals, have an "inside-

out" lymph node. It seems to work just as well as the conventional lymph nodes found in other mammals. T cells in the pig also circulate completely differently from those of other mammals. They enter lymph nodes in the conventional way through high endothelial venules. However they leave the lymph node not through the lymphatics but migrate directly back into bloodstream through the high endothelial venules of the paracortex.

Camel Immunoglobulins
The camel (*Camelus dromedarius*) has three IgG subclasses IgG1, IgG2, and IgG3. One of these, IgG1 has a conventional structure. The other two subclasses, IgG2 and IgG3 are heavy chain dimers that have no light chains. Despite the absence of light chains these molecules can bind a variety of antigens suggesting that light chains contribute minimally to antigen binding. Camels from both the old world (*Camelus bactrianus*) and the new world (*Lama pacos, L. glama*, and *L. viguna*) also possess a high proportion of these heavy-chain immunoglobulins.

Ruminant T Cells
Ruminants are unique in that unlike humans or rodents, CD4-CD8- T cells form a very high proportion (fifteen to thirty percent) of the peripheral blood lymphocytes in young ruminants. (This can be as high as eighty percent in newborn calves.) Most of these double negative cells have γ/δ antigen receptors and specifically express the unique surface molecule, WC1+. Thus the circulating T cells in ruminants ($\gamma/\delta+$, WC1+, CD4–, CD8–) are very different from the T cells found in the blood of humans and mice ($\gamma/\delta+$, WC1–, CD4+, CD8–). These WC1+ T cells are also found in high numbers in epithelia such as the skin and intestinal wall. Sheep γ/δ T cells are similar. When lambs are born, γ/δ T cells can account for as much as sixty percent of peripheral blood T cells, but this drops as the animals grow older.

Immunity in the Newborn
Perhaps the most significant difference seen among mammals is in the way their newborns are protected. The route by which maternal antibodies reach the fetus is determined by the structure of the placenta. In humans and other primates, the placenta is hemochorial. That is, the maternal blood is in direct contact with the trophoblast. This type of placenta allows maternal IgG but not IgM, IgA, or IgE to transfer to the fetus. Maternal IgG freely enters the fetal blood and the newborn human infant will have circulating IgG levels comparable to those of its mother.

Dogs and cats possess an endotheliochorial placenta. In this case, the chorionic epithelium is in contact with the endothelium of the maternal capillaries. In these species only five to ten percent of IgG may transfer from the mother to the puppy or kitten, but most is obtained through colostrum.

The placenta of ruminants is syndesmochorial. That is, the chorionic epithelium is in direct contact with uterine tissues, whereas the placenta of horses and pigs is epitheliochorial, and the fetal chorionic epithelium is in contact with intact uterine epithelium. In animals with these types of placenta, the passage of immunoglobulin molecules across the placenta is totally prevented, and the newborns of these species are entirely dependent on antibodies received through the colostrum.

Colostrum represents the accumulated secretions of the mammary gland over the last few weeks of pregnancy together with proteins actively transferred from the blood stream under the influence of estrogens and progesterone. In domestic mammals, it is rich in IgG and IgA with a little IgM and IgE. The predominant immunoglobulin in the colostrum of most of the major domestic animals is IgG, which may account for sixty-five to ninety percent of its total antibody content; IgA and the other immunoglobulins are usually minor components. As lactation progresses and colostrum changes to milk, differences emerge between species. In primates and humans, IgA predominates in both colostrum and milk. In pigs and horses IgG predominates in colostrum, but its concentration drops rapidly as lactation proceeds, and IgA predominates in milk. In ruminants, IgG1 is the predominant immunoglobulin class in both milk and colostrum.

All the IgG, most of the IgM and about half of the IgA in bovine colostrum are derived from serum. In milk, in contrast, only thirty percent of the IgG and ten percent of the IgA are so derived, the rest are produced locally in the udder. Colostrum also contains secretory, IgA.

Absorption of Colostrum

Young animals that suckle soon after birth take colostrum into their intestine. In these young animals, the level of protease activity in the intestine is low, and is further reduced by trypsin inhibitors in colostrum. As a result, colostral proteins are not used as a food source but instead reach the small intestine intact. Colostral IgG then binds to specialized Fc receptors on the intestinal epithelial cells of newborns (FcRn). This receptor is a MHC class Ib heterodimer containing a large α chain and β2-microglobulin. Once bound to FcRn, IgG is actively taken up by epithelial cells through pinocytosis and passed through these cells into the bloodstream. Newborn animals thus obtain a transfusion of maternal immunoglobulin.

The period for which the intestine is permeable to proteins is quite short. In general, permeability is highest immediately after birth and declines rapidly after about six hours, perhaps because the intestinal cells that absorb immunoglobulins are replaced by a more mature cell population. Unsuckled, newborn animals normally possess no immunoglobulin in their serum. Once they suckle, the absorption of colostral immunoglobulin immediately supplies them with serum IgG at a level approaching that found in adults.

As lactation proceeds, the secretions of the mammary gland gradually change from colostrum to milk. Milk is rich in IgA. Thus when a young animal suckles it receives significant amounts of IgA. This IgA is protective in the intestine and thus protects young animals against enteric infection. Thus naturally suckled animals of all species suffer from significantly less diarrheal disease than young animals weaned early.

SUMMARY

All animals, regardless of their evolutionary complexity require protection against microbial invasion. In general, invertebrates rely exclusively on innate immune mechanisms. Vertebrates, in contrast, use both innate and specific adaptive immune mechanisms. Thus typical invertebrates such as insects possess a complex mixture of lectins that can bind to microbial carbohydrates, opsonize them, and promote destruction by aggressive phagocytic cells. This is enhanced by an effective inflammatory response and the prophenoloxidase pathway. More advanced invertebrates such as the chordates, while relying on innate immunity, show evidence of the appearance of precursors of the specific adaptive immune system.

The first animals to utilize a specific adaptive immune system incorporating MHC molecules for antigen presentation, immunoglobulins, and TCRs generated by gene segment recombination are the cartilaginous fish. Subsequent evolution simply refined the process. Thus, there is a move from the early multilocus arrangement of immunoglobulin genes to the mammalian arrangement involving few C genes and multiple V genes. There are changes in the structure of immunoglobulin heavy chains and hence in the class of immunoglobulins produced by each species. Probably one of the most significant changes was the need for mammals to adapt to the immunological challenges of bearing live young and the consequent need to prevent immunological attack on the mammalian fetus.

Even within mammals there are some interesting and important differences between species such as the sites of maturation of B cells and differences in the ways by which antibody diversity is generated. However, given the very strong selective pressure exerted by infectious diseases, it is apparent that all animals living must have effective and efficient mechanisms to defend themselves again microbial invasion.

SUGGESTIONS FOR FURTHER READING

1. Bartl, S., D. Baltimore, and I.L. Weissman. "Molecular Evolution of the Vertebrate Immune System." *Proc. Natl. Acad. Sci. USA* 91 (1994):10769–10770.
2. Du Pasquier, L., J. Schwager, and M.F. Flajnik. "The Immune System of Xenopus." *Ann. Rev. Immunol.* 7 (1989):251–275.
3. Hanley, P.J., J.W. Hook, D.A. Raftos, et al. "Hagfish Humoral Defense Protein Exhibits Structural and Functional Homology with Mammalian Structural Components." Proc. *Natl. Acad. Sci. USA* 89 (1992):7910–7914.
4. Kluger, M.J. *Fever, its Biology, Evolution and Function*. Princeton, NJ: Princeton University Press, 1979.
5. Marchalonis, J.J., and S.F. Schluter. "Immunoproteins in Evolution." *Dev. Comp. Immunol.* 13 (1989):285–301.
6. Warr, G.W., K.E. Magor, and D.A. Higgins. "IgY: Clues to the Origins of Modern Antibodies." *Immunology Today* 16 (1995):392–398.

QUESTIONS

1. If most vertebrates can function well without possessing either IgA or IgE, are these immunoglobulins of any use?
2. On what basis are the phagocytic cells of invertebrates considered to be analogs rather than homologs of vertebrate phagocytes?
3. Why do birds and mammals apparently not require kidney-associated lymphoid tissue? Might this have something to do with an adaptation to a terrestrial environment?
4. What is the evidence that supports the proposal that IgM evolved before IgG?
5. Justify the existence of the Bursa of Fabricius. Why might it be found only in birds?
6. How significant is the fact that the genes for some proteins of the immune system, which are well recognized in mammals, such as Thy-1, have also been found in some invertebrates?
7. The development of the bone marrow is associated with adaptation to a terrestrial existence. Comment on possible reasons or advantages for this.
8. It has been suggested that insects do not need an immune system since they are short-lived and can adapt very rapidly to pathogenic microorganisms. Is this a valid argument? If not, why not?

ANSWERS

1. This question supposes that vertebrates that lack IgA or IgE are defenseless on body surfaces. In fact these animals use other immunoglobulins such as IgY for this purpose. The evolution of new immunoglobulins such as IgA and IgE means that these surface defenses are more efficient.

2. Phagocytosis is a property of most cells. They will take up particles if optimally stimulated under the right circumstances. What is important in the defense of the animal body is the existence of "professional" phagocytic cells. Cells whose major function is to be phagocytic. In the case of vertebrates these professional cells are derived from bone marrow precursors and are largely found in blood. In the case of most invertebrates these phagocytic cells are not restricted to the bloodstream and originate from a variety of different sources.

3. Quite simply because they use their bone marrow to act as a source of these cells, birds and mammals do not need kidney-associated tissue. Clearly the function of the kidney changed as vertebrates moved from water to air. One of these changes was the need for enhanced water retention. It is difficult to see, however, any connection between the functions of filtration and water retention and production of lymphoid cells.

4. There are two types of evidence that support this. One is quite simply that IgM is found in less evolved vertebrates such as cartilaginous fish in the absence of, or in cases where IgG is found in small amounts. Second, analysis of the amino acid sequences of immunoglobulins shows a branching pattern that points to IgM being a less evolved molecule and they likely ancestor of IgG.

5. There is growing evidence to suggest that many vertebrates including some mammals possess some form of lymphoid organ at the exit from the digestive tract. This may serve to block invasion of the body from the rear! Just as likely, it may be that the bursa is simply yet another intestinal lymphoid organ that happens to be found close to the cloaca. Certainly some mammals such as lambs and piglets use their intestinal lymphoid organs as a site for B cell development. The bursa is not all that unique.

6. This supports, by molecular evidence, the fact that vertebrates originated by evolution from the higher chordates. It would be incredibly strange if all the molecular structures of vertebrates originated anew. The dichotomy between vertebrates and invertebrates is probably nowhere as great as our arbitrary classification schemes suggest.

7. It is not clear why bone marrow should actually be within bone. Obviously solid bones would be very heavy and making them hollow does not reduce their strength. Thus something had to fill the available space! It is unclear why lymphoid tissues and hematopoietic tissues should be located in this tissue. It is possible that macrophages needed for bone remodeling accumulate here and by extension, these can be used to trap circulating foreign particles. Lymphocytes would follow to initiate immune responses to the foreign antigens. Hematopoiesis is not, of course, restricted to the bone marrow.

8. This is the paradox of small, short-lived animals. Can they do life's essential tasks such as reproduce themselves before pathogens can kill them? This is an invalid argument since even small invertebrates cannot reproduce or mutate at a rate approaching that of bacteria. Insects do protect themselves by means of an effective innate immune system.

Pathogenicity and Virulence

Lola Winter

INTRODUCTION
FACTORS MEDIATING
  ADHERENCE TO HOST
  CELLS
  Adhesins
  Host Cell Receptors
INVASION OF HOST CELLS
PREVENTION OF PHAGO-
  CYTOSIS
  Antiphagocytic Surface
    Structures
  Antiphagocytic Cytotoxins
SURVIVAL WITHIN THE
  PHAGOCYTE
  Interference with the
    Generation of Oxidative
    Metabolites
  Prevention of Phagosome
    Maturation and Phago-
    some–Lysosome Fusion
  Escape from the Phago-
    some
SIDEROPHORES AND IRON
  ACQUISITION
TOXINS
  Endotoxins
  Exotoxins
  Superantigens
R FACTORS and PATHO-
  GENICITY ISLANDS
SUMMARY
SUGGESTIONS FOR
  FURTHER READING
QUESTIONS
ANSWERS

INTRODUCTION

Any microorganism that is able to infect a host and produce disease is a pathogen. Microorganisms vary in their ability to produce disease; some organisms such as *Vibrio cholerae*, the agent of cholera, or *Yersinia pestis*, the cause of plague, are able to produce disease in normal healthy hosts. These bacteria are thus overt pathogens and must be distinguished from those organisms which function as opportunists and produce disease only when a break in the host's normal defense mechanisms enables them to become established. Included in this latter group of opportunists are members of the normal flora such as *Escherichia coli*, *Staphylococcus aureus*, and certain fungi such *Candida albicans*, as well as some free-living bacteria such as *Pseudomonas aeruginosa* and *Legionella pneumophila*.

Whether disease ensues as a result of a host's encounter with a pathogen is dependent upon both the condition of the host and the particular characteristics of the microorganism. Those characteristics that contribute to the ability of a microorganism to produce disease are referred to as virulence factors. Most bacterial and fungal pathogens have many such factors, and although some have been identified, it is still not known in all cases precisely how each factor functions in the production of disease. It is known, for example, that enterotoxigenic *E. coli* adheres to the lining of the small intestine and produces a potent enterotoxin, which is absorbed by the intestinal epithelial cells. This toxin produces an increase in the concentration of intracellular cAMP, which results in an increase in secretion of electrolytes into the intestinal lumen and an outpouring of water; the end result is diarrhea. Both the enterotoxin and the ability to adhere are coded for by plasmids carried by the bacterial cell. If the bacterium is cured only of the adherence plasmid, it cannot produce

265

disease, even though enterotoxin is still produced. Unable to adhere, this organism can no longer maintain itself in the intestinal tract. The small amount of enterotoxin produced in transit may be insufficient to be harmful or may be inactivated by intestinal secretions. If cured only of the plasmid coding for enterotoxin, the *E. coli* adheres, but again, no diarrhea results because the toxin is not produced. The pathogenesis of this particular disease is thus very well understood. By contrast, *S. aureus* produces many virulence factors and causes many different disease syndromes, but as yet, there is a very incomplete understanding of how each factor functions in pathogenicity. Our understanding of virulence factors of other pathogens ranges between these two extremes. This chapter will present information on virulence factors that have been grouped according to their modes of action.

FACTORS MEDIATING ADHERENCE TO HOST CELLS
Adhesins

Infections are initiated on the surfaces of the mucous membranes or through breaks in the skin. Most infections actually begin on the mucous membranes of the respiratory, gastrointestinal or urogenital tracts. In these environments, the potential pathogen must first adhere to the host cell. Adherence prevents the microorganism from being flushed away in mucus secretions and renders it less susceptible to the effects of enzymes and secretory IgA. If disease is to result from the effects of a toxin, such as that of enterotoxigenic *E. coli*, close adherence of the bacterium assures that the toxin will be delivered in high concentrations directly to the host cell. If the organism is invasive, as is *Salmonella typhi*, adherence must occur before penetration of host cells is possible.

The observation that some microbes affect particular hosts and selectively attach only to certain cells within these hosts suggests that adherence is a specific process. There are indeed distinct structural moieties on the surfaces of microbes, termed adhesins, which mediate adherence by binding specifically, much like a key in a lock, to receptors on the host cell surface. Fimbriae, outer membrane proteins, and the lipopolysaccharide (LPS) of Gram-negative bacteria, fibrillae on streptococci, flagellae, capsules, and even exotoxins may function in adherence.

Fimbriae, also referred to as pili, are tubular filaments, 7.5 to 10 um in diameter that are made up of repeating protein subunits. Fimbriae have been identified in many different species including *E. coli, Pseudomonas aeruginosa, Bordetella pertussis, Neisseria gonorrhoeae, N. meningitidis*, and *Haemophilus influenzae* (Figure 14.1).

Fibrillae are hairy surface appendages on the cell wall of streptococci (Figure 14.2) which are composed of lipoteichoic acid and proteins. There is evidence that the lipoteichoic acid as well as two proteins, M and F, function as adhesins but to different host molecules. *Mycoplasma pneumoniae* attaches firmly to host cells of the respiratory epithelium via a surface protein located on a specialized terminal structure. Opacity proteins of the outer membrane (*N. gonorrhoeae*), flagella (*Campylobacter jejuni*), LPS (*Shigella flexneri*), and glycocalyx (*P. aeruginosa*) have also been identified as having a role in adherence.

There are many different factors that can function as bacterial adhesins. Moreover, it is now realized that many bacteria make use of not just one but several of these factors. Most strains of *N. gonorrhoeae* can adhere both by fimbriae and opacity proteins. Strain 9 of this species has been shown to express four different isogenic fimbrial variants simultaneously. Uropathogenic *E. coli*, which adheres to the epithelial cells of the urinary tract by means of P fimbriae, also has the ability to adhere by means of other surface molecules. Multiple adhesins have been demonstrated

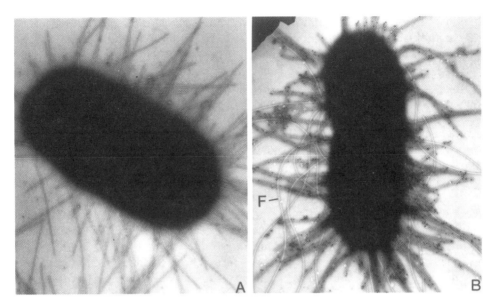

Figure 14.1.   Electron micrograph of stained *E. coli* showing (A) fimbriae and (B) fimbriae and flagella. Fimbriae are the structural adhesins of Gram-negative bacteria. Flagella (F) are the organs of motility of bacteria. (Source: Knutton et al. *Infection and Immunity* 55:86–92, 1987. With permission from the American Society for Microbiology.)

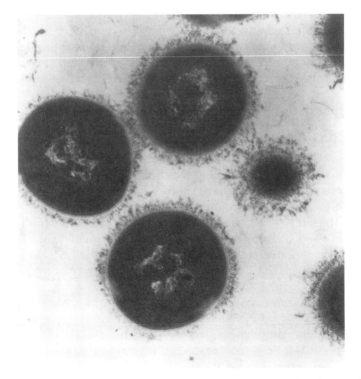

Figure 14.2.   Electron micrograph of group G streptococci showing abundant surface fibrillae (magnification: 60,000x). (Source: A.L. Bisno. *Infection and Immunity* 55:753–57,1987. With permission from the American Society for Microbiology.)

in many other species, including *V. cholerae*, *H. influenzae*, and *B. pertussis*. Bacteria that are able to utilize different adhesins may be better able to evade the defense mechanisms of the host.

Some microorganisms such as *N. gonorrhoeae* and *E. coli* have the genetic ability to alter the molecular composition of a particular adhesin as well as to switch the type of adhesin expressed. The expression of a particular fimbrial adhesin is regulated by a response to environmental stimuli such as temperature and chemical gradients and is under the control of bacterial genes located either on the chromosome or on a plasmid. These genes can undergo "phase variations" which result in alterations in fimbrial states.

Fungi too have adhesins. The WI-1 surface antigen is a cell wall adhesin found on the surface of the blastoconidia of *Blastomyces dermatiditis*. It mediates attachment to macrophages by binding to the complement receptor CR3. Analyses has shown that the WI-1 antigen contains multiple copies of a twenty-five amino acid sequence tandemly. This sequence is highly homologous to the invasin of *Yersinia*.

The importance of adhesins as virulence factors has been demonstrated by comparing the virulence of mutants which have lost the ability to express an adhesin to that of the parent strain. Such comparisons have been made with a number of microbes including *E. coli*, *N. gonorrhoeae*, and *H. influenzae* and have confirmed the role of adhesins in virulence. In addition, treatments which interfere with adhesion, such as the use of antibodies specific for the adhesin, or enzymes which remove the adhesin, result in the reduction of the microbe's pathogenicicty.

While it is generally held that adherence is a prerequisite for infection and the production of disease, there are some situations in which this characteristic is detrimental to the microorganism. Study of urinary tract infections with *Proteus* in rats revealed that the presence of fimbriae was required for establishment of infection in the urinary tract, but that these same fimbriae enhanced phagocytosis of the organism when it entered the bloodstream. Those species that can undergo phase variation to suppress adhesins may therefore have a distinct survival advantage in systemic infections.

Host Cell Receptors

Adherence is a complex process involving specific components not only of the microbial cell but also of the host cell to which the adhesins bind. *In vitro* work with cell and organ cultures has helped to identify some of the receptors. This was done by treating cells with various enzymes or adhesin analogues and then testing for adherence. Thus, it has been shown that the minor subunits of the fimbriae of *B. pertussis* bind Vla-5, a receptor found on monocytes, and the major subunits of the fimbriae bind to sulfated sugars which are found in the respiratory tract. The P adhesin of uropathogenic *E. coli* binds to sialosyl galactosyl globoside and disialosyl galactosyl globoside, glycosphingolipids which are expressed in human kidney tissue. Work with viruses has shown that many molecules that have an important role in normal biological functions of the host serve as viral receptors. It is known, for example, that the complement receptor CR2, present on B cells and certain other body cells, serves as the receptor for the Epstein-Barr virus. The CD4 molecule on T lymphocytes has a crucial role in the response to foreign antigens but has also been shown to be a receptor for the human immunodeficiency virus, the agent of AIDS.

The classical work with enterotoxigenic *E. coli* in swine has shown that host receptors are under genetic control. *Escherichia coli* expressing the K88 antigen, a fimbrial protein, adhere to the intestinal epithelial cells of swine while *E. coli* expressing K99 antigen adhere only to bovine cells. The observation that some swine were resistant to infection by *E. coli* K88 suggested the possibility of breeding for resistance. The resistant swine were shown to lack the K88 receptor, which is coded for by an autosomal dominant gene. In humans, P fimbriated *E. coli* are the most frequent agents of urinary tract infections in females. Certain individuals are more susceptible than others to these infections, as is indicated by the recurrent nature of their infections. It has been suggested that uropathogenic strains of *E. coli* bind more readily to the urogenital epithelial cells of susceptible women. It is known that the P fimbriae of *E. coli* bind to glycolipid receptors on the host cell; an increased concentration of these receptors could account for the higher incidence of infection in certain women.

In addition to naturally occurring receptors, new receptors may be expressed on host cells under certain conditions. For example, an increased adherence of *S. aureus* has been demonstrated to cells which are infected with Influenza A virus. Group B streptococci have also been shown to adhere preferentially to virus-infected cells. Some bacteria release enzymes that break down host tissue, thereby exposing new receptor sites, which aid in their spread. *Pseudomonas aeruginosa* produces a protease which breaks down host fibronectin, a high-molecular-weight glycoprotein present on the surface of many cells. This pseudomonad cannot adhere to fibronectin, but can adhere to the cell structures exposed upon its removal. *Aspergillus* species are ubiquitous in the environment but disease in the healthy host is extremely rare. It has been shown that this agent binds readily to laminin, a cellular component exposed after tissue damage. This may explain in part why aspergillosis is a particular problem for patients undergoing chemotherapy or radiation therapy.

INVASION OF HOST CELLS

Once adherent to host cells, some pathogens, of which *V. cholerae* represents a classic example, maintain a strictly extracellular habitation, while others prefer to live within selected host cells other than polymorphonuclear leukocytes (PMN) and macrophages, the co-called "professional phagocytes." Life within host cells affords protection from a potentially hostile environment and access to a nutrient-rich cytoplasm. To achieve this end, several intracellular microbes have evolved ways of inducing their endocytosis by nonphagocytic cells of the host. Proteins which adhere to the host cell, activate host cell signals, and mediate the use of host cell machinery to allow entry of the bacteria into the cell are called invasins. The invasins of *Listeria*, *Yersinia*, *Salmonella*, and *Shigella* have been identified within recent years using *in vitro* cell culture systems.

Listeria monocytogenes induces its own endocytosis by epithelial cells via an 80kD surface protein, internalin A, that binds to E-cadherin, a cell adhesion molecule that normally functions as a receptor for one of the integrins. The binding of internalin to its receptor initiates a "zippering" of the host cell membrane around the bacterial cell and the subsequent internalization of the microbe within a host membrane-bound vesicle. Internalin B, another member of the internalin family, enables *L. monocytogenes* to enter hepatacytes. The receptor for this invasin has not yet been determined.

Yersinia enterocolitica and *Y. pseudotuberculosis* induce their endocytosis by epithelial cells by means of an outer membrane protein, invasin. Invasin binds to a family of beta 1 integrins, which are receptors for extracellular matrix proteins such as fibronectin. As with *Listeria*, the binding of invasin signals the host cell to "zipper" the bacterium within a host cell membrane. Experimental work has shown that the internalization of both *Listeria* and *Yersinia* requires host cell signal transduction mechanisms that induce actin polymerization.

The invasion of epithelial cells by *Shigella* involves three proteins, IpaB, IpaC, and IpaD for which the host receptor is not yet known. Binding of these invasins initiates an intense local polymerization of actin and myosin that results in "ruffling" of the membrane with the formation of pseudopods, which engulf the bacteria. This process is referred to as macropinocytosis. *Shigella* lyses its vacuole using the ipaB protein and then utilizes host actin to be propelled through the cytoplasm. It is known that *Shigella* makes use of host cadherins to spread from cell to cell, but the exact mechanism is not yet clear.

Three proteins, SipB, SipC, and SipD, are also involved in the endocytosis of *S. typhimurium* but the host cell receptors have not been identified. As with *Shigella*, ruffling of the membrane occurs soon after invasion and the bacteria are internalized within membrane-bound vacuoles by macropinocytosis. These salmonellae do not spread from cell to cell but remain in the vacuole and multiply until lysis of the host cell.

PREVENTION OF PHAGOCYTOSIS
Pathogens must be able to withstand attack by PMNs and macrophages, the professional phagocytes, whose job it is to rid the body of invading organisms by ingestion and destruction. There are several ways by which microbes thwart this process.

Some pathogens, exemplified by *S. pneumoniae*, *H. influenzae*, and *N. meningitidis*, are classified as obligate extracellular parasites because they are readily killed within phagocytes. Prevention of phagocytosis is therefore crucial to the survival of extracellular parasites within the host, and this is accomplished primarily by the presence of antiphagocytic factors on the microbial surface.

Antiphagocytic Surface Structures
Several kinds of surface molecules can serve to prevent phagocytosis, including adhesins, such as the streptococcal M protein, and certain O polysacccharide sugars such as abequose which is found on the LPS of *S. typhimurium*. However, the great majority of antiphagocytic factors are structures outside the cell wall that are referred to as capsules (Figure 14.4).

Most capsules are polysaccharide in nature, but the capsule of *Bacillus anthracis* is a homopolymer of D-glutamic acid, while *Campylobacter fetus* and *Aeromonas salmonicida* (a pathogen of fish) possess surface proteins in an ordered formation that are designated S-layers. The majority of capsules are sufficiently thick to permit their demonstration by conventional microscopy using positive or negative staining techniques. However, the capsules of certain pathogens are so thin that their presence can be established only by electron microscopy or antibody binding techniques such as immunofluorescence. These are referred to as microcapsules and are exemplified by the Vi antigen of *S. typhi* and the monomolecular S-layer of *C. fetus*.

That encapsulation does enhance virulence has been shown clearly in work with *S. pneumoniae*, which demonstrated that unencapsulated, isogenic variants had little ability to cause disease. Further work with these bacteria suggested that not only the presence and the size of the capsule but also its composition determined virulence. Investigations with group B streptococci, which are important pathogens in the newborn, have revealed that the sialic acid component of the capsule has a high affinity for protein factor H which enhances enzymatic degradation of C3b bound to the bacterial surface, and thereby prevents the activation of complement by the alternate pathway. The K1 capsule of *E. coli*, as well as the type B capsule of *N. meningitidis*, are also composed of homopolymers of sialic acid and function in an identical manner. The M protein on the fibrillae of Group A streptococci serves not only to mediate adhesion but also to impede phagocytosis by binding factor H. In contrast, the microcapsule of *C. fetus* prevents the deposition of C3b on the bacterial surface. Capsules also serve to block access of complement to bacterial or fungal cell walls, which contain various molecules capable of causing activation of complement by the alternative pathway. While capsules do increase the negative charge on the surface of microbial cells and thereby tend to repel contact with phagocytes, it is believed that the most important antiphagocytic function of the capsule is to prevent the activation of complement.

Encapsulation does not, however, always serve to benefit the invading microorganism. While capsules may protect microbes invading the bloodstream, their presence may also block the function of adhesins and thereby hinder attachment to mucous membranes. It has been shown, for example, that the hyaluronic acid capsule of *S. pyogenes* hinders both the attachment of phagocytes to the bacterial cells and also the adherence of the bacteria to the oral epithelial cells of the host. Encapsulation has also been shown to diminish the ability of *S. pneumoniae* to adhere to pharyngeal epithelial cells.

It was noted previously that the ability of an organism to modulate the expression of adhesins could influence its ability to survive in the host. In like fashion, the ability to shed or express capsules as situations change can also be an important factor for microbial survival. This is well exemplified by the formation of a glycocalyx, an exopolysaccharide slime layer, which is characteristic of *P. aeruginosa*, *S. aureus*, and some other bacteria when growing in colonies under certain environmental conditions (Figure 14.3). These structures are similar to capsules but have a less ordered morphology. The slime layer of *P. aeruginosa* has been identified as alginate, a glycolipoprotein of the cell wall. The production of slime enables the bacterial cells to adhere to the host cells and to each other, resulting in the formation of adherent microcolonies. These slime-covered microcolonies do not bind antibody specific for the organism's cell wall or complement, and therefore become resistant to phagocytosis. Penetration of antibiotics is also reduced by microcolony formation so that cells in the center of a colony may thus be protected from the antimicrobial effect of antibiotics. The observation that mucoid strains of *P. aeruginosa* (composed of bacteria within a slime layer) are commonly isolated from hosts with abnormal microbial clearance systems but with a properly functioning immune system (for example, humans with cystic fibrosis), while nonmucoid strains are found in immune compromised hosts (burn patients), has suggested that slime formation could be an adaptation to the environmental pressure of the immune response. Viridans streptococci, which are often found in vegetative cardiac lesions, are also protected by a glycocalyx. This observation offers a reasonable explanation for the poor clinical response of patients with this form of heart disease to antibiotic therapy despite the fact that the infections are caused by antibiotic-sensitive strains of the microbe.

LIVERPOOL
JOHN MOORES UNIVERSITY
AVRIL ROBARTS LRC
TEL. 0151 231 4022

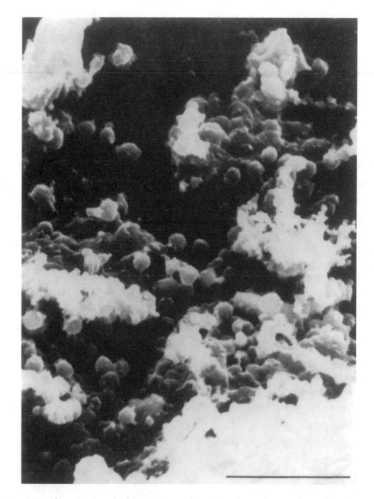

Figure 14.3.   SEM showing staphylococci enveloped in their glycocalyx. These bacteria grow-ing on the plastic surface of a cardiac pacemaker persisted in spite of aggressive antibiotic therapy. (Source: J.W. Costertonaud, and J.J. Marrie. *Medical Microbiology* Vol. 3. Edited by C.S.F. Easman et al. Figure 10. Academic Press, London, 1983.)

Cryptococcus neoformans is the only fungus known to have a capsule (Figure 14.4). The large polysaccharide capsule is essential for virulence since experimental work has shown that acapsular mutants are avirulent in mice. In addition to its role in impeding phagocytosis, the great quantities of capsular antigen shed into the se-rum are thought to bind antibody. This bound antibody is then no longer available to function as an opsonin for the intact organism.

Antiphagocytic Cytotoxins
Bacteria and fungi make use of mechanisms other than surface structures to pre-vent phagocytosis. Many organisms secrete exotoxins that interfere with chemo-taxis (the attraction of phagocytes to the site of the invading microbe), impair phago-cytosis, or kill the phagocyte. *Pseudomonas aeruginosa* secretes a protein that im-pairs chemotaxis and also inhibits lysosomal fusion once phagocytosis has occurred. Several strains of this bacterium also produce a leukocidin, a protein that damages

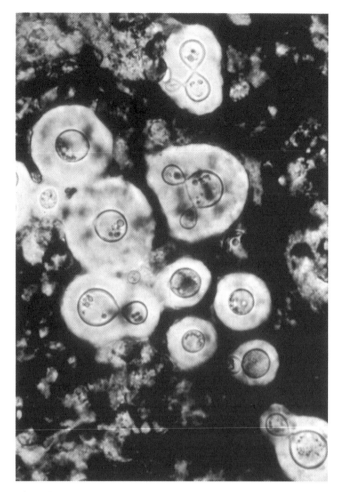

Figure 14.4. India Ink preparation of *Cryptococcus neoformans* showing the budding yeast cells surrounded by large capsules. (Source: Dr. John Timoney, Dept. of Veterinary Science, Gluck Equine Research Center, University of Kentucky, Lexington, Kentucky.)

the cell membrane of leukocytes, resulting in leakage of essential nutrients and cell death. Exotoxin A, produced by most clinical isolates of *P. aeruginosa*, is similar in action to diphtheria toxin and is lethal to human macrophages.

The staphylococci, more commonly the virulent strains, produce several cyto-toxins that act on a variety of cells. The staphylococcal hemolysins kill both eryth-rocytes and leukocytes, while the leukocidin is cytotoxic only for leukocytes. Though there is evidence that the hemolysin can function to impair both chemotaxis and subsequent lysosomal fusion, the actual significance of these toxins in production of disease is not yet clearly defined. However, the production of a leukocidin by strains of *E. coli* correlates well with their virulence.

Group A streptococci produce two exotoxins, streptolysins S and O, which kill leukocytes, erythrocytes, and macrophages.

Recent studies have demonstrated that upon contact with phagocytic cell sur-faces *Yersinia* spp. are induced to secrete several Yop proteins that are transferred into the cytoplasm of the phagocyte. The Yop proteins prevent phagocytosis by inactivating the function of the actin cytoskeleton and blocking crucial signal trans-duction pathways.

SURVIVAL WITHIN THE PHAGOCYTE

In contrast to the obligate extracellular parasites that have evolved means of preventing phagocytosis, there are the intracellular parasites that have developed resistance to the killing mechanisms used by phagocytes, and as a consequence are able to survive and multiply within the phagocyte.

The ingestion of a microorganism by a phagocyte results in the formation of a phagosome, and if the microbe had been appropriately opsonised, as with IgG antibodies, an oxidative burst occurs. If the phagocyte is a macrophage that had been activated by IFN-gamma, the formation of reactive nitrogen intermediates (RNI) is also induced. Under normal conditions the phagosome fuses with lysosomes to form a phagolysosome. The microbicidal systems of the phagocyte are contained within the phagosomes and lysosomes. Any microorganism that has the ability to interfere with these processes therefore enhances its chances of intracellular survival.

Research work in recent years has demonstrated that successful intracellular parasites utilize a variety of methods to combat phagocytes. The principal categories of virulence factors that enhance intracellular survival are described below.

Interference with the Generation of Oxidative Metabolites

Binding of the Fc receptor by an opsonizing IgG antibody triggers phagocytosis and initiates the oxidative burst with the generation of superoxide anion. Superoxide anion is metabolized to yield several highly reactive oxygen intermediates (ROI) including hydrogen peroxide, singlet oxygen, and hydroxyl radicals that are lethal to most microbes. The lysosomes of PMNs and monocytes contain myeloperoxidase that converts hydrogen peroxide and chloride ion to hypochlorous acid, another potent antibacterial product. The functional importance of ROIs is attested by persons with chronic granulomatous disease whose phagocytes lack the ability to generate an oxidative burst. These individuals suffer from an increased incidence of infections with staphylococci and a variety of Gram-negative rods and fungi.

Microbes have evolved different mechanisms to avoid the lethal effects of ROIs. *L. monocytogenes* (an agent of infant meningitis) is one of a number of pathogens that produce superoxide dismutase, which inactivates the superoxide anion. *C. neoformans* grows to large numbers in brain tissue where it utilizes the catecholamines to produce melanin. Melanin scavenges ROIs such as superoxide anion and singlet oxygen, thus rendering phagocytised yeast cells more resistant to killing within PMNs. *Mycobacteria* possess glycolipids that also function as scavengers of ROIs. One effect of YopH, a tyrosine phosphatase of *Yersinia* spp, is to inhibit the Fc receptor-mediated oxidative burst. *Legionella* spp. also produce a phosphatase that blocks superoxide production and another cytotoxin that blocks neutrophil oxidative metabolism.

Other intracellular pathogens avoid the effects of ROIs by arranging their uptake into phagocytes through alternate pathways that do not trigger the oxidative burst. *Salmonella typhimurium* and *Yersinia* spp. accomplish this by utilizing the same invasins to enter professional phagocytes that were described for their invasion of other cell types. Another large group of intracellular pathogens, including *L. pneumophila*, *M. tuberculosis*, and *M. leprae*, *Histoplasma capsulatum*, *Leishmania ma-*

jor, and *L. donovani*, bind abundant $\overline{C3b}$ and $\overline{C3bi}$ and thus ensure their uptake into phagocytes via complement receptors CR1 and CR3, respectively. Phagocytosis mediated by this process fails to evoke an oxidative burst. However, the CR3 receptor has been shown to have a second binding site specific for a lectin, and binding through this site does trigger an oxidative burst. This explains why the promastigotes of *L. major*, which bind the CR3 lectin receptor, are readily killed within macrophages while metacyclic promastigotes, a later developmental stage that binds only the CR1 receptor, are resistant to killing.

In addition to the recognized role of ROIs in microbial killing, recent work in mice has demonstrated the great importance of RNIs against many intracellular pathogens including *M. tuberculosis*, *L. major*, *Toxoplasma gondii*, and *L. monocytogenes*. One of the effects of macrophage activation by IFN-gamma is the induction of nitric oxide synthase (iNOS) which catalyzes the formation of nitric oxide, utilizing the terminal guanadino nitrogen atom of L-arginine. TNF-alpha also plays an essential role by triggering the interaction of iNOS with a required cofactor. Nitric oxide is a powerful microbicidal agent, and its metabolites peroxynitrite and nitrosothiol are even more potent. The mechanisms whereby microbes inhibit the formation of RNIs are not well understood although enzymes that inhibit the oxidative burst would also inhibit the generation of peroxynitrites since superoxide anion is required for the conversion of nitric oxide to peroxynitrite. Interference with the formation of IFN-gamma or with activation signals induced by IFN-gamma would prevent the synthesis of iNOS and TNF-alpha. It has been demonstrated recently that YopB of *Y. enterocolitica* suppresses the production of TNF-alpha, and that *L. major* selectively inhibits the capacity of macrophages to synthesize IL-12, a cytokine required to induce the formation of IFN-gamma by natural killer cells and T cells.

Prevention of Phagosome Maturation and Phagosome-Lysosome Fusion
A phagosome formed through a conventional process of phagocytosis undergoes sequential steps of maturation which culminate in fusion with surrounding lysosomes to form a phagolysosome. Early phagosomes contain products of the oxidative burst and have a pH close to 6, allowing optimal function of the highly bactericidal cationic peptides (defensins) and cationic proteins. At later stages the pH drops to less than 5.5, forming acid conditions ideal for the function of lysosomal enzymes. Lysosomal constituents begin to be transferred across cell membranes of late phagosomes and attain their highest concentrations upon formation of the phagolysosome.

A few pathogens such as *Coxiella burnetii* and certain *Leishmania* spp. are fully capable of surviving within phagolysosomes. Acid fast organisms such as *Mycobacteria* and pathogenic *Nocardia* spp. are also very resistant to enzymatic damage because of their lipid-rich cell walls.

In some instances bacterial products can exert direct inhibitory effects on phagolysosomal fusion. Phagocytized *B. pertussis* release an adenylcyclase which stimulates increased production of cAMP by the phagocyte. The cAMP stabilizes lysosomal granules, thereby inhibiting fusion. Work with mutants lacking the ability to produce this enzyme has demonstrated its importance in virulence. Adenine and guanosine monophosphate that are produced by virulent strains of *Brucella abortus* are believed to inhibit phagolysosomal fusion and thus enhance intracellular survival. It has been demonstrated that both the strongly acidic sulfonated glycolipids of the *M. tuberculosis* cell wall and the ammonium ions released by that organism within the phagosome inhibit fusion with lysosomes.

It is the consensus view that for most pathogens, survival and replication within macrophages require residence in specialized phagosomes that do not undergo normal processes of maturation. Uptake into such vacuoles is in turn dictated by the ligand-receptor interactions that induce phagocytosis. This ability of pathogens to manipulate phagocytosis to their own advantage has already been mentioned in connection with evasion of the oxidative burst. *Salmonella typhymurium*, once internalized through macropinocytosis, is located in an atypically large phagosome. It may then rapidly induce apoptosis of the macrophage or live within the phagosome, aided by the activation of a number of genes coding for novel antigens that act as virulence factors enhancing intracellular survival. Some of their effects are to confer resistance to oxidative metabolites and cationic peptides and to inhibit the processing and presentation of these novel antigens to T cells. The mode of replication of *Salmonella* within macrophages remains to be clarified.

In a manner similar to *S. typhymurium*, *M. tuberculosis* and *M. avium*, *L. pneumophila*, and *Chlamydia* spp. all induce their uptake into specialized phagosomes that fail to acidify and do not fuse with lysosomes. Internalization of *L. pneumophila* and *C. psittaci* occurs by a remarkable complement-dependent process termed "coiling phagocytosis" in which a swirl of pseudopodia coils around the bacterium and engulfs it. The distinctive features of these phagosomes are maintained through active processes directed by the parasites. For example, *M. tuberculosis* prevents acidification of its vacuole by secretion of ammonium ions and by preventing formation of the proton pump in the phagosomal membrane. A common feature among these parasites is their ability, by mechanisms that are still very incompletely defined, to co-opt host cell transport systems so as to ensure delivery into the phagosome of nutrients required for their survival and growth.

Escape from the Phagosome

Some microorganisms make use of yet another means of thwarting the phagocyte. They escape from the phagosome into the cytoplasm of the host cell before lysosomal fusion occurs. Once in the cytoplasm they are safe from destruction and have access to the nutrient-rich medium of the cell. *L. monocytogenes*, *S. flexneri*, and several species of *Rickettsia* utilize this pathway. Whereas little is known of how the phagosome-dwelling parasites are eventually released from the macrophage, the mechanisms whereby *L. monocytogenes* and *S. flexneri* escape the phagosome, are transported through the cytoplasm and gain entry into adjacent cells have been studied extensively in recent years.

Phagocytized *L. monocytogenes* releases a cytolytic exotoxin, listeriolysin O, that disrupts the phagosomal membrane following its activation at pH 5.5. Other microbial enzymes, including two types of phospholipase C and a lecithinase, are believed to have subsidiary roles in membrane lysis. Within the cytoplasm *Listeria* replicate rapidly for two to three hours and then become surrounded by actin filaments that are organized at one end to form a polar tail. Continued deposition of actin at the polar tail pushes the bacterium through the cytoplasm at a remarkably rapid rate. At the cell periphery pseudopod formation is induced, and the pseudopod, with *Listeria* inside, is ingested by a neighboring cell. The double layer of cell membranes is then disrupted by bacterial cytolysins, releasing *Listeria* into the cytoplasm to repeat the cycle. A bacterial surface protein, Act A, induces polymerization of actin but another, as yet unidentified bacterial factor, is required to control the formation of the polar tail and thereby enable directional movement through the cytoplasm. *Salmonella flexneri* uses very similar modes of phagosome disruption, actin-dependent movement, and cell to cell spread. As previously noted, the invasin IpaB lyses the phagosome. The *Shigella* protein IcsA mediates both actin deposition and formation of the polar tail.

SIDEROPHORES AND IRON ACQUISITION

Free ionic iron is present in the body fluids of animals, but only in very low concentrations. Most of the iron is either sequestered inside host cells, in association with functional molecules such as hemoglobin or myoglobin, or captured extracellularly by the glycoproteins lactoferrin and transferrin, which have a high iron-binding affinity. Lactoferrin is found primarily in mucosal secretions and milk, while transferrin is found mainly in blood and lymph. In response to a microbial infection, the host reduces the amount of iron bound to transferrin by transferring it to iron stores. Bacteria and fungi, however, require iron for their metabolism; the survival of the invading microorganism therefore depends upon its ability to scavenge iron from its environment.

Many bacteria and fungi produce siderophores, low molecular-weight compounds that can acquire iron from the host's iron-binding proteins. This ability to scavenge iron has been demonstrated in many species, and has been shown to enhance the virulence of invading bacteria. Experiments have shown that virulence is greatly diminished in certain mutants that have lost the ability to obtain iron. Early work with *Y. pestis* showed that not even 100 million cells of a mutant that had lost the ability to acquire iron were lethal for test animals, whereas as few as 100 cells of the parent strain killed the host.

Salmonella, *E. coli*, and *Klebsiella* produce enterochelin, an iron-chelating agent that can obtain iron from transferrin. This compound is only produced when iron concentrations are very low. It has been demonstrated that the virulence of an enterochelin-defective mutant of *S. typhi* can be increased 600-fold by addition of enterochelin to a suspension of the organism prior to injection into test animals. Pyoverdin, the siderophore of *P. aeruginosa*, has also been shown to enhance the growth of this bacterium *in vivo*.

Some bacteria, which apparently do not produce their own siderophores, have specific surface receptors that enable them to make use of the chelators produced by other species. This has been observed in the campylobacters, shigellae and some salmonellae. Pathogenic *Neisseria* have their own iron acquisition system consisting of two membrane associated iron-binding proteins, which are regulated by the concentration of iron in the environment. Although most species of bacteria obtain iron from the host's glycoprotein storage molecules, there is evidence that some are also able to acquire it from hemin. *Vibrio cholerae* has two types of iron sequestering systems: a siderophore and a surface protein that binds hemin and hemoglobin. *Escherichia coli* provides another example. The hemolysin of *E. coli* lyses red blood cells, thus releasing heme, which stimulates the growth of bacteria. Iron obtained by this method can permit development of fatal infections in individuals who have free blood in their abdominal cavity.

TOXINS
Endotoxins

Patients suffering from Gram-negative septicemias show a variety of effects, including fever, hypoglycemia, intravascular coagulation, and shock. It has been known for many years that these signs are referable to the endotoxin common to all Gram-negative bacteria but found nowhere else in nature. Endotoxin has been identified as a structural component of the bacterial cell wall and is composed of a complex of LPS and outer membrane proteins. LPS consists of three basic units. An interior lipid A molecule is bound to an oligosaccharide core, which is bound in turn to the O polysaccharide side chains that project outward from the bacterial cell surface. The hydrophobic lipid A forms an integral component of the outer membrane. Results obtained with mutants defective in various phases of LPS synthesis, as well as from chemical dissociation of the molecule, have established that most of the toxic effects of endotoxins are due to lipid A.

Most work to date on the characterization of LPS has been performed with *E. coli* and *Salmonella*. In these bacteria, O polysaccharides are composed of repeating oligosaccharide units that differ in chemical composition among strains, thus accounting for the diversity of O serotypes. Virulent strains invariably possess O polysaccharide. This holds true for bacteria of most other Gram-negative genera but there are exceptions, such as *N. gonorrhoeae*, *B. ovis*, and *B. canis*, in which virulent strains lack O polysaccharide.

From distant evolutionary times eukaryotic organisms have evolved mechanisms for recognizing and reacting swiftly to the ubiquitous LPS molecule because it signified the presence of potentially dangerous Gram-negative bacteria. Most LPS molecules are potent activators of complement by the alternate pathway, thereby unleashing the formation of products that function to induce the inflammatory response ($\overline{C3a}$, $\overline{C5a}$), to opsonize bacterial cells ($\overline{C3b}$, $\overline{C3bi}$) and to kill Gram-negative bacteria directly by producing lesions sequentially in the outer and inner cell membranes ($\overline{C5b,6,7,8,9n}$, the membrane attack complex). Professional phagocytes, both PMNs and macrophages, have a surface receptor (CD14) that binds LPS. LPS bound to CD14 acts as a powerful activator of PMN and macrophage function, resulting in the secretion of a variety of cytokines that induce inflammatory and immune responses, and enhance the capacity of the phagocytes to kill intracellular and extracellular pathogens. These responses are normally of great benefit to the host, but under conditions of exposure to massive quantities of LPS, as occurs in Gram-negative septicemias, a systemic hyperreaction occurs that is often fatal.

On their part, Gram-negative pathogens have evolved structural modifications to counteract their vulnerability to the complement system. Inhibition of activation of the alternate complement pathway by various capsules and by abequose in the O polysaccharide of *S. typhymurium* has been mentioned. In other instances complement activation occurs, but the bacterium escapes destruction by the membrane attack complex. For example, some *Salmonella* strains possess unusually long O polysaccharide chains that function as steric barriers to the insertion of the membrane attack complex into the outer membrane. *N. gonorrhoeae* and certain pathogenic strains of *E. coli* possess outer membrane proteins that either prevent the insertion of the membrane attack complex or cause its rapid release.

Exotoxins

Endotoxins were so named by early investigators because they are contained within the bacterial cell, rather than being secreted. Exotoxins were defined as secreted products of microbes that damage host cells directly or interfere with host cell metabolism. Molecular and genetic characterization of exotoxins revealed that they are enzymes, often coded by genes located on plasmids or bacteriophages.

While these enzymes are beneficial for the microbes that produce them, some of them are extremely toxic for the host. In fact, the exotoxins of the *Clostridia* are the most potent biological poisons known. It is notable that the normal modes of existence of *Clostridia* are as commensals in the intestinal tract or as soil saprophytes. Their production of systemic diseases such as tetanus or gas gangrene must therefore be viewed as a biological accident. Fortunately, powerful exotoxins such as those of *C. tetani* or *Corynebacterium diphtheriae* can be converted into toxoids which are very effective vaccines.

Exotoxins that function as virulence factors by interfering with phagocytosis or by disrupting phagosomes have already been described. Other important examples will be discussed in this section.

Proteases of *P. aeruginosa* break down fibrin and elastin connective tissue between cells, thus enabling the bacteria to spread more readily through the tissue and at the same time causing the release of nutrients that enhance bacterial growth. These enzymes also inactivate complement and cleave IgG antibody molecules.

Both virulent streptococci and staphylococci produce kinases that enhance the spread of the microbes by dissolving fibrin clots and inhibiting the clotting of plasma. Hyaluronidase, also associated with virulence in both streptococci and staphylococci, enhances dissemination of infecting microorganisms by breaking down the intercellular mucopolysaccharide hyaluronic acid which "cements" cells together. Virulent strains of staphylococci also produce coagulase which causes deposition of fibrin around the invading cocci, thus reducing their accessibility to phagocytes.

Collagenase produced by the anaerobe *C. perfringens*, an agent of gas gangrene, breaks down collagen in connective tissue. Lecithinase, another enzyme produced by this bacterium, lyses host cells. The resulting destruction of tissue creates an anaerobic environment for the growth of the bacteria and enhances their spread.

Several important pathogens produce proteases that specifically cleave IgA1, a subclass of human IgA. IgA is the most important immunoglobulin isotype mediating protection at mucous surfaces. These enzymes act upon the hinge region of IgA1, splitting the molecule into Fab and Fc fragments which inactivates its function almost completely. IgA proteases have been identified in *N. gonorrhoeae*, *N. meningitidis*, *H. influenzae*, *S. pneumoniae*, *S. sanguis*, and *Bacteroides*, and are believed to contribute to the virulence of these organisms. However, such proteases have also been isolated from the nonpathogenic microbes constituting part of the normal flora.

Coccidioides immitis produces a 60kD serine protease which is associated with the cell surface of both mycelia and spherules and is believed to function in the release of the endospores from the spherule. However, in the host this enzyme degrades elastin, collagen, and immunoglobulins IgG and IgA.

Some bacterial toxins are composed of two subunits: fragment B, the carrier, and fragment A, the enzymatic unit responsible for toxicity. After the binding of fragment B to a specific host receptor the entire complex enters the cell via receptor-mediated endocytosis. Once inside the endosomal vesicle, the units are separated and fragment B enables fragment A to pass through the endosome membrane into the cytoplasm where it exerts its toxic effects.

Diphtheria toxin, an example of an A-B toxin, is produced by *C. diphtheriae*. The toxin is a single-chain polypeptide which catalyzes the transfer of adenine diphosphate dinucleotide from nicotinamide dinucleotide to elongation factor 2, resulting in inhibition of protein synthesis. Diphtheria formerly caused very high morbidity and mortality among young children, but since the incorporation of diphtheria toxoid into the Diphtheria-Pertussis-Tetanus (DPT) vaccine the incidence of this disease has been drastically reduced. Other A-B toxins include Shiga toxin of *S. dysenteriae*, exotoxin A of *P. aeruginosa*, tetanus toxin of *C. tetani*, and botulinum toxin of *C. botulinum*.

Enterotoxins are those exotoxins that exert their activity in the gastrointestinal tract, producing symptoms such as nausea, vomiting, and diarrhea. Certain strains of *E. coli*, *S. aureus*, *Salmonella*, *Shigella*, *Vibrio*, and *C. perfringens* produce enterotoxins. Enterotoxin production may take place in contaminated food, as is the case with staphylococcal enterotoxin, or in the gastrointestinal tract as occurs with *Salmonella* and the other agents. Though the mechanisms of action vary, the end results are similar.

Superantigens

Superantigens are composed of a group of bacterial and viral proteins that can form a direct bridge between antigen presenting cells and T cells by binding directly first to MHC Class II molecules and then to T cell receptors bearing a specific subset of V beta chains. Antigens that are conventionally processed and presented will interact with about one in 10,000 T cells, but superantigens bypass this procedure and can stimulate up to twenty percent of the T cell population. This excessive T cell response results in the production and release into the bloodstream of massive quantities of IL-2 and other proinflammatory cytokines, which can lead to shock and death of the host. Included in this group are the enterotoxin of *Staphylococcus*, the exfoliative toxins, the toxins of Toxic Shock Syndrome, and also the pyogenic toxins of both staphylococci and streptococci. It is thought that tissue destruction resulting from the inflammation induced by these superantigens enables the bacteria to multiply to greater numbers and to be more easily spread.

R FACTORS AND PATHOGENICITY ISLANDS

Plasmids carrying genes for antibiotic resistance known as R factors were first observed in the genus *Shigella* in 1959. These plasmids are readily transferable by conjugation to bacterial cells of the same species as well as to cells of different species and genera and can confer resistance to many antibiotics.

Many bacteria of the normal flora carry R factors, but they present no problem until the prolonged or improper use of antibiotics selectively enhances the survival of drug resistant clones, making further therapy difficult if not impossible. The recent isolation of bacteria resistant to all classes of antibiotics poses a serious threat to the future well-being of us all.

"Pathogenicity islands," discovered within recent years, are large segments of DNA carrying multiple virulence traits which have been found at specific locations on bacterial chromosomes. Analysis of the DNA revealed that these segments are "foreign" to the bacterial cell. It is suggested that these DNA segments are acquired either by transduction via phages or by conjugation. Pathogenicity islands have been identified on strains of *E. coli*, *Salmonella*, *Shigella*, *V. cholerae*, and *Y. pestis*. The significance of this discovery is awesome for it reveals that many virulence traits can be acquired in one step, thus converting a commensal bacterium into a pathogen.

SUMMARY

The production of infectious disease is dependent upon the condition of the host and the characteristics of the invading microorganism. Microbial traits that contribute to the ability to produce disease are called virulence characteristics and include factors which enable the microbe to attach to and invade host cells, to resist ingestion by professional phagocytes or to survive the phagocytic process, to interfere with the host's adaptive immune response, to spread within the host and to be transmitted to new hosts. Most pathogenic microbes express many different virulence traits. Some pathogens are also able to alter the expression of these traits in response to environmental pressure.

SUGGESTIONS FOR FURTHER READING

1. Salyers, A.A., and D.D. Whitt. *Bacterial Infections, A Molecular Approach.* Washington, D.C., ASM Press, 1994.
2. Hogan, L.H., B.S. Klein, and S.M. Levitz. "Virulence Factors of Medically Important Fungi." *Clinical Microbiology Reviews* 9, (1996): 469–488.
3. Finlay, B.B., and S. Falkow. "Common Themes in Microbial Pathogenicity Revisited." *Microbiology and Molecular Biology Reviews* 61 (1997):136–169.

QUESTIONS

1. Any organism that is able to infect a host and produce disease is a pathogen. Whether disease ensues as a result of a host's encounter with a pathogen is dependent both upon the condition of the host and the particular characteristics of the microorganism. Give an example to support and illustrate this statement.
2. Give examples of several different methods that microbes use to adhere to host cells. What therapeutic use could be made of this knowledge?
3. Describe the different processes by which microbes evade destruction by host phagocytes and give examples of each.
4. Explain how endotoxin functions as a virulence factor.

ANSWERS

1. The classic example of enterotoxigenic *E. coli* supports and illustrates this statement. In order to produce disease this bacterium must adhere to the lining of the small intestine and produce a toxin which is absorbed by the epithelial cells, causing an increase in intracellular cAMP and the initiation of diarrhea. It was demonstrated that piglets which lacked the specific receptor for the bacterial adhesin were not colonized and did not develop disease. The agent must have both adhesins and toxin; the host must have the receptor for the adhesin.
2. Microbes adhere to host cells by a number of different methods. Many of the Gram-negative bacteria, such as *H. influenzae*, *E. coli*, *P. aeruginosa* and the neisseriae adhere to host cells via fimbriae, also called pili. The fibrillae of streptococci are hairy surface appendages composed of lipotechoic acid and proteins which function as adhesins. The flagella of *C. jejuni*, opacity proteins of the neisseriae, LPS of *S. flexneri* and the glycocalyx of *P. aeruginosa* are all known to play a role in adherence. Knowledge of these adhesins can be used to develop subunit vaccines which will stimulate production of antibodies against the adhesin and thus prevent colonization.

3. Extracellular pathogens must prevent their ingestion by phagocytic cells. Capsules are external surface structures composed of carbohydrate or protein which function to prevent phagocytosis. Many capsules composed of sialic acid have high affinity for protein factor H which enhances the degradation of $\overline{C3b}$ bound to the bacterial surface and so prevents the activation of complement by the alternate pathway. Other capsules prevent the deposition of $\overline{C3b}$ on the bacterial surface or block the access of complement components to the pathogen's cell walls thus preventing complement activation. Glycocalyces function in a similar manner. Some bacteria secrete toxins, such as the leukocidin of *S. aureus*, which interfere with chemotaxis or impair or kill phagocytes. Exotoxin A produced by *P. aeruginosa* kills macrophages and exotoxins of group A streptococci kill leukocytes and macrophages. A different method is used by *Yersinia* spp which secrete several Yop proteins into the cytoplasm of the phagocyte thus preventing phagocytosis by inactivating the function of the actin cytoskeleton and blocking signal transduction pathways. Intracellular parasites have developed ways to resist the effects of phagocytosis by interfering with the generation of reactive oxygen intermediates. *L. monocytogenes* produces superoxide dismutase which inactivates the superoxide anion. *C. neoformans* produces melanin which scavenges ROIs. Other pathogens enter phagocytes in ways which do not trigger the oxidative burst. *L. pneumophila*, *H. capsulatum* and *L. donovani*, as examples, coat themselves with C3b and C3bi and enter via complement receptors CR1 and CR3. Entry via this method fails to generate an oxidative burst. Still another method used by parasites to insure intracellular survival is to interfere with the generation of RNIs. The precise method by which this is accomplished is not known. It is known however, that by interfering with the production of TNF-alpha (*Y. enterocolitica*) or IL-12 (*L. major*), the synthesiss of RNIs is prevented. Other pathogens, the *Mycobacteria* and the *Nocardia*, are resistant to the effects of lysosomal enzymes because of their lipid-rich cell walls and some pathogens just prevent the fusion of lysosomes with phagosomes. For example, *B. pertussis* releases adenylcyclase which causes the phagocyte to produce cAMP. The cAMP stabilizes the membranes of the lysosomes and thus prevents fusion. Yet another way to thwart the phagocyte is to escape into the cytoplasm before fusion occurs. *L. monocytogenes* releases listeriolysin O, a cytolytic toxin, which disrupts the phagosomal membrane allowing the bacteria to escape into the cytoplasm.

4. In some cases bacteria have evolved structural modifications in LPS that enhance their ability to produce disease. For example, the LPS of *S. typhimurium* contains the sugar abequose which inhibits activation of complement by the alternative pathway. *S. typhimurium* and other salmonella strains that produce systemic disease have very long O polysaccharide chains which sterically prevent deposition of the MAC into the outer membrane, thus making the organism resistant to complement killing. LPS activates both the complement system and the functions of neutrophils and macrophages. These responses are normally beneficial to the host in enhancing the production of inflammatory and immune responses that eliminate infection. However, in people undergoing overwhelming infections with Gram-negative bacteria, the amount of LPS in the system becomes so great that the body's response produces harmful effects. The large quantities of C3a, C5a and the proinflammatory cytokines cause intravascular coagulation and vascular collapse (shock) that is often fatal.

INTRODUCTION
UBIQUITY AND SIZE OF
    MICROORGANISMS
SHAPE AND GROUPING
    AMONG PROKARYOTES
SYNOPSIS OF NUTRITION,
    METABOLISM, AND
    GROWTH
    Oxygen Relationships
PROKARYOTIC CELL
    STRUCTURE
    Cell Envelope and the
        Gram Stain
    Cytoplasm, Nucleus, and
        Inclusions
    Glycocalyx, Capsules, and
        Slime Layers
    Flagella
    Pili (Fimbriae)
    Endospores
TAXONOMY AND PHYLO-
    GENETIC RELATIONSHIPS
SOME MEDICALLY
    IMPORTANT BACTERIA AND
    THE DISEASES THEY CAUSE
    Infections of the Skin
    Infections of the Eye
    Infections of the Mouth
    Infections of the
        Respiratory Tract
    Infections of the Gastroin-
        testinal Tract
    Infections of the Urogeni-
        tal Tract
    Generalized Infections
MECHANISMS OF IMMUNITY
    AND RESISTANCE TO
    BACTERIAL INFECTION
    Extracellular Bacterial
        Infections
    Toxigenic Bacterial
        Infections
    Intracellular Bacterial
        Infections
SUMMARY
SUGGESTIONS FOR
    FURTHER READING
QUESTIONS
ANSWERS

15

Bacteria

Patrick R. Dugan

INTRODUCTION

Increased life expectancy in the United States and in many other geographic regions of the world is largely a result of three major factors: (1) improvements in our understanding of nutrition and in the growth and delivery of nutrients resulting from improvements in agriculture and food processing; (2) improvements in our understanding and use of sanitation, particularly water and wastewater treatment, and in personal and public hygiene; and (3) improvements in our understanding, use, and delivery of modern health practices in medicine, medical technology, pharmaceuticals, and vaccines. These improvements have been instituted since the late 1800s, when microbes were first identified as the causative agents of infectious diseases. All of the above improvements are grounded in science, education, and common sense.

However, our successes have contributed to both an increasing population density and an aging population. These, in turn, are associated with a reemergence of bacterial diseases throughout the world. Bacterial infections have become serious complications in the elderly as well as in those who have received organ transplants and treatments for cancer and have AIDS. There is an almost weekly announcement of a new outbreak of food- or water-transmitted disease. Articles in the press on either new emerging diseases or reemerging diseases that were thought to be eradicated or under control, continue to attract our attention. The shift toward economic and political globalization accompanied by greatly increased travel contributes to the spread of disease from one region to another. Increasing concern is expressed about the potential of global or regional warming to cause frost lines to move toward the North or South Poles allowing infectious disease vectors, such as insects, arthropods, and rodents,

283

to carry pathogens to new locations. Microbial pathogens, through natural evolutionary processes, acquire resistance to antibiotics and this exacerbates the problem of infectious disease. Perhaps we have become too reliant on continued rapid development of new technology as the primary strategy for solving problems associated with emerging and reemerging infectious diseases. Revisiting the precepts of sanitation, hygiene, and prevention will aid in preventing disease transmission better than will an overreliance on use of antibiotics to cure diseases once infection has occurred.

We should not forget the old adage that "an ounce of prevention is worth a pound of cure." An emphasis on the fundamentals that govern and control the growth, distribution, and survival of bacteria has been added to this chapter. More information has become available since the previous edition was published and therefore more specific examples of the relationships between bacterial attributes such as structure and metabolism and specific disease processes have been included. Discussion on the increased incidence of intestinal infections, the role of extracellular polymer capsules as virulence factors, and the resistance of bacteria to antibiotics has been added. Vaccines will be given emphasis elsewhere in this volume.

UBIQUITY AND SIZE OF MICROORGANISMS

Microbes are free-living, predominantly single cell organisms that are ubiquitous in nature. One ounce of rich garden soil may contain 60 billion living organisms; yet only about ten percent of the over 2000 identified species of bacteria are known to cause disease. Microbes are too small to be seen with the naked eye; i.e., they require the aid of a microscope or other magnifying device for direct observation. However, large populations of a specific microbe can be cultivated or grown into colonies in the laboratory and then observed directly. For example: a one-ounce yeast cake contains approximately 300 billion individual cells—a number higher than the world's human population—and is observable; whereas a single yeast cell cannot be seen. Consider that it is the summation of all the organisms' physical, chemical, and biological attributes—all of which are conferred by the genetic complement within the cell—that determines whether the cell can live or die in an environment where it arrives.

Most microorganisms are unicellular and have the ability to grow very rapidly in number as well as in size of an individual cell under ideal growth conditions. Growth of bacteria usually refers to increased size of the population. These attributes of being very small, yet having rapid growth, provide many microbes with the capacity to infect other organisms and cause disease. Rapidity of growth is an important consideration in determining the speed with which pathogens produce disease symptoms. A short incubation period and period of morbidity in the diseased host limits the time available between the onset of symptoms and treatment. Rapidity of growth is also an important aid in laboratory diagnosis and where clinical samples are processed by inoculation into nutritionally optimal cultivation media and held under optimum growth conditions for identification.

The size of an organism strongly affects dispersability and transmission of diseases in both air and water. There is a substantial range in size among microorganisms, with the bacteria in the approximate range of 0.2 μm, which is close to the limit of resolution of a standard light microscope, up to hundreds of micrometers in length for some filamentous species. Many bacteria of clinical significance are in the size range of 0.2 μm to 4.0 μm. This is in the range of *colloidal* particles. Particles

Table 15.1. The relative size of some common particles in comparison to some microscopic cells.

Particle or Cell	Approximate Size in Micrometers
sand grain	200 to 2000
pollen grain	20 to 60
human leukocytes	10 to 15
Saccharomyces cereviseae (baker's yeast)	10
human erythrocytes	7.5
mold spores	1 to 10
Escherichia coli (bacterium)	0.5 x 0.8
poxvirus	0.25 x 0.35
tobacco smoke	0.1 to 0.25
retrovirus	0.005

of less than 1.0 μm diameter, including many bacteria, are referred to as of colloidal size and tend to produce colloidal dispersions in water and air (or other gases). Such colloidal particles can remain suspended indefinitely or at least for a relatively long time. Colloidal size limits are somewhat arbitrary and smaller particles are required to form colloidal dispersions in air than in water. In general, the smaller the particle the longer it will remain suspended in either water or air, providing there is nothing else present to alter the size or surface properties of the particles. Sneezing and coughing creates aerosols of those pathogens that may have been present in the mouth or throat of an infected individual; thereby allowing transmission to any other person who breathes the "contaminated air." Opportunity for this kind of disease transmission is, of course, statistically increased by increasing the number of people in a room (e.g., concerts and theaters, sporting events, etc.) and by not "diluting" the aerosol with uncontaminated air, as would be the case during cold weather when windows are less likely to be open. Table 15.1 lists several common particles and their size range.

SHAPE AND GROUPING AMONG PROKARYOTES

There is a phenomenal variety of shapes and groupings of cells among the prokaryotes. Shapes include the forms historically described as: spherical (cocci), cylindrical (bacilli), either straight or curved (vibrio). The organisms may grow singly or in pairs (diplococci or diplobacilli), in chains (streptococci or streptobacilli), in three-dimensional cubes of spheres (sarcinae), or in randomly arranged clusters (staphylococci); in more or less tightly coiled spirals (e.g., spirochaetes), in long sometimes branched filaments (found in *Streptomyces* and *Actinomyces* species, among others), in squares, and in irregular clusters. In addition to those already described, groupings of cells include: rosette clusters, flexible gliding clusters, and tightly packed films. It seems reasonable to assume that any possible form, shape or arrangement of bacterial cells may exist somewhere in nature awaiting discovery.

However, in spite of our continuing discovery of new shapes and groupings of bacteria, the historic descriptions that were based primarily on observations after cells were cultivated in the laboratory under conditions designed to promote maximum growth rates continue to have value both because of their practicality in rapid identification of pathogens and because of an already existing literature that uses

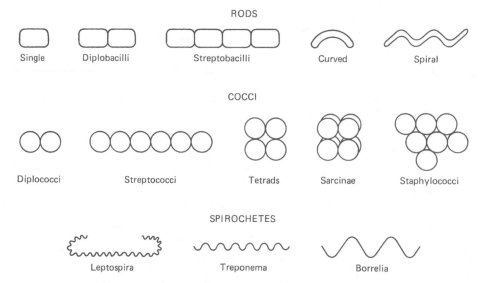

RODS

Single Diplobacilli Streptobacilli Curved Spiral

COCCI

Diplococci Streptococci Tetrads Sarcinae Staphylococci

SPIROCHETES

Leptospira Treponema Borrelia

Figure 15.1. An illustration showing the more common shapes and arrangements of many pathogenic bacteria.

those descriptions. Figure 15.1 illustrates some of the more common shapes and groupings of pathogenic bacteria.

SYNOPSIS OF NUTRITION, METABOLISM, AND GROWTH

Most bacteria consist of about eighty percent water and twenty percent solids and they require moisture to grow. As with all living organisms, bacteria must absorb nutrients, metabolize them in order to derive energy to synthesize new cell structure and then excrete the by-products of metabolism. The cells must have suitable nutritional sources for supplying their requirements for carbon, hydrogen, nitrogen, oxygen, phosphate, sulfur, and several mineral ions such as calcium, cobalt, copper, iron, magnesium, manganese, potassium, sodium, zinc, and others. Most organisms including most bacteria also require additional organic growth factors such as amino acids, proteins, sugars, and vitamins. They require as a nutrient any cellular component they cannot synthesize.

Some bacteria have the capability of synthesizing all of their cellular carbon compounds from carbon dioxide or carbonate and their other nutritional requirements from nonorganic sources, using energy to do so derived either from (A) the oxidation of one of the following nonorganic chemicals: ferrous iron, ammonium, methane, or inorganic sulfur (these organisms are called chemoautotrophs or autotrophs), or (B) light (these organisms are called photoautotrophs or phototrophs).

All of the clinically significant bacteria are *chemoorganotrophs (heterotrophs)*. That is, most of their nutritional carbon must be supplied to them as preformed carbon compounds that contain carbon to carbon chemical bonds; such as are found in amino acids, proteins, sugars, etc., that when metabolized, release energy in a form that can be used by the organotroph.

Briefly, cells take on an oxidizable energy source and release that energy in the form of electrons, through a complex stepwise series of biooxidations known collectively as *intermediary metabolism* (including glycolysis, the tricarboxylic acid cycle, and other pathways). Those electrons, always associated with hydrogen ions, are sequentially picked up and released by cellular compounds such as nicotinic acid dinucleotide (NAD) and flavine adenosine dinucleotide (FAD) in bucket brigade fashion. The NAD and FAD become oxidized and reduced as electrons are transported along the *electron transport pathway*. The final or terminal step transfers the electron to a *terminal electron acceptor* (TEA).

Oxygen Relationships

In obligate *aerobic* organisms the TEA is oxygen and the process is called *aerobic respiration*. This type of metabolism, where oxygen is an obligatory nutrient, is found in all animals and in aerobic bacteria. In some obligate aerobes (e.g., hydrogen oxidizing bacteria), the organism must grow by aerobic respiration but the organism is sensitive to oxygen above about 0.2 atmospheres. These bacteria, known as *microaerophilic*, contain an essential enzyme that is inactivated by oxygen (e.g., hydrogenase). A variation unique to the microbial world is that some bacteria have the capacity to substitute inorganic chemicals (i.e., carbonate, nitrate, nitrite, sulfate) in place of oxygen as their TEA and grow in the absence of oxygen. This process is called *anaerobic respiration*. An additional variation, known as *fermentation*, is found in other microbes that have the capacity to transfer electrons to partially reduced organic compounds in the absence of a complete electron transport system and derive energy from the process. For example, some fermenters are unable to synthesize cytochromes which are essential components of an electron transport system.

During aerobic respiration (electron transport), some highly toxic by-products of oxygen are produced which inhibit any organisms that are not equipped to detoxify them. Two of these by-products of metabolism, superoxide and hydrogen peroxide, can be produced when oxygen reacts with flavoprotein during oxygen respiration. Aerobic organisms contain the enzymes superoxide dismutase, which converts water and superoxide to hydrogen peroxide, and catalase, which converts hydrogen peroxide to water and oxygen; thereby detoxifying the superoxide and hydrogen peroxide. Strict (obligate) anaerobes, i.e., those that are killed or inhibited by traces of oxygen, contain neither superoxide dismutase nor catalase. Some obligate anaerobes, e.g., several species of *Clostridium*, produce superoxide dismutase but not catalase and can tolerate a small amount of oxygen, usually less than one percent partial pressure. Still others, e.g., *Lactobacillus* species, that must derive their energy from fermentation reactions are relatively insensitive to oxygen and are called *aerotolerant* anaerobes. Oxygen tolerant anaerobes are usually fermenters that possess superoxide dismutase but not catalase. *Facultative anaerobes* such as the enteric bacteria, e.g., *Escherichia*, *Salmonella*, and *Shigella* species, have the facility to derive energy from either aerobic respiration if oxygen is present or from fermentation in the absence of oxygen.

Bacteria will grow and multiply until either nutrients are depleted or accumulation of metabolic by-products reaches an inhibitory level. Under ideal conditions the rate of growth of many pathogens can be very high. *Escherichia coli* can divide (double) every twenty minutes. One bacterium can, therefore, double twenty-four times in eight hours, and 2^{24} is equivalent to about 170 million cells generated from a single cell in eight hours.

In addition to nutrient availability and oxidation/reduction potential (Eh), other environmental variables are also important in determining the activity, growth, and survivability of bacteria. Important variables include pH, moisture, osmotic,

Table 15.2. Some fundamental differences between prokaryotic and eukaryotic cells (+ indicates presence and – indicates absence).

Cell Component	Prokaryotic	Eukaryotic
chromosome	circular	linear
ribosomes	70S, exist independently in cytoplasm	80S, attached to endoplasmic reticulum
nuclear membrane	–	+
mitochondria	–	+
mitotic apparatus, meiosis	–	+
cytoplasmic streaming, cytoskeleton	–	+
chloroplasts	–	+
endoplasmic reticulum	–	+
Golgi apparatus	–	+
flagella	simple	complex
cell membrane	generally lack sterols	contain sterols
glycocalyx	extracellular capsule or slime layer	–
cell wall of Eubacteria	contain peptidoglycan	if present, contain cellulose or chitin

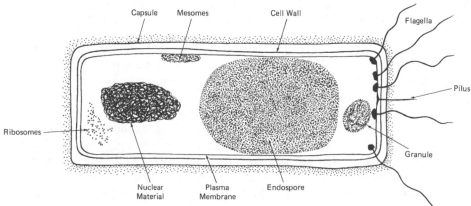

Figure 15.2. Schematic drawing of a bacterial cell showing some of the structural components. Not all of the structures illustrated are present in all bacteria, nor at all times in a given bacterium.

and barometric pressure and presence or absence of electromagnetic radiation (light, ultraviolet, and infrared).

PROKARYOTIC CELL STRUCTURE

Prokaryotic cells are fundamentally different from eukaryotic cells (Table 15.2). Structure is an important consideration because of the involvement of several structural components as factors of virulence, i.e., the ability of the microbe to cause disease. Figure 15.2 is an idealized schematic drawing of a prokaryotic cell showing structural components. It must be emphasized, however, that not all of the components shown are always present in a single species of bacteria. Keep in mind that all bacterial diseases are interactions between prokaryotic and eukaryotic cells.

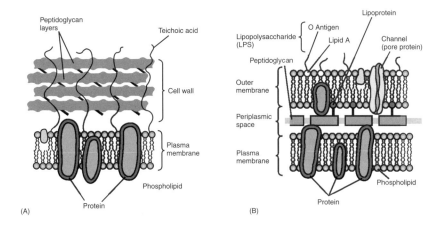

Figure 15.3. Schematic comparison of cell envelope structure and chemical composition of (A) a Gram-positive (+) and (B) Gram-negative (-) cell.

Cell Envelope and the Gram Stain
Long before the chemical structure of bacterial cell envelopes was understood, Hans Christian Gram (1884) observed that some bacteria which had been stained by crystal violet (syn. Methyl violet, gentian violet) retained the stain after the cells were treated with a dilute iodine solution followed by a wash with a dilute ethanol solution. These violet-stained bacteria were called Gram-positive; whereas, bacteria that were decolorized by the alcohol wash were called Gram-negative. Many bacteria are colorless when observed under a light microscope and are frequently stained to improve observation. In the case of decolorized Gram-negative cells, they are generally counterstained with a solution of the red dye, safranin. The chemical basis for differences between Gram-positive and Gram-negative cells is now known to reside in differences in cell wall structure as illustrated in Figure 15.3.

The boundary of the bacterial cell is referred to as the **cell envelope**. It includes the cell wall, one lipid bilayer membrane and, in Gram-negative bacteria, a lipid bilayer outside of the cell wall. These layers contain a variety of components, some of which control the transport of nutrients, including ions, in and out of the cell and also provide protection from changes in osmotic pressure. In addition, some envelop components, e.g., pili, serve as sites for attachment to host cells.

The outer membranes of Gram-negative bacteria are an effective permeability barrier against many external agents that would otherwise be harmful to the bacterium. Polycations such as cationic detergents and some antibiotics (e.g., polymyxins, and cationic leukocyte peptides), as well as chelators (e.g., ethylenediamine tetraacetic acid [EDTA], and sodium hexameta phosphate) remove Ca^{++} and Mg^{++} ions and weaken the lipopolysaccharide (LPS) component, found only in the outer membrane, resulting in loss of permeability control and damage to the bacterium.

Components in cell envelopes are important in host-parasite interactions. LPS is an important virulence factor. For example, *Neisseria meningitidis*, a Gram-negative bacterium, causes the diseases meningitis and bacteremia in humans; sometimes accompanied by septic shock, a process that is induced by LPS from the organism. Many of the proteins and polysaccharides in cell walls are antigenic or act as haptens in immunological reactions. Detection of these antigens often aids in the diagnosis of infections. For example, detection of LPS indicates infection with a Gram-negative bacterium. The lipid A is the part of LPS that is primarily responsible for the endotoxemia that is associated with many Gram-negative bacterial infections. Antibiotic treatment often results in liberation of LPS from the bacteria following their lysis. As a result, clinical endotoxemia symptoms may develop after treatment with antibiotics, also, many commercial foods, bottled water, as well as sterile water used for intravenous applications are routinely analyzed for LPS to assure the absence of these virulence factors.

The LPS which is oriented to the outside of the cell is in contact with the environment. The major surface antigen of all Gram-negative bacteria is the *O-antigen*, which is a side chain that is attached to the outermost core polysaccharide component of LPS. The core polysaccharide, in turn, is attached to the lipid A component of LPS. The lipid A component is embedded in the phospholipid bilayer of the outer membrane (Figure 15.3). Differences in the O-antigen determine the bacterial *serotype*.

The cell wall has a rigid three-dimensional structure composed of cross-linked peptidoglycan, which consists of repeating units of N-acetylglucosamine and N-acetylmuramic acid. These repeating polymeric units are bound together by cross-linked pentaglycine residues. The cell envelopes of Gram-positive cells are structurally simpler than are Gram-negative cell envelopes even though they are generally thicker. In addition to an inner cytoplasmic membrane and a thick peptidoglycan layer, the Gram-positives have an outer glycocalyx or capsular layer. Gram-negative bacteria also have an inner membrane and a second membrane separated by a periplasmic space, providing a higher lipid content in Gram-negative cells (fifteen to twenty percent) compared to that (two to four percent) in Gram-positives. Figure 15.4 is an electron micrograph of a thin section of a Gram-positive bacterium, *Mycobacterium flavum*, and Figure 15.5 is an electron micrograph of an unidentified species of *Pseudomonas*, a Gram-negative bacterium.

Much of the catalytic and metabolic activity of bacteria resides in the membrane surfaces of their cell envelopes. Consider that a cube of one cubic centimeter volume has a surface area of six square centimeters. If that cube was divided into cubes measuring one micrometer, approximately the size of many pathogenic bacteria, the total volume would still be one cubic centimeter but the total surface area would be 60 thousand square centimeters. The enormous surface-to-volume ratio found in bacteria gives them a distinct advantage in their competition with larger organisms for nutrients, accompanied by the inevitable accumulation of by-products. This partially explains why bacteria frequently "out compete" many of the larger cells they attack. The large surface area aides in their secretion also.

Antibiotics are chemical substances that are produced by some microorganisms that either inhibit growth or kill other microbes. The mode of action of the antibiotics *penicillin, cephalosporin,* and *vancomycin,* and their derivatives is blockage of cross-linking of peptidoglycan thereby inhibiting proper synthesis of cell walls in Gram-positive bacteria, resulting in leakage across the wall accompanied by cell lysis. Because animal cells lack these cell walls, antibiotics such as penicillin that act on cell walls are not toxic for animal cells and can be used to treat animal diseases caused by Gram-positive bacteria. However, penicillins are not very effective against Gram-negative bacteria because their cell wall structure is little affected by these antibiotics.

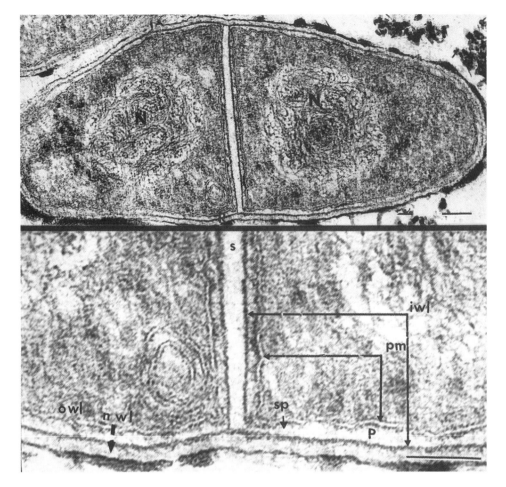

Figure 15.4.   Electron micrograph of a thin section of a dividing *Mycobacterium flavum* cell; a Gram-positive, acid fast bacterium showing the cell wall structure, cell membrane, and nuclear region. From: Reed and Dugan, J. General Microbiology, 133:1389, 1987.

Penicillinase, an enzyme produced by several Gram-positive bacteria including *Staphylococcus aureus*, hydrolyses the beta-lactam ring of penicillin, resulting in penicillin resistant organisms. Development of resistance prompts a continuing need for new and chemically modified antibiotics to circumvent the problem of development of antibiotic resistant organisms.

Cytoplasm, Nucleus, and Inclusions
Cytoplasm is not homogeneous. It has a complex structure which holds the cellular machinery. The ctyoplasm contains all of the substance inside the cell membrane (CM) with the exception of the *nucleus*; which is usually considered to be in a separate nuclear region. In prokaryotes the nucleus consists of a closed circular strand of chromosomal deoxyribonucleic acid (DNA, see Figure 15.4) that is not enclosed in a nuclear membrane. In addition, some cells may contain one to several small (approximately one-tenth to ten percent of the chromosome size) closed circles of

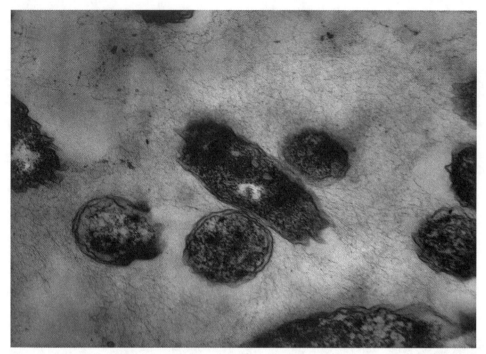

Figure 15.5.   Thin section electron micrograph of an unidentified species of *Pseudomonas*, a Gram-negative bacterium showing the cell envelope and extracellular polymer fibrils that comprise an extensive capsular or slime layer around the cells.

DNA called *plasmids*. Plasmids are independent of the chromosome and carry genetic information that although not critical to the growth of the bacterium, nevertheless often provide useful genetic information. It can be transferred between bacteria of a species and also to related species and even to related genera in some cases. One type of plasmid, known as *Resistance factor (R factor)*, contains coded information that allows the cell to resist substances that would ordinarily be inhibitory. Antibiotic resistance in bacteria often resides in plasmid DNA. R factors have a second part; a resistance transfer factor (RTF) concerned with transfer of the plasmid between cells via the processes of conjugation, transformation, or transduction. R factors are common among species of *Enterobacteriaceae, Pseudomonas*, and *Vibrio* and are responsible for multiple drug resistance in these organisms. Some bacteria also produce plasmid encoded toxic peptides called *bacteriocins* that can kill other bacteria of the same or closely related types. Bacteriocins were first observed in *E. coli* and were called *colicins*. They have since been recognized in many bacteria including Gram-positives. *Episomes* are small circular extrachromosomal DNA containing plasmids, found in the cytoplasm. They confer nonvital properties and may be transferred to other cells by several means. Bacteriophage, sex factors, bacteriocins, and resistance transfer factors are often classed as episomes.

   DNA carries the genetic information to determine heritable properties of an organism (i.e., its *phenotype*). The DNA is initially transcribed into complementary polymers of ribonucleic acid (RNA) in the form called messenger RNA (mRNA). The mRNA subsequently serves as a template for synthesis of protein molecules; a process that is mediated by **ribosomes**. Ribosomes are microparticles composed of protein linked to another class of RNA called ribosomal RNA (rRNA). Ribosomes

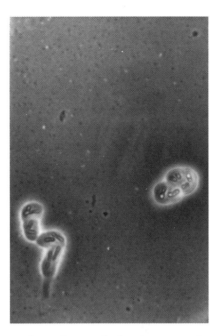

Figure 15.6. Phase contrast photomicrograph showing a capsule surrounding *Pseudomonas* cells; species unidentified.

consist of smaller (30S) and larger (50S) subunits and tend to form aggregates or strands called polyribosomes.

Many antibiotics inhibit bacterial growth by preventing protein synthesis. The antibiotics: streptomycin, neomycin, and kanamycin, bind to ribosomal subunits and thereby prevent the synthesis of protein. The antibiotics tetracycline, chloromycetin, aureomycin, erythromycin, and lincomycin interfere with the transcription of mRNA. Chloramphenicol functions to block peptide synthesis during the association of amino acids with tRNA and rifamycin binds to RNA polymerase and inhibits its function.

Mesosomes are membranous structures found inside the ctyoplasmic membrane (CM) and may arise as an extension of the CM. Mesosomes consist of subcellular particles that are mainly proteins, nucleoproteins, and lipoproteins. In addition, the cytoplasm contains soluble enzymes, nutrients, ions, and waste products that have not yet been excreted. Finally, the cytoplasm of some cells contains storage polymers such a polyphosphate granules and polyhydroxyalkanoate granules.

Glycocalyx, Capsules, and Slime Layers

Most bacteria synthesize insoluble, extracellular polymers that accumulate outside the cell envelope. When these polymers accumulate around single cells or pairs of cells, the structures formed are usually referred to as *capsules* (Figure 15.6); whereas the term *slime layer* is used to describe similar material that is produced in rather copious amounts and surrounds clusters of cells. In some instances extracellular polymer diffuses away from the cells, resulting in increased viscosity of the surrounding liquid medium.

The term *glycocalyx* is sometimes used to describe a mass of polysaccharide polymer that may or may not appear as a contiguous capsule. Some Gram-negative

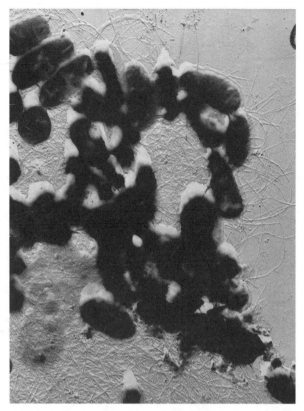

Figure 15.7. Electron micrograph showing extracellular polymer fibrils that comprise slime around *Pseudomonas* cells.

bacteria produce carbohydrate polymer fibrils that resemble alginate or cellulose and have a flocculent growth pattern unlike the dispersed growth pattern of most bacteria, as shown in Figure 15.7. Capsules may be relatively thin and contiguous around the cell or very thick and contiguous or diffuse, depending upon the genetics of the organism, the amount and kinds of nutrients available to the cell, and the chemical composition of the polymer. Different polymers have a greater or lesser affinity for binding water and many other soluble chemicals; binding of chemicals may affect the consistency of the capsular material. Most Gram-negative bacteria have capsules comprised of branched or straight chain polysaccharides or heteropolysaccharides. Capsules of Gram-positive bacteria usually consist of amino acid polymers and may be chemically complex. The capsule of the Gram-positive *Bacillus anthracis* is poly-d-glutamate.

Capsules are very important to the growth, survival, virulence, and potential success of treatment of diseases caused by many pathogenic bacteria. For example, the encapsulated pathogen: *Haemophilus influenzae* is estimated to account for approximately 800,000 human infections per year worldwide, with 145,000 of those resulting in death. Encapsulated *Streptococcus pneumoniae* is estimated to cause 100 million cases of pneumonia per year with 10 million fatal, most in Third World countries. Capsules may interfere with phagocytosis or may prevent activation of complement by the alternative pathway. In addition, capsules are known to concentrate many chemical substances including organic nutrients, toxins, and metal

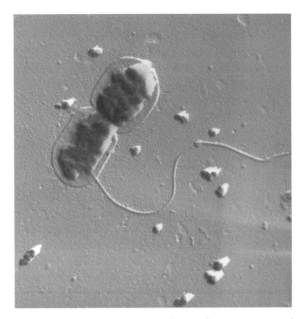

Figure 15.8. Photomicrograph of an unidentified *Pseudomonas* species bacterium showing a single flagellum.

ions from dilute solution. They also aid in cell survival by retarding desiccation when the organism is in a dry environment. The relative nonpathogenicity of noncapsulated strains of *Haemophilus influenzae* and *Streptococcus pneumoniae* attests to the role of capsules in promoting virulence. The capsule is not the only virulence factor of those pathogens, however. It is known that at least three other surface structures contribute to the pathogenicity of bacteria. These are outer membrane LPS, outer membrane protein, and surface pili.

Flagella

Flagella are structures that produce locomotion or motility in those cells which possess them. Not all motile bacteria have flagella. There are other mechanisms of locomotion (e.g., gliding) in some organisms. Flagella are long hollow tubes composed of intertwined fibers of an alpha-helical form of the protein flagelin. These appendages emanate from the cytoplasmic membrane and are anchored by a specialized "hook" embedded in a basal body in the cell envelope. Some bacteria have a single flagellum (monotrichous, Figure 15.8); others have several flagella in a tuft at one location on the cell (lophotrichous); and others have flagella distributed about the entire cell (peritrichous). The arrangement is characteristic of the species and genus. Motility conferred by flagella is a result of their rotary motion; thereby giving directional propulsion to the cell, often in response to chemotactic stimuli.

Pili (Fimbriae)

Pili are very small or fine filamentous appendages that extend outward from some bacteria. They, like flagella, originate in a basal body in the cytoplasmic membrane. Pili occur most frequently on Gram-negative bacilli. They are of two types: (A) the sex pilus that is involved in *conjugation* and allows passage of DNA through the pilus into another bacterial cell, and (B) an attachment pilus that allows bacteria to attach to host cells, especially mucosal cells. Attachment is often necessary for a pathogen to achieve colonization of a host tissue and initiate a disease process. For example, pili of *Neisseria gonorrheae* serve to attach the organism to the urethral mucosa and are an important factor in the organisms' virulence. Vaccines using pilus protein as antigen are being developed for several diseases including gonorrhea and various types of bacterial dysentery.

Endospores

Several bacteria including species of the genera: *Bacillus, Clostridium, Sporosarcina, Sporolactobacillus, Thermoactinomyces,* and *Desulfotomaculum* are capable of producing endospores; an environmentally resistant form of cell that is generated entirely within an actively metabolizing vegetative cell in a process called sporulation. Only endospores from the aerobic *Bacillus* and anaerobic *Clostridium* species are of clinical significance. Endospores are formed when vegetatively growing cells are subjected to a nutritional deficiency causing the vegetative cells to stop actively dividing and instead produce a single complex-walled mature spore within the vegetative mother cell; which eventually lyses and dies. The endospores are highly resistant to extremes of temperature (e.g., boiling water for thirty minutes), desiccation, many chemical agents, radiation, and to physical disruption (e.g., ultrasound, grinding) and may remain dormant for many years. Yet, when optimal nutritional conditions arise, the spores are able to germinate very rapidly to form a new vegetative cell that can either continue to grow and divide vegetatively or again produce a spore, depending upon the environmental conditions. Although spores are not virulence factors, their prolonged survival in the environment increases the chance of infection. The introduction of spores of a pathogen into a susceptible host quickly results in outgrowth of the bacteria. Humans and most of their domestic animals can be infected with spores of *Bacillus anthracis*, the causative agent of anthrax, as well as several species of *Clostridium*, including *C. tetani* (tetanus), *C. perfringens* (gas gangrene), and *C. botulinum* (botulism and food poisoning). Contamination of foods by resistant spores that survive almost indefinitely in soil, dust, and most other materials is the reason that bottled or canned food must be sterilized in retorts, autoclaves, or pressure cookers for a minimum of fifteen minutes at 121°C (250°F) to prevent spoilage or disease transmission. Figure 15.9 shows an endospore in an unidentified species of *Bacillus*. Parenthetically, because of the relative ease of production, storage and dissemination, *B. anthracis* has recently been of concern as a potential biological weapon.

TAXONOMY AND PHYLOGENETIC RELATIONSHIPS

The need for intelligent communication about the large number of vastly diverse organisms has prompted biologists to develop systems of classification. *Taxonomy* is the classification (or grouping) of organisms according to their natural relationships. Hence, a *taxon* (plural *taxa*) is a category. The study of natural relationships or evolutionary history of organisms is called *phylogeny*; i.e., a taxonomic grouping based on heritable or evolutionary relationships. This system of taxonomy leads to construction of a *phylogenetic tree*, which emphasizes branching away from common ancestors due to heritable differences. It does not usually consider adaptations as differences between descendants of a common ancestor.

The word *systematics* refers to evolutionary classification schemes but often tends to include consideration of any possible relationship and difference among organ-

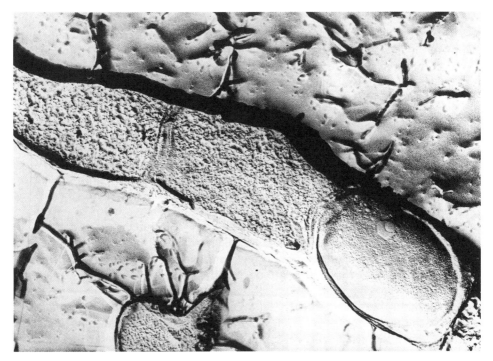

Figure 15.9.   Electron micrograph of a frozen fractured preparation showing an endospore in a *Bacillus* cell; species unidentified.

isms. The term is occasionally used synonymously with taxonomy. *Nomenclature* is the system of names applied to organisms studied in a field of knowledge and the *binomial nomenclature* originally developed by Carolus Linnaeus is used to name all free-living organisms, i.e., all organisms have two names; a capitalized genus name and a lowercase specific epithet which is frequently an adjective.

The relatively recent development of techniques to chemically sequence proteins and nucleic acids has provided the tools necessary to construct phylogenetic and evolutionary relationships among the prokaryotes. Much current taxonomy is based upon similarities and differences of ribosomal ribonucleic acids (rRNA).

To grasp how RNA may be used in taxonomy one must understand the forms in which RNA exists in cells. RNA is found in several configurations and molecular sizes that carry out various functions within cells. Template RNA (tRNA) is an informational molecule, messenger RNA (mRNA) carries information between DNA; the cells' information storage molecule, and ribsomes, replication molecules that are the site of protein synthesis. rRNA is found in particles of ribonucleoprotein, which may exist free in bacterial cytoplasm. rRNA accounts for about fifty percent to eighty percent of the cells' total RNA. Ribosomal RNA consists of polymeric subunits that are described on the basis of separation by sedimentation in a solvent (usually water that contains cesium chloride and other salts) in a gravitational field under highly standardized and controlled conditions in an ultracentrifuge; and expressed as Svedberg (S) units. Actually, a time-saving technique that produces cDNA directly from rRNA in the presence of the enzyme reverse transcriptase, followed by analysis of the cDNA is often used in studies of rRNA.

In bacteria the rRNA is 70S and is made up of submits that include 5S, 16S, and 23S RNA. Those units are completely conserved during cell growth; thus, providing the basis for phylogenetic comparison among the various species, strains, and varieties of bacteria. Eucaryotes contain larger rRNA (80S) than is found in prokaryotes. Eucaryotes also contain subunits of different size, density and shape than bacteria, i.e., with different S values under the same standardized conditions of centrifugation.

There are presently considered to be two distinct *Prokaryotic Kingdoms*: (1) *True Bacteria (Eubacteria)* and (2) *Archaebacteria*; both of which are distinct from a third Kingdom: *Eucarya* (i.e., the eucaryotes), that includes all plants, animals, fungi, ciliates, cellular slime molds, flagellates, and microsporidia. However, some disagreement exists about the taxonomy and spelling as some authors divide the *Eucarya* into four separate kingdoms: (3) *Protista*, which includes water molds, slime molds, protozoa, and primitive eukaryotic algae; (4) *Fungi*, which includes yeast, multicellular molds including some with macroscopic forms; (5) *Plants*, and (6) *Animals*. If the three kingdom taxonomy is adhered to, then the four eukaryote kingdoms would be *Phyla* or *Divisions* within *Eucarya*. Note that the *Protista* and *Fungi* are comprised primarily of microorganisms.

Taxons within the Bacteria include: green bacteria, flavobacteria, spirochetes, purple bacteria, Gram-positive bacteria, cyanobacteria, deinococci, and thermotagales. Archaea taxons include: extreme halophiles, methanogens, and extreme thermophiles.

Although traits such as size, morphology, cellular structure and composition, and similarity of metabolic capabilities no longer are considered to have validity as phylogenetic determinants, they nevertheless continue to have utility as determinants in the identification of causative organisms in clinically important diseases.

SOME MEDICALLY IMPORTANT BACTERIA AND THE DISEASES THEY CAUSE

Many pathogenic bacteria initiate infection by entering the host through the mucous membranes of the oral, respiratory, ocular, gastrointestinal, or genitourinary tract. The other common route of infection is through breaks in the skin. Infection by some bacteria is restricted to the site of entry, while others may disseminate to other sites. In some cases the clinical signs of infection may be widely removed from the original site of initiation of the infection.

The skin is generally an effective barrier against bacterial invasion. A few bacteria, however, can cause infections of the superficial layers of intact skin or even invade lower tissues through the hair follicles in the absence of overt injury. In this case contact with the bacteria is all that is required. However, even with infections caused by these bacteria, a minor break in the skin will greatly increase the chances for the pathogens to pass the barrier.

If the integrity of the skin is broken by wounds, burns, surgery, or animal or insect bites, then a variety of bacterial pathogens, which would not otherwise be able to enter the body, can establish an infection. Wound infections are most often caused by *Staphylococcus aureus* and *Streptococcus pyogenes*, organisms usually living on the skin.

Gas gangrene is an infection caused by the growth of *Clostridium perfringens* or closely related *Clostridium* species. For clostridial infections to develop, wound contamination with endospores and anaerobic conditions for germination and growth are required. The toxins produced by the *Clostridia* are a group of exotoxins and enzymes with a proteolytic activity that literally digest the tissue. If damaged tissue in a wound is removed, anaerobic conditions are unlikely to occur. The predominant gases produced in gas gangrene are due to carbohydrate fermentation and are carbon dioxide and hydrogen.

The term *zoonosis* refers to an infectious disease of humans that was transmitted from diseased or carrier lower animals. Arthropods are the most common vectors for transmitting such microbial diseases. Many zoonotic diseases are acquired through the skin, the arthropod providing passage through the skin while feeding.

Many diseases of the oral cavity are caused by bacteria, especially bacteria that are indigenous to the mouth. These infections are among the most common bacterial infections of man. As the organisms causing them are not highly pathogenic, host factors play a role in whether disease develops following infection.

The respiratory tract also provides a convenient portal of entry for many pathogens. The opportunity for infection is great, as 10,000 liters of air are inhaled by a human each day. Some of the infections remain localized within the respiratory tract, while others may disseminate to adjoining tissues or even disseminate throughout the body becoming systemic infections. Airborne transmission of bacterial pathogens occurs when microscopic droplets containing bacteria are transferred between individuals. A few airborne infections such as Legionnaires' disease are a result of infection with bacteria from the environment; more commonly the organisms are derived from exhalations by infected individuals.

The gastrointestinal (GI) tract is exposed to large numbers of bacteria ingested with food and water and also contains a large indigenous population. Two general types of disease of the tract occur. The first is termed food poisoning and is the result of absorbing toxin produced by the bacteria growing in food. In this type of disease infection or invasion may not occur. The second type of disease is caused by actual invasion of the tissue. It is therefore a true infection. Food poisoning caused by the ingestion of preformed toxins is commonly caused by *S. aureus* or *C. botulinum*, both of which grow in food.

Infections associated with diarrhea are commonly caused by *Salmonella* sp., *E. coli*, *Shigella* sp., or *Vibrio cholera*. *Salmonella enteritis* causes a gastroenteritis that is quite severe and relatively common. *Escherichia coli* is responsible for a *Shigella*-like dysentery, as well as an enteritis similar to that caused by cholera and salmonella bacilli. Pathogenic *E. coli* produce a labile toxin similar in action to that produced by the other Gram-negative rods. *Salmonella typhi* is an example of an invasive bacterium associated with a severe enteric fever.

Infections of the urinary tract often occur with opportunistic pathogens that enter the bladder and kidney. These organisms are most often bacteria of the normal flora of the intestinal tract. Sexually transmitted or venereal diseases are infections with bacterial pathogens that have acquired the ability to be transmitted during sexual acts.

In the following sections of this chapter, we will describe several bacterial diseases grouped according to the organ systems in which they initiate their infections and produce their primary lesions. This is a system of grouping widely used by members of the medical profession as it aids clinical diagnosis. It is a system however which may group together diseases caused by unrelated bacteria. Some diseases moreover affect the entire body, their effect not being limited to a single organ system. These diseases can only be considered to be generalized infections. A compilation of some important pathogenic bacteria is presented at the end of this chapter (Table 15.4).

Infections of the Skin
Acne
Propionibacterium acnes and *Staphylococcus epidermidis* are two of the bacteria that invade the hair follicles in the epidermal layers of the skin. They may not require overt injury to initiate infection. Infection causes excessive secretion by the sebaceous glands at the base of the hair follicles. A pus-filled pimple results. There is some evidence of a cell-mediated immune response. It does not appear to aid recovery. Hormonal disorders associated with puberty appear to be a factor in acne possibly by affecting the skin secretions in such a way as to facilitate microbial survival.

Impetigo
Impetigo is a type of pyoderma caused by infection of the skin with *Streptococcus pyogenes* and then superinfection with *Staphylococcus aureus*. The infection is probably initiated at sites of injury although they may be microscopic. In impetigo, hyaluronidase produced by *S. pyogenes* facilitates microbial spread in the connective tissue underlying the skin. Once infection is started, an humoral immune response occurs. This response does not appear to significantly aid clearance of the infection. The delayed type hypersensitivity response to the bacterial antigens causes itching of the skin which causes scratching which in turn spreads the infection.

Pseudomonas Infections
Extensive burn damage to the skin often permits opportunistic pathogens to infect underlying tissues. *Pseudomonas aeruginosa* is the cause of the most common fatal infection of burn patients. Many *P. aeruginosa* strains are resistant to antibiotics and therefore are a serious threat to the burned patient. Burning may not only damage the integrity of the physical barrier provided by the skin, it also seems to decrease the burned patient's immune response. Healthy humans are rarely infected with *Pseudomonas* species. *Pseudomonas* species are ubiquitous, growing readily as saprophytes in soil and water and become opportunistic pathogens on morbid tissue. (Also see Cystic Fibrosis.)

Infections of the Eye
Conjunctivitis
This is a bacterial infection of the mucous membrane lining the eye socket. Bacterial conjunctivitis is caused by a variety of bacteria: *Hemophilus, Staphylococcus aureus, Streptococcus pneumoniae, Pseudomonas aeruginosa*, and *Chlamydia* sp. are probably the most common. "Pink eye" outbreaks among children are caused by *Hemophilus aegypticus*. The more serious disease, inclusion conjunctivitis, is caused by *Chlamydia trachomatis*. This last organism causes trachoma in which there is an invasion of the cornea itself. Trachoma can cause blindness.

Infections of the Mouth
Dental Caries
The growth of several species of *Streptococcus* on the tooth surface results in lactic acid production. The acid is highly concentrated on the enamel surface because it is released in the glycan polymer produced by the bacteria on the tooth surface. The bacteria implicated are *S. mutans, S. sanguis*, and *S. silivarius*. Diet and dental hygiene are factors along with the bacteria in production of tooth decay. In recent years the incidence of tooth decay in people in the United States has decreased

greatly. The reasons suggested for this include widespread fluoridation of water and widespread use of antibiotics; the causes of the decrease in tooth decay are a matter of active research.

Periodontal Infections
Diseases of varying severity are caused by a variety of bacteria that invade the tissues and the bone supporting the teeth. Gingivitis is caused by species of *Actinomyces*, whereas ulcerative gingivitis or trench mouth is caused by various species of *Veillonella, Fusobacterium,* and *Campylobacterium.* Trench mouth is a disease caused by bacterial synergy since no single species of bacteria alone is able to cause it.

In periodontitis or pyorrhea, there is invasion and destruction of gingival tissue by a mixture of bacteria that includes spirochetes, *Bacteroides* and the bacteria listed above that cause the milder form of gingivitis. The most common causative agents appear to be *Treponema vincentii* and *Bacteroides melaninogenicoccus.* Eventually the growth of the bacteria can erode the bone holding the teeth, resulting in their loss.

General health is a factor in infections of the gums. People who are fatigued or malnourished are much more likely to develop ulcers in their mouths than others. Trench mouth, for example, was first described in soldiers who were fatigued by prolonged service in trenches in the First World War.

Endocarditis
Infections initiated in the mouth and around the teeth may have consequences widely removed from the initial site of infection. One of the most serious is endocarditis. The inflammation of the membrane that lines the chambers and valves of the heart, called the endocardium, is caused by an infection with *Streptococcus viridans. Streptococcus viridans* is part of the normal flora of the mouth which may enter the blood stream as a result of local infection, accidental tissue injury or injury resulting from dental procedures. If the bacteria lodge in the heart, they may produce endocarditis. If the infection spreads to the myocardium or muscle of the heart or seriously damages the heart valves, it may be fatal. Therefore, it is recommended that prophylactic use of an antibiotic effective against Gram-positive bacteria be initiated prior to dental procedures on patients with a history of any heart problem.

Infections of the Respiratory Tract
Whooping Cough (Pertussis)
Pertussis is the formal name of the disease most often designated by the characteristic cough accompanying the disease. It is caused by *Bordetella pertussis* which is a Gram-negative coccobacillus. The virulence factors of *B. pertussis* are the several pertussis toxins, as well as the pili and capsule. Immunization with killed *B. pertussis* bacteria, in a triple vaccine that also contains diphtheria and tetanus toxoids (DPT vaccine), has reduced the incidence of this disease in infants and young children. A factor in pertussis vaccines, however, causes neurologic disorders in a small proportion of children who have received it. This has caused a decrease in use of the vaccine and an upsurge in whooping cough. Attempts are underway to produce a pertussis vaccine free of this undesirable effect.

Diphtheria
The clinical signs of diphtheria are a result of toxin production by lysogenic strains of *Cornyebacterium diphtheriae.* A lysogenic strain is one which has been infected

with a temperate bacteriophage mu, that carries the genetic code for production of diphtheria toxin. Mu integrates with the host bacterium DNA. Only phage-infected lysogenic strains of the bacterium produce toxin and cause diphtheria. The organism is not very invasive and usually only causes a localized infection of the mucosal membranes of the upper respiratory tract; it is from this site that the toxin diffuses and causes damage. The toxin produced is capable of killing most eukaryotic cells. Antibodies to the toxin neutralize it and prevent the disease even though infection may be present and the host becomes a carrier of the organisms. Immunization with inactivated diphtheria toxin effectively prevents the disease.

Scarlet Fever, Streptococcal Sore Throat, and Rheumatic Fever
Scarlet fever is a result of a localized infection of the throat with *Streptococcus pyogenes*. The scarlet rash is caused by an exotoxin secreted by the streptococci which diffuses into the body. An antibody-mediated immunity is developed to the effects of the toxin so that once immunized either from an infection or from immunization with toxoid, the individual does not get scarlet fever again. Unfortunately immunity to the local infection of the throat is not easy to develop, and many people suffer from repeated bouts of streptococcal sore throat. Children who have such repeated streptococcal sore throats often develop rheumatic fever; a serious outcome of such infections. Rheumatic fever is characterized by a complex group of symptoms that include joint pain, fever, and cardiac muscle destruction resulting in a weakened heart. The other major complication of repeated infections with streptococci is poststreptococcal glomerulonephritis that is responsible for a form of renal failure. These serious complications are only caused by hemolytic *S. pyogenes* that belong to the serogroup A. The disease is at least in part autoimmune in nature; the antibodies elicited by the bacteria cross-react with the sarcolemma antigens of the heart muscle resulting in damage.

Pneumonia
Bacterial pneumonia, an infection of the alveoli of the lungs, most often occurs in patients who have an impaired immune system, including the young and the aged. The most frequent causative agent of acute pneumonia is *Streptococcus pneumoniae* which is frequently referred to as the "pneumococcus." It is an encapsulated organism; the capsule of which confers upon it the ability to resist phagocytosis. Pneumococci are often part of the normal flora of the throat and while the host is young or vigorous cause no trouble. Immune serum specific for the capsule permits phagocytosis of the microbe and, when it was introduced in the 1930s as a therapeutic agent, had a dramatic effect upon the fatality rate resulting from pneumococcal pneumonia. Other bacteria that can cause pneumonia are *Haemophilus influenzae*, *Klebsiella pneumoniae*, and *Staphylococcus aureus*. Bacterial pneumonia is today successfully treated with antibiotics, e.g., penicillin for the pneumococcus. Pneumococcal pneumonia is an excellent example of an acute bacterial infection. The elderly as noted above are particularly at risk from this type of pneumonia and frequently die of their infections. The onset of pneumococcal pneumonia is abrupt. Symptoms include a high fever, chills and chest pain. Fluid coughed up from the lungs may be blood streaked, i.e., have a rusty appearance. In response to the lung infection, fluids collect in the air spaces. These fluids contain red blood cells and leukocytes. An X-ray picture of the lungs of an infected individual characteristically shows a congested area within one lobe of the lung. The infection usually clears rapidly as a result of antibiotic therapy.

Streptococcus pneumoniae is a Gram-positive coccus which is usually seen as pairs of lancet-shaped (somewhat pointed) organisms. Once the disease is established, the microbe may be isolated from blood cultures or sputum produced by coughing. When grown in an agar culture medium containing red blood cells, *S. pneumoniae* produces a hemolysin which partially lyses the red cells and causes a greenish color to develop around the microbial colonies. This is an incomplete or "alpha" hemolysis. Like other streptococci, the pneumococcus produces a variety of proteolytic enzymes. However, it is the polysaccharide capsule that is clearly the major virulence factor since it protects the microbes from phagocytosis. Recovery from the infection depends upon production of opsonic IgG antibody against the specific capsular polysaccharide. Type-specific polysaccharides have been developed as vaccines to immunize people in the high-risk populations. While pneumococci may produce over eighty distinct serotypes of capsular polysaccharides, bacterial pneumonias are usually caused by pneumococci of less than one-fifth of the types that are known, and therefore vaccines are composed of a mixture of the types most commonly causing disease.

Atypical Pneumonia

Atypical pneumonias are caused by several very different bacteria including: *Mycoplasma pneumoniae, Legionella pneumophila* and *Chlamydia psittaci*. Mycoplasma lack a cell wall and are not sensitive to penicillin, but can be treated with other antibiotics.

Legionnaires' Disease

Legionnaires' disease was first described in 1976 and eventually the etiologic agent was identified as *Legionella pneumophila*, an inhabitant of contaminated water that may become airborne in aerosols from cooling towers, air conditioners, and plumbing systems where water has previously been heated followed by a prolonged period of stagnation. Apparently sufficient nutrients accumulate in water lines from valve gaskets, etc. to support growth of the organisms. When contaminated aerosols are inhaled, infection may result. The bacteria are probably not free-living in the water, but infect free-living amoebae and ciliated protozoa; where, if they infect amoebae cysts, can survive environmental extremes such as insufficient chlorination, desiccation, and elevated temperature. A second species, *L. micdadei* is also implicated in the disease in immunocompromised patients. Both species are facultative intracellular pathogens which multiply within mononuclear phagocytes following ingestion or inhalation. They have also been observed to multiply in vacuoles of amoebae. Disease production is related to impairment of host defense mechanisms. A heat stable cytotoxin that blocks the oxidative metabolism of monocytes and neutrophils and production of a phosphatase enzyme that blocks superoxide production by neutrophils are implicated in the pathogenesis of the disease. *Legionella* are quite susceptible to erythromycin.

Cystic fibrosis

Cystic fibrosis (CF) is a condition resulting from a genetic defect that predisposes the individual to a chronic course of infection (ten to twenty years) by any of several different opportunistic pathogens including: *Pseudomonas aeruginosa, Burkholderia cepacia (basonym Pseudomonas cepacia)*, and *Stenotrophomonas maltophilia (basonym Xanthomonas maltophilia)*. *Staphylococcus aureus* and *Haemophilus influenzae* appear to be associated with the disease in the young (up to about five years of age); followed after five years of age by a shift in the microflora of major airways to mucoid strains of *P. aeruginosa* and *B. cepacia*, leading to chronic pulmonary infection. During the course of the infection the bacteria, *P. aeruginosa* and *B. cepacia*, appear to go through genetic transition to strains that overproduce the extracellular polymer, alginate, which is the cause of a mucoid condition that impairs the normal mucociliary clearance of foreign substances from the respiratory system. Mucoid-producing organisms also have greater resistance to antibiotics than their nonmucoid counterparts making the chronic condition difficult to treat. The organism can be transmitted from person to person or acquired from the environment. As the organisms are ubiquitous in nature, infection of CF patients is impossible to prevent.

Psittacosis
Psittacosis is also called parrot fever and is caused by *C. psittaci*, which is transmitted from birds to man.

Bronchitis and pharyngitis
Bronchitis and pharyngitis, infections of the bronchial tree of the lungs and of the throat, respectively, are caused by many of the same bacterial pathogens causing pneumonia.

Tuberculosis and Mycobacteriosis
Of the several diseases caused by infections with *Mycobacterium* species; tuberculosis, caused by *M. tuberculosis*, and leprosy, caused by *M. leprae*, have been considered to be the most significant. Several species of mycobacteria that were heretofore considered to be relatively inconsequential, are now being isolated with increasing frequency from diseased patients, and are becoming recognized as important pathogens. The genus *Mycobacterium* contains at least ten species of strictly human pathogens and nine additional opportunistic human pathogens, some of which include identifiable strains. Mycobacteriosis refers to diseases associated with opportunistic pathogens and is not the same disease as tuberculosis.

The *M. avium* complex (MAC) includes both *M. avium*, a parasite of birds, and *M. intracellulare*. Infections by these organisms are common in, but not limited to, immunosuppressed patients including those with AIDS. These bacteria are not usually susceptible to antituberculosis drugs.

The *M. fortuitum* complex (MFC) includes both *M. fortuitum* and *M. chelonae*. MFC organisms grow rapidly compared to other *Mycobacteria*. They are commonly associated with, but not limited to, cutaneous infections following surgical procedures such as insertion of heart valve prostheses and accidental penetrating wounds. Infections have been traced to nonsterile ice used in an operating room and the use of equipment and utensils that were contaminated with nonsterile water, e.g., kidney dialysis equipment.

It is estimated that about 8 million new cases of tuberculosis with approximately 3 million deaths occur each year worldwide. Most are in underdeveloped countries. The incidence of tuberculosis was decreasing annually from the early 1950s; attributable primarily to the development and use of effective drugs such as isonicotinic acid hydrazide (isoniazid), rifampin, and pyrazinamide. However, beginning in 1985, the number of tuberculosis cases began a rise that is correlated with the immunosuppression associated with human immunodeficiency virus infection (HIV) and to an increase in isoniazid resistant strains of *M. tuberculosis*. In AIDS patients, extrapulmonary mycobacterial disease is common and disseminated disease is frequent.

Tuberculosis is an excellent example of an infectious disease in which the response of the host immune system plays a major role in the disease process. The cell-mediated immune response (see chapters 8 and 9) contributes both to resistance to the organism, *M. tuberculosis*, and to destruction of human tissues in the infected area. The interplay of cell-mediated immune activity with other host resistance factors (e.g., genetic background, age, prior exposure, diet) determines whether or not the infection will lead to overt disease.

The primary infection is spread by person-to-person contact. Droplet nuclei produced by coughing or sneezing containing *M. tuberculosis* are inhaled and reach the alveoli of the lungs. Outbreaks have occurred following ingestion of unpasteurized contaminated milk. Cows infected with the bovine strain of the organism may be the source of such contamination. The microbes are phagocytized then multiply slowly in neutrophils and in alveolar macrophages (see chapter 14 for the mechanism). The bacteria may be disseminated through the lymphatic system to the regional lymph nodes and eventually into the bloodstream and to other organs. The original lung lesions may heal if the infection is controlled, or if infection persists, the delayed hypersensitivity response elicited may result in formation of tubercles.

Hypersensitivity, an indication of exposure or infection, can be detected by the tuberculin skin test. Tubercles in the lung are a manifestation of a bacterial pneumonia caused by *M. tuberculosis*, hence the term tubercle bacillus. Following infection the disease may be resolved or the microbe may be spread to other organs of the body and even cause death.

Mycobaterium tuberculosis and related mycobacteria are rod shaped, aerobic organisms rich in lipids especially a Wax D component. Most likely, the lipids of mycobacteria contribute to its maintenance in the host and to its unique staining properties. The Gram stain is not useful for detection or identification of these bacilli. Instead, an "acid fast" stain is used. In this procedure the waxy component prevents the stained mycobacteria from being decolorized by acid alcohol treatment. The ability to retain the acid fast stain is presumptive evidence that the organisms grown from clinical material or found on smears made of sputum specimens are mycobacteria.

Mycobacteria can remain dormant within the tubercles in the lung for long periods; then can become reactivated as a result of malnutrition, stress, or immunosuppression. Tuberculosis is generally a chronic, progressive infection unless treated with appropriate antibiotics over a prolonged period. For example, a recommended treatment regimen is: two months on isoniazid plus rifampin plus pyrazinamide; followed by four months on isoniazid plus rifampin.

Infections of the Gastrointestinal Tract
Food Poisoning and Water Transmitted Intestinal Disease
Food poisoning is a general term referring to gastrointestinal disease caused by ingestion of contaminated food. A distinction is made between toxins produced and released by bacteria growing in food or water prior to ingestion (e.g., botulism, *Staphylococcus* toxins) and ingestion of pathogenic bacteria that subsequently cause an infection of the intestinal tract (e.g., salmonellosis, shigellosis). In the case of

intoxication, onset of disease symptoms can be very rapid (usually two to four hours), and in the case of infection, symptoms occur after progression of the infection (usually twenty-four to forty-eight hours). However, ingestion of large numbers of cells (e.g., 10^{10}) can result in onset of infectious disease in three to four hours. Most waterborne diseases result from drinking contaminated water or inadvertently swallowing contaminated water while swimming.

Food intoxication is caused by a variety of toxin producing strains of various bacteria. These include *Clostridium botulinum* which causes botulism, *Clostridium perfringens*, which causes an enteritis, and *Staphylococcus aureus* which causes staphylococcal food poisoning. All bacteria responsible for food poisoning produce exotoxins that are termed enterotoxins.

There are six strains of *C. botulinum*, differentiated on the basis of the types of toxin each produces. The toxins, designated A, B, E, and F are associated with human diseases; whereas C and D are associated with fowl and cattle disease, respectively. The toxins are rapidly absorbed from the gut and bind to the synapses of motor neurons. As a result of this binding, cholinergic transmission at all cholinergic synapses in the peripheral nervous system is blocked. Type A and Type B neurotoxins block acetyl choline at myoneural junctions which leads to weakening of skeletal muscle followed by paralysis. Death occurs because of paralysis of the respiratory muscles. Ninety percent of the cases of botulism are caused by ingestion of improperly canned food. The endospores of *C. botulinum* found in the soil tolerate oxygen in the air but will not germinate until placed under anaerobic conditions. The spores survive heating in boiling water and the bacteria grow out at neutral pH, establishing a low Redox potential (Eh) between -200 and -400 millivolts in sealed cans.

Sudden infant death syndrome (SIDS) may be caused by growth of the *C. botulinum* in the nonacid environment of the infant stomach and small intestine. The disease is treated by administration of antibodies to the A, B, and E botulinum toxins. Botulinum toxins are among the most potent toxins known.

Food poisoning of a less severe nature than that produced by *C. botulinum* is caused by a type A exotoxin released into cooked meats by *Clostridium perfringes*. Any of seven different heat-resistant exotoxins released from certain strains of *Staphylococcus aureus* growing in food also cause a form of food poisoning characterized by nausea, emesis, and diarrhea. Toxin production is encoded by chromosomal, plasmid or temperate phage genes. The disease is commonly caused by ingestion of foods that either have been contaminated during preparation in the home then improperly stored (not refrigerated) for later use (e.g., potato or chicken salad), or cooked food that has been partially consumed and later improperly stored for a later meal. In the latter case, reheating will not destroy the heat stable toxin and ingestion can result in relatively rapid onset (usually four to eight hours) of intoxication.

Enterobacterial Diarrhea

The family Enterobacteriaceae contains twenty-nine genera and over 100 species of Gram-negative, facultative anaerobic, oxidase negative, nonspore forming, nonhalophilic, nonacid fast, straight rod shaped bacteria, 0.3 to 1.0 by 1.0 to 6.0 μm in size. If they are motile it is by peritrichous flagella. The family contains many animal and plant pathogens that grow optimally between 22°C and 35°C on peptones, protein, several carbohydrates, and polyhydroxy alcohols. Many of the genera within this family have several species, each of which may have several strains and serotypes that produce one or more endotoxins. These toxins may be either heat stable or heat labile. Pathogenic strains are usually identified by detection of a specific virulence factor or of a serotype associated with a virulence factor. Some of these bacteria invade intestinal epithelial cells and stimulate fluid secretion. Some of the toxins produced may subvert multiple host cell processes to elicit secretion by epithelial cells.

Many of these Gram-negative bacteria normally reside in the intestinal tracts of humans and other warm-blooded animals as well as in reptiles. These diarrheal diseases are often spread by drinking water that has become contaminated by the intestinal discharges of humans or other animals that carry the organisms or by ingesting food that has become contaminated by intestinal discharges.

Members of the family Enterobacteriaceae (e.g., *E. coli*, *Klebsiella*, the *Proteus-Providentia-Morganella* group, *Serratia*, and *Citrobacter*) are responsible for forty to fifty percent of the nosocomial infections in the United States. These are infections acquired while in a hospital. They are common for example in elderly patients and others that are immunosuppressed by treatment for cancer or burns, or who have HIV infection. All such immunosuppressed persons are vulnerable to opportunistic pathogens.

It has been recognized that some rheumatoid diseases may arise secondarily from food- and water-transmitted diarrheal diseases. *Yersinia enterocolitica, Y. pseudotuberculosis, Shigella flexneri, S. dysenteriae, E. coli*, and *Klebsiella pneumoniae* all have been found in association with reactive arthritis, septic and aseptic arthritis, ulcerative colitis, and other diseases.

Escherichia coli and Shigella Diarrhea

Several strains of *E. coli* are important producers of diarrheal disease. *Shigella* species, with the exception of *S. boydii*, are usually grouped with *E. coli* because of the close similarity of the toxins they produce.

Enterotoxigenic *E. coli* (ETEC) strains produce both heat labile (LT) and heat stable (ST) enterotoxins that cause a disease known as "traveler's diarrhea" or Montezuma's revenge," in human adults. The genes for production of LT and cholera toxin (CT, see cholera below) are similar with about eighty percent nucleotide homology. Milder "traveler's diarrhea" is much more prevalent worldwide than cholera.

Enteroaggregative *E. coli* (EAEC) produce persistent diarrhea in young children. These *E. coli* strains produce three different toxins; a heat stable (EAST-1), and two different heat labile enterotoxins.

Enterohemorrhagic *E. coli* (EHEC strain 0157:H7) produce bloody and nonbloody diarrhea, hemorrhagic colitis, and hemolytic uremic syndrome. This organism produces *Shigella*-like toxins (SLT-I and SLT-II) in addition to verocytotoxins (VT-I and VT-II). Both SLT and VT toxins are encoded by bacteriophages. The SLT-1 toxin produced by *E. coli* 0157:H7 is essentially identical to the Shiga toxin produced by *Shigella dysenteriae*, type I, and those produced by *Campylobacter jejuni* are somewhat similar to the cholera toxins LT and CT. The toxins have a two-component (A-B unit) structure with neither unit toxic alone. The A unit is responsible for intracellular changes in cyclic AMP levels and the B unit is a pentamer that binds to gangliosides in host intestinal cell membranes.

Enteroinvasive *E. coli* (EIEC) produce dysenteric watery diarrhea. The EIEC strains of *E. coli* produce a plasmid encoded *Shigella* enterotoxin-2 (ShET-2), a cytolethal distending toxin (CLDT); and a cytotoxic necrotizing toxin which is associated with septicemia, urinary tract infections, and enteritis.

Salmonellosis
Several species of *Salmonella*, especially *S. enteritidus*, cause gastroenterocolitis. These *Salmonella* are surrounded by pili that enable them to attach to gut epithelial cells and reproduce there. The enterotoxins they elaborate cause the disease. *Salmonella paratyphi* and *S. typhimurium*, in particular, can invade tissue and cause a bacteremia in addition to gastroenteritis. An epidemic of Salmonellosis occurred in 1985 throughout Illinois and Wisconsin. It was traced to milk that had been contaminated by *S. typhimurium* at a large dairy in Chicago. An outbreak of disease caused by eggs contaminated with *S. enteritis* occurred in the Northeast U.S. between 1985 and 1987.

Typhoid Fever
Systemic infections caused by *Salmonella typhi* usually occur as a result of transmission from asymptomatic human carriers of *S. typhi*, who contaminate food or water. The classical example of a healthy carrier of *S. typhi* was "Typhoid Mary," a cook who infected members of the families who employed her. *Salmonella typhi* invades the intestinal epithelial cells, passing from these into the lymphatic system and then is disseminated throughout the body by the vascular system. Although *S. typhi* is rapidly ingested by neutrophils and macrophages, the bacteria are not killed but rather multiply in these phagocytic cells. Systemic disease including high fever results from the reaction of the body to the widely disseminated organisms. Infection is established in cells in organs such as the kidney, liver, spleen, gall bladder, and the Peyer's patches or lymph nodules of the intestine. It is these infected cells that harbor the *S. typhi* in carriers and serve as the reservoir for the microorganism between epidemics.

Cholera
Cholera remains a major problem in Third World countries and in any area where water supplies are contaminated with domestic sewage. Incidence of the disease increased about 20-fold between 1938 and 1988. The disease is caused by *Vibrio cholerae*, a curved Gram-negative rod that adheres to the mucosa within four to six hours. The cholera toxin of especially virulent strains (*V. cholerae* 01 or 0139) is an A-B subunit toxin (see *E. coli* toxins, above) that stimulates adenylate cyclase production which increases intracellular levels of cAMP. In turn, cAMP initiates secretion of both water and ions from the gut epithelial cells. It is the loss of water and salt that causes the shock characteristic of the disease. Ten to fifteen percent of those infected may die. Treatment is to restore water and electrolyte balance. The patient is made to consume sufficient balanced salt solution to replace the lost water and salt. Endemic infections occur in areas with poor sewage and water treatment facilities. Transmission occurs by contamination of food and water by the diarrheal feces. Between the epidemics the organisms probably survive as harmless parasites of copepods and other animals living in rivers, ponds and estuaries. It is probable that the organism came originally from rivers in northern India.

Vibrio parahaemolyticus is a salt-requiring species that produces a protein toxin called TDH. The diarrheal disease usually results from ingestion of contaminated seafood.

Some Public Health Considerations
Epidemics caused by the spread of diseases via water contaminated by human excreta (cholera, typhoid, paratyphoid, enteric diarrhea, shigellosis, and some virus and protozoan diseases) were common prior to the use of modern water treat-

ment methods. In addition to the spread of disease as the result of ingestion of contaminated water or foods contaminated by polluted water, some diseases are spread by contact. Contact infections of open wounds of bathers, infections of the upper and lower respiratory tract and conjunctivitis are becoming more common as a result of direct contact with contaminated water. Botulism is increasingly being related to polluted water. A localized increase in the presence of *Clostridium botulinum* has been noted in the bottom sediments of lakes where large amounts of organic wastes have accumulated. This anaerobic bacterium produces highly resistant spores and water taken from these locations can be transferred to foods during processing.

In the United States, the number of water treatment plants increased from eighty-three in 1850 to over 4000 in 1900. The first use of chlorine to disinfect a public water supply in the U.S. was in Jersey City in 1908 and was quickly followed by installations in other cities. Water treatment developed primarily as a means of making water potable. The major techniques used in large-scale water purification continue to be coagulation and sedimentation (usually with lime and soda ash), filtration to remove suspended microparticulates, and chlorination to disinfect the water.

The number of deaths from typhoid fever in the U.S. Army dropped from an average of twenty-three per 1000 recruits in 1901 to an average of 2.8 per 1000 recruits ten years later. The drop resulted from improved sanitation. Over the next five years, vaccination further reduced the number to 0.2 per 1000 recruits. Because it is a very effective and inexpensive antimicrobial agent, chlorine in its various chemical forms, including hypochlorous acid, sodium hypochlorite (supermarket bleach), calcium hypochlorite (swimming pool disinfectant) and the chloramines, continues to be the primary means of preventing the spread of water-transmitted epidemic diseases.

Infections of the Urogenital Tract
Urinary Tract Infections
Infections of the urethra or bladder, termed urethritis and cystitis, respectively, can be caused by any one of the Gram-negative bacteria that occur in the intestines. *Escherichia coli* and *Proteus* sp. are the organisms most commonly isolated from individuals with urogenital infections. When the infection progresses into the kidney from the bladder, it may have serious consequences including renal failure and death.

Listeria monocytogenes, a Gram-positive rod, causes a serious type of infection in the urogenital tract because infection with it may result in damage to the fallopian tubes or in pregnant women to infection of the fetus causing fetal abnormality or death.

Vaginal Infections
Vaginal infections occur very frequently. They are often caused by the protozoan *Trichomonas vaginalis* or by the yeast *Candida albicans*. These organisms cause annoying but not serious diseases and are discussed elsewhere in this volume.

Toxic Shock Syndrome
Toxic shock syndrome is caused by a toxin released by certain strains of *Staphylococcus aureus* that contain a lysogenic phage. Although the syndrome has been associated with use of tampons, it also occurs with infection with *S. aureus* at other sites, especially in surgical wounds. The syndrome is essentially an intoxication as the organism grows in some isolated site and elaborates toxin there. The disease occurs

when the toxin diffuses into the surrounding tissues; the organisms seldom invade the tissue however. The condition assumed prominence with the introduction of a new type of highly absorbent tampons. These tampons were sufficiently absorbent that they did not need changing for many hours. The prolonged retention of the blood and secretion soaked tampon provided opportunity for the organisms to grow and elaborate toxin. Surgical wounds also provide sites for microbial growth, for example, around stitches or in gauze or other types of drains which remain in the wounds for fairly long periods.

Gonorrhea

Gonorrhea is the most prevalent sexually transmitted disease and requires direct sexual contact for transmission. The causative agent is the gonococcus, *Neisseria gonorrheae*, which does not survive long outside of infected tissues. The pili of this Gram-negative diplococcus are necessary for attachment to the mucosal cells. There may be some invasion to the subepithelial layer of connective tissue. The gonococcus in not a very invasive organism. It grows mostly in the mucosa of the organs it infects. The resulting inflammation may be quite painful. The organism may grow on the mucosa of the throat and the rectum as well as in the genital organs. Gonorrhea may be spread by asymptomatic carriers or by people with frank infection. It may be a serious disease particularly if it invades the prostate gland or the fallopian tubes. In the latter case it may cause sterility.

Most strains of the gonococcus prevalent today produce a penicillinase and therefore are resistant to the action of penicillin. Newborns receive eyedrops containing a one percent solution of silver nitrate. This agent kills any gonococci that may have entered the eye during passage through the birth canal. The treatment prevents blindness which may result from gonococcal infection of the eye.

Syphilis

Syphilis is another bacterial disease which may be considered to be a disease of the urogenital tract although the disease is not limited to that organ system. Syphilis is sexually transmitted. It is caused by the spirochete, *Treponema palladum*. Transmission requires direct contact with a syphilitic lesion as the organisms cannot survive long in the environment. *Treponema* penetrate the skin or mucous membranes at the contact site where they produce a local ulcer-like lesion called a chancre. The organisms, however, soon spread throughout the body and may in later stages damage the skin, bones, joints, and nervous system. They can also cross the placenta and infect the fetus.

There are three stages of syphilis. The primary stage is marked by a chancre on the genitals or other site of entry. The secondary stage occurs eight weeks later and involves dissemination to numerous parts of the body. There it produces lesions in the skin and mucous membranes which contain treponemes. The tertiary stage occurs many years later and is characterized by damage to many organs, including the aorta and the brain. Patients in the latent periods, i.e., between stages, have no clinical symptoms, and they are not infectious during these periods. No one spontaneously clears infection. An immunity capable of preventing or curing infection does not develop; however, sufficient immunity does develop to bring about healing of the primary and secondary lesions and to produce prolonged latency. There is considerable interest in the development of a vaccine to prevent syphilis but to date success has been minimal. Treatment with antibiotics is however quite successful.

Generalized Infections

While it is possible to consider many diseases to be diseases of certain organ systems, others produce such widespread effects as to require consideration as generalized infections. Syphilis as just noted could be considered a generalized infection although, as a venereal disease, it is usually grouped with the infections of the urogenital tract. The diseases described in the following parts of this section, while perhaps affecting some organ system more than others, produce sufficiently widespread effects as to warrant their consideration in the category of generalized infections.

Lyme Disease

A disease first diagnosed in Lyme, Connecticut, United States, in 1975 is caused by a microaerophilic spirochete, *Borrelia burgdorferi*. Lyme disease is transmitted by the deer tick and is presently the most common vector-borne infection in the U.S., having been diagnosed in all fifty states. It has been recognized as well in several countries in Europe and Asia. The infection is characterized by a distinctive annular skin rash at the site of the tick's bite accompanied by fever and joint pain although *Borrelia* species do not produce any known toxins. From the site of the tick bite, the infection progresses over weeks to months to the nervous system, heart, and large joints, especially the knee where it produces an arthritic condition. The organism is sensitive to amoxicillin, ceftriaxone, doxycillin, erythromycin, and penicillin but resists metronidazole.

It is interesting to note that there is a correlation between the emergence and increased diagnosis of Lyme disease and increases in the deer population in the U.S. The increased population of deer undoubtedly supports corresponding increases in deer tick populations and correlates with decreased deer hunting in the U.S.

Typhus Fever

Several types of typhus fever exist, all of which are caused by *Rickettsia* species transmitted to man by bites of arthropod vectors. There are three common forms of typhus fever in man; i.e., epidemic typhus caused by *R. prowazeki* transmitted by the body louse; endemic typhus caused by *R. typhi* transmitted by the rat flea; and the scrub typhus caused by *R. tsutsugamushi* transmitted by a mite.

Epidemic typhus transmitted between hosts by the body louse usually occurs in people living in unsanitary, crowded conditions. The disease is common in wartime. Lesions occur in the blood vessels of the heart and kidneys. Half of the patients die if untreated. Murine or endemic typhus is transmitted to humans by rat fleas and the disease is similar in nature, but milder than epidemic typhus. In Japan and Korea, humans may become accidental hosts for scrub typhus which is a congenitally transmitted infection of mice. The host responds to rickettsial pathogens with a cell mediated immune reaction which destroys the infected cells.

Brucellosis

Humans are accidental hosts of several *Brucella* species that normally infect farm animals, particularly goats, cows and pigs. This Gram-negative, nonmotile aerobic rod enters its host by many routes. Infection through minor abrasions in the skin, ingestion of food particularly unpasteurized milk and cheese, and infection through the eye are all common routes of infection. Slaughterhouse workers, farmers, and veterinarians are all commonly at risk of this disease. Veterinarians and farmers are infected when they handle aborted fetuses or treat cattle who have aborted as a result of infection. The fever associated with the infection may rise and fall, therefore the disease is called undulant fever. Unless treated, the infection may persist for years. Vaccines have been developed for cattle, but they are not effective for hogs, and they are not used in humans.

Plague

Although this disease is now rare, in the Middle Ages it was responsible for the death of up to twenty-five percent of the human population of Europe. It is caused by *Yersinia pestis*, a pleomorphic rod that is maintained in wild rodents. Man is infected by the bite of fleas which leave the rodents after they have died of the disease. The bubonic form of plague results when rat fleas inject the agent while feeding. In this form of the disease *Y. pestis* becomes localized in the lymph nodes draining the area of the bite. When the nodes become enlarged, they are called buboes. The infection progresses throughout the body. Sometimes the lungs become infected. When this happens, the disease may be spread by aerosols produced by coughing. This form is called pneumonic plague. The disease is readily treatable with streptomycin but if untreated may be rapidly fatal in a high proportion of cases.

Anthrax

Man is an accidental host for *Bacillus anthracis*. Anthrax occurs most often in sheep and cattle. The infection in man is most commonly a result of contamination of breaks in the skin of humans who handle infected meat but also occurs as a result of inhalation of dust containing spores. This form of anthrax commonly occurs in people sorting infected wool and is called woolsorters' disease. Infection also results from ingestion of spores. This is the route of infection most common in domestic animals. The disease is caused by the toxin released by the microbes as they grow, first at the initial site of infection, and then throughout the body as the organisms spread. It is often fatal. The virulence factors are both a capsule and the toxin. Vaccination of domestic animals has reduced the incidence of the disease in them and as a result in man.

MECHANISMS OF IMMUNITY AND RESISTANCE TO BACTERIAL INFECTION

Infections may be intracellular or extracellular, toxigenic or nontoxigenic, and either local or systemic. Most of the available immunological effector mechanisms are induced to some degree by most infections and can be detected during the course of infection. It is however usually only one or two of the induced mechanisms that is primarily responsible for the immunity which develops. In the last section of this chapter the immunological effector mechanisms controlling the various types of infection will be described. The mechanisms associated with each type of infection are summarized in Table 15.3.

Extracellular Bacterial Infections

Bacteria which grow extracellularly often cause rapidly spreading infections with development of large microbial populations and in some cases toxin production. Some toxigenic bacteria however cause severe disease while only forming limited local infections. Some bacteria causing extracellular infections are encapsulated; some are not.

Nonencapsulated bacteria of types causing extracellular infections are seldom very pathogenic. Infection by such bacteria, when it does occur, often follows an injury which breaches the skin or mucous membrane covering the tissues. The in-

Table 15.3. Host defense mechanisms important in resistance to various types of bacterial infections.

Type of Infection	Mechanism
Localized extracellular:	
on or in tissue	Opsonization, complement activation, phagocytosis
on mucous membranes	Blockage by attachment of IgA
Systemic extracellular:	
nontoxigenic	Opsonization, complement activation, phagocytosis
toxigenic	Antibody mediated neutralization of toxin
Intracellular infection:	
in macrophages	Macrophage activation, granuloma formation, action of lymphokines and monokines
in nonphagocytic cells	Granuloma formation, lysis by cytolytic lymphocytes, antibody dependent cell cytotoxicity, action of lymphokines and monokines

fection may be controlled by constitutive opsonins and phagocytosis. If the infection should progress and exceed the capacity of the nonspecific host defense mechanisms, then hopefully inducible immunity develops. In such cases control of the infection is usually by specific IgG antibody, complement activation, and phagocytosis. The opsonized bacteria are ingested primarily by neutrophils.

Many bacteria which cause extracellular infections are encapsulated. The capsules block complement activation by the alternative pathway and thereby prevent phagocytosis. Antibody produced during the inducible response binds to the capsular material, bringing about complement activation and phagocytosis. Bacteria producing extracellular infections usually lack mechanisms to resist killing once phagocytized. The pneumococci, streptococci, and staphylococci are examples of such bacteria. Toxins, if produced, are neutralized by antibody.

Extracellular infections at mucosal surfaces are often controlled by the actions of secretory IgA. This antibody may prevent attachment to mucosal cells and prevent colonization of the mucosa. Secretory IgA, when complexed with the bacteria, can initiate the complement cascade and lysis may result. If phagocytes are present, possibly in exudate produced as a result of inflammation, phagocytosis may take place. Exudates may bring IgG antibody onto the mucosal surface supplementing the actions of IgA.

Toxigenic Bacterial Infections

Strongly toxigenic bacteria provide the host with special problems. The toxins they secrete must be neutralized before they can do harm. Toxin neutralization is often more vital than elimination of infectious bacteria.

Clostridium tetani produces a local infection at the site of an injury. The disease tetanus is the result of an exotoxin which diffuses from the site. Immunization against tetanus is carried out by injection of toxoid; injection of antitoxin alone will prevent the disease from developing. The infection itself is adequately controlled by antibody produced during the primary immune response if the effects of the toxin are blocked by transferred antibody or by antibody produced in the secondary immune response in individuals immunized with toxoid.

Streptococcus pyogenes and *Cornyebacterium diphtheria* in a manner similar to that of *Clostridium tetani* may also produce disease by the actions of exotoxins diffusing from a local site of infection. The clinical signs of scarlet fever, caused by a local infection with *Streptococcus pyogenes*, usually in the throat, and diphtheria, caused by a local infection with *Corynebacterium diphtheria*, also in the throat, are controlled by elaboration of antitoxins. If the toxins are neutralized by antitoxin promptly, the host can usually control the infection later with the aid of opsonic antibody and phagocytosis. The local infections caused by these bacteria are however more severe than those caused by *C. tetani*. People may develop many *S. pyogenes* infections in the throat but develop scarlet fever only once.

Infection with Gram-negative bacteria may result in endotoxemia. Antibodies to endotoxins will precipitate them *in vitro* but do not neutralize their toxicity. The enzymes released by the complement system following its activation effectively degrade endotoxins.

Intracellular Bacterial Infections

Many bacteria and other parasites which normally grow inside of phagocytes are readily phagocytized but have mechanisms to resist destruction once inside. The *Mycobacteria* causing tuberculosis and leprosy are such intracellular parasites. Opsonic antibody which facilitates phagocytosis is of little use in control of such organisms; rather macrophage activation induced in the course of the development of the inducible immune response is a major factor in their control. The chronic granulomatous reaction which results from the delayed hypersensitivity reaction provides a barrier to the spread of the infection. Various lymphokines such as gamma interferon and cachexin (tumor necrosis factor) and the reactive oxygen intermediates and enzymes released by cells activated during the inflammatory process also contribute to control of microbes growing inside phagocytes.

Intracellular parasites growing in nonphagocytic cells may also induce granulomatous reaction. Cytotoxic lymphocytes in the granulomas may destroy the host cells and with them, the parasites. For the cytotoxic lymphocyte to be able to determine which cells are infected, the host cell membrane must however contain parasite derived molecules (Table 15.4).

SUMMARY

A review of emerging and reemerging diseases reveals several major factors responsible for their emergence:

1. The increase and spread of multiple drug resistant bacteria as a result of improper drug use and less reliance on sanitation and hygiene.

2. The increase in incidence and spread of virulent encapsulated pathogens, also partially a result of improper drug use and decreased reliance on sanitation, including in hospitals.

3. The increase in incidence and spread of enteric pathogens via contaminated water and food as a result of population increase exceeding infrastructure development.

4. The increasing number of immunosuppressed hosts as a result of medical transplants and HIV infection.

5. The increase in multiple partner sexual contact without use of protection against disease.

6. Failure of modern society to anticipate and control the health consequences of population increase and of choices in life-style, such as promiscuous sexual activ-

ity, rapid and frequent travel, and increased time spent in crowded, poorly ventilated environments.

The above factors need not be mutually exclusive. All may be exacerbated by the effect of antibiotic use or misuse on the natural selection of multiple drug resistant bacteria and by population growth and density increase accompanied by lapses in the use of known public health measures; particularly sanitation and hygiene practices.

Many diseases are preventable; especially nosocomial infections and those transmitted by contaminated water and food. The frequency of nosocomial cases in particular is reducible through improvements in disinfection, sterilization, cleaning practices, and the use of aseptic technique. In hospitals greater attention should be directed to elimination of locations, objects and materials (fomites) where microbes may grow.

Success in the modern world with its associated life-style of travel and leisure time spent in crowded, poorly ventilated environments such as university classrooms, theaters, and airplanes, has increased exposure to pathogenic microbes. An understanding of the fundamentals of how microbes live, grow, and produce disease can, in many instances, assist in bringing about a decrease in the number of individuals contracting diseases if people use the knowledge to modify their behavior appropriately.

Table 15.4. Characteristics of some important bacteria that cause common diseases.

Organism	Disease	Characteristics
Actinomyces	gingivitis	long slender Gram(+) filaments
Bacillus anthracis	anthrax	Gram(+) aerobic spore forming rod
Bacteroides	trench mouth, gingivitis	Gram(–) pleomorphic anaerobe
Bordetella pertussis	whooping cough	Gram(–) aerobic rod
Borrelia, at least 15 species	relapsing fever	long slender spirochete, tick & body louse transmitted
B. burgdorferi	Lyme disease (borelliosis)	ibid.
Brucella	undulant fever	Gram(–) aerobic rod
Burkholderia cepacia	associated with cystic fibrosis	Gram(–) rod, basonym Pseudomonas
Campylobacter jejuni	gastrointestinal disease	Gram(-) curved rod, microaerophilic
Chlamydia trachomatis	trachoma, lymphogranuloma venerium	Gram(-) coccus
C. psittaci	psittacosis (parrot fever)	ibid.
Clostridium botulinum	botulism, food poisoning	Gram(+) spore forming anaerobe, potent exotoxin
C. tetani	tetanus (lockjaw)	ibid.
C. perfringens	gas gangrene	ibid.
Corynebacterium diphtheriae	diphtheria	Gram(+) rod, requires lysogenic phage
Enterobacteriaceae family	see individual organisms below	All Gram(-) facultative anaerobic, nonspore forming rods, bacteria common in human and animal intestinal tracts
Citrobacter species	upper gastrointestinal infections; nosocomial infections	ibid.

316 • P.R. Dugan

Table 15.4. (continued).

Organism	Disease	Characteristics
Enterobacter cloacae	nosocomial infections	ibid.
E. aerogenes	nosocomial infections	ibid.
Erwinia herbicola	bacteremia, soft tissue infection, implicated in bronchial asthma	ibid., most other species are plant pathogens
Escherichia coli, toxigenic strains	various types of diarrhea, urinary tract, nosocomial infections	ibid.
Hafnia species	intestinal disorders	ibid.
Klebsiella pneumoniae	bacterial pneumonia, septicemia	ibid.
Proteus-Providentia-Morganella group	nosocomial infections	ibid.
Salmonella enteritidis	gastroenterocolitis, salmonellosis	ibid.
S. paratyphi	paratyphoid fever	ibid.
S. typhimurium	paratyphoid fever	ibid.
S. typhi	typhoid fever	ibid.
Serratia marcescens	nosocomial infections	ibid., red pigment (prodigiosin)
Shigella dysenteriae	shigellosis, usually grouped with toxigenic E. coli, similar toxins	ibid.
Yersinia pestis	bubonic and pneumonic plague	ibid., rodent to flea to human transmission
Y. enterocolitica	enterocolitis, ileitis, enlarged lymph nodes	
Fusobacterium species	abscesses of the mouth, upper respiratory, gastrointestinal, gynecological tracts; liver, brain	Gram(–) anaerobic rods frequently with tapered ends. Susceptible to Kanamycin
Haemophilus influenzae	infections of upper respiratory tract, ear; meningitis	Gram(–) small rod
Helicobacter pylori	gastritis	Gram(–) curved microaerophilic rod
Legionella pneumophila	Legionnaires' pneumonia	Gram(–) rods, grow in protozoa and in phagocytes
L. micdadei	Legionnaires' in immunocompromised patients	ibid.
Leptospira interrogans	leptospirosis	a thin spirochete transferred from infected livestock and wildlife to humans
Listeria species	meningitis, fetal infections	Gram(+) nonspore forming rod
Mycobacterium tuberculosis	tuberculosis of lungs and other tissue	Acid fast slowing growing slender irregular aerobic rod
M. leprae	leprosy	ibid.
Mycoplasma	atypical pneumonia	no cell wall
Neisseria gonorrheae	gonorrhea, meningitis	Gram(–) cocci
M. meningitidis	meningitis, bacteremia	ibid.
Propionibacterium acnes	acne	Gram(+) rod
Pseudomonas aeruginosa	opportunistic infections of burns, lungs (CF), skin	Gram(-) aerobic rods

Table 15.4. (concluded)

Organism	Disease	Characteristics
Rickettsia prowazeki	epidemic typhus	very small Gram(-) intracellular rods; transmitted by louse vector
R. typhi	endemic typhus	ibid., transmitted by rat flea
R. tsutsugamushi	scrub typhus	ibid., transmitted by mite vector
Staphylococcus aureus	toxic shock syndrome; boils; toxin is major cause of food poisoning	Gram(+) cocci, opportunistic pathogen
Streptococcus pneumoniae	bacterial pneumonia; meningitis	Gram(+) streptococcus
S. pyogenes	strep throat, scarlet fever; induces rheumatic fever	ibid.
S. mutans, S. sanguis, S. silivarius	dental caries	ibid.
Treponema pallidum	syphilis	very slender tightly coiled spirals
Vibrio cholerae	cholera	Gram(–) curved rod, toxins similar to toxigenic E. coli

SUGGESTIONS FOR FURTHER READING

1. Berkow R., M.H. Beers, and A.J. Fletcher, eds. *Merck Manual of Medical Information*, 1509. Whitehouse Station, NJ: Merck and Co., Inc., 1997.
2. Lewis, K., D.C. Hooper, and M. Ouellette. "Multidrug Resistance: Pumps Provide Broad Defense." *ASM News* 62 (1997):605–610.
3. Sears, C., and J.B. Kaper. "Enteric Bacterial Toxins: Mechanism of Action and Linkage to Intestinal Secretion." *Microbiological Reviews* 60 (1996):167–215.
4. Spangler, J. "Structure and Function of Cholera Toxin and the Related Heat-Labile Enterotoxin." *Microbiological Reviews* 56 (1992):622–647.
5. Stinson, S. "Drug Firms Restock Antibacterial Arsenal." *Chemical and Engineering News* 74 (1996):75, 1996. Available at **http://pubs.acs.org**
6. Verhuel, A.F.M., H. Snippe, and J.T. Poolman. "Meningococcal Lipopolysaccharides: Virulence Factor and Potential Vaccine Component." *Microbiological Reviews* 57 (1992):34–49.

QUESTIONS

1. What is the significance of bacterial endospores to the incidence and transmission of some diseases?
2. What kinds of diseases are likely to be transmitted by contaminated water? Describe the symptoms of those diseases.
3. Why are some emerging diseases so difficult to control?
4. What types of bacteria are major causes of nosocomial infections? How would you reduce the incidence of these diseases?
5. Can you differentiate between bacterial intoxication and infection that is transmitted by contaminated food? Explain.

ANSWERS

1. Pathogens in the genera *Bacillus* and *Clostridium* produce endospores that remain viable for a very long period of time under adverse environmental conditions. Spores of some of the pathogens are able to germinate and grow in certain foods during processing thereby releasing toxins into the food. Subsequent ingestion of the contaminated food can result in serious food poisoning. An example is botulism. Spores of other bacteria can contaminate open wounds resulting in infection and diseases such as gangrene, tetanus or anthrax. (*Any correct example will suffice.*)

2. Diseases of the gastrointestinal tract are likely to be transmitted by contaminated water. Most include severe cramps, diarrhea, and vomiting as symptoms.

3. Many of the emerging and reemerging diseases are increasing in frequency resulting from factors such as: bacterial acquisition of genetic factors that confer resistance to treatment by antibiotics, increased ingestion of water that has been contaminated with pathogens, the spread of encapsulated pathogens causing respiratory infections in immunosuppressed humans, and the spread of venereal diseases via multiple partner sexual contact.

4. Nosocomial diseases are those acquired in a hospital or clinic and include diseases caused by any of the disease causing organisms commonly encountered in those facilities. Diseases commonly encountered in hospitals include bacterial pneumonia and other diseases caused by *Streptococcus* species as well as diseases caused by *Staphylococcus* species. The incidence of nosocomial diseases can be reduced by greater attention to disinfection, sterilization, sanitation, and the use of aseptic techniques.

5. Bacterial intoxication results from toxins produced by some bacteria in contaminated food or water during improper storage. Subsequent ingestion of the food or water containing toxins produces a rapid onset of poisoning without the necessity for establishing an infection. Examples include the intoxications produced by *Staphylococcus aureus* and *Clostridium enteritis*. Enteric diseases caused by some bacteria require ingestion of the pathogen and growth of the organism in the intestinal tract. This process usually requires a longer time span prior to onset of symptoms than does intoxication. Examples include: typhoid fever, salmonellosis, shigellosis, and several other diarrheal diseases.

INTRODUCTION
MORPHOLOGY AND
   STRUCTURE OF VIRUSES
CLASSIFICATION AND
   REPLICATION STRATEGIES
   OF VIRUSES
VIRAL PATHOGENESIS
ANTI-VIRAL STRATEGIES OF
   THE HOST CELL AND
   IMMUNE SYSTEM
ANTI-VIRAL DRUGS
DIAGNOSIS OF VIRAL
   INFECTIONS
IMMUNIZATION AGAINST
   VIRAL INFECTIONS
SELECTED DISEASES
   RESULTING FROM ACUTE
   VIRAL INFECTIONS
Smallpox
Rabies
Polio
Influenza A
SELECTED DISEASES
   RESULTING FROM VIRAL
   INFECTIONS THAT
   RESOLVE OR PERSIST
Measles and Subacute
   Sclerosing Panencephalitis
Warts and Papillomatous
   Tumors
Acute and Chronic Type B
   Hepatitis and
   Hepatocellular Carcinoma
SELECTED DISEASES
   ASSOCIATED WITH
   PERSISTENT VIRAL
   INFECTIONS
Recurrent Herpes and
   Epithelial Cell Carcinomas
Infectious Mononucleosis
   and Malignant
   Lymphomas
Adult T Cell Leukemia/
   Lymphoma and HTLV-1-
   Associated Myelopathy
Acquired Immunodeficiency
   Syndrome
SUMMARY
SUGGESTIONS FOR
   FURTHER READING
QUESTIONS
ANSWERS

CHAPTER 16

The Viruses

Michael D. Lairmore

INTRODUCTION

Viruses infect and cause disease in both plants and animals. They were initially identified as "filterable agents." This terminology developed because viral infections could be produced with fluids which were filtered to eliminate bacteria. This separation is possible because viruses are much smaller than bacteria. Viruses are in fact small packets of protein and nucleic acid that only reproduce inside a susceptible host cell. The proteins of viruses have structural, enzymatic, or regulatory properties. The function of the virion or virus particle is to initiate an infection and promote the replication of more virions by exploiting the environment and enzymes of the host cell.

Viruses have no intrinsic means to generate energy so they must rely totally on the metabolic machinery of host cells to synthesize new viral components. During viral replication, the nucleic acid of the virus which composes its genome becomes active within the infected cell and serves as a template to make copies of itself and to produce new viral proteins. These newly synthesized proteins and genomic elements assemble into new infectious virions that are released by cell lysis or by budding from the host cell. In some cases the viral genome may incorporate into the host cell DNA leading to persistent infections that may lead to many changes in the host cell including cancer. The genetic information in the virus genome and in the host cell determines the outcome of the virus-cell interaction.

MORPHOLOGY AND STRUCTURE OF VIRUSES

The structural proteins surrounding viral genomes are arranged into one of two symmetrical forms called capsids that are either helical or icosahedral in shape. The simplest viruses consist of a rodlike helix or coil of RNA closely associated with structural proteins. There are no known

319

animal viruses lacking an outer envelope and thus naked helical morphology; however, an example of one found in plants is the tobacco mosaic virus. The simplest animal viruses are naked icosahedral viruses such as the parvoviruses. They consist of a DNA or RNA strand within a protein shell called a capsid (Figure 16.1A). The capsid consists of a structure created by the regular arrangement of structural subunits called "capsomeres." Each capsomer is composed of a set of viral structural proteins. The other major forms of viruses are the enveloped icosahedral viruses such as the herpesviruses or the enveloped helical viruses such as the rhabdoviruses (Figure 16.1B and 16.1C). Viral nucleic acid strands with bound proteins generally have helical morphology while viral genomes within a capsid structure also referred to as a nucleocapsid are characteristically icosahedral in morphology.

Nucleic acid genomes of viruses can be either RNA or DNA and be composed of single (ss) or double (ds) stranded units. Single stranded genomes may exist in the plus (+) sense, in which the sequence is identical to that of messenger RNA (mRNA), which can be directly translated into proteins or in the minus (–) sense, in which the sequence is complementary to messenger RNA. In general viruses are very efficient and accomplish replication with relatively fewer proteins then are required by cellular genomes. For example, most RNA viruses encode for less than one dozen proteins. However, the more complex viruses such as the poxviruses may encode around 100 different proteins. The type of nucleic acid and replication strategy of a virus group shapes the methods which must be used to diagnosis the infection and the susceptibility of the virus to specific antiviral agents.

An outer envelope protects many types of viruses. The viral envelope is essentially a membrane derived from the host cell which consists of a lipid bilayer with inserted virus encoded proteins. Such proteins are usually glycosylated by host cell enzymes and appear as "spikes" on the viral surface when viewed by electron microscopy (e.g., Figures 16.1B and 16.1C). Except for some members of the poxvirus family, all enveloped viruses lose their infectivity following extraction of their lipid with ethyl ether. Naked, nonenveloped viruses are unaffected by treatment with ether. Thus, enveloped virus particles are often labile and lose infectivity unless conditions are present to preserve the integrity of the viral envelope. In addition, enveloped viruses are usually more susceptible to detergents that disrupt the lipid envelope.

Viruses may produce "nonstructural" proteins in addition to structural ones. These are usually enzymes involved in the replication of the virus particle. These proteins may include *transcriptases* or enzymes that recognize templates normally utilized by the cell such as RNA-dependent RNA polymerases and "reverse transcriptase" which is used by retroviruses to produce a DNA intermediate from an RNA template. The demonstration of virus-associated enzymatic activity is a method for detection of the presence of viruses in cells.

CLASSIFICATION AND REPLICATION STATEGIES OF VIRUSES

Viruses are classified into a variety of families based on morphologic, structural, and genetic characteristics, including the size, structure, and type of their nucleic acid (Table 16.1). The names of virus families end in the suffix *viridae*, for example paramyxoviridae. Viruses are classified further by the organization and function of their genetic coding and regulatory sequences, and also by the functions of specifically encoded enzymes and protein antigens. These subdivisions are called genera

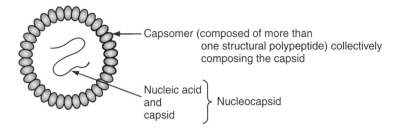

(A) Naked icosahedral
   (e.g., parvovirus, papilloma virus, adenovirus, picornavirus)

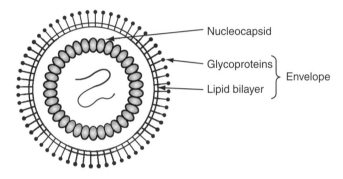

(B) Enveloped icosahedral
   (e.g., herpesvirus, togavirus)

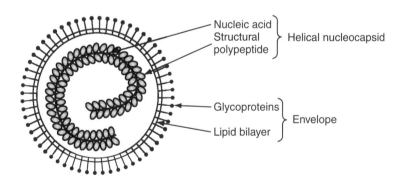

(C) Enveloped helical
   (e.g., paramyxoviruses, orthomyxoviruses (segment), rhabdoviruses)
        (pleomorphic)   (pleomorphic)   (bullet-shaped)

Figure 16.1. Morphology of viruses. Viruses all consist of either a nucleic acid core and a protective coating of protein or in some cases proteins and lipids. Animal viruses may exist in (A) naked icosahedral, (B) enveloped icosahedral, or (C) enveloped helical forms.

Table 16.1. Classification and properties of animal viruses.

Family	Diameter (nm)	CAP	ENV	NA (Size kb)	Examples
DNA viruses					
Parvoviridae	18–25	ICH	N	ssDNA (1.7)[a] linear (+ or –)	Human gastroenteritis viruses, canine parvovirus erythema infectiosum (fifthdisease)
Hepadnaviridae	42–45	ICH	E	dsDNA (3.2)[b] circular (relaxed w/partially SS Region)	Hepatitis B virus, Woodchuck hepatitis virus, Duck hepatitis B virus, Ground squirrel hepatitis virus
Papovaviridae	45–55	ICH	N	dsDNA (5,8)[a] circular (supercoil)	Human, bovine, and rabbit papilloma viruses JC virus (polyomavirus)
Adenoviridae	70–90	ICH	N	dsDNA (30–37)[a] linear	Human adenoviruses
Herpesviridae	120–150	ICH	E	dsDNA (120–220)[c] linear	Herpes simplex I/II, Cytomegalovirus, Varicella/Zoster, Epstein-Barr virus, Herpes virus 6
Poxviridae	200 × 400	Ovoid	C	dsDNA (130–280)[c,d] linear w/covalently closed ends	Smallpox virus, Vaccinia virus, myxomavirus
RNA viruses					
Picornaviridae	20–30	ICH	N	ssRNA (7.5–8.5)[e] linear (+)	Poliovirus, hepatitis A virus, rhinovirus, bovine foot-and-mouth disease
Togaviridae	40–50	ICH	E	ssRNA (12)[e] linear (+)	Rubella virus, Sindbis virus equine encephalitis
Orthomyxoviridae	80–90 (PLM)	HEL	E	ssRNA (13.6)[f] linear (–), 8 segments	Influenza A virus, swine flu virus, avian flu virus
Paramyxoviridae	80–120	HEL	E	ssRNA (18–20)[f] linear (–)	Measles virus, canine distemper virus, mumps virus, Sendai virus respiratory syncytial virus
Rhabdoviridae	60 × 225	HEL	E	ssRNA (13–16)[f] linear (–)	Rabies virus, vesicular stomatitis virus
Filoviridae	180 × 75	HEL	E	ssRNA(12.7)[f] linear (–)	Ebola, Marburg virus

Table 16.1. (concluded)

Family		CAP	ENV	NA	Examples
Bunyaviridae	90–100	HEL	E	ssRNA (13.5–21)^f linear (–), 3 segments	California encephalitis, LaCrosse virus hantavirus
Arenaviridae	80–300	PLM	E	ssRNA (10–14)^f linear (–), 4 large and 1-3 small segments	Lymphocytic chorio-meningitis virus
Coronaviridae	80–160 PLM	HEL	E	ssRNA (27-33)^e, linear (+)	Human respiratory viruses, mouse hepatitis virus
Retroviridae	65–150 COIL	HEL	E	ssRNA (7-10)^g linear (+), (2 copies per virion)	Human T cell leukemia viruses, human immunodeficiency viruses, mammalian and avian RNA Tumor viruses
Reoviridae	70–75 DBL	ICH	N	dsRNA (18-27)^e (10 to 12 segments)	Human reovirus types I, II, and III
Flaviviridae	40–50	ICH	E	ssRNA (10)^e, Linear(+)	Yellow fever virus, bovine virus diarrhea, hepatitis C virus
Caliciviridae	35–40	ICH	N	ssRNA (8)^e	Hepatitis E virus, Norwalk viruses

CAP = capsid morphology: ICH = icosahedral, HEL = helical, PLM = pleomorphic, COIL = coiled, DBL = double layer of capsid proteins; ENV = presence of envelope: E = classical envelope that is ether sensitive, N = naked capsid/no envelope, C = complex outer shell of surface proteins that can be considered an envelope based on sensitivity of some members of this family to ether extraction; however, the better known poxviruses are resistant to ether (e.g., examples in table); NA = nucleic acid (with representative molecular weight in megadaltons): ss = single stranded, ds = double stranded, plus (+) refers to polarity of NA strand being the same as that for naturally occurring mRNA codons, minus (–) indicates that the NA strand is present in the opposite polarity from mRNA. For the replication strategies in footnotes a through g, DDDP = DNA-dependent DNA polymerase, DDRP = DNA-dependent RNA polymerase, RDRP = RNA-dependent RNA polymerase, RDDP/RT = RNA-dependent DNA polymerase/reverse transcriptase; a = uses cellular DDDP and DDRP, b = has ssRNA intermediate (+) strand transcribed by cellular DDRP; this is made into (–) DNA strand by viral RDDP/RT activity which is then converted to a partially completed dsDNA by endogenous viral DDDP, c = virus carries or codes for its own DDDP, d = virus carries or codes for its own DDRP, e = RDRP is synthesized first directly from (+) genomic strand of viral RNA, f = virus carries and codes for its own RDRP to initiate transcription and replication from (–) genomic strand, g = virus carries and codes for its own RDDP/RT enzyme to initiate proviral synthesis (see text for details).

Table 16.2.   Classification of pathogenic animal and human viruses.

Symptoms/Tissue	Viral Pathogen	Virus Family
Respiratory	Influenza A virus	Orthomyxoviridae (RNA)
	Coronaviruses	Coronaviridae (RNA)
	Rhinoviruses	Picornaviridae (RNA)
	Measles virus	Paramyxoviridae (RNA)
	Adenoviruses	Adenoviridae (DNA)
	Smallpox virus	Poxviridae (DNA)
Neurological	Encephalitis viruses	Bunyaviridae (RNA)
	Encephalitis viruses	Togaviridae (RNA)
	Rabies virus	Rhabdoviridae (RNA)
	Measles virus (SSPE)	Paramyxoviridae (RNA)
	Poliovirus	Picornaviridae (RNA)
	Immunodeficiency virus	Retroviridae (RNA)
	Herpes simplex type I	Herpesviridae (DNA)
Gastrointestinal/	Infant gastroenteritis	Reoviridae (RNA)
Viscera	Hog Cholera virus	Flaviviridae (RNA)
	Gastroenteritis virus	Parvoviridae (DNA)
	Smallpox virus	Poxviridae (DNA)
Hepatitis	Hepatitis A virus	Picornaviridae (RNA)
	Yellow Fever virus	Flaviviridae (RNA)
	Mouse Hepatitis virus	Coronaviridae (RNA)
	Hepatitis B virus	Hepadnaviridae (DNA)
	Epstein-Barr virus	Herpesviridae (DNA)
Skin & Mucosal	Rubella virus	Togaviridae (RNA)
Lesions	Measles virus	Paramyxoviridae (RNA)
	Papilloma viruses	Papovaviridae (DNA)
	Varicella (chicken pox)	Herpesviridae (DNA)
	Herpes simplex 1 & 2	Herpesviridae (DNA)
	Smallpox virus	Poxviridae (DNA)
Lymphoid	Measles virus	Paramyxoviridae (RNA)
	Immunodeficiency virus	Retroviridae (RNA)
	Epstein-Barr virus	Herpesviridae (DNA)
Tumors	HTLV-1	Retroviridae (RNA)
Leukemia/Lymphoma	Acute Leukemia viruses	Retroviridae (RNA)
	Epstein-Barr virus	Herpesviridae (DNA)
Mammary carcinoma	MMTV	Retroviridae (RNA)
Cervical carcinoma	Human Papilloma viruses	Papovaviridae (DNA)
Hepatomas	Hepatitis B virus	Hepadnaviridae (DNA)
	Woodchuck hepatitis virus	Hepadnaviridae (DNA)
Polyomas	Simian virus 40	Papovaviridae (DNA)
Myxomas	Rabbit Myxomatosis virus	Poxviridae (DNA)

and end in the suffix *virus* such as the morbillivirus genus of the paramyxoviridae. Viruses in genera are often further divided into viral *species* based on differences in their genomic sequences. For example, canine distemper virus is a member of the morbillivirus genus in the family paramyxoviridae. Some human and animal viruses classified by family are listed in Table 16.1.

Viral pathogens are frequently named after the diseases and the specific symptoms they cause and the tissues they infect (Table 16.2). This is a poor system because in some cases viruses from different families may cause similar disease conditions, and in other cases, viruses of the same family can cause very distinct diseases.

A virus that infects and exerts its main pathologic effect in only one primary target tissue is said to have a restricted tissue tropism. Viruses that infect many different cell types and produce disease in several organ systems are said to have a broad tissue tropism. They may be described as *pantropic*. Viruses that infect and produce disease in a primary target tissue may however sometimes infect other tissues and spread systemically producing secondary disease.

Many viruses are relatively species-specific as is the human poxvirus for example. They cause infection and disease in one or a few specific hosts, whereas others are not species-specific and can infect several species in which they may or may not produce disease. Rabies virus is an example of a virus that is in this category. Viruses produce a wide range of disorders ranging from acute inflammatory disorders to chronic degenerative disorders. Viruses of several families cause cancer or have been implicated as cofactors in the development of cancers.

VIRAL PATHOGENESIS

The cell is the basic unit of biological organization. Most disease processes can be traced to dysfunction in cells. Many aspects of viral pathogenesis result from the superimposition of virus replication on the normal host cell physiology. Cellular malfunctions due to viral infection become manifest when cellular malfunctions disrupt tissue and organ-systems. Many of the fundamental processes involved in viral pathogenesis have been elucidated using cell culture systems and experimental animals. Viruses may cause damage to cells (*cytopathic effects*) in a variety of ways including (1) by causing host cell polymerases to be redirected to viral templates, (2) disrupting cellular DNA during replication of the virus, and (3) disrupting the production of host cell proteins important for maintaining the cell. In all of these situations the virus is exploiting normal cellular mechanisms or resources such as nucleotide pools used in cell replication to produce new virus particles. Disease may result from destruction of the cell or from alteration of normal cell function. Disruption of clearance of respiratory secretions by the movement of cilia is an example of an alteration of cell function. Some viruses like the respiratory syncytial viruses may cause cell membranes to fuse when viral envelope proteins are inserted at the plasma membrane of the host cell. Cell membrane fusion may lead to *syncytial* formation in which numerous cells fuse together forming an enlarged cell with multiple nuclei surrounded by a single cell membrane. Viruses that cause cell membrane fusion may predispose the cell to rupture releasing viral particles or may enhance cell-to-cell transmission of the virus. During the process of virus replication inclusion bodies may form in the cell cytoplasm or nucleus depending on virus type. The herpesviruses produce intranuclear inclusions and the poxviruses intracytoplasmic ones. Inclusion bodies are microscopically visible accumulations of protein or nucleic acid complexes formed during virus replication. These inclusion bodies help pathologists examining tissues microscopically to make a diagnosis of a viral infection.

Viral infection is initiated following virus adsorption, penetration, and uncoating (Figure 16.2). The nucleic acids of DNA viruses, except those of the poxviruses are reproduced in the cell nucleus. Poxviruses are reproduced in the cytoplasm. The nucleic acids of RNA viruses, except for retroviruses and certain orthomyxoviruses such as influenza A virus are reproduced in the cytoplasm. The viral genomic element formed early during viral nucleic acid synthesis acts as a template for synthesis of new viral genomes and messenger RNA transcription and is called the replicative form (RF). The RF gives rise to progeny viral nucleic acids, detected as replicative intermediates in addition to viral mRNA. Translation of viral mRNA

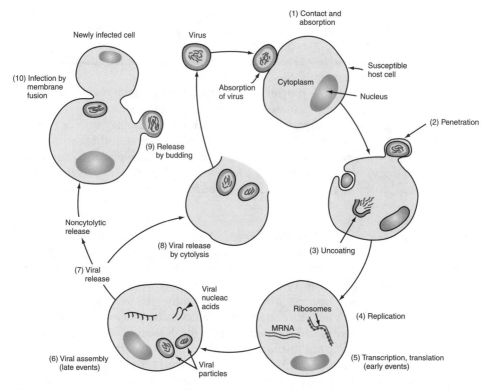

Figure 16.2. Viral replication can be considered to consist of a number of steps. (1) The virus must be absorbed onto the host cell; (2) it must penetrate the cell; (3) it must uncoat inside the cell either in the nucleus or the cytoplasm; (4) it must replicate. In replication there are (5) early events that prepare the cell for virus synthesis and (6) late events that result in production of virus and assembly. Finally, the virus must (7) escape from the cell by (8) causing cell lysis; (9) by budding, or (10) by moving from one cell directly to another through cell membrane fusion.

gives rise to the viral proteins. The processes of assembly, maturation, and release of progeny virions from cells are generally associated with cytopathic effects such as the formation of inclusion bodies, cytolysis, and cell fusion.

Many factors determine susceptibility of cells to viral infection and the resultant pathology. However, the outcome of viral infections in terms of host survival is often governed by the host immune response to antigenic viral proteins (Figure 16.3). Much of the pathology of viral diseases may be due to chronic inflammation in infected tissues and to immunopathologic effects associated with the response of the immune system to infection of cells. Many viruses become latent after infection and produce few if any viral transcripts or viral proteins. Viral latency may be a part of the natural life cycle of the virus or may be imposed on the virus as a result of the host's immune response (Figure 16.4). Latency allows the viral genome to persist in a quiescent or inactive state in the host. Periodic activation may lead to the development of recurrent disease. Reactivation of the genome and production of new virus may contribute to cellular transformation and the development of malignancies. In persistent infections in which a viral genome is relatively limited in expression, the host cell may express few viral antigens and is less susceptible to immune attack. However, in some persistent infections active viral antigen production occurs and such infections may result in tissue injury from the deposition

(1)   Infection Blocking
Virus–neutralizing antibody
Phagocytosis
Complement–mediated lysis

(2)   Fusion Inhibition
Antibody mediated

(3)   Inhibition of Viral Growth in Cells
Interferons

(4)   Destruction of Infected Host Cells
Cytolytic T–cells
Antibody–dependent cell lysis
Killer (K) cells
Natural killer (NK) cells
Macrophages

Figure 16.3.   Host resistance mechanisms. (1) Extracellular virus may be prevented from entering cells by virus-specific antibody. (2) Virus movement from cell to cell by fusion may be blocked by antibody to virus-produced fusogenes in the cell membrane. (3) Interferons and possibly other substances may inhibit viral growth in cells. (4) Virus may be destroyed or prevented from reproducing by destruction of infected host cells.

of immune complexes and complement on the infected cells. Persistent expression of viral antigen by infected cells may also induce cell mediated immune responses and delayed-type hypersensitivity reactions leading to chronic inflammation and tissue damage at the site of infection. A number of viral diseases and their etiologic agents are summarized in Table 16.2. In this table, diseases are grouped by whether the causative virus produces acute, persistent or chronic infection. Various viral diseases are described in a later section of this chapter.

ANTI-VIRAL STRATEGIES OF THE HOST CELL AND IMMUNE SYSTEM
Interferons are a family of proteins produced by host cells in response to a variety of stimuli including viral infection. The formation of double stranded viral RNA within the infected cell induces the formation of interferons. Interferons may induce an antiviral state within many cells in the body. The production of interferons is a basic defense mechanism of animals against viral infections. There are three distinct types of interferons (alpha, beta, and gamma). Alpha and beta interferons bind to specific cell receptors and cause cells to produce proteins that have antiviral properties. For example, 2-5A synthetase causes the activation of nucleases that mediate degradation of viral RNAs. Gamma interferon, which is produced by leukocytes, causes the activation of macrophages and the production of antiviral cytokines which amplify the antiviral immune response.

The immune system has evolved mechanisms against a virus infection that eliminate both extracellular virions and virus infected cells. The most effective responses involve multiple types of immune response. For example, CD8+ cytotoxic T cells and antibody plus complement can recognize and lyse virus-infected cells. The cellular immune response to viral infections includes the actions of natural killer (NK) cells, MHC Class I-restricted CD8+ cytotoxic T lymphocytes (CTLs) and MHC

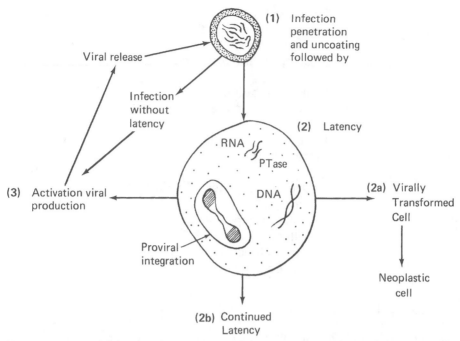

Figure 16.4. Viral latency. After (1) entry into a cell, virus may integrate and (2) become inactive or latent. The virus genome may (2a) cause neoplastic transformation of the cell, (2b) continue latent, or (3) become activated and reproduce.

Class II-restricted CD4+ helper T lymphocytes (Th cells) each functioning independently or in combination as antiviral effector cells. There is an inherited deficiency of NK cells in some persons that may lead to them having extensive and severe virus infections.

NK cells are not virus specific. CTLs however are virus specific. They are a major class of effector cells in antiviral immunity. They have been demonstrated to be effective against most types of virus-infected cells. CTLs play a critical role in the elimination of cells already infected by viruses as well as in restriction of the spread of a virus infection in the body. These effector cells are particularly important during the early phases of many virus infections. However, in some acute lytic virus infections such as influenza or paramyxovirus infections, the replication of the virus may be so rapid that effectiveness of the CTL response may be limited. The contribution of helper T lymphocytes (Th cells) in antiviral immunity is limited, in part, due to the restricted expression of MHC Class II cells. In response to certain viral infections Th cells have been demonstrated to cause some immunopathologic lesions.

Antibodies have the major role in elimination of cell-free virus by neutralizing the infectivity of the virus particle. The mechanisms whereby antibodies make virus particles noninfectious are varied. Antibodies may eliminate infectivity of cell-free virus by aggregation of virus particles. Acting alone or with complement antibodies may alter the structure of the virus particle and neutralize infectivity or may block cell entry at the receptor or at a postadsorption step. Antibodies may also recognize viral antigens on the surface of cells and render the cell susceptible to lysis by the action of complement or CTLs by an antibody-dependent cellular or complement-mediated cytotoxicity process. The importance of complement in controlling viral infections has been demonstrated by the increase in susceptibility of complement-deficient mice to experimental virus infections. Virus particles coated by nonneutralizing antibodies may be cleared from the immune system more effectively than noncoated viral particles. In some cases nonneutralizing antibodies may inhibit the release of virus from infected cells. As noted earlier not all immune responses are beneficial. Antiviral antibody responses in certain circumstances have been shown to potentiate disease by enhancing the entry of virus particles into macrophages via Fc receptors. This is the case for example in Dengue virus infections.

ANTI-VIRAL DRUGS

There are relatively few drugs presently available that are effective against viral infections. The virus-host cell interactions are so intimate that it is difficult to interfere with viral functions and not damage host cell functions. Successful antiviral therapies require drugs that are active against virus-specific targets, such as viral enzymes and regulatory proteins but not against host cell systems. Some may act by stimulating natural intracellular processes that prevent replication and spread of viruses.

Despite the difficulty of the problem some effective antiviral drugs have been developed against herpesviruses and retroviruses. The nucleoside analogue acycloguanosine (Acyclovir) is activated by phosphorylation via thymidine kinase, a herpesvirus encoded enzyme. The phosphorylated analogue acts then to inhibit the activity of the virus-encoded polymerase. Nucleoside and nonnucleoside inhibitors have been developed against retroviral infections as a result of the massive efforts developed in response to the AIDS epidemic (see below). Nucleoside analogues such as azidothymidine (AZT) selectively inhibit reverse transcriptase (RT) and thereby inhibit the replication of the retroviruses including HIV. A variety of nucleoside analogs have been produced to combat HIV infections (e.g., ddI, didanosine). The need for additional antiviral drugs against HIV has been driven, in part, by the ability of retroviruses like HIV to mutate and become resistant to the effects of drugs that have been developed. The introduction of protease inhibitors like nelfinavir has provided additional types of drugs active against HIV infection. These drugs in combination with RT inhibitors have provided new hope in the battle against AIDS. However, before long-term success against HIV is achieved elimination of sites of latent virus production and continued development of drugs against resistant strains will be required.

DIAGNOSIS OF VIRAL INFECTIONS

Diagnostic tests for viral infections are designed to detect the presence of the viral agent or its components or to detect antibodies against the viral agent. Some serologic tests are designed to measure amounts of antibodies against infectious agents in body fluids, usually plasma or serum. The type of test used is chosen dependent on what information is desired and ease of use, cost, number of specimens to be tested, commercial availability, and sensitivity and specificity of the assay. For the diagnosis of human viral infections the test and laboratory procedures used in testing must be approved by a government agency, usually the Food and Drug Administration. The United States Department of Agriculture must sanction tests used in the diagnosis of viral infections of animals. Serologic tests are often performed in conjunction with other tests for detection of viral particles or viral antigens.

There are a variety of tests used by virologists for the diagnosis of viral infections. Enzyme linked immunosorbent assays (ELISA) can be sensitive and specific to directly detect antibodies against viral pathogens in serum or other body fluids. Most ELISAs use solid-phase microtiter plates of polystyrene or polyvinyl plastic that are coated with a "capture" antigen consisting of disrupted virus or synthetic peptides of the viral agent. The serum specimen is allowed to absorb to the capture antigen. Unbound antibody is washed away, and a detector enzyme-labeled antibody directed against the bound antibodies is added. Horseradish peroxidase or alkaline phosphatase are the enzymes most commonly linked to the detector antibodies which are then allowed to react to substrates of the enzyme leading to the production of a colored product. Tests are read optically using spectrophotometry or directly by visual examination.

ELISA can also be used to directly detect viral antigens. Most such procedures use solid-phase ELISA plates, which are coated with a "capture" antibody, to a particular viral agent. The specimen suspected to contain virus antigens is allowed to absorb to the capture antibody. Unbound molecules are washed away, and an enzyme-labeled antiviral antibody called a detector antibody is added. The enzymes, which are linked to the detector antibody, are then allowed to react with a substrate of the enzyme leading to a color reaction if the virus is present in the sample. Tests are read optically using spectrophotometry or visually.

Immunofluorescence assays (IFA) are rapid and inexpensive tests also used to detect antiviral antibodies in serum and other body fluids. Known viral antigens fixed on slides or in infected cell cultures are incubated with the serum sample. Binding of the antibody to the viral antigens is detected by use of fluorscein-labeled antibodies to the serum antibody being sought. IFA may also be adapted to detect viral antigens directly in tissue sections. IFA tests are standard tests for rabies virus in brain sections of animals suspected of having the infection.

Certain types of viruses including influenza viruses have the ability to bind specifically to red blood cells and cause them to agglutinate. Specific antibody inhibition of this reaction is call hemagglutination inhibition. Hemagglutination inhibition tests are used to detect the virus or antibodies against the viral agent in many such infections.

Antiserum specific for a viral agent can be used to prevent the cytopathic affect of the virus in culture. By serially diluting the antiserum being tested, the titer of antibodies in the sample may be estimated. Procedures of this type are called virus neutralization assays. This type of assay is technically difficult to perform and is used only by reference laboratories seeking to differentiate pathogenic viral strains.

The immunoblot assay also termed "Western blot" is performed by first solubilizing a viral preparation such as purified virus particles or virus-infected cells and separation of the mixture of molecules by gel electrophoresis and transfer of viral proteins to membranes. The membrane containing the viral proteins is then treated with antiserum followed by detection of bound antibody using radiolabeled or enzyme-labeled antispecies antibodies. The test allows the detection of antibodies to specific proteins of the virion and is useful to discriminate between infections by closely related viruses and is often used to confirm the results of ELISA tests.

Electron microscopy of viral particles, following in particular preparation by negative staining, has allowed identification of viral agents that are difficult to culture. The advantages of electron microscopy for virus identification include the rapid test time and detection of multiple agents in a single specimen. This technique is particularly useful for detection of enteric pathogens in fecal specimens and in skin lesions such as herpes vesicles. The use of labeled specific antiserum or monoclonal antibodies to the virus may increase the sensitivity and specificity of the test. Such procedures are called immunoelectron microscopy. Nucleic acid hybridization procedures allow the direct detection of viral nucleic acid by nucleic acid probes. Single-stranded RNA or DNA will hybridize by hydrogen bonded base pairing to another single strand of RNA or DNA which has complementary base sequences. For detection of viral DNA the two strands of the target DNA molecule are first separated by boiling, then following some cooling hybridized to ssDNA or ssRNA probes. Hybridization is performed in solution or after the target DNA or RNA is absorbed onto nitrocellulose or nylon membranes. The degree of probe binding and hybridization will depend on how closely the target and probe sequences are complementary and the conditions of the assay. Probes can be labeled with radioactive isotopes such as ^{32}P and binding detected by counting the radioactivity, or they can be linked to proteins or enzymes, which are then allowed to react with a substrate to produce a color reaction. Biotin-labeled probes are commonly used. Southern blot hybridization (named after Dr. Edward Southern) tests for DNA sequences that are cut up by enzymes which cleave the nucleic acid into separate short segments called oligonucleotides. The cleaved components in a sample of nucleic acid are separated by electrophoresis and then transferred onto filter paper and detected with a labeled probe which hybridizes to the sequence of interest. "Northern" blotting of RNA follows similar principles. *In situ* hybridization tests for nucleic acid in tissue samples. The labeled probe is placed on tissue sections that contain the target sequence. This type of test permits the diagnostician to determine which cell in a tissue is infected. In situ hybridization is useful to detect viruses that are difficult to isolate in cell culture.

The polymerase chain reaction (PCR) amplifies the target sequence prior to an attempt at its detection. This procedure permits detection of very small amounts of target sequence and can be applied to small samples of diagnostic material such as a few drops of blood or serum. Heating is needed to melt the DNA, then short specific oligonucleotides called primers are allowed to bind to the strands of DNA flanking the sequence to be amplified. The primers are extended by DNA polymerases, which work at high temperatures. The new DNA strands made by the polymerases are these of the DNA between the primers. The amplification procedure is repeated multiple times to increase the target sequence which is then detected with procedures such as Southern blot hybridization.

Virus isolation remains an important component of procedures used to confirm the identity of viral pathogens. Fluids or tissues likely to contain a viral pathogen are collected and placed in cell cultures capable of supporting the replication of the virus. The procedure can be technically difficult because of the potential for bacterial and fungal contamination of cell cultures used in the procedure. The agent must be detected by procedures outlined earlier in this section. and requires confirmation of the viral agents by specific means (e.g., antigen detection of cultures). The choice of the cell used for isolation is very important. Primary fetal cells are often good hosts, yet they are difficult to maintain. Cell lines are convenient and as a consequence are frequently used for isolation, but it is necessary to establish that they are susceptable to the virus that one is attempting to isolate.

IMMUNIZATION AGAINST VIRAL INFECTIONS
Immunization to prevent infection has been the most important and successful

strategy against virus-induced disease. Immunization has been particularly effective against acute viral infections. Jenner introduced the first effective vaccine in 1798. Cowpox, a natural pathogen in cows was scratched into the skin to create mild lesions in humans. This process immunized humans against the related virulent pathogen, smallpox.

Ideally the antigens in the vaccine should stimulate antigen-presenting cells such as macrophages to promote an immune response against the virus. The generation of an effective immune response requires the expansion of the populations of cells involved in elimination of the virus and the production of memory cells to maintain the immunity. Thus, the ability of a vaccine preparation to promote local cytokine responses or stimulate the expansion of the populations of the appropriate cell type may determine the effectiveness of a vaccine. In general, there are multiple antigenic sites on a virus that promote an immune response. Some of these may be hidden from the immune system in the intact virus particle, but are exposed when the virus replicates in the host cell. Some viruses rapidly mutate these critical antigenic determinants and avoid the immune system. Thus, multiple antigenic determinants are often included in effective viral vaccines. In addition, if the vaccine is designed with multiple epitopes multiple arms of the immune system may be stimulated, both cell-mediated and humoral.

The antigen preparations in a vaccine may have a limited half-life in the body following the injection of a vaccine or be poorly antigenic. This transient response may limit the duration of the immune response. To overcome these problems vaccines are often delivered in combination with substances called adjuvants to prolong the exposure of the antigen to the immune system and increase its immunogenicity. Adjuvants are thus materials mixed with vaccines to increase the immune response to the vaccine. Examples include alum, mineral oils, and muramyl dipeptide. Mechanisms of action of adjuvants include (1) slowing the release or prolonging the retention of an antigen, (2) activating macrophages, and (3) promoting lymphocyte proliferation. Finally, an ideal vaccine should have a wide margin of safety. For example, live attenuated vaccines should not convert to virulence. A vaccine must also be cost effective, its benefits should exceed its costs.

Viral vaccines are of two major types: live attenuated virus vaccines, which may be delivered in the form of a vaccine vector and inactivated vaccines which may be delivered as whole virus or as parts of the virus also called subunit vaccines. Live-virus vaccines consist of nonpathogenic mutant viral strains or viruses such as vaccinia viruses engineered to serve as vectors that express heterologous genes derived from pathogenic viruses. Live virus vaccines are excellent in that they often generate long-term immunity. Some live virus vaccines consist of naturally occurring strains of a virus from a different host species, an example is a form of Marek's disease vaccine which is actually a herpesvirus of turkeys. The turkey herpesvirus is used to protect chickens from the pathogenic virus of chickens and prevents the formation of tumors.

A variety of strategies are used to produce attenuated vaccines including adaptation to unnatural host species by serial passage in unnatural host animals or by serial passage in cell culture. Inactivated vaccines are made of whole virus or components of virulent viruses that have been physically or chemically modified to destroy infectivity. They are generally safe and provide protection, but often provide a shorter-lived immunity than do live attenuated vaccines. Commonly used agents to inactivate viruses in the preparation of a "killed" vaccine include formaldehyde, β-propiolactone, and ethyleneimine.

All vaccines licensed for use are tested for effectiveness and safety. Production of such effective and safe viral vaccines is often difficult as there are a number of potential problems. Vaccine preparations made using animal cells or tissues may contain contaminating viruses. For example, smallpox vaccine may be contaminated with foot-and-mouth disease virus during passage in calves. The scrapie agent related to the "mad cow" agent contaminated louping ill vaccines previously used in England. A source of potential contamination of vaccines is bovine calf serum used in many cell cultures. Another problem is that live viral vaccines can be inactivated if held at room temperature or in warm conditions. This is particularly true in warm climates and in the tropics. Thus, efforts must be in place to maintain the "cold chain" before the vaccine is administered. In general, live vaccines are not used in pregnant women or animals because of potential teratogenic effects.

SELECTED DISEASES RESULTING FROM ACUTE VIRAL INFECTIONS
Smallpox
Smallpox was a common disease of humans in the fifteenth and sixteenth centuries. It was observed in sporadic and epidemic outbreaks with high or low mortality. Jenner developed the first safe vaccination procedure against small pox.

The etiologic agent of smallpox is the variola virus, a large and complex DNA virus (Poxviridae, Table 16.1). It naturally infects man and can also be transmitted to some higher primates. Two distinct forms of the disease occur in man: variola major, with twenty-five to fifty percent mortality, and variola minor (classical smallpox), which has less than one percent mortality. Smallpox is a highly contagious disease spread mainly by inhalation of virus. The virus also infects through breaks in the skin either from contact with pock fluids or contaminated clothing and bedding. Poxviruses survive in the environment because the virion has a protective fibrous protein outer coat.

Smallpox produces an acute infection. After inhalation the virus first multiplies in mucosal cells of the upper respiratory tract and then infection spreads to the regional lymph nodes. A mild transient viremia is followed by infection of the liver, spleen, and lungs. In these organs multiplication continues for about twelve to sixteen days. Few symptoms are present at this stage, and it is thus referred to as the "incubation" period. The secondary viremia that ensues then produces generalized symptoms, including fever, pain, headache, malaise, and rash. Epidermal cells then become infected and the virus multiplies over an additional two-week period. During this phase, there is necrosis of epidermal cells and leukocyte infiltration leading to formation of the characteristic skin pustules, or pocks. Pocklike lesions may also form in the liver and other soft tissues. In nonfatal cases, the skin lesions eventually resolve by "crusting" and scarification, and the infection terminates with the development of permanent immunity.

Variola virus differs from other DNA viruses in that it replicates entirely in the cytoplasm of infected cells. The characteristic cytoplasmic inclusion bodies (Guarneri bodies) contain viral antigens, nucleic acids, and maturing virus particles. Virus production ultimately kills the infected cells and progeny virions are released by cytolysis.

The outer coat of variola virus contains a hemagglutinating protein that mediates virus uptake by cells and it is the main target for virus-neutralizing antibodies. Viral dissemination in the primary viremic phase is prevented by vaccination because vaccination induces virus-neutralizing antibodies. A worldwide vaccination program initiated by the World Health Organization ultimately led to the eradication of smallpox in the present century.

Rabies

In early times, rabid animals and humans were thought to be "possessed." However, by 1804, the infectious nature of the disease was well recognized. In the 1880s, Pasteur attenuated the virus by serial passage in mice of brain homogenates from rabid dogs. The passaged material was used as a postexposure vaccine for persons bitten by rabid animals. In 1903, Negri showed that a filterable agent produced the disease in animals and first demonstrated the characteristic cytoplasmic inclusion bodies of rabies (*Negri bodies*) in neural cells.

Rabies is caused by a bullet-shaped, RNA-containing virus which has been classed with the Rhabdoviridae (Table 16.1). It can infect virtually all mammals and is transmitted in saliva inoculated by the bite of diseased animals. Rabies may sometimes be acquired by inhalation of aerosols in caves inhabited by large numbers of rabid bats. Rabies virus has a worldwide distribution, and there is a considerable reservoir of the virus in wild animals, which frustrates control efforts. The main sources of human rabies infection are unvaccinated pets that contract the virus from wild animals. Most control efforts are directed at the pet population. Attempts to control the infection in wild animals may be possible by use of oral vaccines in bait.

Rabies follows an acute course that causes death in a high proportion of individuals who develop clinical disease. Virus enters a bite wound with infectious saliva and replicates locally in muscle cells and other cells at the site of injury. The incubation period is twenty to sixty days in man. There is little hematogenous spread of rabies virus. Instead, the virus enters nerve endings and travels in the nerves to the central nervous system. Infection of nerves causes the "prodromal" phase characterized by sensations at the site of injury, fever, and changes in temperament. The "excitative" phase correlates with virus multiplication in the brain, and during this phase there is spread of virus through efferent nerves to the salivary glands. Virus multiplication in the salivary glands is associated with symptoms such as difficulty in swallowing and frothing at the mouth. It is from these symptoms that the term "hydrophobia" is derived. The "convulsive" phase is characterized by seizures and terminates in death within three to five days.

The mortality in rabies is probably caused by disruption of vital functions mediated by specific neurons because the lesions detected in the central nervous system at necropsy are not usually extensive. Specific groups of neurons become infected, but the virus does not cause cytolysis of these cells. The virus reproduces in the cytoplasm and matures by budding through the cell membrane. The mechanism of host protection induced by administration of vaccine is not well understood, but it is probably related to cell-mediated destruction of infected cells in the bite wound and the antibody-mediated neutralization of progeny virions before they invade the nervous system. The currently used rabies vaccines consist of inactivated virus derived from cell cultures and they require only a few inoculations to elicit immunity.

The envelope glycoprotein component of rabies virus has a role in the pathogenesis of this disease. The lethal characteristics of rabies virus for mice are determined by a single amino acid in the envelope glycoprotein. Viruses having envelope glycoproteins with isoleucine or glutamine substituted for arginine at residue 333 are attenuated, whereas revertants with arginine at this site are lethal.

Polio

Polio was first described in the eighteenth century. Epidemics occurred frequently until about 1955 when attenuated and inactivated polio vaccines came into wide use. Poliovirus was one of the first viruses propagated in cell culture and its complete crystallographic structure is known today.

Poliovirus is a relatively small, naked icosahedral virus with a single stranded RNA genome. Its family, the Picornaviridae (Table 16.1) includes the rhinoviruses, which cause the common cold, and the hepatitis A virus, which causes acute liver disease. Man is the natural host of poliovirus. The virus infects primarily intestinal mucosal cells but may infect other cells, including neurons. The virus can be transmitted to the chimpanzee, and strains are available that infect mice.

In nature the virus spreads from person to person by ingestion of food and water contaminated with fecal material. The virus is stable in the environment and is not inactivated by the stomach acids. Poliovirus infection in man can be inapparent. This is the most common form of infection. Poliovirus infection can also cause acute mild illness, acute nonparalytic aseptic meningitis, or paralytic poliomyelitis. The paralytic disease results in permanent paralysis and occurs more often in older children. Between 1940 and 1950, improved infant health care practices in developed countries prevented infections of young children. Infection then occurred when the children were older, and there was therefore a greater incidence of paralytic disease.

Early in the infection, poliovirus replicates in the oropharyngeal and intestinal mucosal cells and is shed into the throat and feces. The virus then infects the tonsils and Peyer's patches and the cervical and mesenteric lymph nodes. After seven to fourteen days, a transient viremia develops which is sometimes followed by clinical recovery. In other individuals there is further dissemination of virus to susceptible, nonneural tissues. This gives rise to systemic illness. By fifteen to twenty days, the virus may enter the central nervous system and cause neurologic effects. Virus replication in the central nervous system results in death of neurons. This is fatal in cases of infection of the medullary portion of the brain, but gives rise to variable degrees of paralysis when the infection is in the cortex or spinal cord. Partial or complete recovery from paralysis depends on host factors, such as compensatory muscle hypertrophy and use of alternate efferent motor circuits. Only one to two percent of all poliovirus infections result in central nervous system involvement, but in epidemics, the overall number of individuals with paralytic disease can be quite high.

Poliovirus has a relatively simple method of replication. The virus enters susceptible cells following attachment to cellular receptors, new virus production occurs within the cytoplasm, and cells are lysed to release the progeny virions. The single-stranded RNA genome is plus-stranded, as is cellular messenger RNA. This enables the viral RNA to be translated directly after uncoating. The result of translation is a single large protein which is cleaved into an RNA-dependent RNA polymerase, and also into four polypeptides that form the individual capsomers of the nucleocapsid. The genomic RNA is copied by the viral polymerase into a complementary strand of RNA that serves as the replicative form of the virus. New virions assemble in the cytoplasm within inclusion bodies and are released following cytolysis.

The attenuated Sabin vaccine and the inactivated Salk vaccine contain the capsid proteins of the three major serotypes of poliovirus. Immunity is conferred by the induction of virus-neutralizing antibodies to the capsid proteins. These neutralizing antibodies prevent infection of neurons. Compared to inactivated vaccines, attenuated live vaccines require smaller initial quantities of virus, and viral replication is required for induction of immunity. They must therefore be handled carefully during distribution and use to prevent inactivation and ensure infectivity. The major advantage of the inactivated vaccine, despite the need for larger initial amounts of virus, is that inactivation eliminates the possibility of reversion to the wild type virus.

Influenza A

Flu-like symptoms can be produced by several viruses and by other infectious agents, including bacteria. Influenza imposes a significant disease burden on the population because it occurs in large epidemics every two to four years. The pandemics of 1743, 1889 to 1892, and 1918 to 1919 were widespread and caused particularly serious disease. In the last worldwide influenza pandemic (1918–1919), over 80 million people became ill and there were many deaths. A filterable agent, later named influenza virus, type A, caused the pandemic. Type A influenza viruses are genetically distinct from type B and C influenza viruses and are distinguishable and classified on the basis of serologic differences among their nucleocapsid antigens.

Human influenza A virus is a typical enveloped virus with a helical RNA-containing nucleoprotein (Orthomyxoviridae, Table 16.1). Influenza virus is normally inhaled and multiplies initially in mucosal cells of the upper respiratory tract. There is no viremia phase, but the acute disease is nonetheless associated with general symptoms such as malaise and fever. Virus replication kills mucosal cells and results in necrosis and desquamation of the mucosa. The virus may spread to the lungs where it can cause moderate to severe damage including bronchial necrosis, hemorrhage, and edema. As free virus inhibits the uptake of bacteria by phagocytes, severe secondary bacterial pneumonia may sometimes develop.

The neuraminidase enables influenza virus to penetrate mucous secretions by virtue of its enzymatic activity. Neuraminidase also promotes the release of the virions as they bud from the cell surface. The envelope hemagglutinin serves to attach the virus to cells by binding to cell receptors. The virus then enters the cell in an endosomal vesicle. As the pH of the vesicle becomes acidic, the hemagglutinin changes conformation and allows fusion of the viral envelope with the endosomal membrane, resulting in uncoating and release of the viral nucleocapsid into the cell cytoplasm. Influenza viruses, unlike most RNA viruses, replicate in the cell nucleus rather than in the cytoplasm. The influenza virus has a negative stranded RNA, which is not translated directly by the host cell. Initiation of replication is possible because the virus encodes and packages its own RNA-dependent RNA polymerase. The viral RNA consists of eight different single-stranded segments, each coding for at least one of the major viral proteins. If two strains of influenza A virus infect the same cell, an interchange of entire genomic segments can occur (reassortment). Unlike classical genetic recombination, splicing and rejoining of the nucleic acid is not required in this process. Related influenza A viruses also infect animals of a variety of species, including pigs and many types of birds. These viral strains represent potential pools of genetic material for pathogenic human influenza strains by reassortment of genomic segments between animal and human influenza strains that infect a common host.

At least twelve different hemagglutinin (H) and nine different neuraminidases (N) occur in influenza A. Reassortment gives rise to a large number of HN serotypes. A recombinant type A virus that contained the human type 1 neuraminidase and the swine flu hemagglutinin apparently caused the great flu pandemic of 1918–1919. This process of reassortment is referred to as "antigenic shift." The possibility that the highly virulent "swine flu variant" was present in 1976 led to the vaccination of over 40 million people. However, a swine flu virus which was not highly virulent in man, caused the 1976 outbreak. A pathogenic avian influenza virus that caused human mortality was discovered in 1998 in Hong Kong. Killing millions of chickens suspected of carrying the infection in Hong Kong and surrounding regions apparently eliminated it.

In addition to changes in the set of envelope proteins brought about by antigenic shift, the viral envelope genes can undergo small mutational changes resulting in amino acid sequence divergence in the envelope protein. These changes are called "antigenic drift" to imply that they occur within a given parental HN serotype. The changes in serotype resulting from antigenic drift frequently enable the variants to evade neutralization by humoral antibody to the parent type and may permit reinfection of a previously exposed host.

SELECTED DISEASES RESULTING FROM VIRAL INFECTIONS THAT RESOLVE OR PERSIST
Measles and Subacute Sclerosing Panencephalitis

Measles was first described in the seventeenth century and was shown to be infectious in 1758 by transmission to human volunteers. The disease was transmitted to monkeys in 1911 and, in 1954, Enders isolated and grew the causative virus in cells in culture. The virus belongs to the family of large enveloped RNA viruses referred to as the Paramyxoviridae (Table 16.1). The acute disease caused by measles virus is called rubeola. Rubeola is distinct from rubella or German measles, which is caused by a Togavirus (Tables 16.1 and 16.2). The measles virus is related to the canine distemper virus, the Sendai virus of mice, and the rinderpest virus of cattle. Other members of the Paramyxoviridae include mumps virus and respiratory syncytial virus.

Measles is one of the most infectious diseases known. It is present in respiratory secretions before the development of symptoms. In children it causes an acute illness which may confer sustained immunity. The measles virus multiplies first in the mucosal cells of the upper respiratory tract and in cells in the regional lymph nodes. It is then shed into the secretions and bloodstream. The prodromal phase, characterized by respiratory symptoms, fever, and the presence of red macules called Koplik spots inside the cheeks, occurs when the virus is in the blood. Following the prodromal stage, the virus is disseminated to previously uninfected lymphoid tissues and to basal epidermal cells. Infection of the latter cells results in the measles rash.

Measles virus infection of cells of the immune system, particularly B and T lymphocytes, causes transient immunosuppression. Natural killer cell activity is also depressed during acute measles virus infections but the mechanism of this suppression is less clear. The virus infects numerous cell types where it replicates in the cytoplasm. It is noncytolytic, and matures by budding from the plasma membrane. The virus has a single-stranded, unsegmented RNA of negative polarity which codes for a matrix protein, a nucleoprotein, a phosphorylating protein, a RNA-dependent RNA polymerase, and two envelope structural proteins. One envelope protein is a combined hemagglutinin and a neuraminidase, and the other induces membrane fusion. The neuraminidase hemagglutinating protein mediates attachment of virus to cells while the fusion protein mediates penetration.

In people with measles, multinucleated giant cells are frequently found in respiratory secretions. Antibodies to the neuraminidase hemagglutinating proteins and some antibodies to the fusion protein neutralize virus infectivity; however, only antibodies to the fusion protein inhibit virus-mediated fusion of cells. There is only one serotype of measles virus and therefore a monovalent vaccine is all that is needed. An attenuated strain of the virus is used. Vaccination against measles should not take place before nine months of age. Passively acquired maternal antibody to measles virus normally protects young children from infection, but, for reasons not fully understood, the maternal antibody appears to impede or alter the child's immune response to the vaccine. In such individuals the course of infection may be altered to favor persistent viral infection in lymphoid tissues and the central nervous system. These infections, which can persist for a long time, cause the development of the debilitating condition known as subacute sclerosing panencephalitis. In children with this type of measles infection, there may be progressive destruction of the nervous system, which is ultimately fatal.

Warts and Papillomatous Tumors

A filterable agent was demonstrated to transmit human warts in 1907. Occasionally warts may become malignant. In the 1930s Shope demonstrated that myxoma virus, a papilloma-inducing virus of rabbits, could cause malignant squamous cell carcinoma. He showed that domestic rabbits infected with myxoma virus developed malignancy more frequently than did wild cottontail rabbits and that topical application of certain chemicals increased the incidence of malignancy. Thus, both host genetic factors and environmental agents were shown to act as cofactors in the development of the virus induced malignancy.

Papilloma viruses are small naked icosahedral viruses composed of a capsid and a closed circular, double-stranded DNA molecule with superhelical conformation (Table 16.1). These viruses occur in a variety of mammals. Infection resulting in production of complete virus is generally species-specific. Transmission of virus occurs by contamination of mucosal surfaces or injured skin. The viruses have not been grown in culture and therefore must be obtained from susceptible animals. The bovine papilloma virus is a prototype of this group of viruses.

There are a variety of different serotypes of human papilloma virus differing in their major capsid antigens. Most cause benign warts including the familiar skin wart and the deeply recessed plantar wart. The viral DNA replicates as an episomal element in dermal cells enhancing host cell proliferation and differentiation into keratinized cells. It is during the keratinization process that new viral components are expressed and assembled.

Warts often regress spontaneously, and regression may occur in several locations at once. This pattern of rejection suggests an immune-mediated mechanism. This suggestion is further supported by the observation that rabbits cured of benign papillomas are resistant to subsequent challenge with the virus that caused them.

Papilloma viruses may be transmitted during sexual contact. The mucosal infections which result can be asymptomatic or give rise to characteristic lesions in the ano-genital and cervical areas. Development of papillomas in these areas has been linked epidemiologically with an increased risk of developing genital tumors and cervical carcinomas.

Acute and Chronic Type B Hepatitis and Hepatocellular Carcinoma

Viral hepatitis is a common inflammatory disease of humans and a variety of animal species. A variety of viruses can cause hepatitis or infect the liver as part of their systemic spread and replication. The resulting pathologic lesions may be acute and transient as in Hepatitis A or result in chronic infections and persistent tissue damage (e.g., cirrhosis) or cancer (e.g., hepatocellular carcinoma) as in Hepatitis B infections. In animals the range of viral infections that cause infection or inflammation of the liver is broad and includes such examples as adenoviruses (infectious canine hepatitis), bunyaviruses (rift valley fever in sheep), and retroviruses (equine infectious anemia). In humans hepatitis is most commonly caused by one of five species of viruses named A, B, C, D, and E. However, as in animals the disease is caused by a variety of viruses with the common trait of hepatic tropism (Table 16.1).

Hepatitis B virus (HBV) is a double-shelled structure. It consists of an inner nucleocapsid core and an outer shell of coat proteins with some associated lipids. During infection, hepatocytes produce virions and also noninfectious subviral structures consisting of the outer surface proteins. Blumberg discovered the subviral particles in the mid 1960s, but the virion was not discovered until the 1970s by Dane. There are 10^4 to 10^6 subviral particles for each virion in the blood. Chronic carriers of the hepatitis B virus who have no overt symptoms can have up to 500 micrograms of total viral surface protein per milliliter of plasma.

HBV is of global importance causing infection of over 250 million people. The virus is the primary agent transmitted by bloodborne routes such as needlestick injuries. Chronic HBV infection may be asymptomatic or result in hepatitis, which occurs in approximately five percent of individuals who acquire the infection, or it may cause hepatocellular carcinoma. Until the 1970s, the virus was difficult to study due to a lack of cell culture systems to propagate the virus and the lack of readily available animal models of the infection. The virus is transmitted by sexual contact and by exposure to the virus in contaminated blood or blood products including transmission from an infected mother to neonates at birth. HBV is a member of hepadnaviridae family of viruses. Other members include woodchuck hepatitis virus, ground squirrel hepatitis virus, and duck hepatitis virus. The other viruses provide some useful animal models of the infection in humans.

The modes of transmission and the nature of the liver disease caused by HBV infection vary from region to region. For example, in Western societies, most infections occur in adults as a result of contact with infectious body fluids such as blood or semen. The infection is common among intravenous drug abusers and among male homosexuals, where it is a common venereal disease. The infections are either inapparent or produce acute hepatitis. Recovery follows production of antibodies to the viral surface antigens. Fulminant acute hepatitis may occur resulting in death but this is rare. In contrast, in the Orient and subSaharan Africa the infections occur in the young. Infants mainly acquire infections from mothers who are chronic carriers of the virus.

Infections in the very young often result in persistence of infection throughout the life span of the individual. In persistently infected people, the virus may replicate in the hepatocytes, may exist in a quiescent episomal state, or may be integrated into the host cell DNA. Integrated viral DNA is frequently incomplete and no longer gives rise to new virus, but may still program production of surface antigens. Persistent infection may be asymptomatic or may cause liver inflammation, which frequently results in liver cirrhosis and, after many years, hepatocellular carcinoma.

Hepadnaviruses replicate their DNA by a complex and unique mechanism involving a virally-encoded DNA polymerase having both DNA-dependent and RNA-dependent polymerase activities (Table 16.1, footnote b). Hepadnaviruses make highly efficient use of their small genome for encoding proteins. Virus particles are found in three forms. "Dane" particles are an infectious form of the virus and are 42–47 nm double-shelled particles. 20 nm spheres are present in 10,000 to 100,000-fold excess over Dane Particles and are composed of HBsAg (see below) and host-derived lipid and are noninfectious. Filaments of 20 nm in diameter and variable length are also composed of HBsAg (see below) and host-derived lipid and are noninfectious.

Hepatitis B surface antigen, (HBsAg) is the common antigen on the surface of each form of the virus particles. HBsAg is found in great excess in infected subjects and therefore is used in diagnostic tests for the virus infection. The major structural core protein (C protein or hepatitis B core antigen) is a 21 kD basic phosphoprotein that contains viral DNA and a polymerase called P protein. The pre-S1-region of the viral genome encodes the L protein. This protein is a minor component of proteins produced, but is an important component of the infectious Dane particle and is important in virus assembly. L proteins are thought to contain receptor recognition domains. The S protein makes up the majority of the HBsAg and is produced in abundance.

The virion genome is DNA (3.2 kb) in a relaxed circular, partially duplex strand. The + strand is shorter and more variable in length than the – strand. The genome is highly compact and every nucleotide is used for coding. HBV has some unusual features in its mode of replication: (1) it uses an RNA intermediate called the pregenomic RNA or pgRNA, (2) it uses a reverse transcriptase to convert pgRNA into viral DNA, (3) it uses a duplex DNA form in its infectious particle, (4) more than one type of virus particle is produced, and (5) it converts the relaxed DNA into a covalent closed circular DNA (cccDNA) in the nucleus prior to transcription. Following attachment and entry the virus DNA is delivered to the nucleus and is converted to cccDNA. This process requires repair of the single strand, removal of the 5' terminal structure consisting of RNA and P protein, and covalent ligation of the strands. HBV has two major classes of transcripts, these are genomic and subgenomic. Each contains multiple members. All are capped, unspliced, and polyadenylated. HBV uses both overlapping reading frames and multiple initiation codons thereby making efficient use of its DNA. The hepadnaviral reverse transcriptase pathway is similar to the process of replication in retroviruses. The process of reverse transcription takes place in the subviral core particles.

People with chronic HBV infections have a 100-fold greater chance of developing hepatocellular carcinoma than do noninfected persons. About eighty-five percent of these tumors have DNA integrated in their genomes. The integrated virus DNA is often highly rearranged and contains deletions. The mechanisms of integration are poorly understood and no integrase enzyme has been shown to be present to do the job. The tumor may be formed by direct or indirect mechanisms.

The first HBV vaccine, consisting of plasma-derived surface antigen particles, cost about $100 per person and was too costly for application on a worldwide scale. The surface antigen particles are now produced more cheaply in cultures of yeast into which the viral surface protein gene has been introduced by recombinant technology. All of the vaccines currently available function by stimulating production of antibodies to viral surface proteins. These antibodies neutralize the virus and promote its phagocytosis.

SELECTED DISEASES ASSOCIATED WITH PERSISTENT VIRAL INFECTIONS
Recurrent Herpes and Epithelial Cell Carcinomas

Herpes simplex viruses are responsible for the recurrent "cold sores" many individuals develop on their lips and for similar sores in the genital region. The introduction of the birth control pill and the relaxation of sexual mores in the United States in the late 1960s ushered in the great herpes epidemic of the 1970s. The herpes simplex viruses have also been implicated in the etiology of several human tumors.

The herpes simplex viruses (HSVs) are large enveloped DNA viruses that are members of the Herpesviridae (Table 16.1). The ability to produce latent infections is a property of all members of the Herpesviridae including cytomegalovirus, varicella-zoster virus, and Epstein-Barr virus. In latent infections, the primary symptoms resulting from virus replication resolve and viral genomes become quiescent and persist in only a few cells. In fact, when quiescent, viral genomes and antigens are extremely difficult to detect in host tissues. In latent infections, the virus occasionally reactivates and new progeny virions are produced. Stress may play a role in viral reactivation. Virus reactivation results in the development of recurrent lesions near the site of the initial infection.

Serological and genetic criteria are used to classify HSVs into the two types which occur, HSV 1 and HSV 2. Viruses of the two serotypes cause lesions in different areas of the body because they infect different nerve ganglia and are transmitted by different forms of contact. HSV 1 is usually transmitted orally, while transmission of HSV 2 is usually venereal. Both viruses can infect and produce lesions in both areas, however.

Primary infection with HSV 1 is generally inapparent; however, fifteen percent of infections result in gingivo-stomatitis, with multiplication of virus in oral mucosal cells. The virus also replicates in regional lymph nodes and may cause viremia and disseminated disease. In some cases, HSV 1 causes fatal encephalitis. This results from spread of virus into the brain cortex where it precipitates inflammatory disease. More often the virus enters peripheral nerve endings in the oral region and migrates to the trigeminal ganglion where it becomes latent. HSV 1 has been implicated as a cause of nasopharyngeal carcinoma. HSV II infects mainly the genital or ano-rectal mucosa and ultimately becomes latent in the sacral ganglion. Generalized herpes infections often occur in children born to women with recurrent genital herpes lesions. There is a higher risk than normal of cervical cancer in women who develop recurrent herpetic lesions on the cervix.

The nucleic acids and nucleocapsids of herpes viruses are assembled in the cell nucleus and bud through the nuclear membrane. They acquire their envelope during budding. The mature virion is not directly cytolytic. It spreads from cell to cell by a process of cell fusion or after release by exocytosis. The recurrent lesions on the oral and genital mucosa result from the host immune response to virus released from neural endings.

Replication of Herpesvirus DNA is a complex process. It involves the formation of four types of DNA isomers and the controlled, sequential expression of viral genes. In the latent state, the viral genome may be an episome or may be partially or entirely integrated into the host genome. Only a very few cells in the ganglia become latently infected, perhaps with as few as one viral genomic equivalent per ten neurons. During latency the majority of the genome is not transcribed into RNA. However, at least one of the genes may be expressed at very low levels. The product of this gene may promote the expression of other viral genes and down-regulate its own activity. It may also regulate function of the infected neuron.

Infectious Mononucleosis and Malignant Lymphomas

"Kissing disease" is one name for an acute illness of adolescents and young adults referred to more correctly as infectious mononucleosis. Lymphadenopathy, mild hepatitis, abnormal mononuclear lymphocytes, and large amounts of heterophile antibodies in the blood characterize the disease. Infectious mononucleosis is caused by the Epstein-Barr virus, a member of the Herpesviridae (Table 16.1). Epstein-Barr virus is transmitted with infectious body fluids, most commonly saliva. The virus is lymphotropic, infecting B cells. Primary infection in early childhood is usually asymptomatic, but thirty to fifty percent of individuals infected in early adolescence develop clinical disease. Most people possess antibodies to Epstein-Barr virus, indicating prior exposure, but only about fifteen percent of seropositive persons shed virus in the saliva.

The virus first infects cells of the buccal mucosa or the salivary glands and then infects B cells in pharyngeal lymphoid tissue. The virus then disseminates to B cells throughout the body. After dissemination the virus may continue to replicate or become latent. Lymphocytes carrying the latent viral genome in episomal form become transformed, or immortalized, and can be propagated in long-term culture. In infected people, the proliferation of transformed B cells is limited in most cases by the host immune response, but latently infected cells that do divide serve as a reservoir for the virus. The host defenses to EBV include the actions of natural killer cells, virus-specific cytotoxic lymphocytes, and antiviral antibodies. Most of the abnormal mononuclear cells present in the blood early in the course of EBV infections are cytotoxic lymphocytes, which specifically kill virus-infected B cells. The Epstein-Barr virus causes polyclonal activation of B cells, which results in production of heterophile antibodies that agglutinate sheep red blood cells. Although during the acute phase of infection there is polyclonal B cell activation and activation of virus specific B cells, there is a transient suppression of cell-mediated immunity to many antigens.

Epstein-Barr virus infection is associated with a high incidence of Burkitt's lymphoma in certain peoples of Africa. Host genetic factors may be responsible for the virus is not always present in people with Burkitt's lymphoma who live in other parts of the world. Generalized lymphomas of various types may develop in immunosuppressed people who carry the Epstein-Barr virus. Burkitt's lymphoma in Africans may therefore be a result of immunosuppression caused by other infections. Malaria is often suggested in this context.

Adult T Cell Leukemia/Lymphoma and HTLV-1-Associated Myelopathy

The first demonstration that a viral agent could induce a tumor occurred in 1908. Ellerman and Bang caused leukemia in healthy chickens by inoculation of a cell-free filtrate of blood from leukemic chickens. Since then, leukemia-, sarcoma-, and carcinoma-inducing viruses have been discovered in a number of species of animals. The virion of the leukemia-inducing viruses contains two copies of plus-stranded RNA. In 1964, Temin showed that specific inhibitors of DNA synthesis blocked the replication of these RNA viruses in cultured cells and proposed that their replication required DNA synthesis.

In 1970 Temin and Baltimore independently demonstrated a virally-encoded enzyme that transcribes RNA into DNA. This enzyme, RNA-dependent DNA polymerase, is a reverse transcriptase. Prior to this, it had generally been accepted that cellular and viral DNA was the template for production of messenger RNA. The only known exception to this pattern occurred in the nontumorigenic RNA viruses, which produced their new genomic RNA on their old genomic RNA and transcribed their messenger RNA by the virus-specific, RNA-dependent RNA polymerase.

The replication process in the RNA tumor viruses is unique. The single-stranded viral RNA template is used to produce an initial DNA-RNA hybrid, which is then converted by DNA polymerase into a double stranded DNA linear intermediate. The DNA intermediate integrates into the host cell DNA and is referred to as a "provirus." The provirus is transcribed into both viral messenger and viral genomic RNA. The RNA viruses containing reverse transcriptase were named the Retroviridae (Table 16.1) in recognition of the retrograde flow of genetic information from RNA into DNA. Retroviruses are known to infect a wide variety of animals, including humans, and are associated with certain types of cancer. They may also induce immunosuppressive or immune-mediated diseases, or may exist as stable members of the host germ line.

The first human retrovirus was isolated in 1980 from a T cell line established from a patient diagnosed with cutaneous T cell lymphoma. In retrospect, it is likely that this original patient suffered from adult T cell leukemia/lymphoma (ATL). Subsequently, the virus was isolated from additional patients in the Caribbean, and in the United States.

Like other retroviruses, HTLV-1 has a genome consisting of two strands of positive sense RNA. The viral RNA is reverse transcribed by a virally encoded RNA-dependent DNA polymerase, a reverse transcriptase, and the resulting double-stranded DNA is randomly integrated into the host cell DNA by means of a virally encoded integrase. In the integrated, proviral form, HTLV-1 is transcribed using cellular pol II and this RNA is then transcribed and proteins are assembled using host cell machinery.

The HTLV-1 provirus consists of two long terminal repeats (LTRs) flanking structural and regulatory genes. Like other exogenous retroviruses, the HTLV-1 provirus encodes for structural proteins (*gag*), viral enzymes (*pol*), and envelope glycoproteins (*env*). The HTLV-1 provirus is typical of complex retroviruses containing regulatory genes in the 3' portion of the genome originally called the X or pX region. Genes in the pX region encode for accessory proteins Tax and Rex, which regulate transcription and RNA transport respectively. Tax, a 40 kD protein encoded by a doubly spliced transcript from ORF IV plays a critical role in transcriptional regulation of both viral and cellular genes involved in lymphocyte proliferation. Rex, a 27 kD phosphoprotein, derived from ORF III, regulates the expression of incompletely spliced viral transcripts encoding enzymatic and structural gene products.

HTLV-1 structural and enzymatic proteins are transcribed from a single, nonspliced genome-length mRNA. The gag gene encodes the structural proteins of HTLV-1. The individual proteins are cleaved from a 55 kDa polyprotein precursor yielding the 19 kDa matrix, 24 kDa capsid, and 15 kDa nucleocapsid proteins. The individual structural proteins are cleaved from the polyprotein precursor by the viral protease. Enzymes coded from the *pol* gene include the Mg^{2+}-dependent reverse transcriptase, integrase and RNase H. Viral *env* gene products are translated from a singly spliced 4.3 kb subgenomic mRNA. These gene products are translated as a 61 to 69 kDa glycoprotein, which is subsequently cleaved into a 46 kDa surface protein (gp46) and a nonglycosylated 21 kDa transmembrane protein (p21).

HTLV-1 is a cell-associated virus and transmission occurs through routes which promote lymphocyte transfer between individuals. These routes include breast-feeding, blood transfusion, sexual contact, and intravenous drug use. In the United States, all blood donated for transfusion is screened for seropositivity to HTLV-1. The majority of persons infected with HTLV-1 are asymptomatic carriers with only one in 1,000–2000 persons developing leukemia after a long latent period. The mean age of onset of the disease is fifty-five years, with a 1.4:1 male to female patient ratio. Clinical manifestations of the acute leukemia include general malaise, fever, cough, dyspnea, lymph node enlargement, hepatosplenomegaly, and jaundice. The prognosis of the leukemia is very poor. Mean survival times range from six to twenty-four months depending upon the clinical subtype.

HTLV-1 is also implicated as the causative agent in the neurological disorder HTLV-1-associated myelopathy (HAM) or tropical spastic paraparesis (TSP). HAM/TSP is a chronic demyelinating disease characterized by weakness and spasticity of the extremities, hyperreflexia, and mild peripheral sensory loss. The pathogenesis of HAM/TSP is not fully understood, but it appears to be distinct from ATL. Development of the myelopathy occurs within several years following infection, whereas development of the leukemia normally requires twenty to thirty years. HTLV-1 provirus is polyclonally integrated in the peripheral blood cells of HAM/TSP patients as opposed to mono or oligoclonally integrated with ATL. There are approximately three-times more infected cells in HAM/TSP patients than in asymptomatic carriers, and there are also higher titers of anti-HTLV-1 antibodies in the serum and CSF. It has been suggested that HAM/TSP is an autoimmune disease resulting from immune dysregulation. HTLV-1-infected patients exhibit an increased incidence of a variety of immune-mediated disorders. However, these disorders are less clearly associated with HTLV-1 than ATL and HAM/TSP.

Acquired Immunodeficiency Syndrome

The present AIDS epidemic is a complex phenomenon. Jaffe and coworkers first described the acquired immunodeficiency syndrome in 1981. These physicians observed that sexually active, young adult male homosexuals frequently developed an unusually aggressive Kaposi's sarcoma, normally a rare disease in people of this age group. They also observed many opportunistic infections of types that occur in people in an immunosuppressed state. The syndrome also occurred occasionally in people who had received transfusions, in hemophiliacs, and in intravenous drug users. Evidence accumulated rapidly between 1981 and early 1983 suggesting that an infectious agent was involved, most likely a virus. In May of 1983, a group at the Pasteur Institute in France headed by Montagnier and Chermann published a paper in which they described finding a new retrovirus in a patient with a lymphadenopathy of a type that frequently occurs in patients who will develop AIDS. The virus was called lymphadenopathy-associated virus (LAV) and was eventually shown to be the causative agent of AIDS. The virus is a member of the Retroviridae and is closely related to retroviruses of the lentivirus subgroup, which includes Visna virus of sheep. The AIDS virus has been referred to by many names (e.g., LAV, HTLV-III, ARV) but was officially named human immunodeficiency virus (HIV) in 1986. At present, two viruses, called HIV-1 and HIV-2, are considered to cause AIDS in man. In practice this genus includes numerous viral strains because of the ability of the virus to undergo successive mutations and evolve into new and often more virulent strains.

HIV-1 probably arose in central African and has spread from there to other parts of the world. HIV-2 is presently endemic mostly in West Africa. Most HIV infections occur as a result of unprotected sexual contacts. Injection of contaminated blood and blood products are also a cause of infection. Infection in intravenous drug users results from use of needles contaminated with infected blood. The screening of blood for antibodies to HIV by serologic tests has reduced the frequency of infection in people requiring transfusions.

Following infection, there is a long incubation period. Usually eight to ten years may pass before the development of disease; however, during this time, the virus can still be transmitted. The human immunodeficiency virus is transmitted as free virus or as cell-associated virus; this usually requires that contaminated blood or semen be introduced into the bloodstream of the person at risk. HIV is not transmitted by casual contact with an infected individual.

The envelope of HIV, like that of all retroviruses, consists of a lipid envelope, SU, and TM components. The viral envelope is derived by budding from the cell membrane during the process of viral assembly. The envelope proteins form a dimeric or oligomeric complex held together by nonconvalent interactions, as well as by disulfide bonds. The surface envelope proteins (SU) are the largest proteins in the virus and are externally located. They are the receptors that specifically bind to the cell surface receptor of the target cell such as T cells and macrophages. Variable domains of the SU protein are important as they bring about virus-cell fusion, cytopathic effects, and determine the cell tropism of the virus. The transmembrane protein (TM) is smaller than the SU protein and spans the membrane of the viral particle. Virus fusion to the cell membrane occurs via a series of conformational steps. The gp120 SU protein binds the virus to the CD4 D1 domain. The complex with cellular proteases undergoes a conformational change to form a fusion domain from the leucine zipper domains and the fusion peptide of the transmembrane protein. The fusion domain thus formed inserts into the cell membrane to allow penetration of the host cell.

Chemokine receptors have been identified on cells and are important in that they aid entry of HIV in certain cell types. The first of these coreceptor proteins on host cells was initially called "fusin" and brought about fusion of CD4+ cells that were resistant to fusion and syncytial formation. Fusin (CXCR-4) is a member of a family of chemokine receptors. Recent studies indicate that macrophage-tropic viruses use CC chemokine 5 (CCR-5) as a principal coreceptor and to a lesser degree CCR-3. T cell-tropic viruses can employ CXCR-4. Persons with mutations changing the nature of these coreceptors may be protected from HIV infection or have a slower rate of progression to AIDS. Other receptors for HIV include galactosyl ceramide in glial cells and in some colon cell lines, Fc Receptors, and adhesion molecules on macrophages. These receptors may promote entry into key body sites such as the brain.

After the virus enters the cell, the virus integrates a copy of its provirus into the host genome and maintains a relatively constant and in some cases high level of replication. However, in some persons the virus may remain latent until the host cell is activated or stimulated to divide, usually by exposure to antigens and cytokines.

Human immunodeficiency virus has been transmitted to the chimpanzee, but disease has not occurred in animals of this species. Disease-producing lentiviruses have been identified that infect simians and felines. The pathology of the diseases produced in these animals is being studied in an attempt to obtain knowledge possibly useful in control of the human infection. Through massive research efforts and the application of new biotechnology, HIV has become one of the most studied and characterized viral agents.

The virus causes disease by a variety of actions disrupting normal cell processes. The virus replicates in activated or dividing host cells and, in the case of T cells, may lead to syncytium formation and cell death by lysis or programmed cell death (i.e., apoptosis). The eventual depletion of CD4+ helper cells leads to immunodeficiency, thus permitting opportunistic infections. A severe, often fatal pneumonia caused by *Pneumocystis carnii* a microorganism not usually associated with disease in immunocompetent hosts, is common in AIDS patients. Other common diseases in AIDS patients include diarrhea, thrush (caused by *Candida albicans*) tuberculosis, an endothelial cell cancer, Kaposi's sarcoma, and malignant B cell lymphomas.

Ongoing vaccine trials and newly developed antiviral drug combinations offer hope for the control of the AIDS epidemic in the future. However, until these research efforts produce a "magic" bullet such as an effective vaccine that clearly and easily controls HIV infection the application of well-established public and private preventative health measures to control the spread of the infection is our best hope for controlling the epidemic. These include public education about the best means to prevent the infection such as the proper use of condoms.

SUMMARY
Viruses are obligate intracellular parasites made up of small packets of protein and nucleic acid. The primary function of the virus particle is to initiate an infection and promote the replication of more virions by exploiting the host cell. Viruses have no innate ability to generate energy, so they must rely totally on the metabolic machinery of host cells. Their genomes are made up of either DNA or RNA strands that serve as a template to make copies of it and to produce new viral proteins. Thus, the viral genetic information in the host cell determines the outcome of the virus-cell interaction. The structural proteins surrounding viral genomes are arranged in one of two symmetrical forms called capsids that are either helical or icosahedral in shape. The simplest animal viruses are naked icosahedral viruses. The other major forms of viruses are the enveloped isosahedral viruses. In general, viruses are very efficient and accomplish replication with relatively fewer proteins then are required by cellular genomes. Viruses are classified into a variety of families based on morphologic, structural, and genetic characteristics, including the size, structure, and type of their nucleic acid. Most viruses associated with disease do so by causing disruption of normal cell functions or processes. Particular problems are created by persistent viral infections which may cause tissue injury by promoting inflammatory processes in infected tissues. The diagnosis of viral infections is accomplished in part by tests that detect the presence of virions or their components, or tests that detect antibodies against the viral agent. Once diagnosed viral infections can be treated providing the antiviral drugs used against the infection are active against virus-specific targets, such as viral enzymes and regulatory proteins but not against host cell systems. Immunization remains an important strategy against virus-induced diseases. Improvement in vaccine development, in knowledge of general

mechanisms of how viruses cause disease and even of basic cell function can be obtained by the careful study of virus-host cell interaction in individuals infected with viral diseases.

SUGGESTIONS FOR FURTHER READING

1. Evans, A.S., and R.A. Kaslow. *Viral Infections of Humans: Epidemiology and Control*. 4th ed. New York, NY, Plenum Medical Publishing Corporation, 1997.
2. Fields, B.N., D.M. Knipe, and P.M. Howley. *Fields Virology*. 3rd ed. Philadelphia, PA, Lippincott-Raven Publishers, 1996.
3. Mims, C.A., N.J. Dimmock, A. Nash, and J. Stephen. *Mims' Pathogenesis of Infectious Disease*. 4th ed. San Diego, CA, Academic Press, Harcourt Brace and Company, 1995.
4. Fenner, F.J., E.P.J. Gibbs, F.A. Murphy, R. Rott, M.J. Studdert, and D.O. White. *Veterinary Virology*, 2nd ed. San Diego, CA, Academic Press Inc., 1993.

QUESTIONS

1. Viruses are obligate intracellular parasites? True or False.
2. How were viruses originally discovered?
3. Describe the simplest morphologic forms that viruses may take?
4. Name types of serologic assays used in the diagnosis of viral infections
5. Why are antiviral drugs difficult to produce?
6. Name a mechanism that a cell may use to combat a viral infection.
7. Name two components of the immune response that combat viral infections.
8. What is meant by the term antigenic shift in relationship to influenza infection?
9. What virus family does the etiologic agent that causes measles belong to?
10. What are the etiologic agents of adult T cell leukemia and of AIDS?
11. How does AZT interfere with the replication of the AIDS virus?
12. Name a key property of herpesviruses that allows them to produce persistent virus infections?

ANSWERS

1. True. Viruses require the host cell for their replication.
2. By reproducing diseases of plants or animals by injection of materials that were able to pass through filters which eliminated larger organisms such as bacteria.
3. The simplest virus particles consist of a rodlike helix or coil of DNA or RNA associated with proteins that are either helical or icosahedral in shape. Some are contained in envelopes derived from the host cell.
4. ELISA, IFA, Western blot.
5. Antiviral drugs used against the infection must be active against virus-specific targets, such as viral enzymes and regulatory proteins but not against host cell systems.
6. The production of interferons, is one but not the only mechanism.
7. Production of antibodies against viral antigens and cell-mediated immune mechanisms.
8. The genome of the infuenza virus may undergo reassortment and thereby produce a new antigenic strain capable of evading the immune system or causing more virulent disease.
9. Paramyxoviridae

10. Adult T cell leukemia is caused by human T cell lymphotropic virus (also called human T cell leukemia virus or HTLV-1). AIDS is caused by human immunodeficiency virus, abbreviated HIV.
11. AZT interferes with the process of reverse transcription which is necessary for the virus to replicate.
12. They establish latency in the genome of cells of the nervous system and are not eliminated from there by the immune response against the virus.

The Parasitic Protozoa and Helminth Worms

F.E.G. Cox

OUTLINE
INTRODUCTION
PARASITIC PROTOZOA
  Immunity to Intestinal
    Protozoa
  Intestinal Amoebae
  Intestinal Flagellates
  Intestinal Coccidians
  Protozoa Inhabiting the
    Urinogenital Tract
  Blood-Inhabiting Protozoa
  African Trypanosomes
  New World Trypanosomes
  Malaria
  Toxoplasmosis
  Microsporidians
PARASITIC NEMATODES
  Ascaridid Worms
  Hookworms
  Trichinosis
  Filarial Worms
  Lymphatic Filariasis
  Onchocerciasis
PARASITIC TREMATODES
  (FLUKES)
  Schistosomes (Blood
    Flukes)
CESTODES (TAPEWORMS)
  Pork Tapeworm
  Beef Tapeworm
  Echinococcus Granulosus
    (Hydatid Cyst)
  Fish or Broad Tapeworm
SUMMARY
SUGGESTIONS FOR
  FURTHER READING
QUESTIONS

OUTLINE

Parasitic protozoa and helminth worms cause some of the most intractable diseases mainly in the tropics and subtropics where they affect over half the world's population. The parasites that cause these diseases are highly evolved eukaryotes with complex life cycles often involving a number of stages that are physiologically, biochemically, and antigenically distinct and therefore present difficult targets for immunological recognition and attack. In addition, parasites have evolved a number of ways to evade the hosts' immune responses. The net result is that parasites typically cause long-lasting and chronic infections often accompanied by severe immunopathological changes brought about by the host's often futile attempts to bring the ongoing infection under control. The complexity of the immune response, coupled with the inevitable accompanying immunopathology, makes it difficult to develop immunization strategies and, to date, there is no vaccine against any parasitic infection of humans. As no two parasites evoke exactly the same kind of immune response it is necessary to consider each parasite and the responses to it separately in the quest for ways to prevent infection and to ameliorate the immunological damage caused.

INTRODUCTION

The term parasitism describes any relationship between two organisms in which one lives at the expense of the other and includes infections caused by prions, viruses, bacteria, fungi, protozoa, and helminth worms. However, the word parasite itself is normally only used when referring to the eukaryotes, protozoa and helminths. Protozoa are small single-celled organisms mostly measuring 1–10 μm. Helminth worms are much larger multicellular organisms, measuring 100 μm to 1000 μm or more. Humans are particularly susceptible to infections with parasites and over fifty species of protozoa belonging to twenty genera and over 350 species of helminths belonging to over fifty genera have been recorded from humans. The most important protozoa causing disease in humans fall into one of four major groups: the amoebae (Sarcodina), the flagellates (Mastigophora), the sporozoans (Sporozoa or Apicomplexa), and the microsporidians (Microspora). The parasitic helminths are found among the round worms (Nematodes) and the flatworms (Platyhelminthes) which are either tapeworms (Cestodes) or flukes (Trematodes). All of the organisms commonly called parasites, being eukaryotes, more closely resemble their mammalian hosts biochemically and physiologically than do bacteria and viruses. This presents problems when designing chemotherapeutic compounds and emphasizes the need for vaccines which, so far, have not been forthcoming.

Parasitic protozoa and helminth worms are major causes of mortality and morbidity worldwide although their effects are greatest in the tropics and subtropics where they affect over half the world's population. In addition, some also pose an increasing threat to those suffering from HIV infections anywhere in the world. Parasites cause some of the most important human diseases such as malaria and schistosomiasis, which together afflict over 500 million people in the tropics, and ascariasis that affects some 900 million people worldwide. Parasitic diseases are difficult to control because they often cause long and debilitating infections, largely as a result of the inability of the immune system to keep them in check.

All parasitic infections are accompanied by immune responses which are partially protective but can also cause pathological damage. In order to understand the immune responses involved in parasitic infections, it is best, in the first instance, not to consider them as protozoa and helminths but as microparasites and macroparasites. Protozoa, like viruses and bacteria, are microparasites, which are small and multiply within their vertebrate host, typically causing an infection characterized by a latent period during which the parasites multiply, a period of overt infection, a period of recovery during which the immune response brings the infection under control and, finally, long-term resistance to reinfection. Helminth worms are macroparasites, which are relatively large and do not multiply within their vertebrate hosts. However, the host must protect itself from large infections and reinvasion by infective stages and does so by mounting an immune response that may not be effective against the established worms but does prevent reinfection. Immune responses to protozoa and helminths are, therefore, very different from one another but do have a great deal in common usually being very long lasting and, over a period of years, inducing immunopathological changes that may be more dangerous than the infection itself. This is because parasites have complex life cycles involving stages that are antigenically distinct, occupy different sites in the host and have evolved mechanisms for evading the immune response. In most cases the infection is partially controlled, but if the antigenic stimulus is not removed, the host continues to mount increasingly complex immune responses, some of which may be counterproductive and which the host may try to avoid by damping down the immune response. Parasitic infections are therefore typically long and chronic and accompanied by immunopathological changes and periods of immunodepression to superimposed antigens.

Although the immune responses to parasites are complex, the individual components are relatively simple and are in accordance with the normal rules of immunology and involve the four arms of the immune response, cytotoxic T cells, natural killer (NK) cells, activated macrophages, and antibody, the first three often called cell-mediated immunity and the last humoral immunity. Cytotoxic T cells are seldom involved in parasitic infections. The elucidation of the Th1/Th2 paradigm, roughly corresponding to cell-mediated (Th1) and humoral (Th2) immunity, discussed in chapters 8 and 9, has permitted a detailed dissection of the immune responses in parasitic infections and a vast amount of information about the cytokines involved in these infections has accumulated in recent years. In general, Th1 responses, involving the activation of macrophages by IFN-γ, play a central role in immunity to many parasites in contrast to the central role played by cytotoxic T cells in viral infections and antibodies in bacterial infections. A number of toxic molecules are produced by activated macrophages and these include reactive oxygen intermediates and nitric oxide (NO) that may be involved, directly or indirectly, in parasite killing. Small parasites may be phagocytosed and destroyed internally by these toxic molecules, but, as they are also secreted extracellularly, they can also destroy larger parasites in the vicinity of activated macrophages, especially if the macrophage is bound to the parasite via an antibody bridge. However, these molecules can also damage host cells and their release in excess is a major cause of immunopathology. The balance between Th1 and Th2 responses is absolutely crucial in most parasitic infections.

Antibodies are involved in immunity against parasites by blocking binding to host cells and by neutralization, agglutination, complement activation, and opsonization. IgA protects the mucous surfaces of the gut and respiratory tract and inhibits invasion by agglutinating the parasites or blocking attachment to host cells. IgG and IgM cause agglutination, block entry into cells, and initiate complement mediated lysis. IgE, which is responsible for allergies, is also involved in immunity to helminth infections and a characteristic of such infections is an elevation of IgE levels accompanied by pronounced eosinophilia.

PARASITIC PROTOZOA
Immunity to Intestinal Protozoa
A number of organisms including viruses, bacteria, protozoa, and helminth worms inhabit the gastrointestinal tract. Normally, the mucus layer passively protects the underlying cells from invasion, and there is also a specialized mucosal immune system that provides a first line of defense. However, once an organism has broken through these intestinal defenses it becomes subject to attack by other components of the immune system. Thus, protozoa that merely inhabit the gut do not normally evoke an immune response but can do so if in close apposition to, or between, the cells of the gut wall.

Intestinal Amoebae
Entamoeba histolytica is the only amoeba of clinical importance. It is generally agreed that there are both virulent and avirulent strains of *E. histolytica*. Most infections are due to avirulent strains which, in otherwise healthy individuals, do not result in overt disease. Strains that are virulent can cause amoebic dysentery. The amoeba occurs in two forms, trophozoite and cyst. The term trophozoite refers to any motile and feeding stage of a protozoan and in this case is synonymous with the amoebic form. *Entamoeba histolytica* trophozoites, which are 16–30 μm in diameter and possess a single nucleus, are found only in liquid or semiliquid stools. The cyst, which is the resistant form of the organism, is a round thick-walled structure 5–20

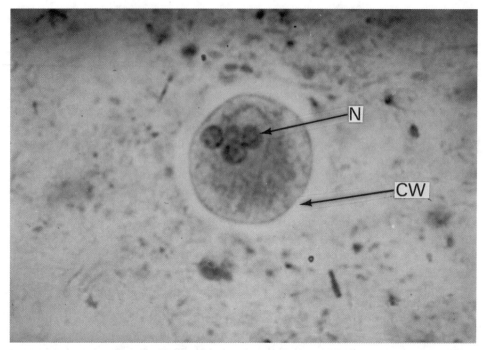

Figure 17.1. An *Entamoeba histolytica* cyst. The mature cyst has four nuclei (N) and a thick cyst wall (CW) that protects it when outside the host.

μm in diameter (Figure 17.1) and is passed in formed stools. The life cycle is simple. Mature cysts, when ingested, excyst in the small intestine giving rise to eight trophozoites that live on the colonic mucosa feeding on desquamated cells and bacteria. Some however may invade the mucosa and after proliferation cause the formation of flask-shaped ulcers (Figure 17.2) causing an infection that is clinically manifest as bloody diarrhea. In some cases the amoebae penetrate the submucosa and disseminate throughout the body. The liver is the organ most commonly involved; such invasion may give rise to multiple or single liver abscesses. Secondary lesions in other organs such as the lungs and brain also occur. The mechanism leading to cytopathology appears to involve three steps. The first is adherence of virulent amoeba to the host cell mediated by an interaction between a lectin on the surface of the amoeba and the appropriate carbohydrate on the target cell membrane. This is followed by a cytocidal process, involving the release by the amoeba of a protein, called an amoebapore, that forms transmembrane pores in the target cell and thus disrupts the cation gradients essential for cell viability. Finally, the lysed cell can be phagocytosed by the amoeba. Most strains of *E. histolytica* are nonpathogenic and live as harmless commensals in the large intestine where they do not elicit any immune response. Immune responses, characterized by the production of specific antibodies, can only be detected after invasion. There is no evidence that recovery from infection induces any protection against subsequent infections, and at the population level, there is no age-dependent decrease in prevalence that could be due to the acquisition of immunity. The absence of acquired immunity may be due to the fact that the amoebae have evolved a number of ways of evading the humoral immune response including the degradation of secretory IgA, resistance to complement lysis, and the redistribution or shedding of surface

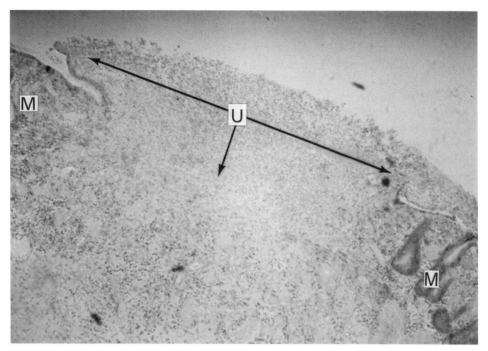

Figure 17.2. Section of intestinal mucosa (M) showing a typical ulcer (U) caused by infection with invasive forms of *Entamoeba histolytica*.

antigens. The role of cellular immune responses is unclear, and there is some evidence that the amoebae can destroy cells of the immune system, as described previously, and this might contribute to the ability of these parasites to evade the immune response. In conclusion, there is little evidence that humans mount an effective immune response against *E. histolytica*. Nevertheless, the fact that recurrences of amoebic ulcers are rare may call for a reappraisal of this statement. It is not known for certain whether or not there is any correlation between amoebiasis and HIV.

Intestinal Flagellates

Giardia lamblia, also known as *Giardia duodenalis* or *Giardia intestinalis*, is usually considered to be a harmless commensal of the small intestine, but it can cause malabsorption and severe diarrhea. Evidence for acquired immunity is circumstantial, but there is usually spontaneous clearance and resistance to reinfection. Epidemiological studies indicate that those living in endemic areas are less affected than visitors, the young are more affected than adults and immunodepressed individuals tend to experience long chronic infections. Secretory IgA is the most characteristic *Giardia*-specific antibody in patients with acute giardiasis, but there is little direct evidence of any IgA antiparasitic effects although specific antibodies occur in human milk and saliva and breast-fed infants in endemic areas seem to acquire some protection. Overall immunity to giardiasis seems to be similar to immunity to a number of bacterial infections in which secretory IgA in breast milk protects the newborn infant until it can produce its own IgA. IgA probably prevents attachment to the villi. *Giardia lamblia* can undergo antigenic variation, but it is not known how this might affect the acquisition of immunity to this parasite. There have been reports of giardiasis in AIDS patients, but this infection is not a major concomitant of HIV infections.

LIVERPOOL
JOHN MOORES UNIVERSITY
AVRIL ROBARTS LRC
TEL. 0151 231 4022

Although the human alimentary canal is parasitized by a number of other flagellates, *Chilomastix mesnili, Dientamoeba fragilis, Trichomonas gingivalis,* and *T. hominis,* these are not normally regarded as important pathogens and virtually nothing is known about any immunological responses to them.

Intestinal Coccidians

Coccidia are important sporozoan infections causing a condition known as coccidiosis in farmed animals, especially fowl bred under conditions of intensive rearing. Humans are infected with three intestinal coccidians *Cryptosporidium parvum, Isospora belli,* and *Cyclospora cayetanensis,* but little is known about the immune responses to any of these. Cryptosporidiosis is an increasingly important disease that is self-limiting and characterized by mild to severe watery diarrhea in healthy individuals but is more persistent and severe and may cause death in AIDS patients. Specific antibodies are found in the serum of infected individuals but nothing is known about their possible relevance.

Protozoa Inhabiting the Urinogenital Tract

Trichomonas vaginalis is the only protozoan that inhabits the human urinogenital tract of men and women in whom it causes vaginitis, an important sexually transmitted disease that persists for long periods unless treated. Epidemiological evidence indicates that prevalence of trichomoniasis does not fall off in older women suggesting that there is little or no acquired immunity. However, secretory IgA antibodies to *T. vaginalis* occur in vaginal secretions but diminish with time and do not appear to protect against reinfection. The reasons why there appear to be no immunity are not clear. *T. vaginalis* has considerable antigenic diversity but whether or not it is capable of antigenic variation is not known.

Blood-Inhabiting Protozoa

Some of the most important protozoan parasites inhabit the human bloodstream. These are the African trypanosomes (*Trypanosoma brucei gambiense* and *T. b. rhodesiense*), the South American trypanosome (*Trypanosoma cruzi*), the malaria parasites (*Plasmodium falciparum, P. malariae, P. ovale,* and *P. vivax*), and occasional infections with *Babesia* spp.

African Trypanosomes

The African trypanosomes, *Trypanosoma brucei gambiense* and *T. b. rhodesiense,* are both subspecies related to *T. b. brucei,* a trypanosome of wildlife and domesticated animals that does not infect humans. The trypanosomes are slender flagellates approximately 3 by 15–32 μm in size. The flagellum arises from a unique DNA-rich organelle, the kinetoplast, and runs the length of the cell body attached to it by an undulating membrane (Figure 17.3). The life cycle involves two hosts, a tsetse fly, *Glossina* spp., and a mammalian host. Trypanosomes in the blood of the mammalian host are taken up by the tsetse fly while feeding, multiplication takes place in the midgut, and the trypanosomes undergo various transformations culminating in the production of metacyclic trypomastigotes in the salivary glands from which they are passed to another mammalian host when feeding. Trypanosomes first multiply in the tissues at the site of the bite, and there may be an initial inflammatory response, but generally the patient remains asymptomatic for several weeks or months. As the trypanosomes proliferate in the blood vessels and lymphatics,

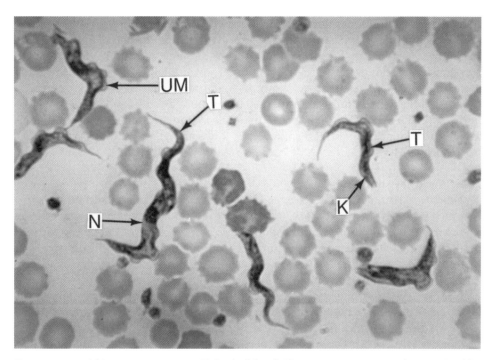

Figure 17.3. African trypanosomes (T) in the blood. The trypanosomes are characterized by the presence of a nucleus (N), kinetoplast (K), and undulating membrane (UM).

the host develops a fever and rash. Meanwhile, the immune system is stimulated and antibodies to the surface antigens of the trypanosome are elicited, and these bring about a drastic reduction in the trypanosome population. However, after about a week, the trypanosome population has again risen and new antibodies appear and the trypanosome population again diminishes, a process that may be repeated numerous times. Eventually some trypanosomes invade the central nervous system leading to coma and death. The antigen to which the antibodies are produced is called the variable surface glycoprotein (VSG), a thick layer covering the entire trypanosome membrane. As antibodies specific for the particular VSG appear, they result in the elimination of about ninety-nine percent of the trypanosome population. Among the remaining one percent, however, some trypanosomes have switched on another VSG gene so that their VSG coat is not recognized by the antibody elicited by the first wave of parasites. As trypanosomes with the new VSG variant proliferate, the immune system is again stimulated, this time to produce antibody that recognizes the new VSG variant. Again the vast majority of the population is eliminated and parasites with yet another VSG specificity are selected out. Current evidence suggests that trypanosomes possess several hundred distinct VSG genes and that these in turn can be recombined to produce an even larger array of VSG specificities. Only one VSG can be expressed at a time, but the precise mechanisms involved in switching from one gene to another are not known. Suffice it to say that these organisms have evolved an extraordinarily effective means of circumventing the host's immune defenses. Evasion of the immune response is also brought about by the parasite's ability to resist complement lysis and to induce a state of immunodepression at least in animal models. Little is known about the acquisition of immunity to trypanosomes in humans, but there is epidemiological evidence that some immunity does develop, albeit slowly, in human populations. The main antibody involved in trypanosome infections is IgM, and the actual killing mechanism involves agglutinating antibodies, lysis, and phagocytosis. The destruction of trypanosomes results in the release of numerous antigens, and toxic factors that circulate in the body giving rise to immune complex-mediated damage. In experimental animals, infection is accompanied by immunodepression to superimposed antigens, but it is not clear what the situation is in humans, whether or not there is any immunodepression and, if so, whether it has any affect on intercurrent infections such as HIV.

New World Trypanosomes

Trypanosoma cruzi, which infects over 150 species of mammals including humans, in which it causes Chagas disease, is confined to South and Central America where it affects some 18 million people. The infection, which is one of the most insidious of all the parasitic diseases, is transmitted by biting bugs and is typically acquired in childhood. The victim usually experiences little more than a localized swelling and fever although in some individuals the infection may be acute and life-threatening. The trypanosomes divide at the site of the bite and circulate briefly in the blood before entering macrophages in which they survive by escaping from the phagolysosome and multiplying in the cytoplasm. Eventually, they escape from the macrophage and invade muscle, particularly cardiac muscle, and nerve cells. The infection is typically lifelong and chronic and accompanied by the gradual destruction of the infected cells giving rise to cardiac failure and loss of control of the digestive system later in life, possibly twenty to thirty or more years later. The mechanisms of pathogenesis involve the autoimmune destruction of host cells, but whether this is initiated by antigens of host or parasite origin is still not known, but some antigens are shared by the parasite and host neural cells and cardiac cells. It might be to the advantage of the parasite to mimic host cells in order to avoid immune recognition, but the inevitable outcome of the possession of shared antigens is autoimmunity which is characteristic of this infection.

Macrophages activated by interferon-gamma represent a major defense mechanism against *T. cruzi*, but the parasite is to a certain extent capable of evading macrophage attack by escaping from the phagolysosome, and the parasites themselves produce a number of products that inhibit the immune response.

Because of the autoimmune component of the immune response to *T. cruzi*, there is little prospect of a vaccine against this infection.

Malaria

Malaria is one of the most important parasitic diseases in the tropics and subtropics where it affects some 350–500 million people killing 2-3 million annually, mostly children in subSaharan Africa. Humans harbor four species, *Plasmodium falciparum*, *P. vivax*, *P. malariae*, and *P. ovale* in order of clinical importance. Several other species infect primates, birds, and reptiles, and there is a high degree of species specificity. The life cycles are complex. While feeding, an infected mosquito injects saliva containing the sporozoites (Figure 17.4A) that travel via the blood to the liver where they enter the hepatocytes and divide by merogony, also called schizogony, a form of division in which the nucleus divides repeatedly, and the cytoplasm becomes partitioned about each nucleus (Figure 17.4B). The end result of this form of multiplication is a meront (schizont), a collection of daughter cells which, on cell rupture, are released

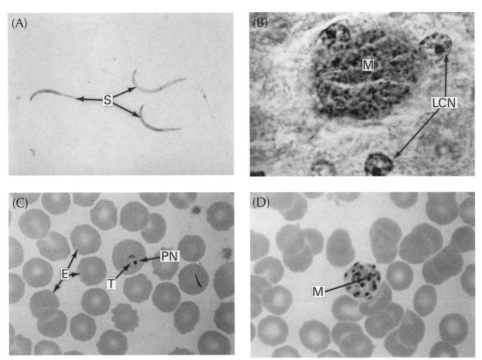

Figure 17.4.   Stages in the life cycle of a malaria parasite *Plasmodium* spp. (A) Sporozoites, the stages injected by an infected mosquito when it bites. (B) Mature exoerythrocytic meront (schizont) in the liver; liver cell nuclei are indicated as LCN. (C) Early (ring) stage of a malaria parasite clearly showing the parasite nucleus (PN) in a newly invaded red blood cell. Uninfected red blood cells are indicated E. (D) Mature erythrocytic meront (schizont) with fully formed merozoites (M) in a red blood cell.

as merozoites into the circulation where they invade erythrocytes. The merozoites attach to the erythrocyte membrane which then invaginates causing the parasite to be internalized within a vacuole where it first becomes a trophozoite before another cycle of merogony occurs (Figure 17.4C,D). Each cycle takes about forty-eight hours for completion, seventy-two hours in the case of *P. malariae*, and results in the production of about eight to sixteen merozoites. Unless multiple infections occur, the erythrocytic cycles remain in phase, and the new merozoites are released from all the infected erythrocytes at about the same time. Toxins liberated during this process trigger the episodes of chills and fever associated with malaria (the paroxysm). After several asexual cycles, some of the merozoites differentiate into male and female gametocytes. If the infected individual is bitten by an uninfected mosquito, the gametocytes are ingested with the blood meal and mature into the male and female gametes, and fertilization occurs in the mosquito's stomach. The resultant zygote differentiates into an ookinete which passes to the external surface of the stomach wall were it becomes an oocyst within which a further cycle of multiplication occurs resulting in the production of many elongated sporozoites. The sporozoites migrate to the mosquito's salivary glands from which they are transmitted to another individual at the next feeding. In the case of *P. vivax*, some of the parasites in the liver may remain dormant and are later stimulated to complete their life cycle and give rise to a new batch of merozoites. Such relapses can occur repeatedly over a period of several years after the initial infection.

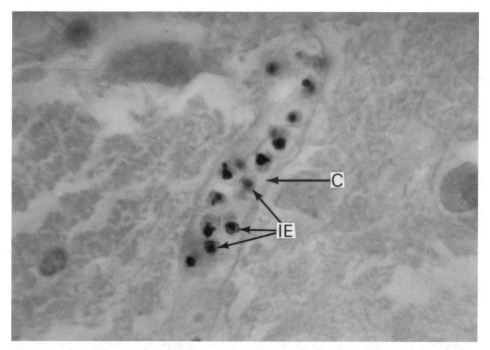

Figure 17.5. Postmortem section of the brain from a case of cerebral malaria showing infected erythrocytes (IE) of the malaria parasites, *Plasmodium falciparum*, blocking a capillary (C).

Infection with *P. falciparum* is associated with higher case-fatality rates than are infections with other *Plasmodium* species. The severe clinical manifestations frequently seen in *P. falciparum* infections are due in part to the sequestration of infected erythrocytes in the capillary bed. Erythrocytes infected with older *P. falciparum* trophozoites and meronts exhibit electron-dense knobs on their surfaces. These knobs bind to venous endothelial cells resulting in the sequestration of infected cells in the capillaries of the heart, lung, kidney, spleen, and, most importantly, the brain (Figure 17.5). This phenomenon is responsible for the fact that, contrary to the situation in *P. vivax*, *P. falciparum* meronts are rarely found in blood smears.

The spleen plays an important role in the host's defense, and splenectomy can markedly diminish the host's ability to control the infection. The exact role of the spleen is unknown, but it has been suggested that it may be involved in the clearance of infected erythrocytes from the circulation.

Susceptibility to malaria is genetically determined. Negroes are usually more resistant to *P. vivax* than are people of other racial groups because they lack a molecule on the red cell required by *P. vivax* merozoites for penetration into erythrocytes. Individuals with sickle hemoglobin are more resistant to *P. falciparum* infection than are individuals without the sickle cell trait, and persons with glucose-6-phosphate dehydrogenase deficiency and thalassemia are likewise more resistant to *P. falciparum*. This could account for the prevalence of these genetic variants in geographic areas endemic for *P. falciparum*.

The immunology of malaria has been extensively studied, and it is known that there is a gradual build up of immunity over a period of many years. However, this immunity quickly fades and is largely strain specific. Immunity to malaria can, therefore, be considered to be the rule although it is often incomplete and may take many years and numerous exposures to the bite of infected mosquitoes to develop. The malaria parasite is relatively free from attack while it is intracellular, so the only stages that are susceptible are the sporozoites circulating in the blood, merozoites liberated from the liver into the bloodstream before they invade the red blood cell, and merozoites released from red blood cells. Sporozoites are obvious targets for immune attack. The sporozoite possesses an immunodominant protein surface coat, called the circumsporozoite protein (CSP) that elicits a strong antibody response. However when exposed to antibody, the surface molecules cross-link and the sporozoite sheds the coat and escapes. It is now thought that the shedding of the coat may be a mechanism enabling the parasite to evade the immune response by putting up a powerful 'smoke screen' that deflects the response away from more important targets. Once in the liver, the parasite is relatively safe from immune attack, but there is evidence that there is a cytotoxic T cell response to the early stages in the liver, and this might reduce the number of meronts that subsequently develop.

The erythrocytic stages are responsible for the disease and they are obvious targets for attack, and many of the antigens involved have been characterized and cloned. A number of important antigens vary between strains of parasites and some undergo antigenic variation so it is very difficult for the host to mount an effective immune response. The actual mechanisms involved in immunity are not at all clear but seem to involve the inhibition of erythrocyte invasion by merozoites. The sexual stages are also very important, as they are susceptible to antibody attack when they are taken up by a mosquito together with antibodies in the serum, and this reduces subsequent transmission.

A major problem in malaria is that all the stages in the life cycle are antigenically distinct, and the acquisition of immunity involves a number of separate processes that must be controlled in terms of place, magnitude, and duration. Much of the pathology is associated with misdirected immune responses, for example, some of the symptoms of cerebral malaria are caused by macrophage products elicited as part of the immune response, and these cause blockage and sludging of blood in capillaries and affect the signalling pathways in the brain leading to coma and other cerebral symptoms. Macrophage products are also probably involved in the hypoglycemia and anemia associated with malaria.

The control of malaria would be facilitated if a vaccine against malaria could be developed, but despite a vast amount of effort, we still do not have a vaccine mainly because, as pointed out above, the malaria life cycle is very complex and includes a number of biochemically and immunologically distinct stages. Possible targets for vaccines are shown in Figure 17.6. Sporozoites are obvious targets, as they are the first stage to enter the body, and a vaccine would prevent infection by blocking the next stage in the liver. Part of the circumsporozoite protein (CSP) of the sporozoite has been used in recombinant and synthetic vaccines, but despite promising early trials, the CSP on its own has not turned out to be a good vaccine candidate. There is currently some interest in vaccines against the forms in the liver, but these are only at the experimental stage. Blood stages are also potential targets because they cause the disease. Several *P. falciparum* antigens are currently being considered as candidate vaccines, but the only vaccine that has undergone extensive field trials is SPf66 developed by the Colombian biochemist Manuel Patarroyo. Spf66, a synthetic vaccine consisting of a polymer of three merozoite antigens, was approved by the World Health Organization (WHO) and has undergone extensive trials in

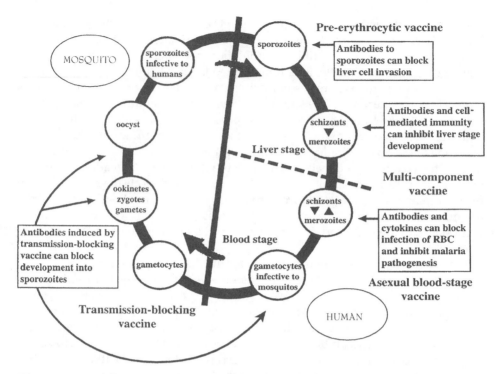

Figure 17.6. Diagrammatic representation of the life cycle of a malaria parasite showing possible targets for vaccination. Courtesy of the World Health Organization.

natural populations of adults and children. The results of these trials have been disappointing as the vaccine seems to be least effective in the most susceptible group, young children in subSaharan Africa, where the vaccine is most needed.

Other vaccines currently being considered target the sexual stages and the toxic molecules produced when the merozoites are released into the bloodstream. In the long run, it will probably be necessary to have a multipronged approach using vaccines incorporating a number of malaria antigens from different stages in the life cycle. Some of these multivalent vaccines are now undergoing experimental trials.

Finally, although the immune response to malaria involves a number of different immunological responses, there is no evidence of any correlation between malaria and AIDS.

Toxoplasmosis

Toxoplasma gondii is a parasite of cats which can be transmitted to virtually all warm-blooded animals including humans. It is probably the most common parasite in the world and about one-third of the world's population will be infected sometime in their lives. *T. gondii* is a sporozoan, like the intestinal coccidia and malaria parasites, and has a complex life cycle. The infection begins when infective stages, from cat feces or infected meat, are ingested. From the gut, the parasite invades macrophages in which it survives by preventing phagosome-lysosome fusion and undergoes rapid division which, after a short time, slows down and the parasites transform into slowly dividing forms that remain dormant in cysts mainly in the brain. If the infected individual is subsequently immunocompromised in some way, the parasites in the dormant cysts may become activated and cause a fulminating infection. In humans, most infections are benign or inapparent, but if the parasite passes across the placenta, it can seriously damage the fetus. *Toxoplasma gondii* infections are also now becoming serious concomitants of AIDS. Most individuals acquire the infection relatively early in life and recover and become immune to reinfection. Acute infections are characterized by specific IgM and chronic or recovered infections by IgG. Parasites coated with antibody are either prevented from invading macrophages or are unable to prevent phagosome-lysosome fusion if they are successful. Although parasites can survive in normal macrophages, they are killed by interferon-γ activated macrophages, therefore the most important cells involved in immunity to toxoplasmosis are macrophages. Whatever the mechanism, the ability to mount an effective immune response is very important in humans given the fact that many of the world's population will be infected at some time and those that are immunoincompetent (e.g., the fetus) or immunodepressed are at risk from a fulminating infection. Toxoplasmosis is now regarded as an important concomitant of AIDS.

Microsporidians
Microsporidiosis, caused by at least seven species belonging to five genera, is a rare but increasingly recognized condition in immunologically compromised patients particularly those suffering from AIDS. As the condition is virtually unknown in immunologically competent individuals, there is obviously some immune response that keeps these infections under control, but definite evidence that this is the case, or what the mechanisms are, is lacking. Apart from the epidemiological evidence, most of what is known comes from animal and *in vitro* studies which might not be relevant to what happens in humans. However, what is apparent is that perturbation of T cell function is a major cause of immunological failure leading to microsporidiosis, but as T cells are central to so many immunological responses, it is difficult to draw any firm conclusions about the nature of natural or acquired immunity to microsporidiosis in humans.

PARASITIC NEMATODES
Most nematodes are free-living organisms but nearly fifty species are known to parasitize humans. Typically, nematodes are cylindrical with tapered ends and are not segmented, the digestive tract is well developed with the mouth at the anterior end, the sexes are separate, and the female is usually larger than the male. For convenience, the more important nematodes of humans can be broadly categorized as intestinal or filarial, the latter being those that live in the tissues and blood and are transmitted via some kind of arthropod host.

Ascaridid Worms
The largest and most common nematode of humans is *Ascaris lumbricoides*. The adults are substantial in size, males being 0.3 cm by 15–30 cm and females 0.5 cm by 20–35 cm. The life cycle involves only one host, the human. Adult females residing in the gut release their eggs which pass from the body with the feces and are subsequently consumed usually on unwashed vegetables. The eggs hatch in the small intestine and release larvae that penetrate the gut wall and enter the lymphatics from which they are transported via the blood to the lung where they molt, enter the alveoli, migrate up the respiratory tract to the pharynx, are swallowed and mature in the

jejunum. The average worm load is about six adults, and even a few dozen worms seldom cause any marked symptoms, and the infection is usually self-limiting unless reinfection occurs. However, with repeated infection, an individual may become sensitized to worm antigens and may subsequently respond allergically to the migration of larval forms through the body. The ascaris allergen is probably the most potent parasite allergen known and this helps to explain why sensitization occurs so frequently upon repeated reinfection. Although the sensitized host responds allergically to the larvae regardless of where they are located, the serious manifestation of this phenomenon occurs in the lungs, a condition referred to as ascaris pneumonitis. From age-prevalence studies it appears that there is some degree of acquired immunity to *Ascaris* and, although the actual mechanism(s) involved is not known, it is widely believed that it involves the destruction of larvae while they are migrating through the tissues possibly by the binding of eosinophils to the worm surface, via an IgE bridge, and the release of toxic substances onto the worm with the consequent destruction of its external cell membrane.

Another disease that can occur in humans is visceral larval migrans caused by accidental infection with ascaridids of dogs and cats (*Toxocara canis* and *Toxocara cati*). These have life cycles similar to that of *Ascaris lumbricoides*. When ingested by humans, *Toxocara* eggs hatch but cannot develop into adult worms and continue to migrate throughout the body until they finally die. During this migration, larval antigens elicit various immune responses, including the production of IgE antibodies, resulting in eosinophilic granulomas around the larvae. Visceral larval migrans is most commonly seen in small children because of their closer association with cats and dogs and greater opportunity to ingest infective eggs.

Hookworms

The principal hookworm species infecting humans are *Necator americanus*, *Ancylostoma duodenale*, and *Ancylostoma ceylonicum* which is rarer. The adult worms are relatively small, approximately 0.3 by 10 mm, the females being slightly larger than males. The anterior portion of the worm is sharply flexed, creating the appearance of a hook (Figure 17.7A), hence the name of this group of helminths. Mature adults in the intestines mate and the females produce eggs that are deposited in the soil with the feces. The eggs hatch and produce free-living larvae which, under appropriate conditions (ample moisture and temperatures above 10°C), feed on bacteria and organic material in the soil. Eventually these larvae mature into infectious larvae which, upon contact with exposed parts of the body, penetrate the skin, enter capillaries, and are carried to the lungs from whence they migrate to the pharynx, are swallowed, and mature into adults in the intestine. In the case of *A. duodenale*, eggs ingested before reaching the soil can hatch and mature into adults in the intestine without going through the migratory phase in the lungs. In the intestine, the worms anchor and feed on the mucosa for up to five years, and the primary cause of pathology relates to the feeding habits of the adult worms in the intestines. The powerful muscular pharynx of the worm sucks mucosal tissue into the mouth (Figure 17.7B), and this sucking action continues until the mouth reaches the muscularis of the intestinal wall. The worm then releases itself and finds a new site to continue its feeding routine, but the vacated site continues to ooze blood for some time before clotting occurs. Since worm loads may reach several thousands in an individual, heavily infected persons can develop severe anemia. Reinfections, by virtue of the continual exposure of the host to larval antigens, stimulate the immune system and elicit the production of antibodies that react with migrating larvae. Epidemio-

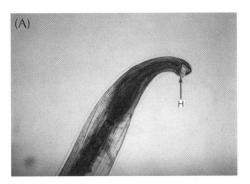 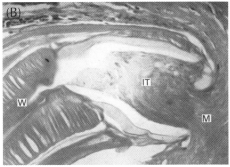

Figure 17.7.   (A) Anterior part of the human hookworm, *Necator americanus*, showing the hooked shape (H) from which the common name of this nematode is derived. (B) Section of intestine showing the attachment of a hookworm (W) and the ingestion of host tissues (IT) by the hookworm.

logical evidence suggests that individuals can develop some degree of immunity, but the actual mechanism(s) involved is not well understood but is likely to be directed against the migrating immature stages of the parasite given the fact that immunity to a related dog hookworm, *Ancylostoma caninum*, can easily be induced using attenuated larvae. Humans can also become infected by the larvae of the dog (and cat) hookworms that cannot complete their life cycle but do migrate in the skin for some time and may elicit allergic reactions, giving rise to cutaneous larval migrans (also known as creeping eruption).

Trichinosis

Trichinosis is caused by infection with the nematode worm, *Trichinella spiralis*. The adult worms, which can infect virtually any carnivorous mammal, are quite small, about 1.5 mm by 0.04 mm for the male, and 3.5 mm by 0.06 mm for the female. The life cycle is simple with the same individual serving as both the intermediate host and definitive host. When infected muscle (containing encysted larvae) is ingested, the larvae are released in the small intestine and invade the mucosa where the worms mature. The females then migrate deeper into the mucosa to deposit larvae that gain access to the lymphatics and the blood. The larvae burrow into the fibers of striated muscle and then encyst (Figure 17.8). The symptoms produced depend on the number of worms ingested and may occur in phases corresponding to the periods of intestinal invasion, migration of larvae, and encystment in muscle. Clinical findings usually consist of diarrhea, muscle pain, fever, weakness, and eosinophilia, and death may result in severe infections. As for most other nematode infections, the mechanisms involved in immunity to *T. spiralis* in humans is unclear. The migrating larvae secrete a number of antigens that elicit both cellular and antibody responses, and some of these are responsible for the formation of granulomas, consisting of macrophages, lymphocytes, eosinophils, and neutrophils that eventually encapsulate the worm. Adult worms in the gut may be affected by IgE-mediated changes in gut physiology that result in the dislodgement of the worms but not in their death.

Filarial Worms

Human filariasis is caused by infections with several species of nematode worms, the females of which produce larvae that are released in the body of the host, often

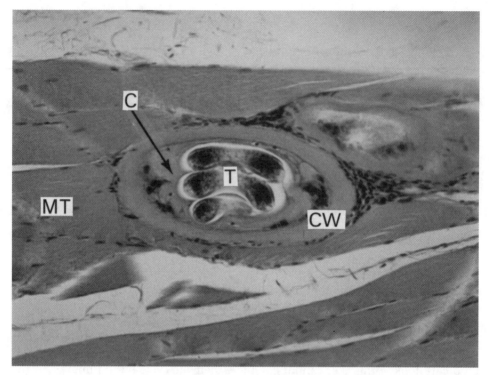

Figure 17.8. Cyst (C) of the nematode *Trichinella spiralis* (T) in muscle (MT). The thick cyst wall (CW) is also shown.

in the blood, until taken up by an arthropod vector. The most important manifestations are lymphatic filariasis and onchocerciasis. In lymphatic filariasis, caused by *Wuchereria bancrofti*, *Brugia malayi*, and *Brugia timori* and transmitted by mosquitoes, the adults live in the lymphatics, and the disease is characterized by lymphatic blockage resulting in swelling of the limbs, scrotum and other parts of the body causing the condition known as elephantiasis. In onchocerciasis, caused by *Onchocerca volvulus* and transmitted by blackflies belonging to the genus *Simulium*, the adults live in skin nodules, and the disease is characterized by blindness.

The life cycles of all filarial worms are basically similar. The infection begins when infective larvae are deposited on the skin by the insect vector when it feeds, enter the body via the bite, migrate around the body, grow, moult, and mature into male and female adults. The female produces larvae, called microfilariae, that are taken up by the insect vector, when it feeds. In the vector new infective larvae develop and the cycle is repeated.

Lymphatic Filariasis
In lymphatic filariasis, some individuals show no signs of infection, others harbor large numbers of microfilariae in their blood (microfilaraemia) but show few signs of disease, while others harbor few microfilariae but show severe pathological changes. Adult worms in the lymphatics live for ten years or more, indicating little immunity to primary infections. However, the female produces millions of microfilariae that are capable of eliciting immune responses, and many of these

larvae die, thus it seems that any immunity generated is directed against microfilariae and newly invading larvae. Little is known about the actual mechanisms of immunity and immunopathology in humans. As mentioned previously, some individuals appear to harbor no microfilariae and exhibit no pathological changes despite intensive exposure to infection in endemic areas. These people, known as 'endemic normals,' show no signs of any acquired immune responses although their lymphocytes are capable of responding to filarial antigens suggesting that they have been exposed to infection. What this actually means is not clear but suggests that these individuals are genetically nonsusceptible. Most infected individuals harbor large numbers of microfilariae but show no obvious signs of pathology. These individuals have low levels of specific antibodies, poor cell-mediated responses and are unable to clear their parasitemias. In the third category, both antibody and cell-mediated immune responses are elevated, and individuals harbor few microfilariae but exhibit severe pathological changes such as lymphatic blockage (elephantiasis), fever, and other symptoms. In the fourth category, there are high levels of eosinophils and exaggerated IgE responses, and individuals exhibit a condition known as tropical pulmonary eosinophilia (TPE). From epidemiological studies, it seems that there is a good correlation between the clearance of parasites and the development of pathological changes and that this is age related suggesting that pathology may be associated with an immune response involving increases in eosinophilia and IgE.

During the course of an infection, the adult worms in the lymphatics appear to be unaffected by the immune response, but some protective immunity develops against the microfilariae in the blood or larvae newly introduced by a mosquito. The killing of filarial larvae seems to involve IgG, IgE, eosinophils, macrophages, and neutrophils that adhere to the surface of the larva via an antibody bridge, while toxic substances are secreted onto the surface of the worm. The most important antibodies involved in protection are IgE, but IgG antibodies are involved in pathology and could be involved in the kind of destructive lesions seen in elephantiasis. In summary, it appears that filarial worms are able to evade the immune response and to establish a state of concomitant immunity which may protect against reinfection but can also generate immunopathological processes such as those occuring in schistosomiasis.

A vaccine against lymphatic filariasis is not a realistic possibility given that most people infected do not suffer any adverse effects and that severe pathology is probably immunologically mediated. In any case, there are good, cheap, and effective drugs against both the adult worms and microfilariae.

Onchocerciasis

Onchocerciasis is caused by infection with the filarial nematode, *Onchocerca volvulus*, transmitted by the blackflies belonging to the genus *Simulium*. The infective larvae injected by the sandfly mature to adults, which live for nine to fourteen years, in subcutaneous connective tissue, muscle, or fibrous nodules. Females produce 700 to 1500 microfilariae per day many of which do not survive but those that do migrate to the skin, eyes, and other organs where they survive for six to twenty-four months. Most infected individuals are asymptomatic but others suffer from damage to the skin, eyes, and lymphatics. The eye lesions often result in progressive loss of vision and blindness. There are similarities with lymphatic filariasis. Among those infected are the 'endemic normals,' who are apparently unaffected, those who harbor large numbers of microfilariae but who are hyporesponsive to worm antigens, and those showing considerable signs of pathology. The 'endemic normals' may have some innate immunity. Over a period of one to two years after infection, a number of immunological changes occur; some hyporesponsive individuals do not return to immune responsiveness whereas others do, and this is accompanied by rises in the levels of IgG and IgE. During the period of restored immune responsiveness, living adult worms and microfilariae are not affected. However, dead parasites evoke strong immune responses, and these contribute to the pathology characteristic of onchocerciasis including inflammation around dead adults in the nodules and microfilariae in the skin and eyes. The most severe skin reactions are associated with the condition known as sowda, a localized dermatitis in which the skin becomes swollen and the associated lymph nodes greatly enlarged. Sowda is correlated with high levels of antibody and few microfilariae in the lesions themselves. It is still not known whether immune responses cause the death of the worms or are caused by the release of internal antigens following the death of the worms. Treatment with the drug diethylcarbamazine, which kills the larvae, is often accompanied by strong skin reactions, called Mazzotti reactions, and this supports the second hypothesis.

Newer, well-tolerated drugs constitute the basis of current control programs, and the WHO predicts the eradication of onchocerciasis, so in the long term, there is no need for a vaccine.

PARASITIC TREMATODES (FLUKES)
The trematodes, commonly known as flukes or flatworms, are generally hermaphroditic and have a flattened, leaflike appearance. They possess two suckers and an abbreviated digestive tract. All require a mollusc as an intermediate host. Depending on the fluke species, adults may reside in various organs of humans including the intestine, liver, lung, or blood vessels. Clinically, the blood flukes (schistosomes) are the most important and these are discussed further below.

Schistosomes (Blood Flukes)
Schistosomiasis is caused by infection with several species of the genus *Schistosoma* of which the most important are *S. mansoni*, *S. japonicum*, and *S. haematobium*. These large worms, 15 to 20 mm in length, live in the lumen of blood vessels associated with the intestine or, in the case of *S. haematobium*, in the bladder. Schistosomes have complex life cycles involving a human host and a snail (Figure 17.9). The infection in humans begins when free swimming schistosome larvae called cercariae (Figure 17.9C) penetrate the skin, where they develop into schistosomula. These remain in the skin for three to four days before being carried in the bloodstream first to the lungs and then to the portal system and thence to their final sites in mesenteric or bladder blood vessels. Here the worms mature into males and females that pair for life and attach to the walls of the blood vessel where they may live for five years or more (Figure 17.9D). During this time the female worm produces millions of eggs (Figure 17.9A). Some of these are passed out in the feces or urine into freshwater where the eggs hatch releasing a ciliated larva, called a miracidium (Figure 17.9B), that finds and invades a suitable snail within which two generations of multiplication occur culminating in the production of large numbers of cercariae larvae that emerge and infect a new host.

Immunity to schistosomiasis in humans does occur but is slow to develop. Most

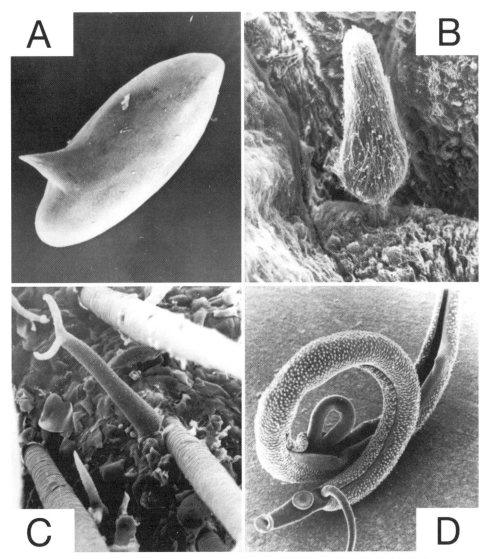

Figure 17.9. Scanning electronmicrographs of stages in the life cycle of the blood fluke *Schistosoma mansoni*. (A) Egg showing the characteristic spine that assists in the penetration of host tissues. (B) Miracidium larva entering a snail. (C) Cercaria, the free living infective larval stage entering the skin. (D) Pair of adults showing the female lying within a groove formed by the male. Courtesy of Dr. Harvey Blankespoor, Professor of Biology, Hope College, Holland, Michigan.

of what we know has come from studies on *S. mansoni*. On penetrating the host's skin, part of the outer surface, or tegument, is shed and a new tegument formed. The tegument absorbs a number of host molecules, including red blood cell and histocompatibility antigens, that effectively disguise the worm as its host, so it is able to travel through the body and to live in its final immunologically exposed site unrecognized hence its ability to survive for five years or more. However, the worm produces a number of molecules that are immunogenic and elicit antibody responses as do eggs produced by the female worm that do not reach the outside world but are deposited locally or are carried around the body and deposited in the liver.

Some antigens are common to the egg, larval, and adult worms. In response to the presence of these antigens, the host mounts a series of immune responses that are ineffective against the disguised adult worms but are effective against subsequent invading larvae, a phenomenon known as concomitant immunity. This prevents superinfection but, when the adult worms die, the host once again becomes susceptible to reinfection. On a second or subsequent challenge, the newly arrived larvae are extremely vulnerable to immune attack before they have acquired any host antigens. The immune response involves many factors, and the actual mechanisms vary from host to host, but the most important components are IgE and eosinophils and IgG or IgE and macrophages. IgE binds to the schistosomulum and eosinophils bind to the IgE and release toxic molecules that disrupt the tegument and allow the eosinophils to penetrate and strip off the tegument causing the death of the worm. Macrophages can also bind to the worm via IgG and release toxic molecules, including NO, onto the surface of the worm also facilitating its destruction. A number of other mechanisms, some involving neutrophils and platelets and complement-mediated killing, have also been suggested. There is some controversy concerning the actual site where the larval worms are killed, and it is not known for certain whether this takes place in the skin or in the lungs.

The live eggs in the tissues are also recognized as foreign, and the immune responses elicited against them bring about the formation of granulomas resulting in gross pathological changes culminating in fibrosis of the liver. Similarly, eggs deposited in the bladder eventually lead to immunologically mediated calcification.

The development of a vaccine against schistosomiasis is a real possibility, and the idea is to bypass the primary infection and to induce an immune response that is effective against newly invading cercariae. This can be done in experimental models and irradiated, but not killed, cercariae have been used to protect cattle against *Schistosoma mattheei*. This method would not be acceptable in humans, but a number of schistosome antigens are currently undergoing trials for safety and immunogenicity.

Individuals subject to repeated infection with cercariae become sensitized and manifest local allergic reactions around the burrowing parasite. Outside the tropics, including northern United States and Canada, humans may become infected with cercariae from bird schistosomes. These schistosomes cannot complete their life cycle in humans, but repeated exposure can sensitize an individual, and fresh contact with cercariae elicits the allergic manifestations responsible for the condition commonly called 'swimmers' itch.'

CESTODES (TAPEWORMS)

Tapeworms are common parasites in temperate as well as tropical countries. The worms are flat and ribbonlike in appearance, hence their name, and live as adults in the intestines of their mammalian hosts. The adult consists of a head or scolex (Figure 17.10) which attaches to the intestinal mucosa by means of suckers (and in some species, also with hooks), and a segmented portion, the body, made up of proglottids (Figure 17.11) resulting from the continuous production of new segments just behind the scolex. There is no digestive tract, and nutrients are absorbed directly by the worm from the contents of the intestinal lumen. Each proglottid possesses both male and female reproductive organs and is self-fertilizing. The gravid proglottids, containing numerous eggs, eventually separate from the body and are passed with the feces.

LIVERPOOL JOHN MOORES UNIVERSITY
LEARNING SERVICES

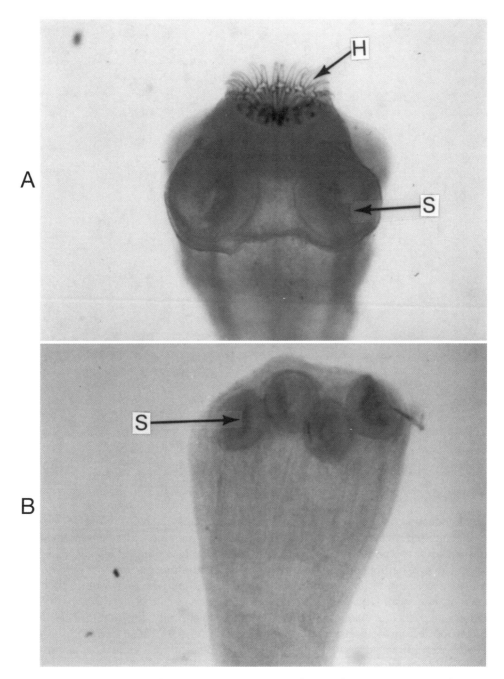

Figure 17.10.   Scolices of the tapeworms (A) *Taenia solium* and (B) *Taenia saginata* showing hooks (H) and suckers (S).

Pork Tapeworm

The adult worm, *Taenia solium* (Figure 17.10A), can reach 2 to 8 meters in length. Gravid proglottids are passed in feces and release eggs that are subsequently ingested by pigs, hatch in the intestine, enter the blood and are transported to muscles where they develop into cysticerci, the larval form of the organism (Figure 17.12).

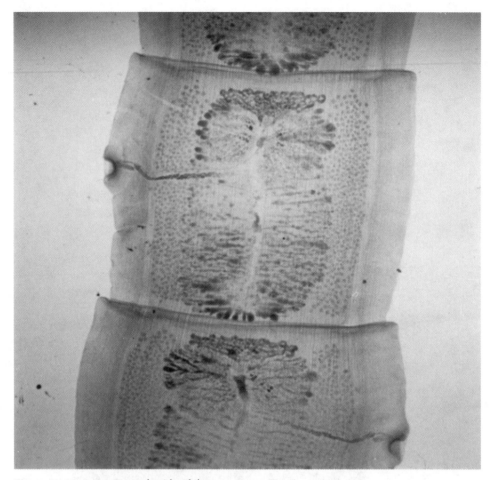

Figure 17.11. Mature proglottids of the tapeworm *Taenia saginata*.

Upon ingestion of uncooked, infected pork by humans, the bladder of the cysticercus is digested away, and the scolex attaches to the intestine wall where it develops into an adult worm. Regardless of the number of cysticerci ingested, an individual almost always harbors only one adult worm in the intestine; the reason is not known. Most infected individuals exhibit no symptoms and may be unaware of the presence of the worm. However, if a human ingests the eggs these can hatch and develop into cysticerci throughout the body. These eventually degenerate and calcify, but if located in the brain or other vital organ, they can cause severe disease or death. Very little is known about immunity to the adult stages of *T. solium* in humans although spontaneous recoveries have been recorded. It is thought that there might be some concomitant immunity directed against the invading larval stages. The cysticerci, on the other hand, do elicit immune responses characterized by the production of specific antibodies and cellular responses. How the parasites survive immune attack is not known.

Beef Tapeworm

The adult worm, *Taenia saginata* (Figure 17.10B), is approximately 4 to 25 meters in length. As in the case of *T. solium*, if the cysticercus in the tissues of cattle is ingested

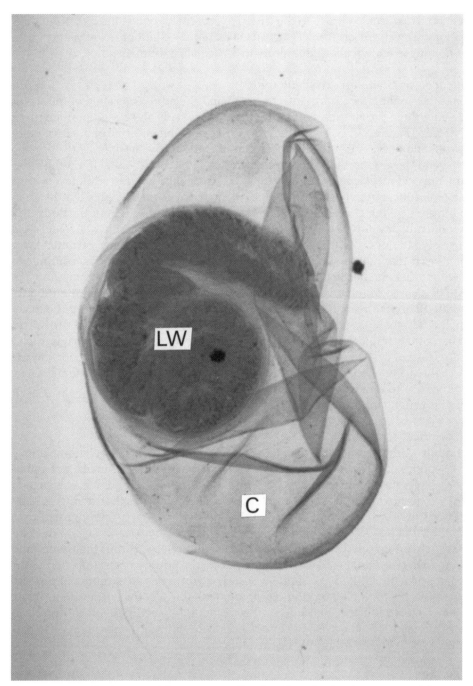

Figure 17.12.   Cysticercus of the tapeworm *Taenia solium* that has been removed from muscle tissue showing the larval worm (LW) and the cyst (C).

by a human, hatching occurs in the intestine and adult worms develop. Gravid proglottids release eggs in the feces that are then ingested by cattle in which they develop into cysticerci in the tissues. As for *T. solium*, the human host usually harbors only a single adult worm, and its presence generally induces little or no signs of infection. However, contrary to the situation seen in *T. solium*, the risk of humans developing cysticercosis from *T. saginata* is extremely slight or nonexistent. Virtually nothing is known about immunity to *T. saginata* in humans.

Echinococcus Granulosus (Hydatid Cyst)

This is the smallest tapeworm infecting humans, the adult consisting of the scolex plus only three proglottids (immature, mature, gravid) and has a total length of only 5 mm (Figure 17.13). The adult worm resides in the intestine of dogs (or other canines) and releases eggs in the feces that, if ingested by sheep or cattle, become larvae and develop in the tissues into forms called hydatid cysts. If, on the other hand, infected meat is ingested by a dog, the larvae develop into adult tapeworms in the intestine. Humans are infected accidentally by ingesting eggs that hatch in the intestine giving rise to larvae that are disseminated throughout the body and subsequently develop into hydatid cysts. Most are located in either the liver or the lungs. Hydatid cysts, which consist of an outer cyst wall, an inner germinal layer that gives rise to numerous scolices, and the fluid filling the cyst, may continue to grow for years and become life-threatening. Clinical symptoms are comparable to those of a slow-growing tumor. The parasite elicits cell-mediated and antibody-mediated immune responses. These seem to be ineffective in resolving the infection, but it is not known how the parasite evades the immune response. Treatment consists of the surgical removal of the hydatid cyst but care must be taken to prevent release of cyst contents during surgery since severe allergic reactions to the fluid contents may occur. Furthermore, each scolex or fragment of germinal tissue can give rise to a new hydatid cyst. To prevent such complications, formalin or iodine is usually injected into the cysts during surgery.

Fish or Broad Tapeworm

The adult worm, *Diphyllobothrium latum*, is about 3 to 10 meters in length. Unlike *Taenia* species, the gravid proglottids do not pass out in the feces intact, but generally disintegrate and release their eggs into the intestinal lumen. If the eggs gain access to fresh water, they hatch and release ciliated embryos that are ingested by copepods in which the larva encysts. If the infected copepods are ingested by a fish, the larvae penetrate the intestinal wall and enter various tissues. When infected fish are ingested by humans, the larvae are released from the tissues and adhere to the intestinal wall where they mature into adult worms. Infection in the human is usually limited to a single worm. The worm has an exceptional propensity to absorb vitamin B_{12} and thus competes with the host for this nutrient. When dietary factors limit the ingestion of this vitamin, this competition can result in anemia in the host, otherwise the infection may be entirely symptomless. There is not thought to be any immunity against this tapeworm.

SUMMARY

This is by no means a comprehensive account of immunity to parasites but the discussion of the selected parasites should serve to indicate the range and complexity of some of the immune responses involved and to explain the basis of much of the pathology associated with parasitic infections. The various problems raised should also explain why the development of vaccines against parasitic infections has been so difficult.

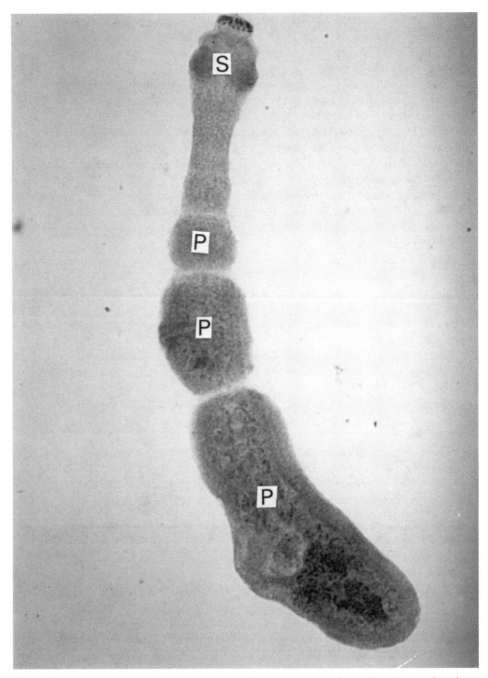

Figure 17.13. Mature form of the tapeworm *Echinococcus granulosus* showing proglottids (P) and scolex (S).

SUGGESTED READING

1. Behnke, J.M., ed. *Parasites, Immunity and Pathology*. London: Taylor and Francis, 1990.
2. Boothroyd, J.C., and R. Komuniecki, eds. *Molecular Approaches to Parasitology*. New York: Wiley Liss, 1995.

3. Clark, I.A., and K. Rockett. "Nitric Oxide and Parasitic Disease." *Advances in Parasitology* 37 (1992):1.

4. Cox, F.E.G., and F.Y. Liew. "T-Cell Subsets and Cytokines in Parasitic Infections." *Immunology Today* 13 (1992):445.

5. Cox, F.E.G., and D. Wakelin. "Immunology and Immunopathology of Human Parasitic Infections." In *Topley and Wilson's Microbiology and Microbial Infections, Vol. 5: Parasitology*, 57–84. 9th ed. London: Edward Arnold, 1998.

6. Davies, D.H., M.A. Halablab, J. Clarke, F.E.G. Cox, and T.W.K. Young. *Infection and Immunity*. London: Taylor and Francis, 1998.

7. Facer, C.A., and M. Tanner. "Clinical Trials of Malaria Vaccines: Progress and Prospects." *Advances in Parasitology* 39 (1997):2, 1997.

8. Freedman, D.O., ed. "Immunopathogenic Aspects of Disease Induced by Helminth Parasites." *Chemical Immunology* 66 (1997): Basel: Karger, 1997.

9. James, S.L. "Role of Nitric Oxide in Parasitic Infections." *Microbiological Reviews* 59 (1995):533.

10. Kierszenbaum, F. *Parasitic Infections and the Immune System*. San Diego: Academic Press, 1994.

11. Liew, F.Y., and F.E.G. Cox, eds. "Immunology of Intracellular Parasitism." *Chemical Immunology* 70 (1998). Basel: Karger, 1998.

12. Liew, F.Y., and C.A. O'Donnell. "Immunology of *Leishmaniasis*." *Advances in Parasitology* 32 (1993):161.

13. Mauel, J. "Intracellular Survival of Protozoan Parasites with Special Reference to *Leishmania* spp., *Toxoplasma gondii* and *Trypanosoma cruzi*." *Advances in Parasitology* 38 (1996):1.

14. Riffkin, M., H-F. Seow, D. Jackson, L. Brown, and P. Wood. "Defence Against the Immune Barrage: Helminth Survival Strategies." *Immunology and Cell Biology* 74 (1996):564.

15. Wakelin, D. *Immunity to Parasitic Infections: How Parasitic Infections are Controlled*. 2nd ed. Cambridge: Cambridge University Press, 1996.

16. Warren, K.S., ed. *Immunology and Molecular Biology of Parasitic Infections*. Oxford: Blackwell Scientific Publications, 1993.

QUESTIONS

1 Describe the ways in which parasitic protozoa and helminth worms evade the immune responses of their hosts.

2 "In parasitic infections, the disease begins with the immune response." Discuss this statement.

3 Review the current status of vaccines against parasites.

4 Why is it important for immunologists to understand the life cycles of parasitic protozoa and helminth worms?

ANSWERS

1. Parasitic protozoa and helminths are extremely versatile eukaryotes with complex life cycles. In order to survive they have evolved numerous ways to counteract hostile environmental and immunological conditions. Some parasites use their complex life cycles to minimize the possibilities of immune attack by moving from site to site, for example the malaria parasites and schistosomes, while others, such as the intestinal nematode worms actually hide by moving to the comparative safety of

the alimentary tract. *Toxoplasma gondii* evades immune attack by migrating to the brain, an immunologically privileged site free from immune attack. Malaria parasites have the most complex life cycles of all the parasites and occupy successively the bloodstream, the liver, the bloodstream, red blood cells, the bloodstream, red blood cells and the mosquito gut. The different stages in the life cycle are antigenically distinct so the immune response is always chasing a moving target. In addition, malaria parasites exhibit a degree of antigenic diversity not seen anywhere else. Most parasites have evolved specific, and sometimes unique, ways either to avoid eliciting an immune response or escaping its consequences. *Entamoeba histolytica* is able to degrade IgA and to resist complement lysis and also to shed surface antigens that have been bound by antibodies. The African trypanosomes undergo antigenic variation in such a way that when one population of trypanosomes is mowed down by the immune response another population with a completely different surface coat emerges and this process is repeated indefinitely. The malaria parasites and *Giardia lamblia* also undergo antigenic variation. Some parasites can survive in macrophages, for example the New World trypanosome *Trypanosoma cruzi* escapes from the phagolysosome into the host cell cytoplasm while *Toxoplasma gondii* prevents phagosome-lysosome fusion and multiplies in the phagosome. Sharing antigens with the host is another way to avoid recognition by the host and this method is exploited by *Trypanosoma cruzi* and the schistosomes. Schistosomes acquire host antigens when they enter the host and these subsequently protect them from immune attack. Most helminth worms can survive in their hosts for many years, for example the larvae of the filarial worms. How these parasites evade the inevitable immune responses is not known. The long term consequences of the continual antigenic stimulation without any diminution of the antigenic load often leads parasites to down-regulate the immune responses. This is very clearly seen in the case of African trypanosomiasis. Such mechanisms can be advantageous to the parasite but can leave the host open to attack by other pathogens.

2. Most parasitic infections are long and chronic and this is due in part to the ability of the parasite to evade the host's immune responses. However, parasites are highly immunogenic and elicit a range of immune responses some of which are protective, some are neutral while others are counterprotective and may cause serious immunopathological changes. Immunopathology is characteristic of most parasitic infections and, in most cases, this involves some kind of autoimmune reaction. In the African trypanosomes, the parasites are killed releasing antigens that bind to host tissues, causing autoimmune lysis, or circulate resulting in the formation of antigen-antibody complexes which lodge in various tissues. In the case of *Trypanosome cruzi*, the antigens shared by the parasite and host result in autoimmune destruction of nerve and muscle cells often many years after the infection began. Malaria parasites induce autoantibodies reactive against uninfected red blood cells resulting in anaemia. Inappropriate inflammation is also characteristic of many parasitic infections. Malaria parasites sequester in the brain and elicit the production of a number of inflammatory cytokines that can lead to cerebral malaria. In toxoplasmosis and onchocerciasis inflammatory responses in the eye can cause visual disturbances and blindness. There is some evidence that the lymphatic blockage associated with lymphatic filariasis is immunologically mediated as the most severe symptoms are associated with the strongest immune responses. The pathology of schistosomiasis is unique. The adult worms produce antigens that elicit immune

responses that are ineffective against the adult worms which are immunologically invisible because they are coated with host antigens. However, schistosome eggs deposited in the liver and other tissues are subject to immune attack and become surrounded by immunologically-mediated granulomas that can lead to the death of the host. One other aspect of immunity to helminth worms is that they all characteristically elicit high levels of IgE and eosinophilia leading to a number of allergic reactions.

3. There are no vaccines against any of the parasitic diseases of humans. There are a few against parasites of veterinary importance but they are not really very satisfactory. The main problem is that parasites are structurally and biochemically complex and elicit a range of immunological responses only some of which are protective. In addition, parasites have evolved a number of ways to evade the immune response either by avoiding eliciting the response in the first instance or by counteracting its effects. Numerous attempts have been made to develop vaccines against parasites particularly as many of the other methods of control, including the use of drugs, have become ineffective. Some parasitic infections, such as *Entamoeba histolytica* and *Giardia lamblia* do not require a vaccine because they do not present serious health risks to most of those infected. Intestinal nematodes and the filarial worms that cause onchocerciasis can be treated very effectively with drugs and also do not require a vaccine. In other cases, a vaccine is unlikely to be effective, for example it is difficult to envisage a vaccine against the African trypanosomes, because of the ability of the parasites to undergo antigenic variation, and a vaccine against *Trypanosoma cruzi* might actually precipitate autoimmune disease instead of preventing it. Most progress has been made in developing a vaccine against malaria, a disease that urgently requires such an approach. There have been a number of human trials involving sporozoite antigens and various blood cell antigens. The most extensively tested vaccine has been a synthetic one based on 3 blood stage antigens. This vaccine, known as SPf66, has been extensively tested but after some initial success was found to be disappointing when given to children in regions of high transmission where the vaccine is most needed. The current approach to a vaccine against malaria is to use a cocktail of antigens derived from the different stages in the life cycle. From the veterinary viewpoint, there are vaccines, based on irradiated larvae, against the lungworms of sheep and cattle. There are also commercial or widely used vaccines based on attenuated lines of *Eimeria* spp., the case of coccidiosis in chickens, *Toxoplasma gondii* in sheep and *Theileria* spp., the cause of lymphoproliferative diseases in cattle. An irradiated larva vaccine against the dog hookworm, *Ancylostoma caninum* has been abandoned in favor of drug treatment. None of the living vaccines would be acceptable for use in humans. Current approaches involve the use of molecular techniques to target particular antigens but, although there have been some experimental successes, the realistic possibility of a commercially available vaccine against any parasite of humans is a distant prospect.

4. Most parasites have complex life cycles involving successive stages that are biochemically and immunologically distinct and which often occupy different sites in the body and sometimes a vector which transmits the parasite from host to host. It is therefore essential when contemplating the design of vaccines, or methods to ameliorate immunopathological damage, to know exactly where the parasite is, what stage it is in, and what antigens it is expressing at that stage. For example, a vaccine against the sporozoite of the malaria parasite will not be effective against

the blood stages and vice versa. It is also important to know when a parasite is unlikely to be affected by the immune response, for example when it is in an immunologically privileged site or in the gut or even if it has escaped from the human host into its vector. Finally, a thorough knowledge of the life cycle can reveal whether or not the development of a vaccine is feasible. A knowledge of the life cycles should therefore prevent a vast amount of wasted effort and the possibility of doing more harm than good.

18

The Fungi

Lola Winter

INTRODUCTION
CLASSIFICATION OF
  MYCOTIC DISEASES
  Superficial Mycoses
  Subcutaneous Mycoses
  Systemic Mycoses
  Opportunistic Mycoses
LABORATORY DIAGNOSIS
THERAPY
SUMMARY
SUGGESTIONS FOR
  FURTHER READING
QUESTIONS

INTRODUCTION

Fungi exist in nature mainly as saprophytes. Only about fifty of over 200 thousand known species of fungi have been identified as pathogens of humans and animals. Humans are very resistant to fungal disease, and although exposure to fungal conidia occurs daily, we are well protected by both the innate and adaptive immune responses as long as they are functioning properly. Within the last decades, the incidence of mycoses has increased greatly. This is not due to any increased virulence on the part of the fungi but rather to an increase in the number of hosts who are immunologically compromised and are therefore more susceptible to fungal disease.

CLASSIFICATION OF MYCOTIC DISEASES

Fungal diseases have been classified according to the tissues and organs affected and the range of clinical manifestations.

The superficial mycoses are those conditions which involve the superficial layers of the dermis. The most common agents involved in these diseases are the dermatophytes. These agents, able to colonize hair, skin, and nails, are readily transmissible from host to host by direct contact or through fomites. Though the diseases they cause are very annoying and cosmetically unappealing, they do not pose a threat to the life of the host.

The subcutaneous mycoses involve tissues located beneath the dermis. These diseases usually result from the direct implantation of the agent through a break in the skin. Nodular lesions develop subcutaneously which will eventually ulcerate and drain. These conditions can be painful and disfiguring but they are amenable to treatment and rarely become systemic in the otherwise normal host. These mycoses are transmitted only by direct inoculation.

The deep mycoses refer to diseases in which internal organs are affected. Because most of these conditions follow inhalation of the agent, respiratory distress is a common primary manifestation of such diseases. Though some of the agents do seem to have predilections for particular sites, systemic dissemination of the agent can bring about involvement of any organ system. Agents causing deep mycoses include *Histoplasma capsulatum*, *Blastomyces dermatiditis*, and *Coccidioides immitis*. These mycoses, characterized by an insidious onset and chronic nature, can occur in the previously healthy host. A vigorous inflammatory response to the fungal antigens accounts for a large part of the resulting pathology. The agents are all dimorphic; they exist in the environment in the mycelial phase and undergo phase transformation to become yeast forms in the host. These fungi are also associated with endemic areas, specific geographic areas where the incidence of infection is high and disease is more often seen. Opportunists such as *Aspergillus*, which is ubiquitous, and *Candida*, which is part of the normal flora, are able to cause systemic disease only in the severely compromised host.

Superficial Mycoses
Dermatophytosis
Cutaneous infection involving the skin, hair, and nails is the most common manifestation of disease caused by the dermatophytes, which belong to the genera *Microsporum*, *Trichophyton* and *Epidermophyton*. These fungi are unique because they are able to utilize keratin as a source of energy. The dermatophytes have been grouped according to their more natural environmental habitat. Geophilic dermatophytes such as *Microsporum gypseum* are able to survive in the soil for extended periods of time and retain their infectivity. Zoophilic dermatophytes such as *Microsporum canis* have become dependent on animal hosts which then serve as sources of dissemination. These agents have limited capacity to survive in the environment. The anthropophilic agents such as *Trichophyton mentagrophytes* have become dependent on humans. Although most of these agents do have a preferred host, cross-species infections can occur and in unusual hosts can result in diseases of greater severity but of shorter duration.

The skin is well protected against colonization by dermatophytes by its function as a physical barrier, its low moisture content, and the presence of normal bacterial flora which compete for iron and may also secrete antifungal chemicals. Fatty acid secretions within the skin, and the constant desquamation and proliferation of the epidermal layer are additional factors that contribute to resistance to dermatophytic infection.

On the other hand, factors which predispose to these infections include increased moisture or glandular occlusion in the skin, underlying diseases such as Cushing's disease, hematologic malignancies, and prolonged systemic corticosteroid therapy. There is no evidence that antibodies play any role in eliminating infection; in fact, chronic infections are often accompanied by increases in antibody titers. The observations that secondary infections with the same agent resolve faster and that nude mice with no T cell function are unable to clear infection with *Tricophyton mentagrophytes* suggest that the cell-mediated immune (CMI) response plays a critical role in resolution. *Trichophyton* species have been shown to activate complement by the alternative pathway, resulting in chemotaxis of polymorphonuclear leukocytes (PMN) to the site of infection. There, these play a role in controlling disease.

Dermatophytic infection is initiated by the deposition of fungal elements onto the skin, hair, or nails. These infectious units either gain a foothold and grow or are

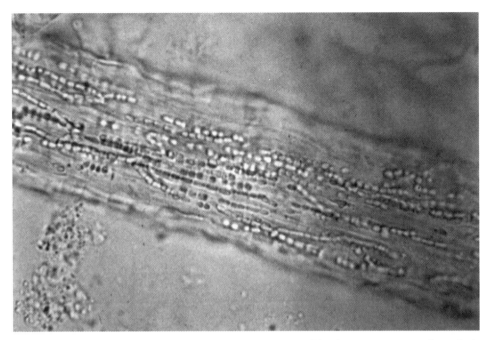

Figure 18.1. KOH preparation showing arthroconidia and hyphae growing on a hair shaft. (Source: Dr. John Timoney, Dept. of Veterinary Science, Gluck Equine Research Center, University of Kentucky, Lexington, Kentucky.)

lost. Friction, abrasion, and moisture enhance the ability of the fungi to colonize. Conidia germinate and form hyphae which invade the tissue and hair follicles and then fragment, resulting in the production of arthroconidia (referred to as microconidia) (Figure 18.1). The microconidia germinate and produce more hyphae and the cycle continues until the infection is resolved. Infected hair grows out thick and brittle. Circular red skin lesions expand with healing in the center. To the early workers, this characteristic growth of the lesion suggested the presence of a worm growing within the skin, hence the name, ringworm. The periphery is the active area of fungal growth and of the host response to the fungal irritants. This inflammatory response results in the overproduction of keratin which causes the scaliness and thickening of the skin characteristic of these infections. Infection is almost always limited to the stratum corneum although the intense itching and scratching may result in the development of secondary bacterial infections.

Ringworm in children is usually manifested by lesions on the head, tinea capitis, or on the body, tinea corporis.

Athlete's foot, tinea pedis, caused by *T. mentagrophytes*, is the most common fungal infection in the United States. At any one time about sixty-five percent of the population is experiencing active infection, and it is estimated that one to three percent of the population are carriers. Stress has been shown to predispose to active infection.

Although many of these conditions are self-limiting, antifungal drugs, both oral and topical, which are effective in therapy may be used.

Subcutaneous Mycoses

Sporothricosis

The agent *Sporothrix schenkii* is a common soil saprophyte. It is found in higher concentrations in environments enriched with spaghnum moss or other organic

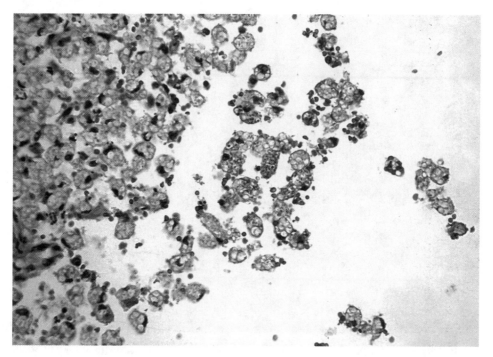

Figure 18.2.   H & E stained preparation showing yeast cells of *S. schenkii* within macrophages. (Source: Dr. John Timoney, Dept. of Veterinary Science, Gluck Equine Research Center, University of Kentucky, Lexington, Kentucky.)

matter. *Sporothrix* is a dimorphic fungus, which grows as mycelia in the environment but grows as a yeast in the host. Soil contamination of a scratch or direct implantation via a puncture wound introduces the agent to the host. The initial lesion at the site of entry heals, but weeks or months later an ulcerated lesion develops at the site of inoculation. This is followed by the development of painful nodules and abscesses along the path of lymphatic drainage, referred to as the cording effect. With resolution of the disease these nodules will ulcerate and drain.

At the cellular level, it has been demonstrated that the tiny (2 to 3 μm in diameter) yeast cells which result from phase transition of the conidia from the mycelial environmental growth are ingested by macrophages (Figure 18.2). In time activated macrophages are able to eliminate the infection. *In vitro* work with peritoneal macrophages has shown that the cell surface polysaccharides of the yeast cell, galactomannan and rhamnomannan, inhibit phagocytosis. It is also possible that the alkaline phosphatase activity associated with this fungus functions in virulence by inhibiting the production of superoxide by neutrophils and macrophages. Other enzymes associated with virulence include Proteinase I and II, which degrade human stratum corneum.

This condition is successfully treated with potassium iodide and rarely becomes systemic in the immunocompetent host.

Systemic Mycoses
Histoplasmosis
Histoplasma capsulatum is a dimorphic fungus which has, unfortunately, been improperly named. The appearance of a capsule in stained preparations, which led to this name, is an artifact of the staining process.

The fungus exists in the mycelial phase in the environment. Conidiophores produce both microconidia and macroconidia which become aerosolized. The microconidia, about 5 μm in diameter, are the infectious units. The larger tuberculate shaped macroconidia are characteristic of the fungus and aid in its dispersal and identification but because of their large size are not a source of infection for humans or animals.

Microconidia of *H. capsulatum* enter the host via the respiratory tract and undergo phase transformation to yeast morphology (blastoconidia) sometime after exposure to body temperature in the lungs. It is not yet known how long it takes for this transformation to occur. The alpha-1,3,glucan in the cell wall of both the microconidia and the blastoconidia attaches to the CD18 adhesins on macrophages and PMNs. Attachment is followed by ingestion and phagolysosomal fusion. Although the PMNs are not able to kill the microconidia, *in vitro* work suggests that they are fungistatic. However, multiplication of the blastoconidia continues within the phagolysosomes of the alveolar macrophages. Experimental work has shown that the blastoconidia are able to raise the pH of the phagolysosome; this renders the hydrolases much less effective. The blastoconidia also alter the oxidative burst of the macrophage by failing to induce production of reactive oxygen metabolites. Protected within these defectively functioning macrophages, the blastoconidia continue to multiply and spread throughout the body. Resolution of the disease is dependent upon the proper functioning of the CMI response with the secretion of cytokines that cause the activation of macrophages, so that they are able to kill or control the reproduction of the ingested blastoconidia. Nitric oxide has been identified as the effector molecule in this killing. The development of granulomas that contain the agent is also dependent upon the CMI response. Any depression of the CMI response at a later time may result in the reactivation of conidia sequestered within the granulomas. Evidence indicates that antibodies play little if any role in immunity to this disease.

Histoplasma exists predominantly within endemic areas where the incidence of infection in the population can be very high. Such areas are found around the Ohio and Mississippi river valleys in the midwestern and southern parts of the United States. Although *Histoplasma* is not a pathogen of birds, it is found in high concentrations in bird feces, which supply the enriched environment needed for its growth. It is also carried in the intestinal tract of bats and is found in high concentrations in bat caves. Exposure to bat caves, bird roosts, and chicken yards in these endemic areas therefore increases the risk of infection.

Exposure and subclinical infections are common in endemic areas. Different studies have revealed that from fifty to ninety-five percent of the population in these areas show evidence of infection as revealed by a positive reaction to the delayed type hypersensitivity (DTH) skin test. Clinical disease occurs in only a small percentage of those infected, and respiratory disease is the most common manifestation of clinical histoplasmosis. In otherwise healthy individuals, this disease is self-limiting. Progressive, disseminated histoplasmosis can occur in individuals who have been exposed to a large inoculum or who are unable to mount a CMI response. This explains why the disease poses a particular problem with AIDS patients.

Antifungal therapy is available for the control of this mycosis but its effectiveness is very dependent upon the underlying health of the host and the stage of the disease at the time therapy is initiated.

Although there is no evidence for the transmission of *Histoplasma* from host to

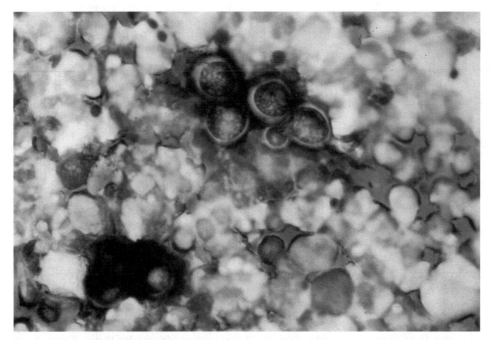

Figure 18.3.   Wright stained preparation showing large blastoconidia of B. dermatiditis. (Source: Dr. Julia Blue, College of Veterinary Medicine, Cornell University, Ithaca, New York.)

host among humans, there is a recent report of direct transmission from dog to dog. In this case it is believed that the yeasts, which were shed in the feces, urine, and saliva of one diseased dog were ingested or inhaled by a kennel mate which subsequently developed histoplasmosis.

Blastomycosis
Blastomyces dermatiditis is another dimorphic fungus, the agent of blastomycosis, which is very similar in its manifestations to histoplasmosis.

Infection is initiated by the inhalation of mycelial microconidia. These microconidia are phagocytosed and killed by both alveolar macrophages and PMNs, but if the inoculum is large and some escape killing phase transformation occurs with the production of large (5 to 20 μm in diameter), broad based budding yeast cells with a double refractile wall (Figure 18.3). The yeast cells are much more resistant to the effects of phagocytosis due to their large size, thick cell wall, and their ability to depress the generation of the peroxidase microbicidal system. The alpha-1,3,glucan of the cell wall has been associated with increased virulence though at this time how it does this is not known. It has been demonstrated experimentally, however, that mutants which have low levels of this carbohydrate are less virulent. A 120kD protein known as WI-1 has recently been isolated from the yeast phase of *Blastomyces*. This protein functions as an adhesin by binding to the CD14 receptors on macrophages, thereby enhancing phagocytosis. It has been suggested that the abundant alpha-1,3,glucan of the more virulent clones masks this adhesin thereby allowing the yeasts to escape recognition by macrophages and disseminate more readily. Perhaps this is another example of the ability of a pathogen to alter its phenotype in response to environmental pressure.

Blastomycosis is endemic in the south-central, southeastern, and midwestern

United States. Though the agent has only rarely been isolated from the soil, epidemics have been traced to point source exposures. Environmental microfoci of the fungus are believed to be soil areas of acidic pH with a high organic content and abundant moisture.

The use of a new, more specific skin test for blastomycosis has shown that in endemic areas infection rates are high but disease is rare. Pneumonia is the most common manifestation of disease. A normal host can often resolve the disease even without therapy. In the compromised host, dissemination occurs to any organ system but most frequently to skin and bone. As with histoplasmosis, a CMI response that induces the formation of granulomas is critical for resolution of the disease. Therapy is effective but only if administered early in the course of the disease to immune competent hosts.

Coccidioidomycosis

Coccidioidomycosis is caused by the dimorphic fungus, *Coccidioides immitis*. This agent is endemic in the southwestern United States, an area characterized by a hot, dry climate. Mycelial growth occurs in rodent burrows where the soil is moist and enriched by animal droppings. After periods of heavy rains the arthroconidia, formed by fragmentation of the hyphae, are carried to the surface and aerosolize upon drying. Arthroconidia are the infectious units which are inhaled by the host. Upon entry into the lung, phase transformation to a spherule takes place. Spherules grow to large sizes, 20 to 80 µm in diameter. Cytoplasmic reorganization occurs within the spherules resulting in the formation of hundreds of endospores, 3 to 4 µm in diameter, which are released upon rupture of the spherule. Each endospore develops into another spherule, thus, continuing the cycle.

The cell walls of the arthroconidia, endospores, and spherules activate complement by the alternate pathway. Although PMNs are able to phagocytize the opsonized arthroconidia and endospores, only about twenty to thirty percent of those ingested are killed. The spherules are too large to be phagocytized, but PMNs are able to damage such large fungal structures by a process of extracellular degranulation that is triggered by contact with the phagocyte cell membrane. However, the spherule escapes damage, perhaps because of its extracellular glycoprotein covering that prevents access of the PMNs to the spherule wall. The development of a CMI response with the activation of macrophages and the formation of granulomas is essential for resolution of this disease.

Skin tests for DTH have indicated that about a third of the population in endemic areas is infected with this agent; clinical disease occurs in about forty percent of those who are infected. Signs can include mild respiratory distress, meningitis, bone and joint infection, skin and soft tissue lesions, and, more rarely, widespread dissemination. The incidence of disease is highest among the very young and the very old, those infected with HIV, and others who are otherwise immunologically compromised. The success of antifungal therapy follows the same pattern as that for *Histoplasma* and *Blastomyces*.

Cryptococcosis

Cryptococcus neoformans has a worldwide distribution. It is found in very high concentrations in pigeon manure, which supplies the creatinine needed for its growth. Though it has both a mycelial and yeast phase in the environment, it is believed that the blastoconidia of the yeast phase (0.6 to 3.5 µm in diameter), are the infectious agents which dry up, aerosolize, and are inhaled. Initial respiratory disease may be mild and unrecognized or progress to pneumonia and meningitis.

A glucouronoxylomannan capsule made both in the environment and in the host is the undisputed virulence factor of *C. neoformans*. It functions *in vivo* to inhibit phagocytosis (see chapter 14). Work with avirulent, gene deleted, acapsular mutants has proven the importance of the capsule in virulence. Purified capsular carbohydrate incubated with acapsular mutants was shown to impair phagocytosis of the mutants. The capsule is also believed to be involved in the depression of several macrophage functions including generation of the respiratory burst, production of cytokines, and presentation of antigen. Virulent cryptococci also produce melanin, which functions *in vivo* to scavenge reactive oxygen intermediates including superoxide anion and singlet oxygen and thereby enhances survival in phagocytes. The production of melanin may explain, in part, why these fungi multiply so well within the central nervous system. The brain contains an abundance of catacholamine which is used by the cryptococci for the production of melanin. The production of D-mannitol, which scavenges both OH- radicals and reactive oxygen intermediates, also contributes to virulence.

The cryptococcal capsule is also a potent activator of complement by the alternate pathway, and complement is very important in innate resistance to disease through its chemotactic and opsonic functions. Due to the resistant nature of the fungal cell wall, the membrane attack complex is not effective against these agents. It has been shown experimentally that IgG2 antibodies specific for the capsular polysaccharide are effective opsonins. However, the concentration of these antibodies that is induced in natural conditions of exposure is generally insufficient to mediate opsonization. Cryptococci can survive and multiply within nonactivated macrophages, but human alveolar macrophages that have been activated by IFN gamma secrete cationic proteases that kill encapsulated cryptococci. This is consistent with clinical evidence that a properly functioning CMI response is critical for resolution of this infection, since the incidence of disease is highest among those with underlying defects in this arm of the immune response.

Systemic spread to the central nervous system results in life-threatening meningitis, which is the most common manifestation of disease caused by *C. neoformans*. Disseminated infection less frequently involves the skin and skeletal system. Although cryptococcal pneumonia in an otherwise healthy individual can resolve without treatment, antifungal therapy is essential for the immune compromised host and any host with meningitis.

Though the agent is widespread in the environment, disease is rare. There is no reliable DTH skin test for epidemiological surveys, but the presence of antibodies in a large percentage of individuals suggests that the occurrence of infection is commonplace. In several studies eighty-nine to ninety-eight percent of volunteers tested had antibodies to *C. neoformans*, yet none of them had a history of disease. Most overt disease occurs in the compromised host, in particular those with diminished T cell function. Paradoxically, twenty to thirty percent of patients with cryptococcosis have no underlying disease. Whether these cases result from exposure to unusually large inocula is not known.

Opportunistic Mycoses
Aspergillosis
The genus *Aspergillus* includes many species, but most disease in humans is caused

by *Aspergillus fumigatus*. The aspergilli are common saprophytes which produce hyphal growth both in the environment, where they are ubiquitous, and in the host. Despite daily exposure to aspergillus conidia, invasive aspergillosis occurs only in the severely compromised host. Either a lack of PMNs or improperly functioning PMNs predispose the host to life-threatening aspergillosis. Neutropenia is in fact the greatest single risk factor for invasive aspergillosis and occurs primarily in patients undergoing immunosuppressive chemotherapy or radiation therapy for cancers or transplants. Antifungal therapy is attempted in these cases, but the prognosis is generally poor due to the underlying condition of the host.

The small conidia of *Aspergillus* (2 to 3 μm in diameter) are inhaled and readily reach the lungs. There the alveolar macrophages form the first line of defense. These phagocytes are able to prevent the germination of the conidia and also to kill them. If a large inoculum is inhaled and some conidia are able to elude the defenses of the macrophages, PMNs phagocytize and kill the germinating conidia by the products of both the respiratory burst and lysosomal degranulation. Germinating conidia which escape the PMNs produce hyphae, but these are susceptible to the products of extracellular degranulation of the PMNs. If these first lines of defense are in any way depressed, invasive disease results.

It has been observed that the conidia of this fungus bind to both fibrinogen and laminin. In fact, receptors for these host constituents have been identified on the conidial cell wall. Because chemotherapy and radiation therapy damage host epithelial tissue with a resulting increase in the accessibility of both fibrinogen and laminin, it has been suggested that the ability of *Aspergillus* to bind to these substrates is a virulence factor that enhances invasiveness of host cells.

Proteinases and cytotoxins have also been isolated from these fungi but their role in pathogenesis has yet to be proven.

Candidiasis

Organisms of the genus *Candida* are a part of the normal flora of humans. Candida yeasts can be found in the gastrointestinal tract where in the stressed host they may cause the disease thrush, and also in the female reproductive tract where their overgrowth results in vaginitis. Of the many species within this genus, *C. albicans* is most commonly associated with disease. Blastoconidia are the most common commensal form of the organism, but blastoconidia, as well as hyphae and pseudohyphae, have all been associated with invasive disease. Disease manifestations range from the more benign, chronic, superficial skin infections to life-threatening systemic disease.

Broad spectrum antibiotic therapy, indwelling canulas, chemotherapy, and hyperalimentation exemplify important conditions that predispose to candida infections. In addition, defects in T cell function predispose to skin infections, while neutropenia or any defects in the function of neutrophils, such as those manifested in chronic granulomatous disease or myeloperoxidase deficiencies, predispose to systemic disease. Severely immune compromised individuals are also predisposed to disseminated disease.

Properly functioning PMNs, which are able to phagocytose and kill invading conidia, form the first line of defense against these agents. Hyphae and pseudohyphae are killed extracellularly by both oxidative metabolites and cationic proteins. PMNs stimulated by gamma interferon or TNF alpha are more effective in elimination of fungal elements. Mannan in the fungal cell wall activates the alternate complement pathway and contributes to host defense by enhancing PMN chemotaxis.

Several virulence factors have been associated with *Candida*. Its ability to adapt to a changing environment by altering its phenotype contributes to its ability to invade tissues, evade the immune response, and develop resistance to antifungal drugs. A definite role in virulence has been established for the fungal enzyme aspartyl proteinase. Mutants unable to produce this enzyme, which functions in both adherence and invasion, have been shown to be avirulent.

The role of the humoral immune response is still unclear, though the observation that mice deficient in B cells are no more susceptible to this fungal disease than normal mice suggests that antibodies are not important in defense. Experimental work has shown that the proliferation of Th1 cells with the production of IFN gamma and TNF alpha is critical for resisting systemic disease, whereas the proliferation of Th2 cells results in progressive disease.

LABORATORY DIAGNOSIS

Accurate and rapid identification of the agent is crucial for the containment or resolution of the disease. The two basic approaches to identification include the direct demonstration of the agent and the demonstration of specific antibodies.

The demonstration of the agent can be very effective in the rapid identification of a fungus since fungal morphology is distinctive. Moreover, since a number of fungal agents have a unique morphology, direct examination of a clinical specimen can often give a definitive diagnosis. For example, the observation of broad-based budding yeast cells in the sputum of a patient with pneumonia, who had lived in an area endemic for blastomycosis, is considered diagnostic for *B. dermatiditis*. The presence of encapsulated yeast cells in an India Ink preparation of the cerebrospinal fluid of a patient with meningitis confirms the presence of *C. neoformans*.

Skin scrapings taken from a patient with scaly lesions can be treated with a potassium hydroxide preparation which clears extraneous tissue and renders the fungus more readily observable when examined microscopically. The presence of hyphae and arthroconidia in the specimen identifies the agent as a dermatophyte but does not define its genus.

Several fungal stains, such as periodic acid Schiff and Gomori's methanamine silver are also very useful in demonstrating fungi in clinical specimens. For example, the observation of large spherules in a stained exudate of a draining skin lesion from a patient from Arizona identifies the agent as *C. immitis*. However, the observation of hyphal elements in a stained specimen of sputum from a patient with pneumonia establishes only a fungal etiology of the infection since most of the common opportunists, such as *Aspergillus*, grow in the host in hyphal morphology. In this case culture would be needed for further identification.

Other tests have been developed to determine the presence of fungal antigens in fluid specimens. The latex agglutination test is used to detect the polysaccharide antigen of *C. neoformans* in spinal fluid. Radioimmune assays have been developed for detection of histoplasma antigens in urine and serum. Immunofluorescent staining is also used for the detection of fungal antigens.

Detection of antibodies by tests such as complement fixation, latex agglutination, and immunodiffusion have generally not proven to be very useful in diagnosis, in part because fungal diseases occur more commonly in hosts who are in some way immune compromised. Also, cross-reactions are common since fungi share many antigens. Although a recently developed sandwich enzyme immunoassay was shown to have a specificity of 100 percent in identifying *Blastomyces*, its sensitivity was only eighty-eight percent, so a negative result could not be taken as definitive. Serological testing should be used only as an adjunct to other diagnostic tests and for epidemiological surveys.

Culture, and in some cases phase conversion, both of which can take several weeks, may be necessary to confirm the identity of an agent. DNA gene probes, which identify specific RNA sequences unique to a particular fungus, have been developed to identify some agents, thereby establishing the diagnosis more quickly.

THERAPY

Since the discovery of the effectiveness of amphotericin as an antifungal drug in 1955, other drugs have been developed to treat systemic mycoses. Most of them target the ergosterol component of the fungal cell memebrane, though by two different mechanisms.

Amphotericin B is an example of the polyenes, a group of antifungals which bind to ergosterol and alter the permeability of the membrane, causing death of the fungus. Unfortunately these agents also bind to a lesser extent to cholesterol in the host cell membrane, producing similar damage to the host cell. Consequently these agents cause considerable host toxicity, especially nephrotoxicity. Although amphotericin B is still very effective in therapy against many of the systemic mycoses, resistance to the drug is developing. Usage of this drug is also restricted because it is not yet available in an oral form and must be administered intravenously.

The azoles, ketoconazole, itraconazole, and fluconazole are a newer class of antifungal drugs which inhibit an enzyme needed for the synthesis of ergosterol. They are fungistatic and produce less host toxicity than the polyenes. These drugs are available in the oral form.

Flucytosine, effective against yeast, and griseofulvin, effective against dermatohytes, both function by inhibiting nucleic acid synthesis.

In all cases therapy must be initiated early in the course of the disease and must be continued for a long period of time (months).

Recent work has demonstrated the effectiveness of chitin synthesis inhibitors such as lufenuron in the treatment of coccidioidomycosis. Other efforts are underway to target the topoisomerases of the fungi.

SUMMARY

Although we are exposed to fungal elements daily, we are very resistant to fungal disease. Proper functioning of both the innate and the adaptive immune responses are essential for our resistance to mycotic disease since fungi possess many different virulence factors that enhance their invasiveness and survival in the host. The current increase in the incidence of fungal disease is due to the growing number of immune compromised hosts in the population. Laboratory identification of the fungal agent can be made by direct microscopic observation or by the demonstration of fungal antigens in the specimen. Serological testing is of limited use in the diagnosis of mycotic disease but is useful for epidemiological surveys. Antifungal drugs are available for therapy. Unfortunately all of these drugs produce some toxic side effects, a problem compounded by the fact that all fungal therapy is long term.

SUGGESTIONS FOR FURTHER READING

1. Hogan, L.H., B.S. Klein, and S.M. Levitz. "Virulence Factors of Medically Important Fungi." *Clinical Microbiology Reviews* 9, no. 4 (Oct. 1996):469–488.

2. Ajello, L., and R.J. Hay, eds. *Topley and Wilson's Microbiology and Microbial Infections, Vol. 4: Medical Mycology,* 9th ed. London: Arnold, 1998.

QUESTIONS

1 Explain why the incidence of fungal disease is increasing. Give two specific examples to support your answer.
2 Fungal therapy is very effective is controlling fungal infections but serious problems are frequently associated with it. Using one of the common antifungal drugs as an example, explain these problems.
3 Explain what is meant by the following terms and give an example for each: dimorphism, phase transformation, endemic areas, conidia, spherule.
4 In general, CMI responses are of critical importance in the resolution of fungal infections. What observations give support to this statement?
5 How is the fungal agent of disease identified?
6 Identify at least three well-documented virulence factors of fungi and explain how each of them functions in the pathogenesis of the disease.

ANSWERS

1 The incidence of fungal disease is increasing due to the increased number of immune compromised individuals in the population. People on immune suppressive therapies, chemotherapy or radiation therapy for cancer or organ transplants, people suffering from AIDS, and any others who are immune compromised are all predisposed to fungal disease. The incidence of both histoplasmosis and cryptococcosis is especially high among individuals with AIDS. Aspergillosis is a serious threat for people who are neutropenic, a condition commonly brought about by radiation or chemotherapy. Candidiasis also is more commonly seen among hosts with underlying disease.
2 Therapy for fungal disease is available and is generally effective. However, there are problems associated with therapy. All of the fungal drugs are toxic for the host due to the drugs' effects on the cholesterol of the host cell membrane. Since the drugs must be given for long periods of time, i.e., months, there is a greater chance that toxic reactions will develop. Amphotericin B, which is a very good fungal drug must be given IV and is associated with nephrotoxicity. Drug resistance to fungal drugs is also developing.
3 Dimorphism refers to the characteristic of certain fungi to exist in two different morphological states, a mycelial phase in the environment and usually as a yeast phase in the host or when grown at 37°C. Examples are: *C. immitis* which grows in the host as a spherule, *B. dermatiditis*, *H. capsulatum*, and *S. schenkii* which grow in the host as yeasts.
Phase transformation refers to the conversion of the fungus from the conidia of the mycelial state to the yeast (or spherule) morphology found within the host. This ability to undergo transformation is a virulence trait because the resulting cells are much more resistant to host responses. The fungi listed above all undergo phase transformation.
Endemic areas are identified geographical areas in which the incidence of a particular fungal infection is higher than in other areas. These areas are environmental niches which better support the growth of a particular fungus than other localities.

B. dermatiditis is endemic to the areas around the St. Lawrence River, in Wisconsin, and in southern central states. *H. capsulatum* is endemic to the states of the Ohio-Mississippi River Valley area. *C. immmitis* is endemic to the states of the southwest. Conidia are the asexual reproductive units of the fungi. They are produced from mycelial growth and also by budding of the yeast cell (blastoconidium). Conidia from the mycelial growth of the dimorphic fungi are the infectious units which are inhaled and undergo phase transformation to the yeast morphology.

The exception is *C. immitis*; the conidia of this fungus transform into spherules in the host. Spherules are the asexual reproductive units of *C. immitis* in the host. The inhaled conidia from the mycelial phase undergo phase transformation to spherules in the 37°C environment of the lungs. These units grow to 20–80 μm in diameter. Endospores are produced within the spherule and released when the spherule ruptures. The spherule is covered by a fibrillar network which may function to limit access of PMNs.

4 Clinical evidence supports the importance of the CMI in resolution of most fungal diseases. This evidence includes the increased incidence of severe histoplasmosis in AIDS patients, the observation that the immune competent host is able to control blastomycosis, coccidioides, and cryptococcosis but that these diseases become systemic in the host with an improperly functioning CMI response.

5 The fungal agent of disease can be identified by observation of the agent in a clinical specimen in a KOH or stained preparation, or by immunofluorescent staining. Tests to detect the presence of fungal antigen in the host include the latex agglutination test for *C. neoformans*, radioimmune assay for *H. capsulatum* in urine and serum, and immunifluorescent staining for fungal antigens. Serological testing for the presence of fungal antibodies is of limited value in diagnosis, as such antibodies are widely present in healthy persons.

6 The capsule of *C. neoformans* functions to impede phagocytosis. It is believed to depress the respiratory burst of macrophages, and depress the CMI response. It has been shown that acapsular mutants are avirulent.

Candida's ability to adapt to a changing environment by altering its phenotype not only allows it to keep a step ahead of the immune response, but also to invade tissues and to develop resistance to antifungals. A proteinase functions both in adherence and in invasion and a cell wall mannan is immune suppressive.

The thick cell wall of the blastoconidia of *B. dermatiditis* is a virulence factor due to its increased resistance to the effects of phagocytosis. It has been suggested that the glucan of the cell wall functions to mask the adhesin which binds the blastoconidia to macrophages thereby allowing the yeasts to escape recognition by these phagocytes. The spherule of *C. immitis* is surrounded by a fibrillar, glycoprotein matrix which is believed to limit access of phagocytes to the cell. The large size of the spherule also precludes phagocytosis. The blastoconidia of *H. capsulatum* raise the pH of the phagolysosome thereby rendering the hydrolases much less effective. They also fail to induce reactive oxygen metabolites.

Immunization

Michael F. Para, Susan L. Koletar and Carter L. Diggs

INTRODUCTION
GENERAL PRINCIPLES
  Active Immunization
  Passive Immunization
HOST RESPONSE TO
  VACCINATION
  General Features
  Determinants of Response
    to Vaccines
COMPLICATIONS
  RESULTING FROM
  VACCINATION
  Risk/Benefit Evaluation of
    Vaccine
VACCINE DEVELOPMENT
  AND PRODUCTION
  Introduction
  Types of Vaccines
CHALLENGES IN VACCIN-
  OLOGY
SUMMARY
SUGGESTIONS FOR
  FURTHER READING
QUESTIONS
ANSWERS

INTRODUCTION

The practice of vaccination, the artificial induction of immunity to disease, is based on a long history of accumulated observations and experimentation. As early as the sixth century, long before firm knowledge of immunologic and infectious processes existed, physicians of the Sung Dynasty tried to prevent severe smallpox (variola) by intranasal inoculation of crusts of active lesions from mild cases. Centuries later, *variolation*, the practice of inoculating susceptible persons with material from people with mild variola infections became popular. While this procedure was relatively effective, occasionally complications and spread of disease would occur. The modern era of immunization began in 1796, when Edward Jenner noticed that milkmaids who had cowpox were immune to smallpox. Jenner took advantage of this observation and inoculated children with the vesicular fluid from cowpox (vaccinia) lesions. He was able to induce protection against smallpox without danger of inducing smallpox. As this practice of *vaccination* became widespread during the nineteenth century, smallpox was gradually controlled. Two centuries after the introduction of vaccination and after an aggressive global immunization program, the World Health Organization (WHO), in 1980, declared smallpox to be completely eradicated.

Since the eighteenth century, a large number of immunizing agents against a variety of diseases have been developed and are currently available. Although none have served as the basis for eradicating a disease as has smallpox vaccination, many have had a major impact on the epidemiology of the infectious diseases they were designed to control (Table 19.1). As a tribute to Jenner's use of cowpox virus to prevent smallpox we have adopted the term *vaccination* as a general term for agents used to immunize

393

Table 19.1. Numbers of cases of somes infectious diseases occurring in the United States before and after introduction of vaccines for the disease.

	Reported Cases		
	Before Introduction of Vaccine		After Introduction of Vaccine (1999)
Disease	Number	Year	Number
Diphtheria	206,939	(1921)	1
Pertussis	265,269	(1934)	6,031
Tetanus	601	(1948)	33
Measles	894,134	(1941)	86
Mumps	152,209	(1968)	352
Rubella	57,686	(1969)	238
Paralytic Polio	21,269	(1952)	0
HiB	20,000+	(1984)	33

against disease. In this chapter, we will discuss the general principles of vaccination, the types of vaccines available, development and production of vaccines, and future prospects for development of vaccines.

GENERAL PRINCIPLES

Any disease to which a human or other animal may develop an immunity which protects against subsequent infection is a candidate for control by vaccination. Attainment of the immune state can be by active or passive means. Active immunization is based on the premise that administration of an appropriate immunogen will stimulate the afferent arm of the immune system to provide immune effector agents (cells or molecules capable of immune attack) which will protect the recipient against disease if exposure to the virulent agent occurs. Useful vaccines will do this without themselves causing significant disease. Passive immunization involves the administration of specific neutralizing or opsonizing antibodies or other immune effector molecules to protect against known or probable exposure. (Passive immunization with cells is not currently practical because of transplantation immunity against cells derived from a donor of a different histocompatibility haplotype [see chapter 11].) For the most part, this process depends on the availability of protective antibodies which must have initially been generated by an active immune response, but recent studies have demonstrated the protective effect of passively administered recombinant cytokines.

Active Immunization

To be an effective vaccine, the immune response which follows active immunization must protect against subsequent infection or disease. The mechanisms by which this occurs are either by blocking infection or interfering with a disease-causing process. The two critical factors in determining the antigenic composition of a vaccine are the appropriateness of its chemical composition to the molecular targets of the invading agent (i.e., the inclusion of protective epitopes) and polymorphism in the antigenic structure of the molecules which are the targets of the immune response in the pathogenic organism.

Protective Epitopes

Immunizing agents, including vaccines used to prevent disease, are often comprised of multiple antigens each of which may have multiple specific antigenic

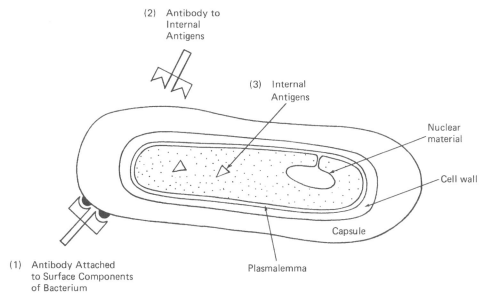

Figure 19.1.   Diagram of a bacterium showing location of antigens inducing immunity. Most beneficial responses are directed against surface components of parasites (1). Internal antigens (3) may induce an immunological response; however, the response generally contributes little to the defense against infection. This is because the effector system of immunity such as antibody or cytolytic T cells react with the surfaces of living parasites. Reaction with internal components (2) only takes place after the parasite is already dead and has disintegrated. Such reactions are useful however in clearance of debris and thus contribute to recovery.

sites or epitopes. These are defined by both the sequential molecular and the conformational macromolecular arrangements of the immunogen. Not all epitopes are equivalent in their ability to induce a protective immune response. Antigens can either be external and exposed on the surface of the microbe or internal and not exposed. Since it is the surface of the microbe which first interacts with the host, the external antigens are usually the antigens useful for vaccination (Figure 19.1). In this situation, the humoral or cell-mediated immune response induced by the vaccine results in products which inactivate the parasite's pathogenic potential. For example, the influenza virus has both external antigens such as the hemagglutinin and neuraminidase molecules which are exposed on the surface of the virus and internal antigens such as the matrix protein or nucleoprotein which are not exposed. While the internal antigens do induce antibodies during infection, only antibodies to the external antigens are capable of neutralizing the infectious virus and preventing infection. However, while protective immune responses are primarily directed against external antigens, not all external antigens induce protective responses. For instance, antibodies to the hemagglutinin molecule of influenza are much more effective at preventing infection than are antibodies to the neuraminidase molecule.

Antigenic Polymorphism

If a vaccine is to prove useful, the immune response to it must be appropriate to control the disease caused by the pathogen. One must select an antigen with antigenic sites which are present on the pathogen to be controlled. In some cases a single antigen is sufficient. For example, the hepatitis B vaccine includes only a single antigen but it has an epitope which is shared by all hepatitis B viruses. In other cases it is necessary for the vaccine to include multiple immunogens representative of antigens in many strains of the organism. This is the case with the pneumococcal capsular polysaccharide vaccines which induce opsonizing antibodies specifically directed against each of the various polysaccharides included in the vaccine. The currently available pneumococcal vaccine includes capsular antigens from twenty-three pathogenic serotypes of the organism and thus induces protection against all of the bacterial strains that provided antigen for the vaccine.

A vaccine, even if at one time adequate, may provide suboptimal protection if there are antigenic changes in the pathogen population. Loss of utility may result from "antigenic drift" of the microbe. This occurs frequently with the influenza virus since this microbe has the inherent ability to undergo antigenic changes secondary to point mutations of the genes programming production of the surface hemagglutinin and neuraminidase molecules. The frequent antigenic changes in the influenza virus are the basis for the inclusion of many viral strains in the vaccine. Even with the inclusion of many viral strains in the influenza vaccine, it is still necessary to constantly change its composition to keep up with changes in the virus.

An even more difficult situation is presented by organisms that undergo antigenic variation during an infection in a single host individual. African trypanosomes and malaria parasites are examples. The genome of these organisms encodes a wide repertoire of surface antigens which are expressed separately in individual microbial cells in the population. When an immune response is induced by the major population resulting in its elimination, a small, previously subimmunogenic population grows up to perpetuate the infection. This process is repeated many times, often killing the host before the repertoire is exhausted. In part because of this phenomenon, successful vaccines have not yet been developed against these pathogens.

If living attenuated vaccines are used, they often generate a wide variety of antigens which will induce a broadly reactive immune response that reacts with antigens in a variety of strains of the pathogen. The cowpox virus which served as a vaccine to protect from smallpox is an example of a living agent that protects against a heterologous infection. Live vaccines which elicit humoral and cell-mediated immune responses against many different antigens and multiple epitopes are often broadly protective.

Passive Immunization

Passive immunization, unlike active immunization, depends on the administration of preformed antiodies such as antitoxins to confer immediate, albeit temporary protection. This approach is useful when exposure has already occurred (postexposure prophylaxis) or when there is either inadequate time to allow for effective active immunization before exposure or there is no active vaccine available (Table 19.2). Passive immunization is most useful if given before disease symptoms occur; it cannot reverse damage already done.

Passive immunization occurs naturally through transplacental transmission or passage in breast milk of a mother's antibodies to her fetus. It is only the very young who can assimilate antibody through the digestive tract. In older individuals administration of antibodies must be by injection. These antibodies may be in the form of antisera derived from various types of animals which have been immunized with specific pathogens or toxins. While these heterologous sera have some

Table 19.2.   Globulin preparations available for passive immunization.

Product	Indications for Use
Standard human immune serum globulins Intramuscular preparation	Prevention of Hepatitis A, Measles, Polio, and Rubella
Intravenous preparation	Supplementation of people with Immunoglobulin Deficiencies and people with Idiopathic Thrombocytopenic Purpura
Specific human immune serum globulins Antibody to Hepatitis B Antibody to Rabies Antibody to Tetanus Antibody to Varicella-zoster	Prevention of Hepatitis B Prevention of Rabies Prevention or treatment of Tetanus Prevention of Chickenpox

use when administered preexposure or very early in the disease course, the hypersensitivity reactions which result from the administration of heterologous protein frequently outweigh the benefits to be derived from their administration.

In the 1940s, immune serum globulin prepared from pooled human plasma became available. It was and continues to be used in the prevention of infectious hepatitis, measles, rubella, and poliomyelitis. Immune serum globulin is often given to pregnant women who have contact with children infected with rubella. The antibodies protect the fetus from infection which is a common cause of birth defects.

Immune serum globulin is a sterile solution containing antibodies from human blood; it is a fifteen to eighteen percent protein suspension derived by cold ethanol fractionation of pooled plasma. For years, immune serum globulin was available only as a preparation for intramuscular injection. This is because the ethanol precipitation procedure used for fractionation aggregates the immunoglobulin yielding clumps which can activate complement, and cause a shocklike condition when given intravenously. Intramuscular administration keeps the aggregates in the muscle but allows single immunoglobulin molecules to enter the circulation. The main problem with this is that only 10 to 20 milliters can be comfortably administered by the intramuscular route.

New techniques for separating gamma globulin from plasma which do not cause aggregation of antibodies have been developed more recently. These immunoglobulin preparations can be administered intravenously so that large volumes and high levels of antibodies can be given. In fact, physiologically normal levels of immunoglobulin can now be achieved in patients who completely lack the ability to generate their own antibodies.

Human origin immune globulins directed against specific diseases have been developed. These specific immune globulins are prepared from donors with high antibody titers against specific diseases. For example, individuals who have just recovered from varicella-zoster (shingles) will provide high titer antibody to that virus. Homologous antibody preparations are available for use in the prevention of tetanus, rabies, hepatitis B, and varicella-zoster infection of man for example.

Veterinarians use homologous sera to protect animals that have been exposed to various infections or which will be at immediate risk. For example, dogs taken to shows or housed in boarding kennels if they have not been immunized against distemper will be given canine origin antidistemper serum. Any horse that is injured or that undergoes surgery receives equine origin antitetanus serum.

HOST RESPONSE TO VACCINATION
General Features
The induction of a protective immune response depends in most cases on the interaction of both B and T cells. This is the case with live vaccines such as those for prevention of measles. Some vaccines, however, can initiate B cell proliferation and antibody production without the involvement of T cells (see chapter 8). Such vaccines are based on T-independent antigens, usually polysaccharides; examples are capsular polysaccharide vaccines against pneumococci.

The clonal expansion and activation of lymphocytes of the various subsets result in the production of multiple types of effector systems. There may be multiplication of B lymphocytes with production of immunoglobulin directed against the antigenic determinants in the vaccine. The mechanisms of action of antibodies include direct neutralization of toxins (as in control of diphtheria), opsonization of pathogens (as in control of pneumococcal infections), complement-dependent microbial lysis (as in meningococcal infections), neutralization of viral infectivity (as in control of hepatitis B infection), and antibody-dependent cellular toxicity (as in the control of *Salmonella typhi* infections). Any or all of these effector mechanisms can in theory operate individually or collectively depending on the nature of the pathogen, the stage of the immune response, and other factors. Initial immunization also induces memory cells which promote a rapid secondary immune response at the time of exposure to the pathogen.

Activation of T lymphocytes by the vaccine may bring about a broad range of responses, which in part, are related to the antigen's ability to activate specific T cell subsets. T cells can influence B cell activity or can act directly through cell-mediated immune responses. One mechanism of action of T cells is the production of lymphokines which stimulate macrophage function. T cell-mediated immunity is particularly important in vaccines against intracellular microbes.

Artificially induced immunity may not be complete, and even with generally functional vaccines, one cannot always assume that protection has developed after immunization. One way of evaluating the immune response following injection of vaccine is the measurement of circulating antibodies to the antigens in the vaccine. The process of development of antibodies is called *seroconversion*. In some instances, the presence of circulating antibodies correlates well with development of protection. This is the case with hepatitis B and rubella vaccines. Antibody levels, however, do not tell the whole story. If there is a strong immunologic memory response, protection may exist in the absence of detectable antibody. For example, following vaccination with agents such as live attenuated measles and rubella vaccines, there will be an initial IgM antibody response, followed by a rise in IgG antibody titers. Over time, the antibody titers will fall, and although they may fall to undetectable levels, when infection occurs there is a rapid response by the memory cells. In such situations there is a prompt increase in IgG antibodies specific for the virus and protection from disease. The mere presence of antibody, however, may not be sufficient to assure protection from disease, but rather a minimum level of antibody may be required. Such is the case if immunity to tetanus is to be induced by injection of tetanus toxoid.

Determinants of Response to Vaccines

Many factors determine the nature and extent of the response to immunization. These attributes of the vaccine include the physical, chemical, and conformational state of the antigenic agent, i.e., its antigenicity and other factors including the route and timing of administration and the condition of the host at the time of immunization.

The route of administration influences the nature, extent, and duration of the immunologic response to the vaccine. The inactivated poliomyelitis vaccine (Salk vaccine), for example, is injected into the muscle while the live, attenuated polio vaccine (Sabine vaccine) is administered orally. The Salk vaccine induces systemic IgG antibodies against polioviruses. In individuals given this type of vaccine, poliovirus can infect the intestines but the spread of virus to the brain and spinal cord through the bloodstream is blocked by the neutralizing IgG antibodies. On the other hand, the Sabin vaccine induces both system IgG and local IgA antibody production in the gastrointestinal mucosa. This type of vaccine therefore not only blocks dissemination of the virus but also prevents significant infection of the gastrointestinal tract by pathogenic polioviruses.

Timing of vaccination in relation to anticipated exposure is important in disease control by immunization. To have optimal efficacy, vaccines must be administered far enough in advance of potential exposure to permit immunity to be induced. In general, it takes one to three weeks for full development of the immune response following vaccination. Further, the induced immunity and resulting protection may wane with the passage of time, requiring the administration of "booster" immunizations to maintain adequate protection. Knowledge of epidemiologic factors is thus crucial in deciding appropriate timing of vaccine administration. Immunization against influenza is most efficacious if the vaccine is administered in late autumn or early winter just prior to the influenza "season." Similarly, the schedule for routine childhood immunizations against measles, diphtheria, whooping cough and scarlet fever for example is based on the prevalence of those diseases in childhood. Immunization is usually done before enrollment in school where concentration of children in classrooms favors infection.

A factor which significantly affects the response to immunization is the overall condition of the vaccine recipient. Endogenous factors such as age, genetic makeup and general health status, and exogenous factors such as intercurrent infection, nutritional status, and medication are all important. Vitamin A deficiency has been especially clearly demonstrated to interfere with host defense. Satisfactory response to immunization requires the recipient to be in an immunocompetent state. Those individuals with reduced immunocompetence, whether it be from an infection, hereditary defects, or treatment with immunosuppressive drugs, not only have poor immune responses but may also be at increased risk from the immunizing agent. This is especially true if live, attenuated vaccines are used. The attenuated agent may reproduce without restraint and disease may be produced by the vaccine in the immunosuppressed individual. Introduction of vaccine into individuals incubating a disease or infection during the period when the immune response to the vaccine is developing may also result in severe disease. Living attenuated vaccines should not be given to pregnant individuals for the fetus may be infected and damaged.

In summary, many factors must be taken into account when developing recommendations for immunoprophylaxis. The recommendations must be based on the

Table 19.3.   Routine childhood immunizations.

Age	Immunization
Birth	Hep B
2 mos.	DPT, IPV, Hep B and HiB
4 mos.	DPT, IPV, and HiB
6 mos.	DPT, Hep B, and HiB
15 mos.	DPT, IPV, HiB, MMR, and Var
4–6 yrs.	DPT, IPV, MMR
14–16 yrs.	
every 10 yrs.	Td

DPT – Diphtheria and tetanus toxoids combined with pertussis
IPV – Injectable polio vaccine
MMR – Measles, mumps, rubella
HiB – *Haemophilus influenzae*, type B
Td – Tetanus and diphtheria (adult type)
Hep B – Hepatitis B
Var – Varicella

potential for exposure to particular pathogens, the probable times of exposure and the consequences of such an exposure. The severity of the disease to be prevented must be balanced against the dangers of immunization and the discomfort and costs of immunization. The availability of a vaccine or toxoid must also be considered. The routine childhood immunizations in the United States are directed at the usual childhood diseases which occur there, such as measles, mumps, rubella, poliomyelitis, diphtheria, pertussis, tetanus, and *Haemophilus influenza* infection (Table 19.3). Immunization for segments of the population are based on expected risk factors. Veterinarians and animal handlers receive prophylactic preexposure rabies vaccines; travelers and military personnel may be immunized against plague, yellow fever, and cholera. Elderly people may be immunized against influenza and pneumococcal pneumonia. Occupational hazards and life-style habits are thus important factors in planning immunization programs (Table 19.4).

COMPLICATIONS RESULTING FROM VACCINATION
Immunization is not completely free of problems. As noted previously, immunologically incompetent individuals may develop infections and disease following injection of attenuated live vaccines and fetuses in pregnant individuals may also be adversely affected by these agents. Inactive or killed vaccines simply have no effect in immunologically incompetent individuals.

On some occasions the disease against which the vaccine is used may be induced by the vaccine. This occurred with some of the early Salk polio vaccines in which not all the virus was inactivated during vaccine production. Idiosyncratic reactions may occur following immunization. The Guillain-Barré syndrome which occurred following the swine influenza vaccination in 1976 is an example.

Allergic responses to vaccine components, independent of any protective responses, may result in immunologic disease in the vaccine recipient. Hypersensitivity reactions occurred following immunization with the original rabies vaccine prepared by Pasteur. This vaccine was composed of rabbit nervous tissue infected with rabies virus. After treatment to inactivate the virus, the entire preparation of nervous tissue was inoculated. The neural tissue in the vaccine produced an immune response which cross-reacted with host neural tissue and damaged the re-

Table 19.4. Vaccines for specific situations or groups.

Vaccine	Target Group
Influenza	Health care personnel Immunocompromised patients Patients with chronic diseases Persons over 50
Pneumococcal Polysaccharide	Immunocompromised persons Persons with splenic dysfunction/asplenia Chronic alcoholics Patients with chronic diseases Those over fifty years of age
Rabies	Veterinarians, animal handlers, dogs, cats
Cholera, Plague, Yellow Fever	Persons traveling to infected regions

cipient's nervous system. Damage to vaccine recipients as a result of hypersensitivity to immunizing agents has also occurred following administration of killed measles vaccine. Occasionally this vaccine induced incomplete humoral immunity, and, following infection by the measles virus, a cell-mediated hypersensitivity sometimes developed which caused a severe atypical measles syndrome.

Risk/Benefit Evaluation of Vaccine
Although vaccination is associated with some risk of adverse side effects, the benefits derived from immunization in most cases far outweigh the risks. Table 19.1 clearly illustrates the benefits. Some permanent disabilities or deaths have been attributed to vaccination. Although any undesirable effects are unfortunate, the decision to vaccinate is in most cases clearly the best choice for individuals at risk.

VACCINE DEVELOPMENT AND PRODUCTION
Introduction
Development of vaccines for human use can be divided into the following stages: discovery, design, production process development, pilot production, characterization and specification, quality assurance, preclinical safety evaluation, and clinical and field testing (Phases I, II, III). If the candidate vaccine passes study in these areas, then registration, introduction, and postmarket surveillance follow (Phase IV). The process is regulated in the United States by the Food and Drug Administration (FDA). Vaccines for nonhuman animals go through similar types of evaluation but are regulated by the Department of Agriculture.

The discovery phase consists of the collection of fundamental knowledge and information about the disease and the pathogen to permit a rational approach to the design of a vaccine. Typically, the data collected in the discovery phase provides an understanding of the pathogenesis and epidemiology of the disease, the structure and function of the pathogen and as much information as possible about the host-parasite interaction. Application of current vaccine development technology requires that the molecular structures of the antigens involved, as well as the genes determining these structures, be completely known.

While those designing vaccines take into account the knowledge available, vaccine design is still a very empirical process. The decision of which immunogens to prepare is often through a laborious process based on subjective judgments of the value of scant data. There is no assurance that the preliminary evaluation of the candidate vaccines selected will prove them to be promising enough for further testing. Evaluation of candidate vaccines is different from the hypothesis-driven research conducted during the discovery period, as it is oriented towards evaluation of a product rather than collection of more general information about a disease. The type of research used for production of candidate vaccines depends on the problem at hand, but currently is most often one using a molecular biological strategy for making a product.

Once a design concept is selected for candidate antigen production, the production process development phase is instituted which seeks to determine if the design concept is valid. Currently this phase is often concerned with issues such as the amount of recombinant protein expressed or produced by the system being used. The genes producing the antigen may have been introduced into bacterial, yeast, insect, or mammalian cells, or the antigen may have been made by a peptide synthesizer. The integrity of the product, whether or not it is expressed intact or whether it is truncated, whether or not it is glycolsylated and the consequences thereof, etc., must be determined. Then it must be determined how the product can be adequately purified. In this phase the feasibility of a scaleup of the process from the laboratory bench to the pilot production plant is undertaken.

The U.S. Code of Federal Regulations specifies that vaccines for human use be made under rules called collectively, "Good Manufacturing Practices." Thus, a system for the development and maintenance of records which will enable the precise documentation of the production process of the pilot vaccine lot as well as the conditions under which production was carried out must be instituted. Factors to be fully monitored include the microbiological and chemical condition of the air, water, reagents, and equipment in the production and purification suites. When the vaccine is finally prepared, sealed in a vial, usually with an adjuvant (see below), and ready for clinical use, production is complete.

Following chemical and microbiological characterization of the vaccine and after its quality is assessed to assure that the specifications for the vaccine are met, it may be released for preliminary testing. All lots of the vaccine must meet the specifications laid out.

Among the preliminary tests are ones for safety. Safety is assessed by appropriate tests in laboratory animals. Depending on the vaccine, and especially the adjuvant used (see below), these tests might be simple and involve only a few mice and guinea pigs or involve relatively large numbers of nonhuman primates.

Human evaluation of a vaccine is preceded by the filing of an investigational new drug (IND) application with the FDA. In this application a detailed description of the vaccine and of its production and characterization is given. Much additional information is also required in this application. It must include a clinical protocol describing the proposed studies, and an indication of approval by a duly constituted Institutional Review Board (IRB) which has examined the protocol for scientific and ethical adequacy.

The initial clinical studies (Phase I) are carried out on a small number of people and are designed to begin the study of the safety of the vaccine for humans. Phase II studies expand safety evaluation and may, if feasible, gather information relevant to the efficacy of the vaccine. Phase III trials are typically much larger and assess vaccine efficacy.

Registration of a vaccine takes place when the officials of the FDA are satisfied that exhaustive studies have demonstrated that the vaccine is well characterized, can be manufactured reproducibly, and is safe and efficacious. At this point, the vaccine can be manufactured and marketed. Following introduction, surveillance continues to uncover previously undiscovered safety hazards as well as for continued assurance of efficacy. It is also at this point that the true effectiveness of the vaccine on the incidence of the disease is established.

Adjuvants

In addition to the antigenic components to be described below, vaccine preparations usually contain other constituents, some active and some inert. Among the most important are adjuvants, i.e., agents which increase immunogenicity. Adjuvants are proving to be especially important in recombinant subunit vaccines which as a group tend to be poorly immunogenic. It is now appreciated that bacterial whole cell vaccines may owe at least a portion of their immunogenicity to naturally occurring materials such as lipid A which act as natural adjuvants. Their particulate nature may also be a contributing factor, since the immune system processes particulate and soluble antigens differently. Currently, the only adjuvant licensed in the United States is alum. Alum consists of either aluminum hydroxide or aluminum phosphate and is an insoluble substance with the property of adsorbing protein to its exposed surfaces. The efficacy of alum in promoting the immune response is poorly understood, but may be related to the concentration on the particles of alum of many molecules of antigen, thus presenting to the immune system particles covered with multiple epitopes. As occurs with cellular vaccines, so with alum-containing vaccines, the persistence of antigen at the injection site due to the decreased solubility of the complex may also play a role in increasing immunogenicity.

The limitations of alum are becoming more appreciated as research on recombinant vaccines proceeds. Adjuvants have been used routinely in laboratory animals to enhance the immune response, but the best of these, known as Complete Freund's Adjuvant (CFA), is quite toxic and cannot be used in humans. In fact its use in laboratory animals, especially nonhuman primates, is currently discouraged. However, a number of adjuvants have been tested in humans and are available for formulation in investigational vaccines for evaluation in humans. These agents can be divided into several major categories: oil/water emulsions, bacterial products, polymeric compounds, and detergents which are used alone or in combination. Oil/water emulsions may be prepared with either an oil or water continuous phase with the opposite phase dispersed, thus yielding oil in water and water in oil categories. The efficacy of the two categories has been reported to be different depending on the specific antigen studied. Bacterial products, usually chemically modified, are often used in oil/water formulations. Currently the most commonly used adjuvant in these studies is lipid A which has been partially dephosphorylated (monophosphoryl lipid A), a process which markedly reduces toxicity. Another compound of bacterial origin which has adjuvant properties is muramyl dipeptide. Muramyl dipeptide is a constituent of tubercle bacilli which are themselves constituents of CFA, which is also an oil/water emulsion. Polymer adjuvants are usually charged and adsorb antigen according to their charge. Polymer adjuvants also enable presentation of the

Table 19.5. Examples of types of immunogens available for active immunization.

Type of Vaccine	Disease Prevented
Live, unattenuated vaccines	Anaplasmosis, babesiosis, hog cholera
Live, attenuated vaccines	Measles, mumps, rubella, polio, yellow fever, tuberculosis, anaplasmosis, babesiosis, hog cholera
Killed or inactivated vaccines	
Whole organisms	Cholera, pertussis, plague, influenza, polio, hog cholera
Subunits of organisms	Influenza, hepatitis B
Soluble capsular polysaccharides	Pneumococcus, meningococcus, *Haemophilus influenzae*
Recombinant DNA type vaccines	Hepatitis B, malaria* (sporozoite)
Toxoids	Diphtheria, tetanus
Synthetic polypeptide vaccines	*S. pyogenes* infection, foot and mouth disease, cholera, malaria* (sporozoite and blood stage)

* Still in testing stage.

antigen as a part of a particle with low solubility. A detergent adjuvent under active investigation currently is a purified fraction of saponin, a natural plant product which has been recognized as an adjuvant for many years. The purification process fraction seeks to minimize toxicity while retaining adjuvanticity.

In addition to the actions described above, adjuvants clearly modulate cytokine production. Different adjuvants tend to favor one or another aspect of the immune response, such as proliferation of TH1 versus TH2 CD4+ T cells in mice. Since control of different diseases requires activation of different immune effector mechanisms, direction of the immune response through application of adjuvant technology is a much sought after goal. In fact a young science of immune chemoregulation is emerging. However, the most profound and useful results of knowledge to be gained by this type of study are in the future.

Types of Vaccines

Although the account above is of problems associated with recombinant development methodology for vaccine production, vaccines currently in use for active immunization are mostly produced by other means (Table 19.5). Vaccines may consist of suspensions of live attenuated microbes, of killed, inactivated microbes, of fractions of microbes, or of microbial products. Live vaccines generally evoke a durable immunologic response much like that resulting from natural infection. The currently available measles, mumps, and rubella vaccines are live attenuated agents. Living agents engender good immunogenicity because their growth results in continuous formation of antigen and prolonged antigenic stimulation. In addition, a broad spectrum of microbial antigens is presented to the immune system. If the organisms are intracellular pathogens, the method of presentation favors the development of cell-mediated immunity (see chapter 8). As infection is induced by the attenuated agents, the immunity generated resembles that resulting from natural infection. There is extensive stimulation of the immune system by the antigens produced by the infection; consequently live vaccines usually require just one dose to induce protection.

Killed or inactivated vaccines which consist of whole organisms include the traditional cholera and pertussis vaccines; those which consist of components or subunits of an organism include hepatitis B and the new "acellular" pertussis vaccines. Vaccines made from soluble capsular polysaccharide material include those against pneumococcal pneumonia and meningococcal meningitis. Vaccines prepared from microbial products include the toxoids which are prepared by modification of bacterial exotoxins to make them nontoxic. Toxoids are used for prevention of diphtheria, scarlet fever and tetanus.

As a rule, to achieve strong immunity with toxoids and killed vaccines multiple doses of vaccine must be given. To maintain adequate protective antibody levels for prolonged periods, booster injections are frequently required.

Live Vaccines

Attenuated-type vaccines have been classically produced by growing the pathogens in an "unnatural" host, by growth in culture or by some other procedure which would select for mutant forms of the pathogen. Viruses have also been attenuated by being selected for inability to grow well at temperatures present in the host but able to grow at lower temperatures, a process called *cold-adaptation*. The desired end result of these processes is selection of a microbe with decreased virulence and pathogenicity but capable of inducing an immune response capable of protecting against the naturally occurring organism. Until recently, the attenuation process was entirely by trial and error. An organism was repeatedly passaged in the unnatural host or other selective environment, then tested for virulence and antigenicity. As the science of molecular genetics is now providing information about the specific genes responsible for virulence and antigenicity, site-directed mutagenesis is being employed to produce microorganisms which lack only the genes responsible for virulence.

Inactivated Vaccines

Microbes to be used in inactivated vaccines may be inactivated by subjecting the pathogens to heating, by treatment with chemical agents such as formaldehyde, methanol, or beta-propiolactone, or by irradiation. As with attenuation, the goal of inactivation is to block infectivity yet preserve the major antigen determinants which induce the protective immune response.

Toxoids

Toxoids, as previously mentioned, are detoxified bacterial exotoxins. Soluble toxins, most notably from diphtheria and tetanus-causing organisms are converted to toxoids by treatment with formalin and moderate heating. Though no longer toxic, toxoids have the ability to stimulate antitoxin formation. Immunization with toxoids protects by blocking the disease-causing process rather than by preventing infection by the microbe. To prepare toxoids for use as vaccines, they are usually precipitated by alum which serves as an adjuvant. The primary immune response to most toxoids is generally very good, and anamnestic increases are appreciable when booster injections are given.

Subunit Vaccines

While both attenuation and inactivation have produced many satisfactory vaccines, there are still many diseases for which vaccines do not exist, and many currently available vaccines produce undesirable side effects. In the continuing search for new vaccines and for improvement in existing vaccines, procedures for production of useful fractions of microbes are being sought. Vaccines which consist of fractions of microbes are called *subunit vaccines*. Subunit vaccines may be fractions of the infecting organism which are biochemically purified or may be produced by recombinant DNA technology. Since subunit vaccines do not contain actively replicating material, the risk of inducing infection is eliminated. They also lack microbial nucleic acids which may be potentially carcinogenic. One of the first successful subunit vaccines for use in man is that for prevention of hepatitis B infection. It contains only purified hepatitis B surface antigen, the portion of the virus which elicits neutralizing antibodies. In one type of this vaccine, the antigen is derived from the plasma of chronic hepatitis B carriers; in another it is produced by genetically modified plasmid bearing yeasts. The efficacy of both types of this vaccine has been well documented in controlled trials.

The polysaccharide capsules of encapsulated organisms such as pneumococcus, meningococcus, and *Haemophilus influenzae* are the virulence factors for those microbes. At one time these vaccines were prepared from whole inactivated microbes. The soluble components of the capsules from these bacteria, however, have been shown to evoke type-specific protective responses as strong as those induced by the whole microbe. The polysaccharide capsule vaccines now in use induce antibodies which protect the recipient by enhancing phagocytosis of the organisms. These vaccines are used primarily to protect people in high risk groups, such as the old and the young. A recently developed subunit vaccine consists of a conjugate of *Haemophilus influenzae* type B polysaccharide with diphtheria toxoid. The protein toxoid serves as a carrier for the *Haemophilus* capsular polysaccharide, greatly improving its immunogenicity in infants. This vaccine provides good protection against invasive hemophilus infection in young infants who as a group respond poorly to the unconjugated capsular antigen.

Recombinant DNA technology has great promise as a means of producing subunit vaccines. The process requires isolating the gene for the antigen, inserting that gene into a plasmid or other suitable carrier, introducing the complex into some host cell such as a bacterium, a yeast, or a mammalian or other animal cell which will express the gene. After the desired material is produced, it must be isolated from the culture or cell in which it is produced.

The recombinant hepatitis B vaccine is an example of a subunit vaccine produced by these procedures. The Food and Drug Administration licensed the recombinant hepatitis B vaccine produced in cultures of the bread yeast *Saccharomyces cerevisiae* in July 1986. Hepatitis B vaccine derived from plasma and the recombinant vaccine have the same efficacy.

Another example of a currently available genetically engineered vaccine is that for immunization of piglets against enterotoxigenic strains of *E. coli*. These bacteria secrete an enterotoxin which is responsible for severe diarrhea. The toxin consists of two subunits, an A subunit which is responsible for the toxic activity and a B subunit which is responsible for binding the A subunit to the intestinal epithelium. Following cloning of the toxin gene, the A subunit sequences were deleted, and the B subunit gene was transferred into *E. coli* K12. The result was that the genetically altered *E. coli* K12 produced a purified B subunit which, when collected from the culture, was an excellent toxoid.

Infectious Agents as Carriers of Genes for Antigen Production
While recombinant DNA technology is proving to be a useful means for producing

subunit vaccines such as those described previously, in general these products produce immunity only equal to that of conventional inactivated vaccines. To obtain the type of immunity that results from the prolonged antigenic stimulation associated with infection, genetically modified microbes are being produced. The vaccinia virus is a popular agent for this work. Genes programming the production of the desired antigen are inserted into the virus. The modified virus is then used as the vaccine.

The concept is an attractive one. An attenuated live carrier, for example a virus or bacterium which can infect but not harm the host, is engineered to express an added gene. When it produces infection, this recombinant microbe will then evoke long-lasting immune responses directed at both itself and the additional antigens. Vaccinia virus has been found to have a fairly broad capacity for accommodating foreign DNA without losing its infectivity. Vaccinia virus recombinants carrying genes for hepatitis B surface antigen, influenza virus hemagglutinin, herpes simplex virus glycoprotein D, the gp120 surface antigen of the AIDS virus (HIV), and the parasite causing falciparum malaria have been reported. The malaria vaccine, which contained genes encoding for seven different antigens, was tested in a human challenge trial and showed some promise of efficacy.

An avirulent *Salmonella* strain has also been tested as a carrier of genes producing antigens for immunization against infection by a variety of other microbes. This system has been used to induce immunity to infection by virulent strains of *Salmonella*. The avirulent *Salmonella* has also been used as a carrier for a plasmid-encoded gene for production of a toxin of *Shigella sonnei* as well as a carrier of the gene coding for the B subunit of the toxin of enterotoxigenic *E. coli*.

Use of the heterologous recombinant carriers is still in its infancy, and field testing will be required to fully evaluate their safety and efficacy.

Synthetic Antigens

Though not a new concept, the production of synthetic polypeptide vaccines has become more feasible with the advent of the techniques of molecular genetics. It was demonstrated many years ago that short polypeptide fragments of the protein coat of tobacco mosaic virus could block inactivation of the virus by antiserum. Subsequent studies showed that a hexapeptide from one fragment, when coupled to bovine serum albumin, would induce production of virus specific neutralizing antibodies.

The first step in developing synthetic polypeptide vaccines is identification of relevant "protection-inducing" antigens and epitopes. Next, the amino acid sequence is determined, and the critical epitope is then synthesized chemically. The polypeptide, when attached to an appropriate carrier, induces production of antibody with specificity to the primary amino acid sequence. Induction of a protective immune response is not solely related to the primary amino acid sequence of an antigen however. Antibodies to conformational determinants of the antigen expressed on the native pathogen may also be important. Though no synthetic polypeptide vaccines have been approved for use, some have been tested in man under controlled conditions.

Genetic Immunization

This recent approach to vaccine development has received considerable attention because of its potential for revolutionizing the entire field. A gene coding for a relevant antigen is inserted in a plasmid containing a viral promoter which enables expression in a mammalian system. Purified plasmid is injected into the individual to be immunized and produces the gene product *in situ*. This endogenously released antigen then induces an immune response. This system could potentially greatly accelerate vaccine development since the often rate-limiting step of production process development could be greatly shortened; recombinant protein expression technology is circumvented reducing production process development to construction of the plasmid. Purification process development is minimized since the purification process is the same for all plasmids regardless of the antigen gene inserted. If a genetic vaccine was developed to the point of registration and large-scale manufacture, it is likely that it could be produced at less expense than its recombinant protein counterpart. For these reasons, the approach is under active investigation. Protection from experimental infection of immunized hosts has been demonstrated in laboratory animal systems (for example, rodent malaria), and initial clinical trials of investigational HIV, influenza, and malaria vaccine in human volunteers have already taken place. Obstacles to development of the approach include a lack of knowledge of how to optimize the immune response to genetic vaccines and how to modulate the type of immune response obtained. Route of administration (intramuscular or intradermal) appears to be an important determinant of whether the response is predominantly humoral or cellular, but no useful general rules have emerged in this regard. A persistent concern is that the foreign DNA could become integrated into host DNA resulting in insertional activation of oncogenes and subsequent development of neoplastic disease. Another type of problem would arise if foreign antigen were to be incorporated in the membrane of the infected cell; cell-mediated immunity directed against the host cell could result in cell death. These concerns will continue to be evaluated. Only time will tell whether or not the potential of genetic immunization will be realized; but this and other emerging technologies insure that the next several years will be an exciting period in vaccine development.

CHALLENGES IN VACCINOLOGY

In spite of the enormous benefit of vaccination programs in terms of the prevention of morbidity and mortality, much work is needed in order for the full potential of vaccines to be realized. No registered vaccines exist for a number of diseases, such as HIV/AIDS and malaria, which are major public health problems globally. Improved vaccines are also needed to replace current products with suboptimal efficacy and ones with unwanted side effects.

Some diseases have not yielded to ongoing vaccine development efforts. There are many reasons for this, prominent among them is the unsolved problem of the pathogenesis of the diseases they produce and the limited engagement because of market considerations by commercial vaccine developers who have both the most advanced technological knowledge and facilities and the resources required. However, unless a clear pathway to a commercially viable product is apparent, industry will not commit resources; the full cost of development of a vaccine can easily reach $100 million or more. With this situation, "orphan" vaccine development must be pursued using public funding until evidence of commercial viability can be demonstrated.

Even when vaccines are available, they are often not delivered to populations at risk. The WHO-sponsored "Expanded Program of Immunization" (EPI) has done much to increase vaccination coverage rates in the underdeveloped world, but much work is still needed to reach optimal rates. Measles, for which there is an excellent vaccine, still kills more than one million people annually. International organizations are hard at work to improve vaccine delivery systems.

In spite of these difficulties, the well recognized superiority of prevention of disease over curative measures, both in terms of cost effectiveness and in terms of its impact on the well being of those being cared for, dictates continuing efforts to develop new vaccines and to improve vaccine delivery. The exciting new technological possibilities being introduced with increasing frequency will add further impetus to the endeavor to prevent infectious diseases.

SUMMARY

Progress in vaccine development has been characterized by simplification and purification of immunogenic agents; materials not needed for immunization are deleted from the vaccine. Attempts are made to increase antigenicity through use of more effective adjuvants. Attempts are also being made to develop vaccines for diseases for which no vaccines exist such as malaria and human immunodeficiency virus (HIV) infection. As our body of immunologic knowledge expands and our technologies become more sophisticated, new vaccines, based for example on simple synthetic peptides, may become a reality. Immunization is, and will remain, our major tool in the prevention of disease in man and animals.

SUGGESTIONS FOR FURTHER READING

1. Committee on Infectious Diseases. American Academy of Pediatrics. *Report of the Committee on Infectious Diseases*. 19th ed. Evanston, Illinois, 1982.
2. Recommendation of the Immunization Practices Advisory Committee (ACIP). "General Recommendations on Immunization." *MMWR* 32 (1987):1.
3. Anderson, D.C., and E.R. Stieham. "Immunization." *JAMA* 258 (1987):3301.
4. Bart, K.J., W.A. Orenstein, and A.R. Hinman. "The Current Status of Immunization Principles: Recommendations for Use and Adverse Reactions." *J. Allergy Clin. Immun.* 79 (1987):296.
5. Liew, F.Y. "New Aspects of Vaccine Development." *Clin. Exp. Immunol.* 62 (1985):225.

QUESTIONS

1 What is the goal of vaccine development? Describe the history of vaccine development.
2 Outline the types of immunization.
3 What is an epitope?
4 How many epitopes may be present on a pathogen and where must they be located on a pathogen to be useful in inducing immunity?
5 List the types of vaccines.
6 List and discuss complications resulting from vaccination.
7 Explain the concept of risk-benefit analysis in vaccine usage.

ANSWERS

1 The goal of vaccine development is to obtain the purest preparation of the critical immunologically active materials with minimal contamination by nonessential

materials. The objective is to assure an appropriate antigenic stimulation and to minimize the likelihood of undesirable side effects. The earliest vaccines were composed of live, wild-type organisms; most conventional modern-day vaccines, however, consist of either live attenuated or inactivated forms of microorganisms. Vaccines are currently being developed which take advantage of recent advances in immunology and molecular biology. Genetic engineering and chemical synthesis procedures show great promise as methods for vaccine production. The products produced by these techniques may prove to be advantageous in terms of good antigenicity, high specificity, and low ability to induce hypersensitivity.

2 Immunization may be active or passive. In active immunization the individual being immunized is exposed to the antigenic agent and develops the immunity as a result. In passive immunization the individual being immunized receives the protective immunogenic products produced by some other immunized individual. Passive immunization may be natural or artificial. Natural passive immunization occurs when a fetus receives protective immune agents across the placenta from its mother or when the newborn ingests colostrum or first milk within a few hours of birth. Artificial passive immunization occurs when an individual receives pre-formed protective immune agents by injection during the course of treatment or administration of prophylaxis by a physician or veterinarian.

3 An epitope is a particular site on an antigenic molecule that is recognized by the immune system. It may be a sequential structure determined by the sequence of monomers in a macromolecule, or conformational, in which case it is a shape formed by the folding of the chain of monomers in the macromolecule.

4 There are usually many epitopes on a pathogen, in fact, even most macromolecules may have a number of distinct epitopes. In general the epitopes important in inducing protection are those on the surfaces of the pathogen. They are usually portions of molecules the pathogen uses to protect itself from the host defenses, as for example, capsular materials.

5 Vaccines may consist of living attenuated microorganisms or of killed or inactivated organisms. The noninfective types of vaccines may consist of the inactivated whole intact pathogens or of components of the agent such as capsules or pili for example. Products of the pathogen, such as toxins in inactivated form, i.e., toxoids, are also used as vaccines. Some living vaccines are genetically altered organisms of various types, for example, genetically altered vaccinia virus altered to carry genes for plasmodial antigens may be used as a vaccine for malaria some day. The components of subunit vaccines may be obtained from the pathogen directly or produced by other genetically modified organisms. For parasites that are difficult to culture this latter technique is useful.

6 Vaccines are by definition antigenic, they may therefore induce undesirable allergic reactions in some recipients. Toxic components in some vaccines may cause pathology as for example has occurred in some individuals given pertussis vaccines. Vaccines may be unstable and lose potency if not stored properly or used before spontaneous decomposition even if stored properly. Vaccines given to individuals incubating the disease of concern may aggravate the disease. Vaccines only work well in individuals with a healthy immune system. In immunoincompetent individuals inactivated vaccines may have no effect and living attenuated vaccines may actually cause disease.

7 All types of immunization carry some risks as well as potential benefits. One must balance the benefits against the risks when deciding to immunize. This can consist

of evaluating the probability of injury to the individual by vaccination against the probability of sickness and death from the disease in question. If the probability of infection is low or the disease in question mild, one may decide vaccination is not worthwhile. We do not for example vaccinate everyone against rabies routinely but do vaccinate those at higher risk of infection such as veterinarians and animal handlers. Pertussis vaccination has had a fairly high incidence of undesirable effects, people therefore resisted continuing its use and as a result there was a resurgence of pertussis infections with many serious effects. It is doubtful that abandoning vaccination was really a good course of action in this case.

Risk and benefit to the individual being immunized is one consideration. Somewhat more difficult, particularly in an individualistic society, is weighing the collective benefit of mass immunization against the possibility of harm to small numbers of individuals in the population. For all risk-benefit analysis one needs good statistical data on the results of the previous use of the vaccine and the consequences of the infection in the absence of vaccination. Just analysis of good data is not all however; the analysis of risk versus benefit is in part made on the basis of moral and ethical considerations and thus our decisions are in part based on our belief system. In a heterogeneous society such as ours, with beliefs ranging from christian science to scientific humanism, consensus may be hard to reach.

CHAPTER 20

INTRODUCTION
IMMUNOLOGICAL TESTS
  Precipitation
  Precipitation in a Gel
    Matrix
  Agglutination
  Neutralization
  Complement Fixation
  Radioimmunoassay (RIA)
  Fluorescent Assay
  Enzyme-Linked Immuno-
    sorbent Assay (ELISA)
MONOCLONAL ANTIBODY
  PRODUCTION
SUMMARY
SUGGESTIONS FOR
  FURTHER READING
QUESTIONS
ANSWERS

Immunological Tests for Diagnosis of Disease and Identification of Molecules

Frank Petersen

INTRODUCTION

To recognize that an antibody exists, a corresponding antigen must be identified. To do this a method of detecting the reaction of antibody with antigen is necessary. A variety of methods have been devised for this purpose. Primary reactions, which depend only on antibody binding to the antigen, are the basis of immunofluorescence, ELISA, and radioimmunoassay procedures. Secondary reactions which depend on formation of a lattice yielding insoluble immune complexes and possibly on postbinding conformational changes within the antibody molecule for completion of the reaction are the basis of precipitation, agglutination, and complement fixation reactions.

IMMUNOLOGICAL TESTS
Precipitation

Precipitation is one of the oldest methods for detecting antigen-antibody interaction and remains widely used today. In 1935 Heidelberger described the precipitin curve (Figure 20.1). Precipitation results from the formation of an insoluble complex when soluble antibody reacts with soluble antigen. When the number of antigenic sites is roughly equivalent to the number of antibody sites available, a zone of equivalence or zone of optimal proportions results, yielding a three-dimensional lattice-like structure, and precipitation is maximal. If antibody is in excess, the lattice does not form; if antigen is in excess, a precipitate may form but then will redissolve.

In the mixture of antigen with an antiserum, several different antibody molecules can bind to each antigen molecule and cause lattice formation. The chemical interaction between antibodies and antigens involves such forces as hydrogen bonding, electrostatic attraction, hydrophobic bonding, electron cloud bonding, and bonding by van der Waals forces.

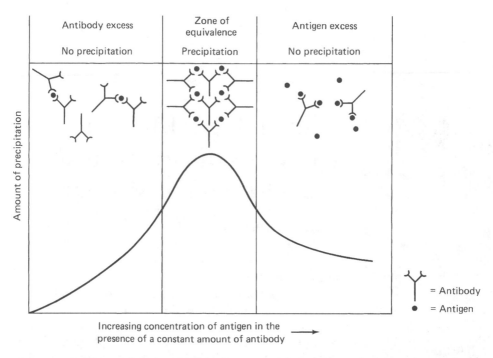

Figure 20.1.   The precipitation test. Maximum precipitate forms at the zone of equivalence where the proportions of antibody and antigen are optimum to produce a large lattice that is insoluble. The amounts of precipitate in antibody or antigen excess are smaller than at the zone of equivalence. In these zones many complexes are too small to be insoluble and for precipitate to be formed.

The principle of immunoprecipitation is used in turbidimetric and nephelometric assays. In these assays the antigen-antibody complexes are measured in suspension by the percentage of light transmitted or by the degree of light scattered, respectively. These assays are useful for the precise measurement of the amounts of a wide variety of proteins in the serum, including the immunoglobulins and complement components.

Precipitation in a Gel Matrix
Immunoprecipitation may be carried out in an agarose gel matrix. The earliest technique, that of Ouchterlony or double diffusion precipitation, is a qualitative test. In this test a visible line of precipitate forms between wells, one containing specific antibody and the other the antigen. If samples are placed in adjacent wells cut in a gel, the precipitin lines which form may reveal immunological identity, partial identity, or nonidentity between the samples in the wells (Figure 20.2). The double-immunodiffusion assay, which yields valuable formation about similarities and differences among different antibody and antigen preparations, is a simple test which to carry out requires nothing more than a glass slide, Pasteur pipette, agar, and phosphate-buffered saline.

Immunoelectrophoresis (IEP) is a separation of antigens by their electrophoretic mobility as well as by diffusion in a gel. Other procedures which are modifications of the precipitation reaction include two-dimensional IEP, crossed IEP, and counter IEP. These are all qualitative procedures. As immunoelectrophoresis is a method

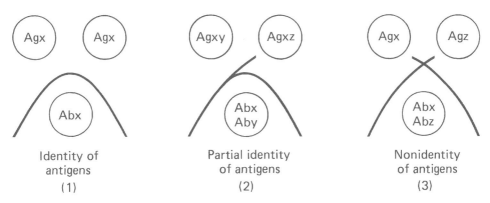

Figure 20.2.   Diagrammatic representation of a double diffusion precipitation reaction in gel. If the antigens in the two antigen-containing wells (Agx) are identical (1), a single line forms. If the two antigens are partially different (Agy, Agz), a spur forms (2). If the two antigens are completely different (Agx, Agz), the two precipitation lines simply cross (3).

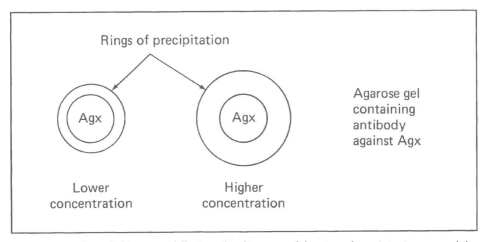

Figure 20.3.   In radial immunodiffusion, the diameter of the ring of precipitation around the antigen (Agx) containing well is proportional to the antigen concentration. The procedure can therefore be used to determine the concentration of an antigen in a solution of the antigen.

that combines the technique of agarose gel electrophoresis with the highly specific antigen antibody reaction, it gives in one procedure information on the electrophoretic mobility of antigen molecules being tested and on their antigenic nature.

There are also a number of quantitative assays based on the principle of precipitation of antigen-antibody complexes in gels. In radial immunodiffusion (RID) and rocket electrophoresis, antibody is incorporated into an agarose gel. Quantitation in both tests is based on the distance from the point of application the antigen migrates into the antibody-containing gel before precipitating. In RID the precipitate forms a ring around the sample well. The antigen diffuses into the antibody containing agar; precipitation occurs where the proportion of antigen to antibody is optimal. A series of antigen standards of known concentration are used to obtain a calibration curve and to determine the amount of antigen in the sample (Figure 20.3). In rocket immunoelectrophoresis the antigen is forced into the gel by an electric current (Figure 20.4). Rocket immunoelectrophoresis is a rapid method suitable

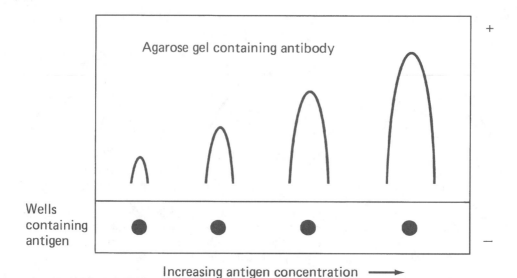

Figure 20.4.   In rocket immunoelectrophoresis, the antigen is forced into the antibody-containing agarose gel by an electric current. The size of the peak of precipitation is proportional to the amount of antigen placed in the well. If standards containing known amounts of antigen are run simultaneously, samples can be evaluated to determine antigen concentration by comparison of the size of the precipitation peaks produced by the unknown samples and the peaks produced by the standards.

for measuring antigens which move toward the positive pole on electrophoresis. Both rocket immunoelectrophoresis and radial immunodiffusion techniques are used in assays for serum proteins. IgG, IgA, and IgM can be quantitated by RID; however, this method is too insensitive to detect IgE in the very low concentrations at which it occurs in serum.

Agglutination

Agglutination is an assay based upon the same principles as precipitation, but in it the antigen is a colloidal particle in suspension. Agglutination is widely used for blood typing. Agglutination, like precipitation, occurs in two stages. Antibody first reacts with antigenic determinants that are part of the large structure, such as red cells or bacteria (sensitization), and then forms bridges between antigenic determinants on adjacent cells to yield grossly visible clumps (agglutination). When antibody is in excess, a phenomenon known as the prozone may occur. In blood group work, for example, reactions of high titer antibodies with their antigens may appear to be weak or negative when undiluted serum is used but become strong with diluted serum. This is because while antibody binding does occur outside of the zone of equivalence, a lattice does not form and clumping cannot therefore occur. The process of formation of a lattice during agglutination is similar to the process which occurs in precipitation.

Precipitation reactions can be converted to agglutination reactions by absorption of the soluble antigen onto erythrocytes, polystyrene or latex spheres, bentonite or starch granules. Latex particles coated with IgG, for example, are used as the antigen in agglutination tests for diagnosis of rheumatoid arthritis.

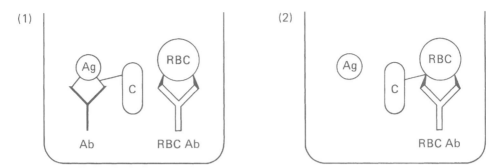

Figure 20.5. These diagrams indicate the basis of the complement-fixation test. If antibody is present in the serum being tested, it binds to the antigen. The complement that is available is then bound and is not available to lyse the red cell indicator system (1); if antibody is not present in the serum being tested, the complement is not bound in the test system and is available to lyse the antibody-coated red blood cells in the indicator system (2).

Neutralization

Neutralization is widely used in work with viruses. The technique of neutralization can be used to detect the reaction of an antigen, in this case, virus, with antibody when no precipitation can occur, as, for example, if the virus is present at low levels in the sample. A sample possibly containing a virus known to be lethal for cells in a culture is divided, one part is mixed with a known antibody against the virus, and the other with normal serum. The mixtures are added to cultures of the cell, and the cultures are observed. If virus is present in the sample, the cells are killed in the tubes receiving the sample and normal serum, but the virus is neutralized in the portion of the sample receiving the known antibody, and the cells are not killed.

Neutralization of toxin by antitoxin is also done. For example, toxin neutralization occurs *in vivo* when an individual exposed to *Clostridium tetani* is injected with antitoxin as part of the prophylaxis of tetanus.

A type of neutralization is also used in blood group work. Soluble blood group substances can be added to a serum containing multiple antibodies to neutralize one or more of them. This allows easier identification of the remaining unneutralized antibodies.

Complement Fixation

Complement fixation, resulting in lysis, is a valuable laboratory technique. (See chapter 9 for the complement activation sequence.) Antibody may be detected by its ability to bind complement in the presence of an appropriate antigen. Red cells coated with antibody are used as indicator cells. If antibody is present, the complement is bound to the antigen-antibody complex formed and is not available to bind to the antibody-coated red cells and the red cells do not lyse (Figure 20.5). Complement fixation is the basis of the lymphocytotoxic tests for detection of histocompatibility antigens (HLA). In this technique, living lymphocyte suspensions are exposed to antisera and complement. If the lymphocytes possess antigen corresponding to the antibody used, complement is fixed, and the cells are lysed. Cells damaged by the fixed complement are penetrated by an added stain, commonly eosin or trypan blue, while undamaged cells are not. By this reaction, cell surface antigens on lymphocytes can be identified.

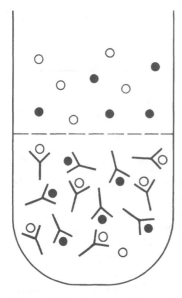

O = Antigen in patient serum

● = Radiolabeled antigen

Y = Antigen–specific antibody

Figure 20.6.   In competitive radioimmunoassay, a radiolabeled antigen is added to the sample. This radiolabeled antigen directly competes with the unlabeled antigen for the antibody added. The amount of labeled antigen in the precipitate is inversely proportional to the amount of unlabeled antigen in the sample.

Lysis, *in vivo* and *in vitro*, requires antibody, antigen, and complement. The complement does not have to be from the same species of animal as the antibody. Complement is fairly unstable; it is less stable than are antibodies. Because of this, fresh sera will often lyse bacteria (bacteriolysis) or red cells (hemolysis) but aged or heated serum may only cause agglutination. The lytic reactions due to fixation of complement are an important part of the immune defense mechanisms.

Radioimmunoassay (RIA)
Some clinically significant proteins occur at concentrations too low to be detected by immunoprecipitation methods. In 1960 Yalow and Berson introduced radioimmunoassay (RIA) which is a sensitive and specific technique. This method permits measurement of very low concentrations of any material to which an antibody can be raised. Sensitivity results from the low levels of radioactivity which can be measured. The specificity of the assay is determined by the specificity of the antibody to which the radioisotope is coupled. A more specific antibody is usually required for RIA than for precipitation assays.

Radioimmunoassays are of two types: competitive RIA and sandwich RIA. In the competitive RIA (Figure 20.6), radiolabeled antigen is added to the sample in which you are attempting to measure unlabeled antigen. An antibody specific for the antigen is added. After washing the precipitate to remove unbound radiolabeled antigen, the radioactivity in the precipitate is measured with a gamma counter. The percent of label in the precipitate is inversely proportional to the amount of unlabeled antigen present in the sample. In this form of the RIA, competition between labeled and unlabeled antigen forms the basis of the test.

Competitive binding procedures can also be based on competition between labeled and unlabeled antibodies. Determination of the proportion of a known

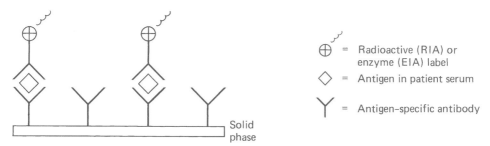

Figure 20.7.   The sandwich radioimmunoassay uses a solid phase to which specific antibody is attached. The specimen that may contain antigen is added and allowed to react; then the surface is washed to remove any unbound antigens. Radiolabeled antibody is then added. After time is allowed for reaction, the unbound labeled antibody is washed away and the bound label counted. The amount of label that is bound is directly proportional to the amount of antigen in the sample. The same basic procedure is used in the enzyme-linked immunosorbent assay; the only differences are the substitution of an enzyme for the radiolabel and the use of a chromogenic substrate and color detection instead of a radioisotope counter for determining the amount of binding that occurs.

amount of labeled antibody bound in the precipitate permits calculation of the amount of unlabeled antibody that was present. For use in these tests, antibody must be labeled with a suitable radionuclide without destroying its specificity.

The sandwich RIA generally uses a solid phase to which specific antibody is fixed (Figure 20.7). The specimen, for example, patient serum, which may contain the antigen, is added to the vessel on the walls of which the antibody is fixed, then a radiolabeled antibody specific for the antigen is added. After washing to remove unbound antibody, the radioactivity retained is counted with a gamma counter. The amount of radiolabel bound is directly proportional to the amount of antigen in the sample.

The sandwich technique is useful because with it one can detect either antibody or antigen. If antigen is used to coat the solid phase, then antibody can be detected by use of a labeled second antibody, such as antihuman globulin, directed against the antibody of concern. If antibody is used to coat the solid phase, then antigen can be detected. In this case the radiolabel is linked to antibody. In tests for hepatitis B antigen in serum, for example, the sandwich technique is used. Unlabeled antibody to hepatitis B antigen is fixed to a solid phase and the suspect serum added. If the antigen is present in the serum, it combines with the antibody on the solid phase; then when radiolabeled antibody is added, it will attach to the bound antigen. After washing away unbound radiolabeled antibody, the amount of radiolabeled antibody is determined and is a measure of the amount of antigen which was present in the serum.

Fluorescent Assay

Fluorescent assays are frequently used for the detection of antibodies in serum or antigens in tissue or cells. Fluorescent antibody tests, such as the indirect immunofluorescent antibody assay (IFA), are similar in principle to the indirect EIA. For detection of antigens, a tissue section or cell culture fixed to a slide serves as the antigen. The antigen in the tissue or cell is detected by its reaction with an antibody to which a fluorescent emitter such as fluorescein isothiocyanate (FITC) or rhodamine is attached. This is the direct type of test. An ultraviolet light source is used

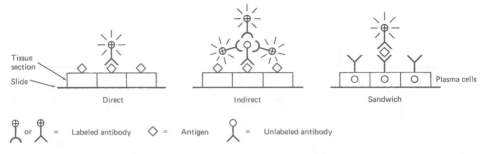

Figure 20.8. The fluorescent labeled antibody test can be done by direct, indirect, or sandwich procedures. The direct test uses a labeled antibody to detect antigen in a tissue section, blood film, or other specimen. The indirect test is used to detect antigens in similar situations but can also be used to detect antibodies. In the indirect test, the detection system uses a labeled antigamma globulin. Where antibody is present in the sample it binds on the antigen, and as a result, the labeled antiglobulin will bind. The sandwich procedure has a more limited use than the other procedures. It is used to detect antibody on, for example, plasma cells. The cell is exposed to antigen, then to labeled antibody to the antigen. The antigen will only bind to cells with bound antibody of the correct specificity, and this in turn determines which cells will bind the labeled antibody.

to excite the FITC, which fluoresces or gives off light of a longer wave length than the exciting ultraviolet light. An ultraviolet microscope or other instrument designed to detect fluorescence permits detection of the bound fluorescent antibody. After the fluorescent-labeled antibody reacts with cellular antigens, for example, the antibody-coated cell becomes visible, usually by emission of a yellow-green light. The immunofluorescent antibody assay allows rapid and easy detection of autoantibodies to a variety of antigens in tissues.

As noted above, the direct FA test for antigen in cells or tissues uses a specific antibody labeled with a fluorescent dye as a detection system (Figure 20.8). In the indirect FA test, a fluorescent-labeled antiglobulin is used to detect unlabeled antibody that is bound to the antigen. The indirect test is more flexible and generally yields a brighter fluorescence than does the direct test.

A third procedure, the sandwich test, detects receptors or antibody on or in the cytoplasm of cells. Antigen is the first reagent, then fluorescent-labeled antibody is added, and the antigen is sandwiched between the two antibodies. Cell surface markers, such as antigen binding proteins (i.e., receptors) of T lymphocytes and immunoglobulins present in and on B lymphocytes, are frequently detected by such fluorescent assays.

Both monoclonal and polyclonal antibodies have been used in fluorescent assays. The choice of which to use depends upon the requirements of the particular assay and the nature of the analysis. For assays in which the most important consideration is specificity, such as separation of T and B lymphocytes, monoclonal antibodies are used. On the other hand, in screening assays where sensitivity is of utmost concern (that is, tests where it is important not to miss any possible positives), polyclonal antibodies are used.

Enzyme-Linked Immunosorbent Assay (ELISA)

The enzyme-linked immunosorbent assay (ELISA) technique is a highly versatile, sensitive, and quantitative procedure that requires little equipment and for which reagents are readily available. It was first introduced in 1971 by Engvall and

Perlmann. The term enzyme immunoassay (EIA) is an alternative name for this type of test and is used for the many variants of the assay. Enzymes such as alkaline phosphatase or peroxidase can be linked to antibody without destroying either the antibody's specificity or the enzyme's activity. The enzyme acts as a label which makes detection of the antibody possible. Both monoclonal and polyclonal antibodies can be used in this type of test. Enzyme labels are cheaper, simpler to measure, and far more stable than radioactive labels. For these reasons, ELISA or EIA assays have in many cases replaced RIA and have done so while maintaining sensitivity and specificity. Many of the assays for hepatitis A and B in use today are based on ELISA. In addition to the use of enzymes in immunoassays, nonenzymatic markers can also be used if they can be conjugated to the antibody (e.g., colloidal gold with silver enhancement, and biotination with avidine).

ELISA tests are specific because of the high specificity of an antibody for its target antigen. In one type of test unlabeled antibodies are bound to a solid substrate, such as the internal surfaces of the wells in a microtiter plate, and these are used to capture the antigen the test is developed to detect. A labeled antibody specific for the captured antigen is then added. Following a sequence of manipulations involving washings, addition of further reagents and incubations, a colored end product is obtained in those wells containing the captured antigens. The amount of color generated by the reaction in a fixed time is directly proportional to the amount of antigen in the sample being tested.

ELISAs can be formatted in several configurations to detect either antibodies, antigens, or haptens. A variety of solid supports may be used. Four types of tests are listed below and will be described further. They are an indirect sandwich ELISA to detect antibodies, a direct antibody-sandwich ELISA to detect soluble antigens, a direct competitive ELISA to detect small molecular weight molecules (i.e., haptens), and an indirect competitive ELISA to detect small molecular weight molecules (i.e., haptens).

Indirect ELISA (iELISA) for Detection of Antibodies
In this type of test, a support matrix such as the walls of plastic microtiter plates is coated with antigen. These antigen-sensitized plates are incubated with the antisera to be tested. Those antibodies specific for the antigen on the plates will bind to the antigen on the plates. Any nonspecific antibodies in the sera being tested are removed by washing. Next an antibody, specific to the antibody being tested for and which is covalently coupled to an enzyme, is applied (Figure 20.9). Washing removes any unbound conjugated antibody, and a substrate for the enzyme is added. The substrate is hydrolyzed if any of the conjugated antibody is bound, and a colored product is generated. Finally, the colored product is detected visually or spectrophotometrically with a microtiter plate reader. The amount of colored product generated is roughly proportional to the amount of specific antibody in the sera being tested. This procedure is used for assaying titers of polyclonal sera and to screen hybridomas for the production of monoclonal antibodies. In this latter case, the solid phase is coated with the antigen of interest, and then culture supernatants from various lymphocyte clones possibly containing the monoclonal antibody of interest are added. Then an enzyme labeled secondary antibody specific for the monoclonal antibody is used to detect any monoclonal antibody which binds to the antigen on the test plate.

An antibody may be used to capture the antigen and bind it to the test plate.

422 • F. Petersen

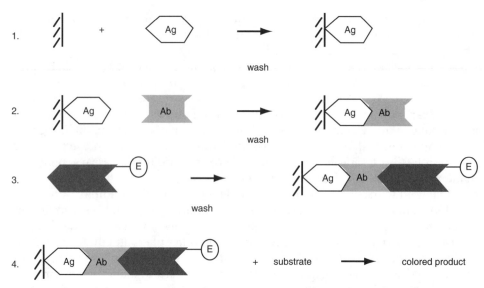

Figure 20.9. The indirect ELISA using an enzyme-conjugated secondary antibody can be used to detect an antibody of interest in a sample being tested. In the test diagrammed, the antigen <Ag> is absorbed directly on the surface of the test vessel (1), the sample possibly containing the antibody (>Ab<) of interest is added (2), the conjugated antibody (<Ab<ᴱ) specific for the antibody of interest is added. If the antibody of interest is present in the sample being tested, it binds to the antigen absorbed to the vessel wall, and then, when the conjugated antibody specific for the antibody of interest is added (3), it binds to the antibody of interest, if it is present. In the final step, substrate for the enzyme is added, and a colored product is generated (4), if the specimen is positive. Washing is required between each step to remove any unbound antigens or antibodies.

Such antibody-sandwich ELISAs may be more useful than the direct sandwich ELISAs for detecting antibody because they are frequently between two and five times more sensitive than ELISAs in which antigen is directly bound to the solid phase. Antibody-sandwich ELISAs are especially useful when screening for specific antibodies in cases when a small amount of specific antibody is available and purified antigen is unavailable. The antibody mediated binding of the antigen of interest assures that only the antigen of interest is bound. This method can be used for epitope mapping of monoclonal antibodies that are directed against the antigen. Figure 20.10 is a diagram of this type of test.

Direct ELISA (dELISA) for Detection of Soluble Antigens
A direct sandwich ELISA (Figure 20.10) is often used for the detection of larger molecules (usually proteins) with multiple antigenic sites. In this type of test, a solid support, such as the wells in a microtiter plate, is coated with an antibody (the capture antibody) specific for an antigenic site on the protein of interest; the antibody attached to the plastic wells in the microtiter plate binds with the antigen of interest (Ag1). Other antigens (Ag2, Ag3, etc.) are not bound and are removed by washing. A detector antibody coupled with alkaline phosphatase, and specific for a second antigenic site on the protein of interest, is then added. After washing the plate, a substrate for the enzyme is added. The enzyme-generated signal, i.e., the colored product of the enzymatic action is roughly proportional to the concentration of antigen captured on the plate.

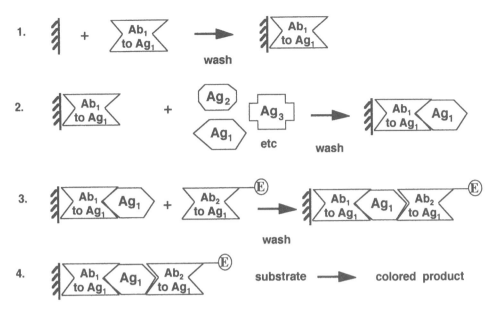

Figure 20.10.   Direct antibody "sandwich" ELISA to detect an antigen of interest. An antibody specific for a site on an antigen of interest is absorbed on the walls of wells in a microtiter plate (1). The sample containing a variety of antigens possibly including the one of interest is added to the wells (2). Antigen of interest if present is bound. A second labeled antibody to the antigen of interest is added to the well (3) after it has been washed to remove unbound antigens. If the antigen of interest was in the sample and was bound, the labeled antibody will bind to it and after washing and the addition of substrate, color will develop (4).

Competitive ELISA
Introduction
Another basic format for immunoassays is the competitive assay. In this assay, a competition between bound and free antigen, or labeled and unlabeled antigen, for available antibody binding sites occurs. This type of assay results in an inverse standard curve; for increasing concentrations of antigen in the sample being tested, a decrease in signal is observed.

Immunoreagents (i.e., monoclonal antibodies) can be developed which specifically bind to small molecular weight molecules (<50 kd) in complex mixtures of molecules such as soil and plant extracts. To produce such reagents, the small molecules (haptens) are bound to a larger carrier molecule before they are used for immunization. These assays have proven to be especially useful in detecting small molecular weight molecules which have only one antibody binding site. The single antibody competitive format has been used to detect such small molecular weight molecules as pesticides, petroleum by-products, and toxins at levels as low as a few parts per billion.

Direct Competitive ELISA for Detection of Small Molecular Weight Molecules
The first direct competitive ELISA was described by van Weemen and Schuurs in 1971. In a direct competitive ELISA, the antibody is immobilized on the solid phase. A preparation of the antigen labeled with an enzyme is a crucial reagent. In the test, binding of the antigen-enzyme conjugate by the immobilized antibody is inhibited by the addition of the unlabeled antigen in the sample being tested (Figure 20.11). Both the antigen conjugate and the unlabeled antigen in the test sample compete

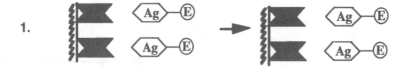

1.

antibody on solid phase binds enzyme-labeled antigen

or

unlabeled antigen contained in sample blocks binding of labeled antibody on solid phase

2.

3.

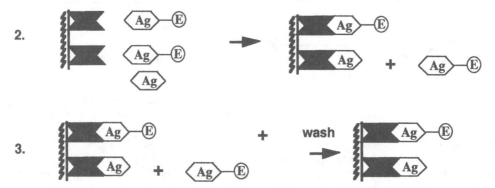

Figure 20.11. Direct competitive, solid phase EIA. A known volume of the unlabeled preparation to be tested and various dilutions of a known preparation of conjugated antigen are incubated on antibody sensitized plates for one hour at ambient temperature. Free antigen in the test sample will compete with antigen-conjugate for antibody binding sites. After washing and with the addition of substrate, color development will occur in direct proportion to the amount of antigen-conjugate bound and in inverse proportion to concentration or unlabeled antigen in the sample being tested. In part 1 of the figure, there is no competition, and all of the available sites bind labeled antigen, while in part 2, unlabeled antigen in the sample blocks one of the binding sites, and a labeled antibody remains free to be removed from the reaction vessel by washing (3).

for binding sites on the immobilized antibody. When after washing the unbound conjugate is removed and substrate is added, color development occurs. The color intensity will be inversely proportional to the concentration of unlabeled antigen in the sample. This assay is used to detect and measure soluble antigens and haptens, and is useful when both a specific antibody to the antigen or hapten and purified or semipurified antigen or hapten are both available.

Indirect Competitive ELISA for Detection of Small Molecular Weight Molecules

In the direct competitive ELISA, as noted above, the specific antibody developed to the antigen or hapten to be analyzed is immobilized on a support matrix, such as the walls of a ninety-six-well microtiter plate. Dilutions of the sample being tested and standard amounts of the enzyme-antigen conjugate are added to the wells. Conjugated antigen and unconjugated antigen in the sample being tested will compete for binding to the immobilized antibody. After washing and when substrate is added, the level of color development will be inversely proportional to the amount of unlabeled antigen in the test sample.

(1) antigen on solid phase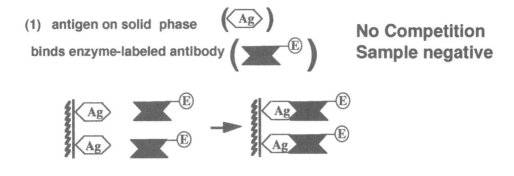

binds enzyme-labeled antibody

No Competition Sample negative

(2) enzyme labeled antibody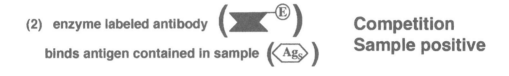

binds antigen contained in sample

Competition Sample positive

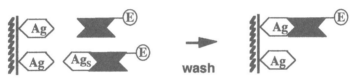

Figure 20.12. Indirect competitive, solid phase EIA. Equal volumes of sample containing unlabeled antigen and of conjugated antibody (1) are incubated on antigen sensitized plates for one hour at ambient temperature. Unlabeled antigen in the sample will compete with the fixed antigen for antibody binding sites (2). Conjugated antibody bound to the free antigen is removed from the reaction vessel by washing before substrate is added. With the addition of substrate, color development will occur in direct proportion to the amount of labeled antibody bound to the antigen fixed on the well walls and in indirect proportion to the concentration of unlabeled antigen free in the sample.

In the indirect competitive ELISA on the other hand (Figure 20.12), the antigen is immobilized on the walls of the microplate wells. An enzymed labeled antibody to the antigen is added along with dilutions of the sample to be tested. The antigen in the sample will compete with the bound antigen on the solid support for binding sites on the labeled antibody. Unbound conjugate will be washed out. Again as with the direct-competitive ELISA, the amount of antigen in the sample will be inversely proportional to the color development.

In all cases, standard curves must be created by testing of known concentrations of the material being tested for quantitative results are to be obtained.

ELISA Formats
Introduction
Many types of surfaces are available for binding reagents to be used in ELISAs including those in or on tubes, microplates, plastic beads, membranes, magnetic particles, latex particles, etc. Each type of surface has advantages which make it

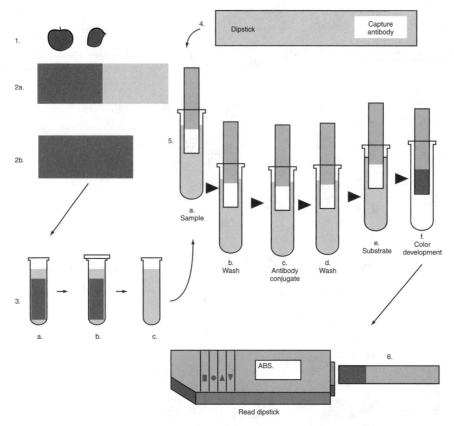

Figure 20.13. Dipstick format for ELISA assay. Figure 20.13 is a flow chart for a dipstick test to determine infection of cranberry bushes with *Phytophthora megasperma*. (1) Obtain cranberry fruit or leaves. (2) Grind fruit or leaves on sandpaper board (2a) with second board (2b). (3) Immerse sandpaper board in extraction buffer (3a), allow extraction to occur (3b), remove sandpaper board (3c). (4) Dipstick with capture antibody. Immerse dipstick into sample, (5a) then wash, (5b) immerse in conjugate, (5c) wash, (5d) immerse in substrate, (5e) wash off unbound products, and allow color to develop (5f). Insert dipstick in reader and read results (6). Color developed will be proportionate to the amount of *P. megasperma* in the fruit or leaves.

more suitable than others for specific applications. In the following section, the types of surfaces to be discussed are grouped under the headings dipstick, microplate, plastic bead, magnetic bead, and latex particles.

Dipstick
The sandwich assay can be adapted to a dipstick matrix. In this format, specific antibodies are absorbed on nitrocellulose pads which are then attached to a plastic dipstick. The dipstick is then cycled through a series of reagent tubes containing first the test sample, then wash solution, antibody-conjugate, wash solution, and finally enzyme substrate. If a chain of ab-ag-ab-enzyme has been formed, the nitrocellulose pad will turn color, the intensity of which is in proportion to the amount of antigen present in the sample. Samples can be read by direct visual examination and quantified by comparison to a color chart; or samples can be inserted into a reflectometer for analysis. Dipstick assays have been widely employed to determine if pathogens are present in plants and if so, the amount present. Figure 20.13

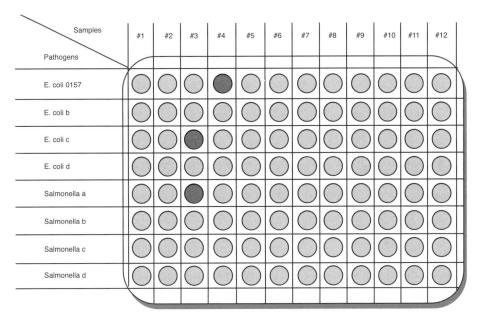

Figure 20.14. Multiwell format for use of the direct ELISA in simultaneous testing of multiple samples for the presence of multiple pathogens. The wells in each of the 8 horizontal rows of a 96 well microtiter plate were sensitized with antibody specific for one of the 8 pathogens listed across top to the right. Twelve fecal samples (i.e., extracts in buffered saline) are being tested in this plate, one sample in each vertical row. Color formation indicates antigen to the pathogen is in the sample. In this particular case, sample #4 contained *E. coli* 0157, and sample #3 contained *E. coli* C and *Salmonella* a. The sequence of steps in the test is (1) antibody specific for the pathogen is absorbed on the plastic in the designated wells. (2) The wells are rinsed. (3) Sample is added. (4) The wells are rinsed. (5) Conjugated antibody specific for the antigen is added. (6) The wells are rinsed. (7) Substrate is added. (8) Color development is observed.

is a flow chart of a dipstick assay for a fungal pathogen of plants (*Phytophthora megasperma*). This particular assay is used to monitor cranberries for infection with this important plant pathogen. A hand-held reflectometer is used in this assay for analyzing the test results.

Microplate

The ninety-six-well format is the standard laboratory assay using a microplate (Figure 20.14). Various steps in the assay can be automated (e.g., plate washing, reagent dispensing, plate reading, etc.) to facilitate the handling of large numbers of samples. Monoclonal antibodies are most commonly used as the diagnostic reagents in these types of tests. One of the most popular versions of the microplate assay uses an enzyme-linked immunosorbent format. In this format the antigen is captured by a layer of specific monoclonal antibodies, and its capture is detected by a second labeled antibody. The first layer of antibodies (the capture layer) is covalently attached to the inside surface of the wells in the polyvinylchloride microtiter plate. The samples suspected of containing the antigen are added to the wells, and the antigen, if present, is captured by the antibodies absorbed to the well walls. Then antibodies which have been tagged with an enzyme are added. The color change indicates the presence of the antigen. This type of assay can be used to process scores of samples simultaneously. It can be automated, and test results can be obtained in one hour or less.

Immunomagnetic Separation

This technique is used to improve the sensitivity and specificity of conventional methods for detecting the presence of microbes in samples. The samples are diluted, and small (<100 µm) magnetic beads coated with microbe specific antibodies are added. The antibody on the beads captures the microbes for which it is specific. The magnetic property of the beads is then used to separate the beads and the attached cells from the broth, and these may be plated out on agar for culture. A conventional culture approach may then be followed to identify any microbe isolated. Alternatively, after the beads are used to capture and concentrate the microbes from a sample suspension, they may be transferred to an agar plate, the plates incubated to produce microcolonies, and the colonies removed by membrane imprint for examination using a chromogenic immunoblot technique for identification.

Tests Using Latex Beads

Introduction

Antibody-coated latex beads can be used in agglutination or ELISA techniques to detect antigen in samples. In addition to simple tube or microtiter agglutination tests which are read visually, several devices have been developed for use of the principle of latex agglutination in tests that can be sold commercially and used by relatively untrained persons. Two tests using latex beads will be described: lateral flow immunoassay, an agglutination procedure, and vertical flow-through immunoassay, an ELISA procedure.

Lateral Flow Immunoassay

In this type of assay, antibodies to the targeted antigen are immobilized in a line on a nitrocellulose membrane. The test sample is placed on a wick which draws it to a pool of latex particles present on the cellulose membrane. If the targeted antigens are present in the sample, they pass along the wick and react with antibody labeled with the colored latex particles. The complex then continues to diffuse along the wick. When, if they are present, they reach the immobilized antibody, they are held there. The immune complexes with the attached latex particles are concentrated by the fixed antibody so that in a positive sample (Figure 20.15) a colored line forms in the test result window. The positive control is a site where a known antigen specific for the antibody-colored bead complex is fixed. If the movement of the reagents is occurring properly, then the antibody-colored bead complex will arrive at the positive control site and be fixed there regardless of whether antigen is present in the sample.

Vertical Flow-Through Immunoassay

The vertical flow-through immunoassay is an adaptation of the ELISA procedure to make it convenient to use in a nonlaboratory setting. To accomplish this, it uses a simple device which eliminates the need for complex washing steps and bulky plate readers. All operations needed to perform the assay take place on the upper surface of an absorbent porous cork bed (Figure 20.16). The bed has a hydrophobic cover with three holes to permit localization of reagents and to direct flow of sample and reagents. The immunological reagents are fixed on latex beads so that they will remain on the surface of the cork bed at the appropriate holes in the mask.

The device is first prepared for the specific use intended. Here we will describe

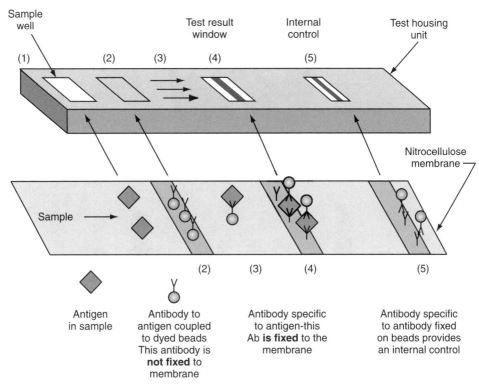

Sample
well

Test result
window

Internal
control

Test housing
unit

(1) (2) (3) (4) (5)

Nitrocellulose
membrane

Sample →

(2) (3) (4) (5)

Antigen
in sample

Antibody to
antigen coupled
to dyed beads
This antibody is
not fixed to
membrane

Antibody specific
to antigen-this
Ab **is fixed** to the
membrane

Antibody specific
to antibody fixed
on beads provides
an internal control

Figure 20.15.   The single step lateral flow immunoassay. The test unit is shown dissembled. When the test is actually run, the nitrocellulose membrane is in the housing. Before the sample is tested, the reagents are placed at the appropriate places on the nitrocellulose membrane which is dried and then pushed into the test housing. In this assay, the sample is placed in the sample well (1), and the products of the reaction with the reagents diffuse along the surface of the membrane toward the antibody dried-bead complex (2). The antigen, if present in the sample, complexes with the antibody coupled to the colored beads forming colored complexes which also diffuse along the membrane (3). The diffusing antigen bearing complexes (3), if present, are trapped by the fixed antibody forming a colored line (4), unbound antibody coated colored beads continue to diffuse along the wick to where they meet the second line of fixed antibody yielding a second colored line (5). This latter reaction is a control indicating that the diffusion process is working. The position of the two types of fixed antibodies on the nitrocellulose membrane must be such that, when the membrane is pushed into the housing, their positions correspond to the positions of the viewing windows.

one of the many uses of the device. In this explanation an antigen in a sample is the target to be identified. Latex beads are coated with antibody to the antigen of interest. A solution of these beads is then placed on the sample hole in the mask. The liquid in which they are suspended is absorbed into the cork bed and the beads remain on the surface in the sample hole. The positive control hole is treated similarly but with latex beads coated with a preparation of the antigen to be detected in the test. The blank hole is similarly coated with beads, but they are covered with an appropriate blocking protein such as bovine serum albumin. After the beads are in place, the fluid chamber is flooded with a blocking solution such as bovine serum albumin which assures that there are no surfaces where immunoreagents may bind nonspecifically. This solution draws through the various holes in the mask and

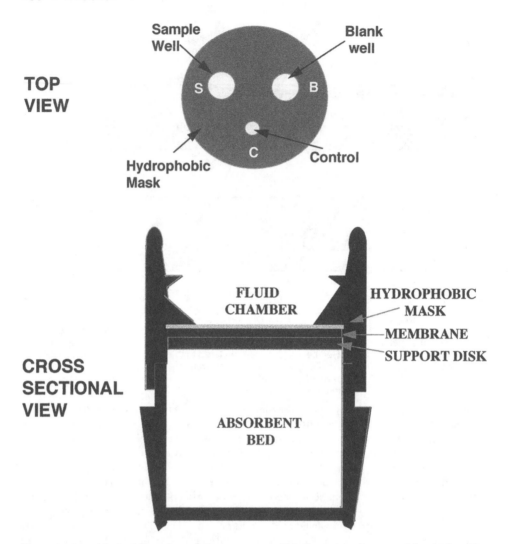

Figure 20.16. Vertical flow-through immunoassay. This figure is a diagram of the device. The absorbent bed takes up reagents and sample that pass through the holes in the hydrophobic mask from the fluid chamber where the sample and reagents are placed. The steps for use of the chamber are described in the text.

enters the cork bed. The device is then stored until dry when it will be ready for use.

To run the test, the sample (possibly containing the antigen of interest) is poured into the fluid chamber. It will pass through the three holes in the mask and enter the absorbent bed. If the sample contains the antigen of interest, it will be bound by the antibody on the beads in the sample hole. It will of course also pass through the blank and sample holes but not bind there. Saline is then put in the fluid chamber and allowed to drain into the cork bed. This is to wash out any unbound sample. An enzyme conjugated antibody specific for the antigen of interest is then placed in the fluid chamber; a saline wash follows and finally substrate is put in the fluid chamber. If the test is working properly and the sample contains the antigen of interest, the sample hole develops color, the internal control develops color, and the blank stays white. If no antigen is in the sample, the sample hole stays white, the positive control hole develops color, and the blank stays white. The development of color is monitored visually.

The vertical flow-through system can be adapted to a competitive ELISA system. Dilutions of the sample being analyzed are each placed in separate devices of the type pictured in Figure 20.16. The units are prepared as for the direct test, then the various dilutions of the sample are mixed with standard amounts of enzyme labeled antigen, and the mixture is put in the fluid chambers of the device. Rinsing and addition of substrate follow. The unlabeled antigen in the sample being tested competes with the labeled antigen for antibody on the beads in the sample hole. If the amount of unlabeled antigen in the sample is sufficient, so much of it will absorb to the antibody in the sample hole that it will block binding of the labeled antigen, and on addition of substrate, no color will develop in the sample hole. If a standard curve has been prepared, then comparison of the colors produced by dilutions of a known standard to the increasing color with increasing dilution of the sample reveals the amount of antigen in the sample.

The volumes of the various solutions applied, the buffers used to suspend the various reagents and the sample, the size of latex particles, and specificity and amount of antibody and antigen used are all critical variables that must be carefully controlled in order to achieve maximum test sensitivity and accuracy.

MONOCLONAL ANTIBODY PRODUCTION

A monoclonal antibody is an antibody secreted by cells of the clones of a single lymphocyte isolated from an experimental animal. Monoclonal antibodies are highly specific because they consist of antibody specific to a single epitope. Monoclonal antibodies are produced by cell hybrids which are made in the laboratory by fusing antibody-secreting cells with immortal cancer cells. In a typical process, a mouse is first immunized with the antigen of interest, then its antibody-producing cells are removed usually from the spleen and fused with mouse cancer cells. The cancer cells impart immortality to the fusion product, the hybridoma, and the spleen cell partner provides the ability to produce and secrete antibodies. The hybridomas are separated into single clones and screened for antibody production. The clones that produce the desired antibodies are retained, and the antibodies are mass-produced and purified (Figure 20.17).

Hybridomas can be frozen and revived at a later time, ensuring the availability of specific monoclonal antibodies over an extended period of time. Monoclonal antibody secreting cells produce a constant supply of uniform reagent; this contrasts with polyclonal antibodies which are the products produced by individual animals and thus are subject to variation.

SUMMARY

Antibodies are fundamental components of the immune system. They serve to fight off invaders by binding specifically with them or their products. The antibodies are produced when a foreign substance enters the system. The usefulness of immunological specificity for identification of pathogens has been recognized for diagnosis of diseases of human and veterinary interest for years. It was realized quite early however that a microorganism contains many antigenic determinants capable of eliciting antibody production, so that following immunization or infection the blood of most animals contains a mixture of antibodies with different specificities. There-

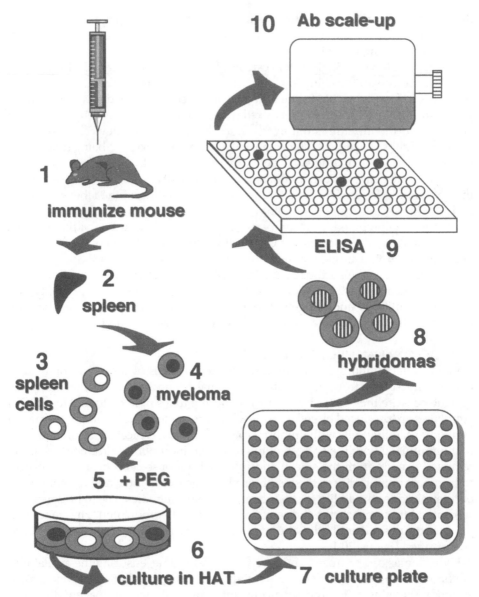

Figure 20.17.   Monoclonal antibody production. (1) A mouse is immunized with the antigen of interest. (2) The mouse is killed, and its spleen or lymph nodes are collected. (3) The lymphocytes in the organs are collected. (4) Myeloma cells from a myeloma cell line are mixed with the spleen cells. (5) They are fused by the action of polyethylene glycol (PEG). (6) The mixture of fused cells, unfused lymphocytes, and unfused myeloma cells is cultured in the presence of hypoxanthine, aminopterin, and thymidine (HAT). Lymphocytes die, as they do not reproduce in culture, and only survive a few days. Myeloma cells die, as they are poisoned by aminopterin. The fused cells survive and grow because the lymphocyte component contributes the metabolic machinery to bypass the toxic effect of aminopterin, and the myeloma component produces reproductive capacity. (7) The suspension of surviving cells is plated out into the microtiter plate at a dilution that puts a single or a very small number of cells in each well. (8) Wells in which growth occurs will contain hybridomas. (9) The fluid in the wells in the culture plate is tested for secretion of antibody to the antigen of interest. (10) Cells in wells secreting appropriate antibody are grown in volume to yield desired antibody.

fore, such polyclonal antibodies can be relatively nonspecific, resulting in cross-reactivity with shared determinants in related and unrelated pathogens and compounds. The development of monoclonal technology which produces antibody specific for a single epitope has made it possible to produce antibody reagents that are highly specific for the targets against which they are produced.

While as noted immunoassay technology has been used in human and veterinary diagnosis for many years, it is only recently that it has found application for detection of hormones and for agricultural and environmental monitoring. The delay in part is the result of delay in developing polyclonal and monoclonal antibodies which target and identify small haptenic molecules in complex matrices such as urine, blood, and soil and plant extracts and the development of procedures for use of such antibodies in tests useful in monitoring hormone levels and in environmental monitoring of pesticides, pathogens, and petroleum products in plants and soil.

Of the methods that are employed for assaying specificity of antibodies and antigens, such as immunoelectrophoresis, double-diffusion, immunosorbent assay (ELISA), complement fixation, and fluorescent assay, all are useful for evaluating polyclonal and monoclonal antisera, but by and large, the double-immunodiffusion assay and immunoelectrophoresis are not useful for evaluation of monoclonal antibodies to monovalent antigens. Precipitation tests and tests using blocking of precipitation as well as ELISA procedures and radioimmunoassay are best for such purposes. Because some tests are better than others for one or another use most laboratories use a combination of techniques, depending upon the nature of the samples received and the results desired. A blood center for example processing blood from donors may use EIA to test for hepatitis B antigen and for antibody to human immunodeficiency virus, agglutination to determine blood type and complement fixation to determine HLA type.

SUGGESTIONS FOR FURTHER READING

1. Abbas, A.K., A.H. Lichtman, and J.S. Pober. *Cellular and Molecular Immunology.* Philadelphia: W.B. Saunders, 1991.
2. Ahern, H. "Immunoassay Techniques Proven to be Outstanding in Several Fields. Tools and Technology." In *The Scientist* 9 (1995): 18–19.
3. Clark, W.R. *The Experimental Foundations of Modern Immunology.* 4th ed. Wiley & Sons, 1991.
4. Kemeny, D.M.A. *A Practical Guide to ELISA.* London: Elsevier Science, 1991.
5. Langone, J.J., and H. Van Vunakis. "Immunological Technique. Part I Hybridoma Technology and Monoclonal Antibodie." In *Methods in Enzymology*, vol. 121. Edited by Sidney P. Colowick, and Nathan O. Kaplan. Academic Press Inc., 1986.
6. Paul, W.E. ed. *Fundamental Immunology.* New York: Raven Press, 1993.

QUESTIONS

1 A competitive ELISA is to be performed on water samples to screen for the presence of Dioxin. From the following spectrometer data, which sample is positive for Dioxen?

Positive Control	Negative Control	Sample A	Sample B	Sample C	Assay Control
0.055	1.120	0.020	1.002	1.202	1.014

2 What is the purpose of the peroxidase in an ELISA test?
3 What would happen in an ELISA if the unbound antibody conjugate was not washed free of the well before the substrate was added?
(a) The ELISA would not develop color when the substrate was added.
(b) The ELISA would develop normally.
(c) All wells would show uniform color development due to the presence of unbound enzyme conjugate.
(d) Both (a) and (b).
4 What would happen if the test sample were omitted from one well of a sandwich ELISA, but all other steps remained the same and were performed properly?
(a) Antianalyte conjugate would not bind and would be removed by washing, and no color would develop in that well.
(b) Antianalyte conjugate would bind nonspecifically to the ELISA well and as a result, color would develop in the well.
(c) The degree of color development would be indeterminant, between positive and negative result.
(d) Both (a) and (c).
5 What are the advantages and disadvantages of monoclonal and polyclonal immunoreagents?

ANSWERS

1 Sample A. In a competitive assay it is the lack of color development resulting in no interference with light transmission which indicates the presence of a positive test.
2 Peroxidase is an enzyme that catalyzes its appropriate substrate. When peroxidase is linked to an antibody, the degree of substrate color development can be correlated with the amount of antigen present in the test sample.
3 The correct answer is (c). Since the enzyme which acts on the substrate is present in all the wells, it would turn all the wells a uniform color whether they were truly positive or not.
4 The correct answer is (a) since no test antigen is present in the well, no antigen is bound and the conjugate cannot bind in the well. Therefore no color would develop and the O.D. value would be the same as a negative control.
5 (a) Monoclonal antibody is highly specific; targets single epitope on an antigen. Polyclonal antibody contains antibodies to multiple epitopes on the antigen.
(b) Only a single type of antibody is secreted by a hybridoma serum. Polyclonal serum contains the numerous antibodies secreted by the lymphocytes of animal's immune system.
(c) Monoclonal antibody purification is easy; as separation of antibody from the components found in the culture medium is generally easy. Purification of polyclonal sera requires affinity purification to separate targeted antibodies from nontargeted antibodies found in the serum.
(d) With monoclonal antibodies there is batch to batch consistency. Each animal and each bleed will produce a different array of antibodies when animals are immunized for production of polyclonal sera.
(e) Hybridoma cell lines can be cyropreserved for future use. The supply of polyclonal sera is finite. Once depleted a new animal must be immunized
(f) The developmental cost for production of monoclonal antibodies is high but scaleup costs are minimal. The developmental cost for production of poly-chlonal sera is low but each batch is distinct.

Epidemiology, Disease Transmission, Prevention, and Control

Gabriel A. Schmunis

INTRODUCTION
TERMINOLOGY
EPIDEMIOLOGICAL
  INVESTIGATION
EPIDEMIOLOGICAL
  SURVEILLANCE
  Data Collection, Collation,
    and Analysis
  Decision-Making for
    Action
  Dissemination of
    Information
INFECTIOUS DISEASES
INFECTIOUS ORGANISMS
EMERGING AND RE-
  EMERGING DISEASES
THE HOST
THE ENVIRONMENT
TRANSMISSION MECH-
  ANISMS
PREVENTION AND
  CONTROL
SUMMARY
SUGGESTIONS FOR
  FURTHER READING
QUESTIONS

INTRODUCTION

Infectious diseases caused by bacteria, viruses, and parasites are a significant cause of morbidity and mortality all over the world. No person has been, or is, exempt from being infected by one or several disease-causing organisms. People travel widely today, those from developed countries for pleasure and business and those from undeveloped countries to better their lives or to escape war and civil disorder. Diseases caused by viruses, bacteria, protozoa, and metazoa are carried to their new homes by migrants and can be picked up by travelers and carried home by them. The worldwide spread of the human immunodeficiency virus (HIV) from its origin in Central Africa should be a lesson to us all that no regions or groups can remain safely separate from the rest of the world's populations and their problems.

Epidemiology was originally considered as a branch of medical science that deals with epidemics. Therefore, its main focus was communicable diseases. Through the years, the definition of epidemiology has been expanded, and now could be defined as the study of the distribution and determinants of disease occurrence in specified human populations. The application of epidemiological findings to the control and prevention of health problems is a natural extension of epidemiology. The field covered by epidemiology has been broadened to include the study of the distribution and determinants of accidents and of genetic and physiological conditions in human populations as well as infectious processes.

Descriptive epidemiology concerns the occurrence of diseases, and their causative agents, in time, place (geographical location), and population (sex, race, age, occupation, and social class). Analytical epidemiology examines and tests associations or hypothesized causal relationships.

435

It identifies and measures risk factors and the health effects of specific measures that may influence disease occurrence. Experimental epidemiology involves stating a hypothesis, developing an experimental model that allows for manipulation of one or several factors, and then noting the effect of the manipulation. One could for example study the effectiveness of isolation or administration of a certain drug on the incidence of diseases such as tuberculosis, meningitis, or malaria.

Epidemiologists use a reasoning process based on biological inferences derived as a result of observation of disease occurrence in population groups. Epidemiologists integrate the concepts and methods of other disciplines such as statistics, sociology, and biology into their field. By using such multidisciplinary methods, they are usually able to establish the etiology of a specific disease or group of diseases. Epidemiological studies may provide the basis for the evaluation of the efficacy of disease preventive procedures and public health practices as well as of health services. Epidemiological methods can be applied to the study of any disease or condition, acute or chronic, infectious or noninfectious, communicable or noncommunicable, and to the study of health as well.

This chapter will describe the role of epidemiology in establishing the status of diseases in populations, the burden that diseases constitute for human populations, and how diseases spread. The focus will be on infectious diseases.

TERMINOLOGY
Any deviation of the health status of an individual, human, or animal from normal may be considered a disease. Those diseases that occur at a usual, continuous, persistent low level in a human or animal population in a given geographical area are called endemic or enzootic diseases, respectively. A sudden increase in the number of cases of a disease above its expected incidence is called an epidemic, or an epizootic if in an animal population. Epizootiology is the name sometimes used to describe patterns of disease spread in nonhuman animal populations. A gradual increase in the occurrence of a disease beyond the endemic level, but still not of epidemic proportion is called hyperendemic. When an epidemic affects an extremely high number of individuals distributed worldwide, it is called a pandemic. A similar situation occurring in an animal population is called a panzootic.

Animal diseases capable of transmission to humans are called zoonosis. In humans such diseases are called zoonotic diseases. History provides examples of pandemics, both zoonotic and not. The influenza pandemic of 1918 killed 20 million people and was spread directly from person to person, while the bubonic plague epidemic of the fourteenth to sixteenth centuries that killed one-third of the population of Europe was a zoonosis, a disease of rats transmitted to humans by fleas.

There are several basic indicators that epidemiologists take into account when measuring and analyzing the health status of a population. Both mortality and morbidity figures for example show effects of a disease in a population. Of the two, mortality is the more severe outcome of a disease. In developed countries where data are available, mortality is easy to measure in an accurate manner and is therefore valuable. In third world countries, however, its value is diminished, as it is often difficult to establish the cause of death, or deaths are simply unrecorded. The mortality rate, also called the death rate, estimates the proportion of the population that dies during a specific period. Morbidity in contrast expresses any departure, subjective or objective, from a state of physiological or psychological well-being. It may be measured as the number of persons who are ill; the number of illnesses that the individuals experienced; and the duration of the illness in an individual. Incidence is the number of new events or cases of a disease in a given population group during a certain period of time. The incidence rate indicates the rate at which new events occur in a population; the numerator is the number of new cases in a defined period while the denominator is the number of individuals exposed to risk during the period. If the period is a year, the figure is called the annual incidence rate.

The prevalence of a disease is the number of instances of the disease in a given population at a designated time. When used without qualification, prevalence indicates a situation at a point in time (point prevalence). On the other hand when qualified by the word "rate," the term changes somewhat. The prevalence rate indicates the total number of individuals who have a disease during a particular time, divided by the population at risk of having the disease at that specific period of time. The main problem in considering the value of this indicator is defining the population that serves as the denominator.

EPIDEMIOLOGICAL INVESTIGATION

As mentioned before, an epidemic is the occurrence, in a population or community, of a group of cases of a disease in excess of the usual number of cases. When the incidence of a disease in a specific population, or during a given period of time in one geographic area, exceeds the usual frequency of that disease for that same population, that is indicative of the need for an epidemiological investigation. The result of an evaluation of risk factors may also indicate the need for an epidemiological investigation.

Usually, the observation that something abnormal is happening will depend on the sagacity and training of the health personnel. However, in order to determine whether the suspicion is true, that is, to confirm that the incidence exceeds the usual frequency, it is necessary to compare the recent incidence with the incidence observed previously. Therefore, in order to characterize the existence of an epidemic, it is important to be aware of the usual frequency of the disease in the same area, in the same population, and at the same time of the year. However, it is necessary to determine that the increase in the number of cases does not depend on an increase in surveillance, improved training of health personnel, or better diagnosis.

The minimum number of cases that signals the existence of an epidemic will vary according to how the disease is perceived by the affected population and by those making the study. Perception is influenced by the nature of the disease and the infectious agent, the type and size of the population exposed, the susceptibility of the population to the disease, and the place and time of the occurrence. As the epidemic takes its course and the number of affected people increases, the number of susceptible ones decreases, and as a result, the epidemic wave tends to disappear (Figure 21.1).

It is also usual to speak about the existence of an outbreak. This can be defined as an episode in which two or more cases of the same disease are somehow related. The relationship among the cases may be the time of onset of symptoms, the place where they occurred, or the characteristics of the sick people, such as their age, ethnic group, or occupation.

On some occasions, the potential existence of an outbreak or an epidemic warrants the implementation of an epidemiological investigation. There are certain general circumstances that signal when an investigation should be undertaken.

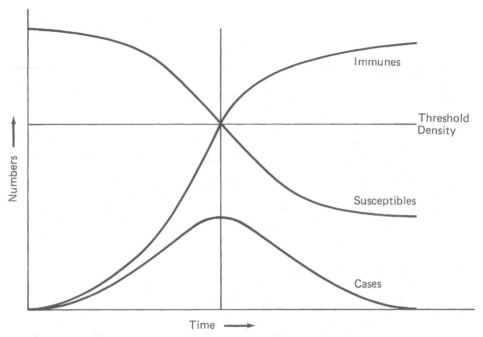

Figure 21.1. Diagrammatic representation of the course of an epidemic wave in terms of numbers and cases, numbers of susceptibles, and numbers of immunes. As the epidemic proceeds, the number of susceptibles decreases, and the number of immunes increases. The peak of the epidemic wave occurs at the threshold density of susceptibles.

First an investigation should be undertaken when the disease is a priority in the country or in a given geographical area. When this is the case, all suspicious cases must be investigated recognizing that the programs for control may be at stake, and the potential for spread of the disease is a significant danger for the population. Second, an investigation should be undertaken when the number of cases exceeds the usual frequency in a specific population group. The objectives of investigating an outbreak of disease are to identify the cause of the outbreak and the method of transmission of the disease. The epidemiologist must define the extent of involvement in terms of time, place, and population. The ultimate purpose of the investigation is to obtain data on which to decide what new or additional measures must be taken to control the outbreak and to prevent further infection from occurring.

In cases where a control program is underway, an investigation should be initiated as soon after the report of new cases is received or when the examination of the data reported to the epidemiologist suggests the need for application of new control or preventive measures. Even when multiple cases of a disease appear in a population which has had a common exposure to an etiologic agent, the outbreak may not be reported if each case is seen by a different health worker. In such a situation no association among the cases may be made. To prevent the failure to report cases, the epidemiologist must alert the field health workers of the need to report all cases of the condition observed, for if they are reported and observed as a group, there is a better chance of rapidly characterizing the outbreak and rapidly instituting control measures. Study of the pattern of the occurrence of separate cases of the same disease may help identify predisposing host factors. With this information available, new measures may be taken such as ones for removing infection sources or protecting people at risk of exposure to some other predisposing factor.

The epidemiological investigation provides the opportunity to collate information about cases which are temporally related and may as a result reveal the cause, route of transmission, and host and environmental factors associated with the outbreak. Study of this information may suggest an intervention leading to control of the outbreak and prevention of new cases.

The first step in the investigation is the decision that the situation warrants investigation. When dealing with infectious processes, the decision should be made quickly to prevent spread of the disease which will complicate control if a program is instituted. The reporting sources should be consulted. This may involve questioning physicians, health officers, patients, and relatives of patients. It is often useful to examine laboratory reports, hospital records, and records of absenteeism in industries or schools in the affected regions also before making the decision to proceed. Once the decision that there is probably a real problem is made, it is necessary to verify the diagnosis of cases by obtaining clinical histories, examining patients, and obtaining appropriate specimens for laboratory study. A case definition needs to be developed to aid the field worker in deciding which patients are in fact affected by the disease of concern. Development of the case definition and identification of cases is complicated by the variability in the signs of infection brought about by the hosts' immune responses and the effects of treatment. As the investigation proceeds, more patients and their contacts are interviewed, more laboratory samples are studied, and additional efforts are made to identify the infectious agent, determine its mode of transmission, and identify contaminated localities in an effort to determine the factors which contributed to the occurrence of the outbreak.

After sufficient data is collected, it may be possible to do a rough case count to get an idea of the magnitude of the problem. Available data should be arranged according to the time and the place where it was collected, and the population affected. This is an application of descriptive epidemiology. An epidemic curve may be drawn from these data. The shape of the curve may allow for prediction about the course of the outbreak. A spot map of the location of cases where infection occurred may indicate the course of the infection, the existence of a reservoir and a method of transmission of the infection. Data on age, sex, occupation, and socioeconomic status of affected individuals as well as their other characteristics, may reveal information about the disease and its means of spread.

For attack rates to be calculated, the population at risk, i.e., those exposed to the infectious agent, must be identified. In order to identify which population subgroups are at higher risk, it may be necessary to calculate attack rates for different subpopulations. The population at risk may be of a geographical area, such as those using a specific water distribution system or those who work in a certain building or factory or attend a specific school, or live in a specific neighborhood. In some instances the exposed population may be more diffuse and difficult to identify, such as people who ate in a certain restaurant, had contact with a certain commercially distributed food, went swimming in a specific area, or belong to an ethnic or socioeconomic group. For example, investigation of a food-borne disease outbreak may require breaking out of subgroups of those who may have been affected according to the food they ate. Sometimes it is necessary to conduct a survey to determine the population at risk.

As early as the data warrants development of a hypothesis on the source of the infection, the reservoir, the pathogen, the mode of transmission, and the relevant host and environmental factors must be made. The hypothesis should be the simplest coherent explanation compatible with the available data. A control plan should be developed on the basis of the available data.

The epidemiological investigation should continue after control measures are instituted to evaluate the effectiveness of the implemented control measures.

EPIDEMIOLOGICAL SURVEILLANCE

Basic knowledge on the health situation of a population as well as information on any deviation from what is considered normal in a given population is provided by epidemiological surveillance. The World Health Organization (WHO) aids in epidemiological surveillance by collecting data on occurrence of a number of diseases. The WHO for example requires countries to follow the agreed upon International Health Regulations and promptly notify it of cases of plague, yellow fever, or cholera. Regional health workers can draw on the WHO's data banks to aid them in their surveillance programs.

Surveillance activities are crucial for detecting outbreaks or other deviations from the usual situation in a population. The routine observation and analysis of the occurrence and distribution of diseases allow for the timely implementation of prevention and control activities. In order to have any value a timely and effective surveillance must be closely tied to a program of control and prevention. Data collected during surveillance may be used to formulate appropriate new control actions or be used to evaluate and modify actions already instituted.

When planning an epidemiological surveillance program, one must first decide what diseases or conditions are to be the subject of the epidemiological surveillance. To collect data on which to base this decision, one should consult health care personnel in the region to obtain some preliminary knowledge of the problems believed to exist in the region. In the surveillance program itself various basic activities must be carried out. These are (1) data collection, collation and, analysis; (2) decision-making for action; and (3) dissemination of information.

Data Collection, Collation, and Analysis

There must be a clear statement of what data must be collected, by whom, with what frequency, to whom the collected data will be transmitted, and by whom it will be recorded and analyzed. All persons involved in the program must be made fully aware of their roles in data collection, transmission, and analysis. Knowledge of the epidemiology of the disease of concern will aid in formulation of this statement.

Providers of information will be of many types, ranging from health personnel to community leaders and the press. The basic types of information to be collected are morbidity and mortality data. Data from case investigations, reports of epidemics, laboratory reports, population surveys, and studies of animal and vector disease occurrence will also be useful. The proper identification and selection of sources of information will be of great value in determining the distribution and occurrence of the diseases which are to be the subject of the surveillance. Regular reporting by regional health workers may be supplemented by reports from selected hospitals or clinics that are staffed by skilled diagnosticians who can provide information on observations they make.

What data is collected is determined by the characteristics of the diseases for which the surveillance program was initiated. Once collected, data must be grouped and organized into tables, graphs, or maps that can facilitate analysis and interpretation. Analysis involves a process of study of the data in order to establish trends in the progress of the spread of the disease, the frequency of its occurrence, and changes in its behavior. Analysis will identify groups at highest risk, and aid in determination of the most vulnerable points of intervention by control measures.

Decision-Making for Action

As a result of the analysis of the data, the measures for prevention or control most suited to the situation will be formulated as promptly as possible. The more rapidly data is collected and analyzed, the more quickly and effectively prevention and control measures can be implemented.

Dissemination of Information

Dissemination of the information obtained from the survey as well as the information about the measures of control being taken and the results obtained by the control measures is essential to the success of the surveillance and control activities being carried out. Without the enthusiastic collaboration of personnel of the health services, both public and private, epidemiological surveillance cannot be fully accomplished and as a result programs for improving public health will fail.

INFECTIOUS DISEASES

Infectious diseases affect hundreds of millions of individuals every year and have been estimated to account for nearly one-third of annual human mortality worldwide. A report from the World Bank (1993) measured the burden that diseases, as a group or individually, have on the various demographic regions of the world. For this purpose, the measurement took into account the combination of losses from premature death, which is defined as the difference between the actual age of death and life expectancy in a low mortality population, and loss of healthy life resulting from disability. The unit used to measure the global burden of disease was the disability-adjusted life years (DALYs). At the end, the global burden of disease was measured by comparing the DALYs lost from different diseases (Figure 21.2A). For this purpose, the incidence of cases by age, sex, and demographic region was estimated, and then the number of years of healthy life lost was obtained by multiplying the potential duration of the disease until it was cured or ended in death by a severity weight that measured the severity of the disability in comparison with loss of life.

Available data indicate that communicable diseases represent a tremendous burden. This burden was greater in demographically developing countries than elsewhere. On the other hand, noncommunicable diseases were a greater burden in countries with established market economies and the formerly socialistic economies of Europe than in the less developed countries (Figure 21.2B). Acute respiratory infections, diarrheal diseases, tuberculosis, sexually transmitted diseases including AIDS, parasitic diseases, and diseases preventable by vaccination are the most important of the infectious diseases, and they contribute most heavily to the burden produced by communicable diseases. Acute respiratory infections and diarrhea are the infectious diseases that produce the highest burden worldwide. In Africa, malaria produces a disease burden almost as high as that produced by acute respiratory infections (Figure 21.3). The disease burden imposed by infectious dis-

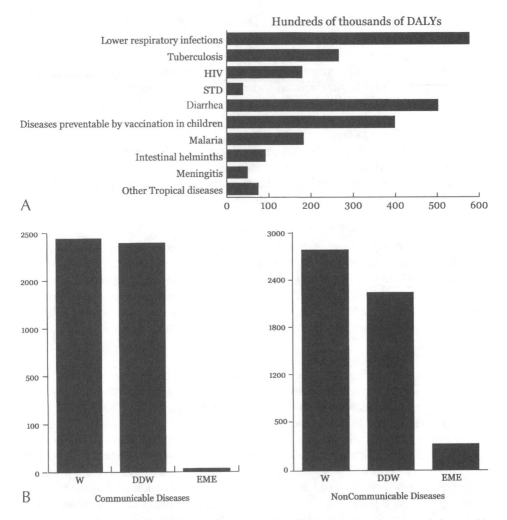

Figure 21.2. (A) Burden of different communicable diseases in females around the world. (B) Burden of communicable and noncommunicable diseases in females around the world in hundreds of thousands of disability adjusted life years lost (DALYs). (W) world, (DDW) demographically developing countries (Low and medium income countries from Africa, America, and Asia including China and India). (EME) established market economies (Australia, Canada, Japan, New Zealand, USA, and Western Europe).

eases varies geographically, as shown by the variation in distribution of losses in different geographical regions measured by DALYs (Figure 21.3).

Age differences in the burden produced by different diseases also exist. As noted above, acute respiratory infections, diarrheal diseases, and malaria are the communicable diseases that produce the highest burden worldwide, but they also are the main cause of death in children less than five years of age.

Data from the early 1990s indicate that a person in one of the least developed countries of the world has a life expectancy of forty-three years while a person in a developed country has a life expectancy of seventy-three years. While life expectancy will increase by the year 2000 up to seventy-nine years in developed countries, even then forty-five developing countries will still have a life expectancy of less than sixty years. About 51 million people died in the world in 1993, 39 million

Hundreds of thousands of DALYs

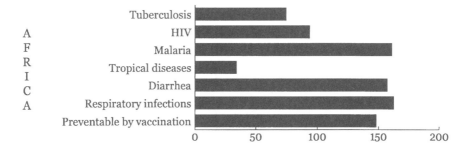

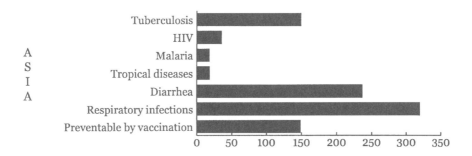

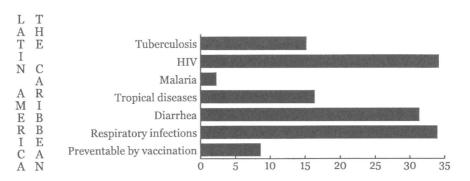

Figure 21.3. Burden of communicable diseases in females around the world by geographical areas.

of them in underdeveloped countries. Worldwide communicable diseases were responsible for about forty percent (20 million) of the total number of deaths. Eighty percent (16 million) of deaths from infectious diseases occurred in underdeveloped countries. Infectious diseases thus impose a tremendous burden to the already precarious health services in the underdeveloped world, where they constitute a serious negative factor for the development of individuals and social groups. They represent at the same time the results and causes of social, educational, political, and economic underdevelopment.

Poverty and its accompanying features, lack of sanitation, malnutrition, illiteracy, and crowding, are major factors in maintenance of infectious diseases but in another sense, infectious diseases are major factors in maintenance of poverty and its accompanying features. Infectious diseases however are not just of importance to those in poverty, for as infectious diseases occur worldwide and spread among people who come into contact directly or indirectly with each other, they are a threat to everyone.

Development of disease is a complex process. It results from the interaction between an infectious organism and a susceptible host. Not all infections result in disease. The organism may already reside inside the host and not cause disease until some change in the host occurs. Such infections are called endogenous infections, and the disease is called an endogenous disease, or it may come from outside, and this is an exogenous infection. Moreover, the chain of events that influence how and when the infectious organism gets in contact with and is introduced into the host is influenced by the environment, involving biological, climatologic, and social factors. Control and prevention of infection requires understanding of these interrelated factors and then finding points at which intervention can interrupt the unfolding chain of events that brings about infection and disease.

INFECTIOUS ORGANISMS
The environment influences human health favorably or unfavorably in many direct and indirect ways. We interact with all living things with which we have contact, i.e., plants, animals, and microorganisms, as well as with inanimate objects. Of particular importance to health are the organisms producing disease, the so-called pathogenic organisms. Pathogenicity refers to the organisms' virulence and invasiveness, factors which determine their capability to produce disease. The higher the virulence, the higher will be the morbidity, mortality, and communicability of the infection and thus the epidemiological importance of the disease caused by the organism.

Many factors are able to influence the role of the pathogen in causing disease. Many but not all of these factors are under the parasite's genetic control. There is in fact a vast variety of genetic and nongenetic factors which determine the ability of an organism to produce disease. Among the many factors influencing an organism's capacity to cause disease are the infective dose of the organism, its physical properties, its host specificity, its ability to undergo antigenic variation, and its ability to elaborate enzymes and toxins.

The infective dose is the number of organisms that must enter a host to cause an infection. It depends on the route and conditions of transmission, as well as the host's susceptibility including the host's immunological status. The physical properties of the organism make it either more or less susceptible to death by desiccation and other environmental affects and determine its ability to survive outside the host in soil or on an inanimate object. Host specificity may limit the availability of suitable hosts. Antigenic variation offers the organism the capability to escape or ameliorate the effects of the host's immune response, while production of certain enzymes and toxins makes the pathogen more able to infect or cause disease.

The ability of a microorganism to disseminate its genetic material to other organisms, for example to transfer plasmids conferring resistance to antibiotics, is a particular problem in the ongoing struggle by humans trying to control disease. Although it was thought that the discovery of antibiotics would solve the problems caused by bacteria in animals or humans, development and widespread dissemination of antibiotic resistant strains has shocked that hope out of existence and given new importance to the use of conventional public health measures to control disease.

In common medical usage not all pathogenic organisms are called parasites. Generally bacteria, viruses, fungi, rickettsia, and chlamydia are not referred to as parasites. The organisms commonly called parasites by people in the medical profession are protozoa and metazoa. To the biologist, however, all of the pathogenic organisms are considered parasites. The protozoa are unicellular organisms that produce, among other diseases, malaria, amoebiasis, giardiasis, leishmaniasis, and trypanosomiasis. The metazoa are multicellular parasites that produce diseases such as trichinosis, schistosomiasis, and ascariasis. The metazoa usually infect their hosts after a stage of free-living development in either soil or water.

The bacteria are unicellular organisms many species of which may produce either local or systemic diseases. Systemic diseases, for example, may involve many organ systems including the respiratory system, the nervous system or the bowel, and may spread widely. Bacteria causing systemic diseases include the mycobacteria, meningococci, salmonella, and shigella. Localized infections, that is ones that do not spread easily from the site of initial infection, are often caused by staphylococci or streptococci.

Rickettsia are small pleomorphic coccobacillary microorganisms that contain both DNA and RNA. Their size is intermediate between bacteria and viruses. In most cases growth only occurs intracellularly and they are disseminated from animal to animal by arthropods. Humans are infected only by accident, but infection may be serious as it is in epidemic typhus, spotted fever, Q fever, and human ehrlichiosis.

Chlamydia are obligate intracellular organisms that have DNA and RNA. There are two species of interest to medicine: *Chlamydia trachomatis* and *C. psittaci*. The viruses are pathogens smaller than those above, have only DNA or RNA, not both, and reproduce exclusively intracellularly. They are the etiological agents of well-known diseases such as measles, rabies, rubella, encephalitis, poliomyelitis, and influenza as well as newly emerging diseases such as AIDS or hemorrhagic fever produced by the Ebola virus. They are often transmitted directly from person to person but may use arthropod vectors in some cases.

The fungi are unicellular or syncytial agents responsible for diseases such as histoplasmosis, coccidiomycosis, tineasis, and blastomycosis. The reservoir in which the fungi are maintained is usually the soil, and in most cases fungal diseases are not transmitted directly from one person to another. Further information on these disease causing agents can be found in chapters 15, 16, 17, and 18.

EMERGING AND REEMERGING DISEASES

According to the Institute of Medicine of the United States of America, emerging diseases are those whose incidence in humans was never high in the past but which have increased in incidence in the last twenty years. Reemerging diseases are those conditions that reappear after a significant decrease in incidence. Figure 21.4 mentions several emerging and reemerging diseases that have been observed in different geographical areas since 1980.

The three diseases, AIDS, cholera, and dengue, are excellent examples of emerging and reemerging diseases. The first is an emerging and the second and third are reemerging diseases. AIDS, unknown until early in 1980, has spread all over the world. On the other hand cholera, endemic in countries of Africa and Asia, has reappeared in 1991 in the western hemisphere after more than eighty years of silence.

Knowledge of AIDS has been widely disseminated by the press. However, even now a great proportion of the population worldwide views AIDS as a plague of male homosexuals and drug users, which is to some degree true in countries located in Europe and North America, but in most others, usually those which are underdeveloped, the disease is a consequence of casual heterosexual intercourse. The long period of eight to ten years during which the infected person is well but can infect others, makes control of HIV infection difficult as healthy carriers do not seek medical care.

Dengue incidence was greatly reduced in the Americas during the 1960s and 1970s. The decline was possible because the dengue vector, the mosquito *Aedes aegypti*, was almost wiped out in Central and South America. In the 1980s, dengue returned with a vengeance and was responsible for an epidemic in Cuba which gave rise to thousands of cases and caused hundreds of deaths. Since then, dengue epidemics have spread steadily in the Caribbean, and in Central and South America.

The general population got to know about the emerging and reemerging diseases through the mass media, which pounded the public all over the world with information on the threat of new and old diseases in the middle 1990s. Ebola in Africa and plague in India dominated the news. Pulmonary Distress Syndrome and its etiological agent, the *Sin Nombre* virus, later recognized as a Hantavirus, were found in the state of New Mexico and attracted great media attention. The same virus was later found in people in Argentina, Brazil, Canada, Chile, Paraguay, and Uruguay. West Nile virus appeared in New York in 1999.

Other new diseases may be added to those already mentioned. There is for example Lyme disease in the U.S., and there are the two diarrheal producing protozoa, cryptosporidia, and cyclosporidia. Cryptosporidia is found all over the world, and cyclosporidia is found only in the Americas. *Escherichia coli* O157:H7 is found in North and South America; drug resistant *Plasmodium falciparum* malaria has appeared in all the countries of the Americas sharing the Amazon basin, in countries of Southern Africa, and in Southeast Asia. Antibiotic resistant pneumococci, staphylococci, enterococci, salmonella, shigella, and *Vibro cholera*, among others, have appeared throughout the world (Figure 21.4).

Specific factors precipitating disease emergence can usually be identified. They are often environmental, ecological, or demographic factors that put people in close contact with unfamiliar pathogens and ones which favor dissemination of the pathogen. The widespread use of chemotherapeutic drugs often without medical supervision increases the likelihood of selection of resistant variants of many bacteria including gonococci, pneumococci, staphylococci, salmonella, shigella and enterococci, and of parasites like the ones causing malaria. Epidemiological studies suggest that the problem of emergence of new diseases and drug resistant strains of existing pathogenic organisms will continue.

THE HOST

Infection is the presence of replicating foreign organisms in the tissues of a host. The host response to the infection will range from subclinical or inapparent to disease. When infectious agents replicate in or on host tissues without clinical or subclinical disease, this is called *colonization*. Contamination, on the other hand, occurs when microorganisms are present on the surface of inanimate objects or on tissues but do not multiply there. A person who is colonized by an organism but shows no

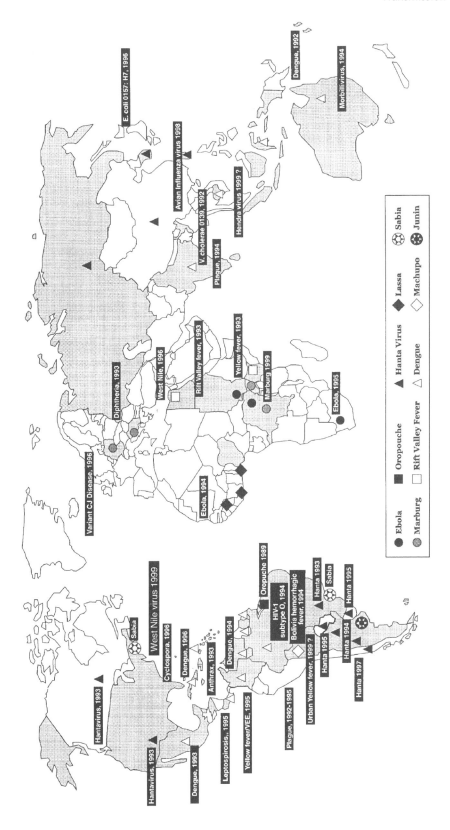

Figure 21.4. Emerging and reemerging diseases in the world since 1980. Geographical distribution.

evidence of disease is called a *carrier*. Carriers may have shown signs and symptoms of the infection earlier and recovered or may never have been made ill by the organism. The carrier state may be short or long term, continuous or sporadic. Disease agents spread by healthy carriers pose more serious problems for disease control than disease agents that infect and cause sickness promptly as the former type of agents can become widespread before people become aware that there is a problem.

The routes by which an infectious agent enters or leaves its host are known as the portals of entry and exit, respectively. The respiratory tract is a common portal of entry for organisms causing, for example, tuberculosis, the common cold and influenza; the genitourinary tract is used as a portal of entry by organisms causing, for example, AIDS, syphilis, and gonorrhea. The gastrointestinal tract provides entry to the organisms causing typhoid fever, hepatitis B, cholera, and dysentery. The skin is a portal of entry generally only if pierced. The organisms enter through preexisting superficial lesions or as a result of stings, bites, or needle wounds. Organisms such as those causing dengue, malaria, and yellow fever, for example, most commonly enter the host through the skin with the aid of agents that pierce the skin.

The placenta usually acts as a barrier protecting the fetus from the mother's infection, but may not always be effective against some disease organisms such as those causing syphilis, rubella, hepatitis, toxoplasmosis, or Chagas' disease.

The portal of exit is usually the same as that used for entry. For example, in respiratory diseases, the airway is utilized as the point of entry when respiratory secretions are passed from one person to another, and as the portal of exit from the person that is the source of the infection. In other diseases the points of entry and exit may be different. In plague the normal portals of entry and exit are the skin with the blood-sucking vector mediating the passage, but sometimes plague switches to a respiratory route leaving the host by the respiratory route and thus becoming pneumonic plague. Many diarrhea causing organisms enter the mouth and leave by way of the anus.

THE ENVIRONMENT

Humans and for that matter other animals are immersed in a physical and social environment. Factors from the characteristics of the landscape to education and economic development have important roles in shaping the patterns of disease in the populations in an area. Although diseases are a worldwide problem, the burdens they produce are different in the different geographical areas of the world. The burdens produced by microbial, viral, and parasitic infections are heaviest in countries having preindustrial social structures. The high incidence of infectious disease in populations of the poorest people in the poorest countries of the world greatly increases social inequalities. (See the section on Infectious Diseases for additional discussion of this subject.)

As noted before, infectious diseases are common in countries with preindustrial social structures. Individuals at greatest risk in such societies are those living in rural areas and urban squatter settlements. Those so affected are primarily the poor, those without access to treated water and sewage or adequate housing and farmers and wage laborers in mining and timber exploitation who are exposed to parasitic diseases as an occupational hazard.

Movement of people is an important feature in the dissemination of disease. The number of travelers is huge. In the early 1990s, 500 million people crossed international borders by plane. In the same period, there were 20 million refugees and 30 million displaced persons. An estimated 70 million persons, mostly from underdeveloped countries, work either legally or illegally in other countries. There are 7 million legal immigrants from Central and South America in the U.S.; more than 400 thousand in Europe and 80 thousand in Australia. Untold others are present illegally. Thousands of refugees migrate from one country to another in Africa every year in order to avoid war and famine.

In the last sixty years, the world has seen migration from the rural to the urban areas in most countries. In the underdeveloped world, this phenomena has increased the problem of overcrowding in cites. The authorities of the overcrowded cites struggle daily to provide their citizens clean water and waste disposal. It is not strange then that diseases like dengue fever, dependent on the presence in urban areas of *Aedes aegypti* mosquitoes, and cholera, spread by fecal contamination of food and water, have returned to the western hemisphere.

Nations that desire national development and that are under pressure from expanding populations are cultivating new lands by opening jungle areas to agricultural development. They are opening new areas for exploitation, extracting natural resources, building hydroelectric dams, and developing many other aspects of their societies. An undesired consequence of many such activities is an increase in the risk of disease, especially malaria and leishmaniasis.

In the course of development, internal migrations occur. These migrations often are determined by the demands of planting and harvesting. Settlers and their families penetrate into jungle areas in which disease vectors abound. Temporary dwellings are constructed that lack even minimum sanitary facilities and place the residents at the mercy of disease vectors. Often the areas into which migrants go lack the most basic health and sanitation facilities, and the most rudimentary programs for education and political and administrative organization. As a result of these conditions, the population is left without protection from disease.

Flood type irrigation systems that are used for growing rice and banana crops as well as poorly built roads, dams, and irrigation canals are often excellent breeding sites for mosquitoes, particularly after long periods of rain. Such conditions should be anticipated during the planning phase of development projects. Epidemiologists should be included on the teams planning road building, colonization, agricultural settlement, livestock raising, and utilization and extraction of natural resources such as oil production and timber exploitation. The epidemiologists on the teams will anticipate and suggest actions to control the various situations induced by development that increase the risk of illness or death from disease. Some problems which planners have not anticipated are epidemics of malaria in South Africa, South America, and Southeast Asia following development. The obvious relationships that have been found by epidemiologists between malaria incidence and environmental change following development call attention to the undesirable aspects of unplanned or not well planned projects.

Climatic factors influence the occurrence and transmission of infectious diseases through multiple direct and indirect effects upon pathogenic microorganisms and their vectors, reservoirs, and hosts. Climate influences the flora and fauna of a region. Such influence is great in vector-borne, viral and rickettsial zoonotic diseases transmitted by arthropods. Murine typhus and the arbovirus diseases including yellow fever and dengue are examples. Climate also influences vector-borne protozoal diseases such a malaria, leishmaniasis, and African and American trypanosomiasis. Much of the climatic effect is mediated by the influence of temperature on the development of the insects that are vectors of these diseases. Development of microorganisms carried by mosquitoes, ticks, and other arthropods is also influenced by the temperature of the microenvironment within their vector hosts. Survival rates of vectors and the rates of multiplication and transmission of microorganisms that infect them are also temperature dependent. Temperature and precipitation are related to the incidence of nonvector-borne infectious diseases such as cholera and leptospirosis also. The epidemic due to hantavirus in the southwest U.S. in 1993 was associated with an increase in the wild rodent population brought about by food availability resulting from the abundant rainfall at the time.

Variation in rainfall can affect disease transmission directly by its effect on the vector population or indirectly by affecting reservoirs or water supplies. Both flooding and drought may have influence on infectious diseases. Using malaria as an example: adequate rainfall with temperatures in the 20 to 30°C range and humidity above sixty percent provides optimal conditions for mosquitoes to incubate and transmit the parasite. Moderate precipitation may fill up breeding sites for Anopheles mosquitoes increasing breeding, while severe rainfall may wash out breeding sites, and low rainfall may restrict the breeding of mosquitoes decreasing the numbers of them.

Flooding can influence disease transmission in a number of ways, most notably by increasing run-off and disturbing breeding grounds and habitats of vectors. The drowning of rodents that are reservoirs for disease may decrease the incidence of disease, while flooding may increase contamination of water with rodent excreta and corpses which can lead to increased transmission by exposing humans to contaminated water.

Wind has been associated with epidemics of meningococcal meningitis in sub-Saharan Africa. It was suggested that the dry, sand-carrying winds caused mucosal damage that facilitated the entry of the meningococci into the body.

TRANSMISSION MECHANISMS
Basically, infectious diseases are transmitted by direct contact, or by indirect contact. The latter occurs when a vehicle such as water or air, or a vector is involved. Infectious agents spread from a source or reservoir to a person directly or indirectly. In direct contact, there is a transfer of the organism from an infected human or animal to another in which the infection may take place. Direct contact (person to person or animal to animal) implies that the infectious source and the susceptible host come into physical contact. This may be by touching, biting, kissing, or sexual intercourse. Infectious mononucleosis is transmitted by kissing, while AIDS, syphilis, and gonorrhea are transmitted by sexual intercourse. Direct transmission also occurs by droplet spray during sneezing, coughing, spitting, singing, or talking. Tuberculosis and the common cold are transmitted by droplet spray. Droplets containing infectious material reaching the conjunctiva or the mucous membranes of the eye, nose, or mouth can cause infection. Droplets are large, 5 μm particles, that travel short distances through the air (<1 m) and settle out quickly.

Vehicle-borne transmission occurs when the infectious organisms are carried by contaminated inanimate objects such as toys, handkerchiefs, soiled clothes, bedding, cooking or eating utensils, surgical instruments or dressings, water or food. Inanimate objects carrying disease organisms are called *fomites*.

Biological products such as blood, serum, plasma, tissues, and organs may serve as vehicles to transmit disease. A wide range of disease-causing agents may be transmitted by such products including hepatitis B or C virus, HIV, and *Trypanosoma cruzi*. Any infection transmitted in this way may be considered a vehicle-borne transmission. It does not matter whether the agent may (like salmonella in food) or may not (like hepatitis A in water or food) have multiplied in the vehicle serving as the transmitting agent.

Food-borne disease causes significant illness in people in both developed and underdeveloped countries. The microorganisms responsible include viruses, bacteria, protozoa, and worms. Morbidity depends on the pathogen, the susceptibility of the infected humans, and the medical care available. Diarrheal diseases have a strong cyclical occurrence. Higher temperatures favor the prevalence of food-borne illnesses caused by pathogens that replicate on foods at high ambient temperatures. Production of staphylococcal toxins, a common contaminant of food is also associated with high temperature. Other bacteria that are food contaminants are *Campylobacter jejuni*, which is acquired by drinking contaminated milk or water or by eating improperly cooked poultry meat, and *Escherichia coli* O157:H7 by eating undercooked meat. Salmonella, Shigella, and *Vibrio cholerae*, as well as *Cryptosporidium parvum*, *Cyclospora cayetanenis*, and *Trichenella spiralis* are also transmitted by food.

Waterborne microorganisms have been estimated to account for almost forty percent of the annual mortality due to infectious disease. They include Salmonella, Shigella, and *V. cholerae*. *Vibrio cholerae*, in addition to being acquired and spread through food, is also spread by bathing in or drinking contaminated water. It remains endemic in India, Bangladesh, and Africa. It has recently caused epidemics in the Americas. In the United States it exists in waters in the gulf coast of Texas, Louisiana, and Florida, Chesapeake Bay, the California coast, and coastal waters to the north. *Vibrio cholerae* occurs in riverine, brackish water, and estuarine ecosystems, being part of the natural flora of plankton and is found in the gut of, and attached to the surface of, both freshwater and marine copepods. Outbreaks in humans seem to be related to plankton blooms associated with warm sea-surface temperatures. The phytoplankton blooms are a food source for the copepods upon which the cholera bacterium thrives. Movement of tidal waters carries the algal blooms and copepods toward land and into rivers, bringing the bacterium into contact with humans who use this water for bathing or as a source of drinking water. *Vibrio vulnificus* is another *Vibrio* that could be found in estuarine waters and from shellfish and occasionally infects man in the U.S.

Cryptosporidiosis is often spread by contact with surface water run-off contaminated by feces of infected cattle. It has caused thousands of infections in the U.S. by contamination of the drinking water supply. *Giardia lamblia* is a diarrhea producing protozoan acquired usually from drinking contaminated water (Figure 21.5). It can cause mild to severe diarrhea. Heavy rain and increased run-off of contaminated water has been related to increased transmission.

Leptospirosis is a zoonosis of rats. Humans acquire the disease through contact with urine-contaminated water. The organism enters the body through broken skin or the mucus membranes of the nose or mouth. Symptoms range from fever and chills to jaundice and kidney damage.

Schistosomiasis is the most prevalent waterborne disease. It occurs mainly in Africa and Asia. In the Americas the most affected country is Brazil. Estimates sug-

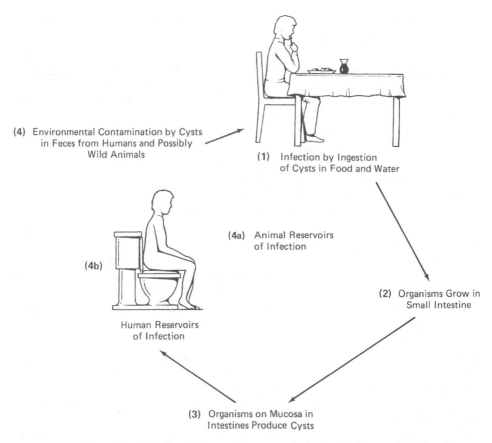

(4) Environmental Contamination by Cysts in Feces from Humans and Possibly Wild Animals

(1) Infection by Ingestion of Cysts in Food and Water

(4a) Animal Reservoirs of Infection

(4b)

(2) Organisms Grow in Small Intestine

Human Reservoirs of Infection

(3) Organisms on Mucosa in Intestines Produce Cysts

Figure 21.5. Life cycle of giardia. This organism enters its host with ingested food and water contaminated with encysted parasites (1). Parasites grow in the intestine (2). Cysts produced are passed in the feces (3). Animal hosts as well as humans may serve as sources of infective cysts (4a&b). Control of the disease thus requires prevention of ingestion of cysts through programs of environmental sanitation. Elimination of wild animal reservoirs of the parasite is not possible.

gest that there are 250 million people infected worldwide. It is acquired by exposure to fresh water containing infected snails (Figure 21.6).

Vector-borne transmission may be by injection of salivary gland fluid during biting (e.g., dengue virus, malaria) or by regurgitation (e.g., *Pasteurella pestis*) or deposition on the skin of feces or other material which can be rubbed into the bite wound or through an area of trauma from scratching or rubbing (e.g., *Trypanosoma cruzi*). Transmission by insects can be mechanical. It is mechanical when the infectious agent is carried on its surface by an insect. Salmonella for example may be carried on the legs of flies.

The vector may harbor the microbe in its body but without multiplication. *Yersinia pestis* is carried by infected fleas, in which it passes through the gastrointestinal tract without change. The transmission is called biological when propagation, cyclic development, or a combination of these is required before the vector can transmit the organisms. Biological transmission implies that an incubation period in the vector is required following infection before the vector becomes infective. An ex-

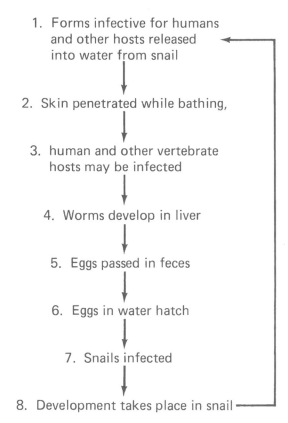

1. Forms infective for humans
   and other hosts released
   into water from snail

2. Skin penetrated while bathing,

3. human and other vertebrate
   hosts may be infected

4. Worms develop in liver

5. Eggs passed in feces

6. Eggs in water hatch

7. Snails infected

8. Development takes place in snail

Figure 21.6.   Life cycle of Schistosoma in water. Infective forms of the *Schistoma mansoni* that are released into water from infected snails (1) penetrate the skin (2). There may be nonhuman reservoirs of infection (3) in some regions. The worms develop in the liver (4). The eggs leave the liver by way of venules. From the venules, the eggs reach the intestine. They are passed from the intestine with feces (5). In water the eggs hatch (6) releasing stages infective for snails (7). After development in the snail (8), stages infective for man are released (1). Those penetrate the skin of people bathing in the contaminated water. Control depends on preventing fecal contamination of water, eradication of snails, preventing bathing in contaminated water, and treatment of infected humans.

ample of this is what happens in the triatomine vectors of Chagas' disease (Figure 21.7). *Trypanosoma cruzi* requires time to multiply in the gut before it is passed in infectious form in the insects' urine and feces. The infectious agent may be passed to succeeding generations as happens with transovarian transmission of some viruses, or it may go from one stage of the life cycle of the vector to another, for example, from egg to nymph to adult.

Airborne organisms enter the air from animals, humans, or inanimate objects, such as soil. Microbe-containing aerosols are responsible for airborne transmission. Microbial aerosols are suspensions in the air of particles, <5 μm in diameter, containing microorganisms. Infectious airborne particles are small bodies formed by evaporation of fluid from droplets emitted by an infected host or are dust particles that may arise from soil, clothes, bedding, or contaminated floors. Such particles may remain suspended in the air for long periods of time, and may retain infectivity or virulence. Microbes in the air are easily drawn into the alveoli of the lungs.

(3) Insect infected by
feeding on infected
animals or infected
humans   Vector, kissing bug

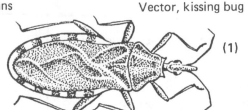

(1) Bite wound or eye
contaminated by rubbing
in of feces deposited
while insect feeds

(2) Infective form of
trypanosme present
in insect feces

Figure 21.7. Transmission of *T. cruzi*, the causative agent of Chagas' disease. Infection by Chagas' disease, causing trypanosomes, occurs by contamination of a bite wound with the vector's feces (1) or by contamination of eye with the contaminated insect feces (2,3). As the vector insect feeds on man or other animals, control measures require prevention of man-insect contact. As a major reservoir of the parasite is present in animals other than man, treatment of human cases may have little effect on the maintenance of the infection.

Most airborne diseases spread through respiratory tract secretions can be carried by the wind or be dispersed within buildings by air-handling systems.

Transmission of tuberculosis and meningococcal meningitis is by airborne droplets and is facilitated by close contact with an infected person. Coccidioidomycosis, an infectious disease of the lungs caused by the fungus *Coccidioides immitis*, is found in the soil of semidesert areas of the western hemisphere. Infection is acquired by inhalation of wind blown spores.

Respiratory syncytial virus causing upper or lower respiratory tract infections and the bacterium *Legionella pneumophila* causing Legionnaires' disease are also airborne. Legionnaires' disease may be spread when the infecting organism, which grows in water in air-conditioning cooling towers and elsewhere in water, is dispersed through the air-handling system of a building.

PREVENTION AND CONTROL

The role of medicine is to promote and preserve health, to restore health when it has been diminished, and to minimize suffering and distress. The object of the epidemiologist is to promote these goals through disease prevention. The goal of prevention programs is to decrease the incidence of disease. It is accomplished by protection of health by the use of personal health measures and encouragement of community-wide efforts for improvement of the environment and maintenance of a safe environment by promoting good nutrition, appropriate use of medical care and of vaccination, and by encouraging high standards of public and personal hygiene. Primary prevention programs are those aimed at preventing disease (reducing incidence) by personnel and community-wide efforts such as immunization and bettering the environment, etc. Secondary programs are those measures available to individuals for the early detection and prompt and effective treatment to correct deviations from the healthy state (reducing prevalence). Tertiary programs consist of the measures used to reduce long-term impairment and minimize suffering (preventing and reducing complications). In fact, primary prevention programs are facilitated by secondary programs, as treatment of cases will reduce sources of infection.

Control measures are operations, the aim of which is to prevent the spread of disease and thereby decrease disease incidence and prevalence. Since the development of infections is multifactorial, designing control measures is complex. Even if one knows the etiology, the route of transmission, the reservoirs and appropriate actions for interrupting transmission, control may be difficult because human behavior and economic and environmental factors all may affect what can be done in the actual situation that exists.

Identification of the most susceptible target as the point of intervention in the chain of transmission of the infectious agent is crucial for the design of an effective control program. If the disease is spread by contact, control measures need to be directed toward people or inanimate objects associated with transmission. When dealing with persons who are the source of the infection, there may be a need for education as well as therapy. Quarantine of individuals carrying the disease may be desirable but is very difficult to effectively carry out. If an inanimate object is involved in transmission, improved disinfection or sterilization methods may be necessary. If airborne infection is involved, effective sterilization of the contaminated air by ultraviolet radiation or other means may need to be instituted. Such an approach is only possible if transmission is occurring in a closed space such as a building. Health education for the general public and specific training for health personnel may be necessary in most cases.

In some instances disease spread may be stopped by eradication of the organisms from the host by treatment. In some situations vaccination will completely prevent the establishment of the pathogen in the host.

It is sometimes possible to interrupt transmission by acting on the reservoir of infection. Rats are controlled to prevent plague in man, for example. The vector of a disease may be a target. Destroying Anopheles mosquitoes by spraying or source reduction or by using a mosquito net to act as a barrier between the mosquitoes and the human host will often prevent malaria (Figure 21.8). If the reservoir is a human, isolation may accompany therapy to prevent spread of infection until treatment is completed.

Control activities may reflect compromises among different intervention measures. Dengue prevention involves control of an urban mosquito, *Aedes aegypti*, at the larval and adult stages. Programs staffed with thousands of employees were able to eradicate this mosquito from several countries of Central and South America in the middle 1960s. Because of lack of continued surveillance, these mosquitoes were reintroduced and the countries were reinfested in the late 1970s. Since then, dengue has spread. Actually, today employing the same tools as were used in the 1960s is impossible for economic reasons. Funds are not available to support thousands of employees going house to house to eliminate breeding sources and spraying for adult mosquitoes. What is now possible is education to obtain the help of the community to implement source reduction by eliminating receptacles containing water that may serve as breeding places, or making them unsuitable as breeding places for the mosquitoes. Vaccination is probably one of the most effective means for control of infectious disease. However, in order to be implemented, a vaccine must be available and an effective delivery system must be in place. The health services system to be used to deliver the vaccine must provide universal coverage and the population must be cooperative. Other elements to be considered are available resources, time constraints, personnel available, and potential com-

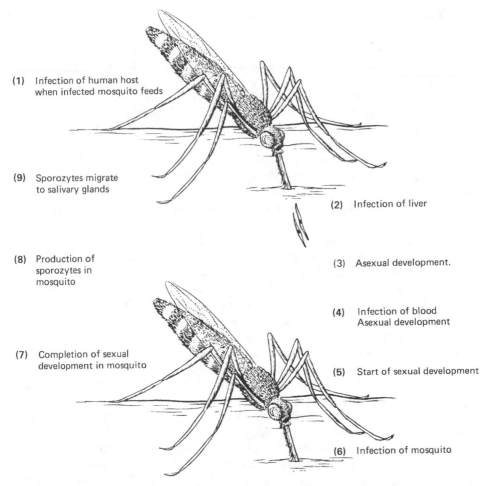

(1) Infection of human host when infected mosquito feeds

(9) Sporozytes migrate to salivary glands

(2) Infection of liver

(8) Production of sporozytes in mosquito

(3) Asexual development.

(4) Infection of blood Asexual development

(7) Completion of sexual development in mosquito

(5) Start of sexual development

(6) Infection of mosquito

Figure 21.8.   The mosquito is the vector of malaria. It injects sporozoites when feeding (1). The sporozoites enter the liver (2) where they develop asexually into meronts (3). The merozoites which develop in the meront in the liver invade red blood cells (4) where they develop asexually. Some of the merozoites become gametocytes (5) capable of infecting mosquitoes (6) in which sexual development is completed (7). When the sporozoites produced (8) migrate to the salivary glands (9), the mosquito becomes infective. Infection may be controlled by reducing the mosquito population, by reducing contact between humans and mosquitoes, and by treatment of humans to prevent infection of mosquitoes. As human malaria has essentially no nonhuman reservoirs other than mosquitoes, control measures are directed to mosquitoes and humans.

plications of the proposed control measures.

In any case, the success of prevention and control activities will depend on many factors including the political will of the public and private sectors in providing financial resources, the dissemination of information by the press, and the community cooperation in implementation of the control programs.

SUMMARY

In spite of an ever-changing epidemiological situation, with its increase in prevalence of chronic diseases and decrease in prevalence of infectious diseases which has accompanied development, the latter still cause substantial burdens in both developed and underdeveloped countries. Established infectious diseases, like tuberculosis or malaria, continue to be prevalent, while new diseases, like AIDS, Lyme disease, cryptosporidiosis, and cyclosporidiosis, have appeared. The list of new diseases is constantly growing. Ebola, hepatitis C, and Guanarito viruses, among others, which were unknown less than twenty years ago, are now being found with increasing frequency. Antimicrobial resistance to antibiotics is also increasing. We now have *Plasmodium falciparum* resistant to antimalarial drugs, and HIV resistant to antiretrovirals. These are a surging threat in both community and hospital settings. Tourism and migration, as well as other social factors, such as social inequality and its companion poverty, facilitate dissemination and transmission of infectious diseases. Such a constantly changing situation requires constant surveillance.

The surveillance of a population for infectious disease provides knowledge of the patterns of occurrence of diseases in the population and of the factors that influence those patterns. Such knowledge is vital to planning an intervention, but many other factors must be considered as well.

In planning an intervention, one must ask and be able to determine if the intervention can do what it is supposed to do. That is, one must be able to judge the efficacy of the intervention. One must be able to estimate the probability that an individual in the target population will benefit from the intervention under the conditions that exist in the target area. The probability that an individual in need will benefit from the intervention under normal programmatic conditions is sometimes difficult to judge. To make these judgments, one needs scientific data obtained by study of the problem, but even with good data available, other factors, primarily political, must be considered. When resources and political commitment are available to support an intervention which technical data indicate will be effective in interrupting transmission, the success is almost assured. At the international level, a good example of a successful program was that for the eradication of smallpox from the world. Another good example, although on a smaller scale, was the eradication of poliomyelitis from the Western Hemisphere. Both were programs based on widescale use of effective vaccines, and both had effective organizations and sufficient resources available.

Data collection can never stop as the health situation is never static. The constant collection of data is necessary for planning and implementation of new public health interventions required to deal with the new situations as they arise and to assess their effectiveness. Surveillance findings make possible timely intervention to deal with the ever-changing environments in which we exist.

For the indefinite future, the cornerstone of prevention and control of disease will remain effective surveillance by health personnel in the field, strong public health laboratories to support the health personnel, good communication networks among field workers, public health laboratories and the public, and the maintenance of a strong public health infrastructure.

SUGGESTIONS FOR FURTHER READING

1. Last, J.M., ed. *A Dictionary of Epidemiology*. 2d ed. New York/Oxford: Oxford University Press, 1988.
2. Benenson, A., ed. *Control of Communicable Disease of Man*. 16th ed. Washington, DC: American Public Health Association, 1995.

3. Colwell, R.R., and J.A. Patz. *Climate, Infectious Diseases and Health. An Interdisciplinary Perspective*. American Academy of Microbiology, 1997.
4. Fletcher, R.H., S.W. Fletcher, and E.H. Wagner. *Clinical Epidemiology. The Essentials*. Baltimore, MD: Williams & Wilkins, 1982.
5. *Emerging Infections*. Washington, DC: Institute of Medicine, 1992.
6. Lilienfield, A.M., and D.E. Lilienfield. *Foundations of Epidemiology*. 2d ed. London: Oxford University Press, 1980.
7. Morse, S.S. "Factors in the Emergence of Infectious Diseases." *Emerg. Infect. Dis.* 1 (1995):7–15.
8. Satcher, D. "Emerging Infections: Getting Ahead of the Curve." *Emerg. Infect. Dis.* 1 (1995):1–6.
9. Schmunis, G.A., and F.J. Lopez Antuñano. "World-Wide Importance of Parasites." In *Topley & Wilson's Microbiology and Microbial Infections, Vol. 5: Parasitology*. 9th ed, 19–38. Edited by F.E.G. Cox, J.P. Kreier, and D. Wakelin, 1997.
10. World Health Organization. *The Control of Schistosomiasis*. WHO Tech Rep Ser 728, 1985.
11. World Health Organization. *Implementation of the Global Malaria Control Strategy*. WHO Tech Rep Ser 839, 1993.

QUESTIONS

1. What is an infection?
2. Mention three emerging diseases that exist in the U.S.
3. When is there a need of an epidemiological investigation?
4. How is an epidemic defined?
5. How is a pandemic defined?
6. What is the meaning of morbidity?
7. What is the difference between prevalence and incidence?

ANSWERS

1. An infection is the presence of foreign replicating organisms in host tissues
2. Three emerging diseases that exist in the U.S. are HIV, hepatitis C, and Lyme disease (there are also others).
3. There is a need of an epidemiological investigation when the number of new cases of a disease in a given period of time in a population of a specific geographical area exceeds the usual frequency.
4. An epidemic is the sudden increase in the number of cases of a disease above its expected incidence.
5. A pandemic is an epidemic that occurs worldwide.
6. Morbidity is an indication of illness.
7. Prevalence is the number of instances of a disease in a given population at a designated time, while incidence indicates the number of new cases in a given population during a certain period of time.

Index

ABO blood group system, 87
  antigens of, 216
Abscesses, staphylococcal, 54
Acellular pertussis vaccines, 405
Acid fast stain, 305
Acid hydrolases, 34
  in azurophilic granules, 33
Acne, 300
Acoleomates, 247
Acquired immune response, subversion of, 8
Acquired immunodeficiency syndrome, 236, 445–446
  antiviral drugs for, 329
  cryptosporidiosis in, 354
  destructive virus of, 3
  gp120 surface antigen of, 407
  HIV virus in, 344–346
  host resistance in, 19
  microsporidiosis and, 361
  toxoplasmosis and, 361
Actinomyces
  characteristics of, 315t
  of mouth, 21
Active immunity, 4f
Acycloguanosine (Acyclovir), 329
Adaptive immune response, 5–6, 10, 262–263
ADCC. *See* Antibody-dependent cell-mediated cytotoxicity
Addison's disease, 182t
Adenoviridae, 322t

Adhesins, 266–268
  blastoconidia attaching to, 383
  preventing phagocytosis, 270
Adhesion
  in hypersensitivity mediation, 190
  at inflamed site, 55
  modulated expression of, 271
Adjuvants, 101
  in vaccine preparations, 403–404
Aedes aegypti, control of, 455
Aerobic respiration, 287
Affinity, 96
  changes in during immune response, 116–119
Affinity constants, 97
Affinity labeling, 94–95
Agarose gel matrix, precipitation in, 414–416
Agglutination, 162, 416
  outcome of, 63t
Agglutination assays, 124–125
  indirect, 125
Agglutinins
  invertebrate, 249–250
  in mononucleosis, 97
AIDS. *See* Acquired immunodeficiency syndrome; Human immunodeficiency virus
Airborne transmission, 299, 453–454
Alexin, 64
Allergens
  ascaris, 361–362

binding to IgE, 119
immunotherapy for, 189–190
Allergic contact dermatitis, 194–195
of hand, 196*f*
Allergic reactions, 181–198
to vaccine, 400–401
Allergic rhinitis, 185
Allergy
definition of, 181
IgE in, 119
immunotherapy for, 189–190
pharmacologic interventions in
treatment of, 190
Alloantigens, 218
Class I and II, 207–208
degree of activation in graft recipients, 214*f*
Allogeneic skin graft rejection, 257
Allografts, 202
donor-specific blood transfusions
and, 217–218
rejection of
acute, immunosuppressive drugs
in, 215
in fish, 254
immunologic mechanisms of,
208–209
in invertebrates, 250
T cell recognition pathways in,
209–211
renal, 203*f*
αβ T cells, 6
Alphaherpesvirus, tumors associated
with, 225*t*
Alum, 101
efficacy of, 403
limitations of, 403–404
Alveolar macrophages, 33, 145
Amino acids
aromatic rings of, 91
on light and heavy chains, 108
sequences of in antigenic proteins, 91
in synthetic polymer immunogenicity, 89
Aminobenzene, 89
Aminopterin, 432*f*
Amoebae, 350
intestinal, 351–353

Amoxicillin, 311
Amphibians
immunity in, 254–256
lymphoid organs of, 2*t*
Amphotericin, 389
Amphotericin B, 389
Anaerobic bacteria, 287
Anaphylatoxins, 167, 193
Anapsids, 256
Ancylostoma
caninum, 363
ceylonicum, 362
duodenale, 362
Angry macrophages, 158–159
Animal diseases, 436
Anthrax, 312
vaccine for, 62
Anthropophilic dermatophytes, 380
Anti-BSA antibodies, 193
Antibiotic resistant disease, 446
Antibiotics
interfering with mRNA transcription, 293
mode of action of, 290–291
protection from, 271–272
resistance to, 284, 444–445
Antibody, 351. *See also* Monoclonal
antibody; Polyclonal antibody
ability to interact with epitope,
111–112
agglutinating, 162
antigen binding of, 89–91
to antigen fragments, 94
antigen recognition of, 91–93
antimicrobial actions of, 162*t*
antiviral effect of, 328–329
B cell production of, 105
B cell receptor binding of, 113, 114*f*
binding sites of, variable regions of,
111*f*
cell-bound, 105
circulation of, 105–106
clonal selection theory of, 66–69
in complement system activation, 53
degradation of, 8
detection of, 119–127
ELISA in, 421–422
discovery of, 64

diversity of, 114–116
evasion of destructive effects of, 8
in fish, 254
formation of
    instructional model for, 69*f*
    in response to vaccination, 398
    side chain theory of, 64–65
four-chain plan of, 109*f*
fragment structures in, 113*f*
generation of, 85
hapten reaction with, 92*f*
humoral, 105
in immune response, 6, 66
    affinity and class changes of
    during, 116–118
immunoglobulin classes and,
118–119
light chains of, 79*f*
measurement of, 75
molecules of, 75*f*
monoclonal, 75–77
nature of, 106–107
in opsonization, 36
secondary and primary, 121
secretion of, 157
specificity of, 68–69, 90–91
structure and behavior of, 74–75
structure of, 107–113
Th2 and B cells in production of, 150
toxin inactivation by, 159–161
variable regions of chains of, 110–111
Antibody-coated latex beads, 428
    in lateral flow immunoassay, 428
    in vertical flow-through immuno-
    assay, 428–431
Antibody-coated microbes, 158–159
Antibody-dependent cell-mediated
    cytotoxicity, 174, 175
    IgG antibody and, 175*f*
    in immune response to Marek's
    disease, 235
Antibody gene structure, 78
Antibody-mediated effector mecha-
    nisms, 158–162
Antibody-producing lymphocytes,
134–135
Antibody-sandwich enzyme-linked
    immunosorbent assay, 421, 422, 423*f*

Antibody-secreting B cells, immortaliz-
    ing of, 119–120
Antibody tests, 388–389
Antigen, 101–102
    adjuvants, 101
    antibody-recognized sites on, 91–95
    B cell binding, 151*f*
    binding sites of, mapping epitopes
    and, 94–95
    binding specificity of in vaccination,
    6–7
    binding strength of, 95–97
    characteristics of, 86–89
    complex, 97
    conformational sites of, 91
    cross-reactivity of, 97–99
    definition of, 85–86
    detection methods for, 127
    extracellular, 71*f*
    gene programming for, 406–407
    hapten-carrier concept and, 89–91
    histocompatibility, 71
    in immune system activation,
    145–153
    measurement of, 75
    nonself, 157
    phagocytized, 146*f*
    processing and presentation of, 136,
    145–146
    response to, 69–70
    routes of administration of, 100–101
    surface, 134
    synthetic, 407
    T cell recognition of, 73*f*
Antigen-antibody complex
    formation of, 85
    free antibody equilibrium with,
    96–97
    gel, 415
Antigen-antibody reactions
    probing of, 94–95
    specificity of, 90–91
Antigen capture assays, 127
Antigen II, 71
Antigen presenting cells, 82, 134–135,
    136
    in allograft reaction, 209–210
    MHC protein on, 93

superantigens and, 280
T cells and, 69–70, 100, 146–147, 148f
types of, 145
Antigen receptor, fish, 252
Antigen-specific receptors
in immune response, 6
in lymphocytes, 5–6
production of, 139–142
Antigenic determinant, 86
Antigenic drift, 337, 396
Antigenic epitopes, 5–6
Antigenic molecules, conformational
and sequential epitopes on, 93f
Antigenic polymorphism, in active
immunization, 395–396
Antigenic shift, 337
Antigenic variation, 444
Antihistamines, 190
Antilymphocyte globulin, 217
Antimicrobial activity, immune serum,
63–64
Antimicrobial peptides, 5
Antimicrobial resistance, 457
Antimicrobial substances
in barrier immunity, 3
secretion of, 27
Antiphagocytic components, 36
Antiphagocytic surface structures, 270–
272
Antiserum
antigen mixture with, 413
labeled, 331
polyclonal, 119
in viral diagnosis, 330
Antitoxin, 313–314
Antiviral drugs, 329
Anurans, 254
immune response in, 256
immunoglobulins in, 255
Apoptosis, 153, 177, 223
Arachidonic acid
in inflammatory response, 56–57
metabolites of, 49f
Archaebacteria, 298
Archosaurs, 256
Arenaviridae, 323t
Armed effector cell, 153
Aromatic ring, 91

Arthroconidia, 381f
of coccidioidomycosis, 385
Arthropods
infestation of, 17
prophenoloxidase system of, 249
in zoonotic disease, 299
Arthus reaction, 193–194
Arylsulfatase, 34
Ascaridid worms, 361–362
Ascaris
lumbricoides, 361–362
pneumonitis, 362
Aspartyl proteinase, Candida, 388
Aspergillosis, 386–387
Aspergillus, 380, 386–387
binding to host cell receptors, 269
Association constant, 97
Athlete's foot, 381
Atopic reagin, 185
Attenuated microorganisms, 62
Attenuated vaccines, 332, 396, 404, 405
polio, 335
Aureomycin, 293
Autocrine factors, 147
Autocrine hormone, 170
Autografts, 202
Autoimmune disease, 68, 88, 181–182
organ-specific, 183
pathogenesis of, 182–184
in rheumatic fever, 99
systemic, 183
types of, 182t
Autoimmunity, 88
Avian influenza virus, 337
Azathioprine, 217, 218
Azidothymidine, 329
Azurophilic granules, 33

B7-bearing cells, 153
B cell receptors
immunoglobulin structure of, 113
minigene segments of, 140t
sequential and conformational
epitopes and, 93
structure of, 114f
B cells
antibody production by, 105, 127–128
antibody synthesis by, 66, 67f

antigen and, 81
antigen binding to, 146, 151*f*
antigen-independent development of, 143*f*
antigen-independent differentiation of, 142
antigen presenting, 145
in birds, 258
clonal expansion of, 116–117
in clonal selection theory, 106*f*
clones of
    antigen selection of, 68*f*
    in immune reaction, 75–76
development of, 138–139
electron micrographs of, 132–133*f*
function and surface markers of, 134*t*
in germinal centers, 137
immature stage of, 142
in immune response, 6, 10, 131, 134–135, 137, 398
inactive, 117
lytic infection of, 233*f*
mature, 142
memory, 117–118
Th2 cell activation of, 147–149
Th2 cells interaction with, 150
Baceroides, intestinal, 21
Bacilli, 285
Bacillus
    anthracis, 312
        characteristics of, 315*t*
    anthraxis, 22
    endospores of, 296
Bacillus Calmette-Guerin, 174
Bacteria, 283–284, 314–317, 445
    antigens inducing immunity in, 395*f*
    cultivation of, 22–23
    disease-causing, characteristics of, 315–317*t*
    encapsulated, 313
    endotoxins of, invertebate protection against, 248–249
    intestinal, 29–30
    lysis of, 418
    mechanism of immunity and resistance to, 312–314
    medically important, 298–312
    nonencapsulated, 312–313
    nutrition, metabolism, and growth of, 286–288
    opsonized, binding of to phagocyte receptors, 35*f*
    oxygen relationships of, 287–288
    parasitic, 13, 14*f*, 17
    pathogenicity and virulence of, 265–266
    preventing attachment to host cells, 161
    prokaryotic cell structure of, 288–296
    shape and grouping of, 285–286
    siderophores of, 277
    size and distribution of, 284–285
    of skin, 20
    structural components of, 288*f*
    superantigenic toxins of, 100
    taxonomy and phylogenetic relationships of, 296–298
    true, 298
    ubiquity of, 284–285
Bacterial infections
    extracellular, 312–313
    intracellular, 314
    reemerging, 283–284, 314
    toxigenic, 313–314
Bacteriocins, 29–30, 292
Bacteriolysis, 162
Bacterionema, 21
Bacteroides
    characteristics of, 315*t*
    melaninogenicoccus, periodontal, 301
    of mouth, 21
BAGE, 241
Band cells, 30
Band of identity, 122
Band of partial identity, 122
Barrier immunity, 3, 10
Basophils
    function of, 34
    Giemsa stained, 33
    hypersensitivity mediators released by, 188–189
    IgE binding to, 119
    IgE-mediated activation of, 187–188
    in immediate hypersensitivity reaction, 187
Beef tapeworm, 370–372

Beta 1 integrins, 269–270
Binding assays, 125–127
Binomial nomenclature, 297
Biodegradability, 88–89
Biological assays, 127
Biological transmission, 452–453
Biooxidations, 286–287
Biotin, microbes synthesizing, 22
Birds
    immunity in, 258–260
    lymphoid organs of, 2t
Blackwater fever, 88
Blastoconidia, 268, 383, 384f
Blastomyces dermatiditis, 380, 384–385
    blastoconidia of, 268, 384f
Blastomycosis, 384–385
Blinking, in host defense, 30
Blood
    antibody circulation in, 105–106
    cells in inflamed area, 54–55
    components of, 106
    proteins of, 51–54
    serum of, antimicrobial activity in,
        63–64
Blood-borne infectious organisms,
    precautions against, 9
Blood flukes, 366–368
    life cycle of, 367f
Blood groups, 87
    antibodies of, 90
    matching, 216
Blood-inhabiting protozoa, 354–356
Blood transfusion, in allograft survival,
    217–218
Bone marrow
    development of, 138
    hematopoietic stem cells in, 114
Bone marrow transplantation, 219
Bordetella pertussis, 301
    binding to host cell receptors, 268
    fimbriae of, 266
Borrelia burgdorferi, 311
Botulism, 160, 305–306
    Clostridium botulinum toxin in, 23–24
    immunization against, 160
    polluted water and, 309
Bovine papilloma virus, 338
Bovine serum albumin, 193, 249
Bradykinin

in inflammatory response, 47, 50f
    mediating inflammation, 52
    source of, 51t
    with tissue damage, 201
Bronchial asthma, 185
Bronchitis, 304
Brucella, 311–312
Brucellosis, 311–312
Brugia
    malayi, 364
    timori, 364
BSA. See Bovine serum albumin
Bubonic plague epidemic, 436
Bunyaviridae, 323t
Burkitt's lymphoma, 342
Bursa of Fabricius, 134
    in birds, 258
Burst-forming unit erythrocytes, 139
Bystander effect, 166

C1 complement, 36
C3 convertase, 164–165
C5 convertase, 164–165
C1 Fc receptors, 164
C genes, 78, 263
c-myc genes, 227
c-onc genes, 227
C-reactive protein
    in inflammatory reaction, 56
    in opsonization, 36
C5a, 34
Ca²⁺-calmodulin complexes, 188
Cachexin, 314
Caliciviridae, 323t
Camel immunoglobulins, 261
Cancer
    aspergillosis in, 387
    cell proliferation in, 82
Candida, 380
    albicans, 14f, 387
        intestinal, 21
        vaginal, 309
Candidiasis, 387–388
Capsids, 319–320
Capsomeres, 320
Capsular polysaccharide vaccines, 405
Capsules, 270–271
    interfering with phagocytosis, 294–
        295

polysaccharide, 272
of prokaryotic cells, 293–295
Carbohydrate-fermenting bacteria,
genitourinary, 22
Carbohydrates
in immune response, 85–86
immunogens, 102
Carbon bonds, 40
Carcinogens, 227
Carriers, 448
Caseous necrosis, 197
Catalase
function of, 34
in phagocytosis, 159
in respiratory burst, 39*f*
Cathepsin G
in azurophilic granules, 33
substrates of, 34
Cathepsins, 34
Cationic antimicrobial proteins, 33
Cationic peptides, bactericidal, 275
C3b complement
activation of, 37*f*
in opsonization, 36
C3b receptors, 161
CD95, activation of, 230–231
CD2 expression, 142
CD40 ligand
expression of in graft rejection, 211–
212
inflammatory T cell expression of,
172
CD marker proteins, 169
CD4+ T cells, 169
antiviral effect of, 328
CD8+ T cells, 169
antiviral effect of, 327–328
CDRs. *See* Complementarity determining regions
Ceftriaxone, 311
Cell-bound antibodies, 105–106
Cell envelope, prokaryote, 289–291
Cell-mediated effector mechanisms,
168–169
antibody-dependent cell cytotoxicity
in, 175
cytolytic T lymphocytes in, 176–177
delayed-type hypersensitivity in,
169–171

macrophage activation in, 169, 171–
174
MHC restriction of cytolytic T cells
in, 177
microbiocidal activity in, 171–174
natural killer cells in, 174–175
tumoricidal activity in, 174
Cell-mediated immunity, 62
in delayed hypersensitivity, 194–197
to feline leukemia, 237–238
in invertebrates, 250–251
with live vaccines, 404
to Marek's disease, 234
outcome of responses in, 63*t*
to parasites, 351
proteins stimulating, 85–86
theories of, 65–66
tumors and, 223–224
Cell membrane fusion, 325
Cells
cycle of, 223
lysis of, 125
specialization of, 66
Cellular immunology, 62–63
major discoveries in, 63*t*
Cephalosporin, 290
Cercariae, 366, 368
Cerebrospinal fluid analysis, 388
Cestodes, 368–372
parasitic, 368–372, 373*f*
CFA. *See* Complete Freund's Adjuvant
Chagas' disease, 14–15*f*
transmission of, 453, 454*f*
Chemical equilibrium, 96
Chemokines
in delayed hypersensitivity, 196
receptors for, 345
Chemoluminescence, 38
Chemotactic factors
in complement activity, 167
host-derived, 34
in hypersensitivity reaction, 190
Chemotaxis, 34
Chicken cholera vaccine, 62
Chlamydia, 445
Chlamydia trachomatis, 300
Chloramphenicol, 293
Chloromycetin, 293
Cholera, 308, 445–446

Cholera vaccine
  inactivated, 404–405
  target groups for, 401*t*
Chromium-51 release assay, 214
Chromogenic immunoblot technique, 428
Ciliated cells, 29
Circumsporozoite protein, 359
Climatic factors, 449–450
Clonal selection theory, 66–69, 77–78, 106*f*
Clostridium
  botulinum
    immunization against, 160
    toxins of, 23–24, 306
    in water supplies, 309
  endospores of, 296
  exotoxins of, 279
  in gas gangrene, 298–299
  perfringens, toxins of, 306
  tetani
    antitoxin injection of, 417
    immunization against, 313
Clotting
  cascade
    with hyperacute graft rejection, 203
    in inflammation mediation, 51–52
  factors
    attracting phagocytes, 34
    in homeostasis, 53–54
  in inflammatory response, 50*f*
  with tissue damage, 201
Cluster of differentiation, 169
CMI response
  in cryptococcosis, 386
  in mycosis infection, 383, 385
Coagulase, 160
  production of, 21
Cocci, 285
Coccidians, intestinal, 354
Coccidioides immitis, 279, 380
Coccidioidomycosis, 385
  transmission of, 454
Coelenterates, 247
Coelomates, 247
Coelomocytes, 249
Cold-adaptation, 405
Colicins, 292

Collagen
  in Hageman factor activation, 52*f*
  in inflammation mediation, 51
Collagenase, 279
  in azurophilic granules, 33
Colloidal particle size, 284–285
Colonization, 446–448
Colony-stimulating factors, 81, 139. *See also* Granulocyte-macrophage colony-stimulating factor
  in inflammatory reaction, 56
Colostrum
  absorption of, 262
  IgA in, 119
  IgG antibodies in, 7
  immunoglobulins in, 261–262
  secretory, 119
Combinational diversity, 142
Commensal relationship, 16
Commensals, 18
Communicable diseases
  burden of, 441–442, 443*f*
  worldwide death rates from, 442–443
Competitive binding procedures, 418–419
Competitive exclusion, 19
Complement
  activation of
    in bacterial infection resistance, 313
    against coccidioidomycosis, 385
    against cryptococcosis, 386
    in response to vaccination, 398
  alternative pathway of, 163*f*
  attracting phagocytes, 34
  biological activities of components of, 164*t*
  cascade, 112
    activation of, 51, 53
    in classical pathway, 164–166
    initiation of, 36
  in cell lysis, 125
  classical pathway of, 163*f*, 191
  components of
    biological activities of, 167–168
    enzymatic cleavage of, 164–166
  discovery of, 64
  in fish, 253

fixation, 164, 417–418
  outcome of, 63t
  in immune response, 5
  regulation of, 168
Complement-mediated effector
  mechanisms, 162–164
  alternative pathway of, 166
  biological activities in, 167–168
  classical pathway of, 164–166
  regulation of, 168
Complement-mediated lysis, 125
  of Gram-negative bacilli, 162
Complement system
  activation pathways of, 52–53
  in inflammation mediation, 51–54
  inflammatory mediators produced
  by, 51t
  in opsonization, 36
  pathways activating, 37f
  with tissue damage, 201
Complementarity determining regions,
  111
Complete Freund's Adjuvant, 403–404
Complexity, 89
Concanavalin A, 252
Congenic mice, 71
  alleles in, 73–74
  production of, 73f
Conidia, germination of, 381
Conidiophores, 383
Conjunctiva, 30
Conjunctivitis, 300
Connective tissue, mast cells of,
  186–187
Constant regions, 112
Constitutive host resistance
  external defense systems in, 27–30
  internal defense systems in, 30–41
Constitutive immune response, 3–5,
  10
Contamination, 446–448
Control programs, 436, 454–456, 457
Coronaviridae, 323t
Corticosteroids, 190
  graft survival and, 217
Corynebacterium
  attenuated strains of, 63–64
  diphtheriae, 301–302
    in healthy humans, 23

host defense against, 314
  of skin, 20
Coughing, 29
Cowpox virus, 61
  immunization against, 332
  in smallpox vaccine, 393–394, 396
Cross-linking, 91, 121
Cross-reactivity
  of antigens, 97–99, 102
  concept of, 61
Cryptococcal capsule, 386
Cryptococcosis, 385–386
Cryptococcus neoformans, 385–386
  capsules of, 272, 273f
Cryptosporidia, 446
Cryptosporidiosis, 354
  transmission of, 451
Cryptosporidium parvum, 354
Cultures, fungal, 389
CXCR-4, 345
Cyclooxygenase pathway, 190
Cyclospora cayetanensis, 354
Cyclosporine A
  for acute rejection, 204
  in clinical transplantation studies,
  216
  in graft survival, 217
Cyclostomes, complement system, 253
Cystic fibrosis, 303–304
Cystitis, 309
Cytokine promoter region polymorphism, 212–213
Cytokines
  in allograft rejection, 208–209
  binding of, 79
  in delayed hypersensitivity, 196
  in graft rejection, 211
  in hypersensitivity reaction, 189–190
  immune induction of, 78–81
  in immune response, 6, 82
    to Marek's disease, 234
  inflammatory T cell secretion of,
  172–173
  mast cell release of, 186
  mimicking of, 8
  natural killer cells and, 174
  receptors for, 139
  T lymphocyte production of, 212
  Th1 cell production of, 147

Th2 cell production of, 149
in tumor immunity, 230–231, 241
types of, 80–81
Cytolytic exotoxin, 276–277
Cytolytic T cells
in cell-mediated immunity, 168, 176–177
generated in mixed lymphocyte cultures, 215*f*
Cytoplasm
of prokaryotes, 291–292
viral proteins produced in, 152*f*
Cytotoxic hypersensitivity, 190–192
Cytotoxic lymphocytes, 314
Cytotoxic response, 63*t*
Cytotoxic T cells, 169
activation of, 150–153, 176–177
antigen-specific, 230–231
antiviral effect of, 327–328
differentiation of, 176*f*, 178
function and surface markers of, 134*t*
generation and detection of, 213–214
in hepatitis B virus immunity, 240
in immune response, 82
to Marek's disease, 234–235
to parasites, 350–351
proliferation of, 176*f*
role of, 135
tumors and, 223–224
Cytotoxins
antiphagocytic, 272–274
in aspergillosis pathogenesis, 387

D gene segment
in birds, 259
coding for B and T cells, 140
random selection of, 142
DAF. *See* Decay-accelerating factor
Data
analysis of, 441
collation of, 441
collection of, 440–441, 457
Decay-accelerating factor, 168
Decision-making, 441
Defense reactions, classification of, 63*t*
Defense systems
external, 27–30
internal, 27, 30–41
Defensins, 5, 275

in oxygen-independent killing, 40–41
Delayed type hypersensitivity, 169–171, 194–197
in bacterial resistance, 314
hallmark of, 170–171
in reptiles, 257
Delayed type hypersensitivity skin test
for coccidioidomycosis, 385
for cryptococcosis, 386
for histoplasmosis, 383
Dendritic cells, 145
in immune response, 137
interdigitating, 145–146
Dengue, 445–446
prevention of, 455
Dental caries, 300–301
Dental plaque, 21
Dermatitis, allergic contact, 194–195, 196*f*
Dermatomycoses, 17
Dermatophytosis, 380–381
Desensitization, 190
Deuterostomes, 247
Diabetes
autoimmune pathogenesis of, 182*t*
juvenile-onset, 88
Diagnostic tests
for fungal infections, 388–389
immunological, 413–433
Diarrhea
bloody, 351–353
burden of, 441–442
enterobacterial, 306–307
Escherichia coli in, 307
microbes causing, 18
organisms causing, 24
parasites causing, 14–15*f*
pathogens causing, 299
Shigella in, 307
transmission of, 451
Diazotization, 90*f*
Diethylcarbamazine, 366
Digestive tract
in constitutive host resistance, 28*f*, 29–30
normal microorganisms of, 20*f*, 21–22
Dinitrophenol, 94

Dinosaurs, immunity in, 258–260
Diphtheria
  cases of before and after vaccine for, 394*t*
  endotoxins in, 301–302
  immunization against, 160
  toxin of, 64, 279–280
  toxoid, 280
  vaccine for, 63–64
Diphtheroids, skin, 20–21
Diphyllobothrium latum, 372
Diplobacilli, 285
Diplococci, 285
Dipstick ELISA assay format, 426–427
Direct binding assays, 121
Disability-adjusted life years (DALYs), 441–442
Disease
  burden of, 441–442
  causes of, 435
  chain of events in, 444
  control of, 454–456
  host selection by, 8–9
  prevalence of, 437
  terminology of, 436–437
Disease vectors, 283–284
Disinfection, 455
Dissemination, disease, 448–449
Distemper virus, 17
Disulfide bonds, 107–108
  inter-heavy chain, 112–113
Disulfide bridges, 118
DJ rearrangement, 140
DNA
  coding for antibody diversity, 114–116
  disruption of, 325
  of prokaryotes, 291–293
  rearrangement, 114
    producing antibody molecules and T cell receptors, 141*f*
  recombination, antibody diversity by, 115–116
  sequences of, 78
DNA gene segments, 140–142
DNA hybridization, 331
DNA viruses
  classification and properties of, 322*t*
  in hepatitis B, 340

  nucleic acids of, 325
  oncogenic, 227–228
  replication of, 333
DNP. *See* Dinitrophenol
DNP-specific antigen binding sites, 94–95
Donor-specific blood transfusions, 217–218
Double diffusion, 122, 123*f*
Double-immunodiffusion assay, 414, 415*f*, 433
Doxycillin, 311
DPT vaccine, 301
DV gene segments, 259
Dynamic equilibrium, 96
Dysentery, amoebic, 351–353

E-cadherin, 269
E-selectin, 190
Ebola virus, 445, 446
Echinococcus granulosus, 372, 373*f*
Echinoderms
  cell-mediated immunity in, 250
  humoral immunity in, 250
Effector cells, 328
Effector mechanisms, 157–178
  antibody-mediated, 158–162
  cell-mediated, 168–176
  complement-mediated, 162–168
Ehrlich, Paul, 64–66, 181
Elastase, 33
Electron cloud bonding, 413
Electron microscopy, 330–331
Electron transport pathway, 287
Electrostatic attraction, 413
Elephantiasis, 364, 365
ELISA. *See* Enzyme-linked immunosorbent assays
Emerging diseases, 8–9, 283–284, 314, 445–446, 457
  geographical distribution of, 447*t*
Encapsulation, 270–271
Endocarditis, 301
Endocytosis, *Listeria monocytogenes*, 269
Endoplasmic reticulum, peptide transport into, 230
Endospores, 295
Endotoxins, 277–278
  antibody inactivation of, 159–161

invertebate protection against, 248–249

Engulfment, 63*t*

Entamoeba histolytica, 14*f*, 351–353
cyst of, 352*f*
mucosal ulcer caused by, 353*f*

Enteritis, 306

Enterobacteria
characteristics of, 315–316*t*
in diarrhea, 306–307

Enterochelin, 277

Enterotoxins, 280
in food poisoning, 306
pathogenicity of, 265–266
superantigenic, 100

Environment, 440, 444, 448–450

Enzyme immunoassay, 421

Enzyme-linked immunosorbent assay, 125–127, 330, 420–421, 433
competitive, 423–425
direct, 422
formats in, 425–428
indirect, 421–422

Enzymes, neutrophil and eosinophil, 33

Eosinophil chemotactic factor, 190

Eosinophil-colony forming cells, 139

Eosinophils
defensive role of, 34
Giemsa stained, 31*f*, 33

Epidemic wave, 438*f*

Epidemics, 436, 437–438
bacterial disease, 308–309

Epidemiological investigation, 437–440

Epidemiological surveillance, 440–441

Epidemiology, 435, 456–457
analytical, 435–436
descriptive, 435
experimental, 436

Epidermophyton, 380

Epinephrine, 190

Episomes, prokaryote, 292

Epithelial cell carcinoma, 341–342

Epitopes, 66, 67
in active immunization, 394–395
antibody interaction with, 111–112
B cell receptors complementary to, 105
conformational, 93*f*, 94

G cell receptor induction and, 93
mapping of, 94–95
monoclonal antibodies directed against, 95*f*
protection-inducing, 407
sequential, 93*f*
shared, 97–98
similarity of, 98–99
T cell, 145

Epizootiology, 436

Epstein-Barr virus, 232, 342
host cell receptors for, 268

Equilibrium constant, 96–97

Equivalence, zone of, 121

Ergosterol synthesis, 389

Erythroblastosis fetalis, 191–192

Erythrocytes, immune complexes on, 168

Erythromycin
interfering with mRNA transcription, 293
for *Legionella* infections, 303
for Lyme disease, 311

Escherichia
coli
adherence to host cells, 266–268
enterotoxigenic, 265–266, 268–269
enterotoxigenic, enteroaggregative, enterohemorrhagic, and enteroinvasive, 307
fimbriae of, 267*f*
growth rate of, 287
hemolysin of, 277
in urinary tract infections, 309
coli K12, 406
coli O157:H7, 446
intestinal, 21

Eubacteria, 298

Eucarya, 298

Eukaryotes, 298
versus prokaryotic cells, 288*t*

Evolution, pathogen, 7–8

Exoskeleton, 248

Exotoxin A, 273

Exotoxins, 159–161, 278–280
antiphagocytic, 272–274
microbial, 161*f*

Expanded Program of Immunization, WHO-sponsored, 408–409
Eyes
    bacterial infections of, 300
    in constitutive host resistance, 28f, 30

Fab fragments, 112–113
Facultative anaerobes, 287
Facultative parasites, 18
Famine, 449
Fas-associated death-domain-like IL-1β-converting enzyme (FLICE), 231
Fas (CD95), 230–231
Fc fragments, 112–113
Fc receptors
    in phagocytosis, 158
    toxin binding to, 160
FcεRI-mediated degranulation, 187–188
Fecal contamination, 449
Feces, bacteria of, 21
Feline immunodeficiency virus, 236
Feline leukemia virus, 225–226, 236, 242
    immunity to, 237–238
    pathogenesis of, 236–237
    resistance to, 237
    vaccines for, 238
FeLV. *See* Feline leukemia virus
Fenton reaction, 38
Fermentation, 287
Fever
    in inflammatory reaction, 55–56
    macrophages in, 46
Fibrillae, 267f, 271
Fibrin
    barrier of, 54
    degradation of, 52
    in inflammatory response, 50f
Fibrinolytic system
    attracting phagocytes, 34
    in homeostasis, 53–54
    in inflammation mediation, 51
    with tissue damage, 201
Fibrinopeptides, 51t
Fibronectin, 36
    activation of, 41
    host cell receptors for, 269–270
Filarial worms, 363–364

Filariasis, lymphatic, 363–365
Filoviridae, 322t
Fimbriae, 266, 267f, 268
    antigens of, 161
    of prokaryotic cells, 294–295
Fimbrial adhesin, 267f
Fish
    adaptive immune system of, 262–263
    immunity in, 251–254
    lymphoid organs of, 2t
Fish tapeworm, 372
FIV. *See* Feline immunodeficiency virus
FK506, 217
Flagelin, 295
Flagella, 267f
    of prokaryotic cells, 294
Flagellates, 350
    intestinal, 353–354
Flavine adenosine dinucleotide, 287
Flaviviridae, 323t
Flavoprotein, 287
FLICE inhibitor proteins (FLIPs), 231
Flooding, 450
Floods, 449–450
Fluconazole, 389
Flucytosine, 389
Flukes, 350, 366–368
Fluorescein isothiocyanate assay, 419–420
Fluorescent assay, 419–420
FOCMA (feline oncornavirus-associated cell membrane antigen), 237, 238
Folic acid, microbe synthesis of, 22
Follicles, 137
Fomites, 450
Food-borne disease, 451
Food handling, 9
Food poisoning, 160
    bacterial toxins in, 299, 305–306
    prevention of, 315
Foreign tissue, rejection of, 201–202
Foreignness, 86–88
Forssman reaction, 97
Framework regions, 110
Free fatty acids, 28
Free oxygen radicals, 251
Fucosidase, 34
Functional immune systems, 10

Fungal disease
  adhesins in, 268
  classification of, 379–388
  diagnosis of, 388–389
  therapy for, 389
Fungal pathogens, 379–389
  parasitic, 14f
  pathogenicity and virulence of,
    265–266
Fungus, 298, 445
  in nature, 379
Fusagen, 77
Fusin, 345
Fusobacterium
  characteristics of, 316t
  of mouth, 21

Galactomannan, 382
Galactosamine, 87
Galactosidase, 34
GALT. *See* Gut associated lymphoid
  tissue
Gamma-globulin, 106, 107f, 397. *See
  also* Antibody
Gammaherpesvirus, 225t, 232
Gas exchange, lung, 28–29
Gas gangrene, 160
  bacteria causing, 298–299
  collagenase and, 279
Gastrointestinal tract infections
  bacteria causing, 305–309
  pathogens causing, 299
  viral pathogens in, 324t
Gel matrix precipitation, 414–416
Gene recombination, 77–78, 79f
  natural selection and, 158
Genetic immunization, 407–408
Genitourinary tract
  in constitutive host resistance, 28f
  normal microorganisms of, 22
Genotypes, immune response, 99
Geophilic dermatophytes, 380
Germinal centers, 116–117, 137
Giant cell granulomatous inflammation, 197
Giardia
  intestinalis, 14–15f
  lamblia, 353
    transmission of, 451
  life cycle of, 452f

Giemsa stained blood films, 31f
Gingivitis, 301
Glandular secretions, 28
Globulins, 74
  alpha and beta, 106, 107f
  preparations for passive immuniza-
    tion, 397t
Glomerulonephritis, 183
Glucose-6-phosphate dehydrogenase
  deficiency, 358
Glucouronoxylomannan capsule, 386
Glucuronidase, 34
Glycerophosphatase, 34
Glycocalyx envelope, 271, 272f
  of prokaryotic cells, 293–294
Glycoprotein envelope, rabies virus,
  334
Glycoproteins
  bacterial endotoxin and, 248–249
  groups A and B, 87
GM-CSF. *See* Granulocyte-macrophage
  colony-stimulating factor
Gomori's methanamine silver, 388
Gonorrhea, toxins in, 310
Goodpasture's syndrome
  IgG antibodies in, 192
  pathogenesis of, 182t
Gorer, Peter, 70–71
Graft-reactive antibodies, screening
  for, 215–216
Graft rejection
  acute, 203–205
  chronic, 205
  clinical strategies for avoiding,
    214–218
  forms of, 202–205
  hyperacute, 202–203
  phenomenon of, 201–202
  in reptiles, 257
Grafts
  host response to, 201–220
  immunosuppressive agents in
    survival of, 216–218
  types of, 202
Gram-negative bacteria, 289–290
  bacteriocins secreted by, 29–30
  capsules of, 294
Gram-positive bacteria, 289–290
  of skin, 20–21
Gram stain, 289–291

Granules
  of basophils, 34
  enzyme content of, 33*t*
  of neutrophils and eosinophils, 33
Granulocyte-macrophage colony-
    stimulating factor, 139
  in graft rejection, 212
  Th1 cell production of, 147
Granulocyte-monocyte colony-
    stimulating factor, 173
Granulocytes
  in fish, 251
  types of, 33
Granuloma formation, 385
Granulomatous disease, 387
Granulomatous inflammation, 197
Granulomatous reaction, chronic, 314
Granzymes, 152*f*, 153, 177
Graves' disease, 182*t*
Guillain-Barré syndrome, 400
Gut associated lymphoid tissue, 136

Haber-Weiss reaction, 38
Haemophilus
  aegypticus, 300
  influenzae
    capsules of, 294–295
    polysaccharide capsules of, 406
Hageman factor
  activation of, 52*f*
  in inflammation mediation, 51
Hair, arthroconidia on, 381*f*
Halide compounds, 38
Halogenation, microbial protein, 40
Hand washing, 9
Hantavirus, 446
  climate and, 450
Haplotypes, 74
Hapten-carrier concept, 89–91
Haptens, 86, 89, 94
  in affinity-labeling antigen, 94–95
  antibody reaction with, 92*f*
  method of attaching to carrier
    molecule, 90*f*
Hashimoto's thyroiditis
  autoimmune pathogenesis of, 182*t*
  pathogenesis of, 183
Hay fever, 185
HBcAg, 240
HBsAg, 238–239, 242

antibodies to, 240–241
  in hepatitis B viral replication,
    239*f*
  Saccharomyces cerevisiae producing,
    240
HBx, 240
Health education, 455
Health practices, 283
Health status, measuring and
    analyzing, 436–437
Heart transplantation, complicating
    factors in, 219
Heavy chains, 107–108, 110
  C region of, 112
  D segments of, 116
  DNA coding for, 114
  DNA recombination of, 116
  folding of, 110
  V segments of, 115–116
  variable regions of, 110–111
Helical viruses, 320
  morphology of, 321*f*
Helminths, 349, 361–373
  eosinophils in defense against, 34
  genera of, 350
Helper T cells. *See* T helper cells
Hemagglutination assays
  direct, 124–125
  indirect, 124*f*, 125
Hemagglutinin, 336–337, 395
Hematopoietic-inducing
    microenvironment, 139
Hemin, 277
Hemocytes, 249
Hemolysin, 273, 277
Hemolytic anemia, 182*t*
  autoimmune, 190–191
Hemolytic disease of newborn,
    191–192
Hepadnaviruses, 340
  properties of, 322*t*
  tumors associated with, 225*t*
Heparin
  in connective tissue mast cells,
    186–187
  in hypersensitivity reaction, 190
Hepatitis
  viral pathogens in, 324*t*
  viruses causing, 24
Hepatitis A virus, 339

Hepatitis B antigen, 419
  core, 240
Hepatitis B surface antigen, 340, 406
  vaccinia virus recombinants
    carrying, 407
Hepatitis B virus, 242
  acute and chronic, 339–340
  carriers of, 406
  host response to vaccination against,
    398
  immunity to, 240
  pathogenesis of, 238–240
  recombinant vaccine for, 406
  resistance to, 240
  transmission of, 339
  tumors and, 227
  tumors associated with, 225t
  vaccine against, 240–241, 396, 397,
    405
  viral DNA replication in, 239f
Hepatocellular carcinoma, 238
  hepatitis B virus and, 339–340
  immunity to, 240
  pathogenesis of, 238–240
  resistance to, 240
  vaccination against, 240–241
Herpes simplex virus, 341
  glycoprotein D, 407
  serotypes of, 341
  types I and II, 341
Herpesvirus, 320, 342
  antiviral drugs for, 329
  DNA replication of, 341–342
  intranuclear inclusions of, 325
  properties of, 322t
  recurrent, 341–342
  tumors and, 227
  tumors associated with, 225t
  of turkeys, 232
  vaccine for, 332
Heteropolysaccharides, 294
HiB, 394t
Hinge region, 112
Histamine
  in basophil granules, 34
  chemotactic for PMNs, 193
  in hypersensitivity reaction, 186,
    190
  prostaglandins and, 50

release of in inflammation, 46–47
  in vasodilation, 167
  in vessel permeability, 53
Histiocytes, 33
Histocompatibility. *See also* Major
    histocompatibility complex
  in immunology, 71–74
  system of, 87–88
  typing, 216
Histocompatibility antigens. *See also*
    Major histocompatibility antigens
  detection of, 417
  in graft rejection responses, 205–208
  in hyperacute graft rejection,
    202–203
  minor, 208
Histocompatibility genes, 70–71
  of major histocompatibility complex,
    205f
  reassortment of, 207f
Histocytes, 145
Histoplasma capsulatum, 380, 382–384
Histoplasmosis, 382–384
  therapy for, 383
  transmission of, 383–384
HIV. *See* Human immunodeficiency
    virus
HIV-1 virus, 344
HIV-2 virus, 344
HLA complex. *See* Human leukocyte
    antigens
Homologous antibody preparations,
    397–398
Honk Kong flu, 337
Hookworms, 362–363
  local injury caused by, 15
Hormonal substances, 78–81
Horror autotoxicus, 88, 181
Horseshoe crab, 249–250
Host -pathogen interactions, 7–9
Host cell polymerases, 325
Host cell receptors
  adherence to, 268–269
  factors mediating adherence to,
    266–269
Host cells
  anti-viral strategies of, 327–329
  disruption of protein in, 325
  invasion of, 269–270

preventing microbe attachment to, 161

Host complement factors, 8

Host defense mechanisms, 312–314

Host factors, 440

Host-graft immunologic response, 201–220

Host immune response, 24, 446–448
  immune evasion strategies and, 7–8
  to vaccination, 398–400

Host-parasite interaction, 13–25, 24
  immunology and, 61–82
  types of, 15–18

Host range, restriction of, 24

Host resistance
  constitutive, 27–41
  effector mechanisms of, 157–178
  to viral infections, 327f

Host specificity, 17, 444
  of parasites, 17

HTLV-1-associated myelopathy, 344

HTLV-1 provirus, 343

Human immunodeficiency virus, 236
  in AIDS, 344–346
  antiviral drugs for, 329
  incubation period of, 345
  with *Mycobacterium tuberculosis*, 304–305
  replication of, 346
  transmission of, 435

Human leukocyte antigens, 71, 87, 205–206
  alloantibodies and, 218
  haplotypes, 206–207
  matching, 208, 216

Humanized animal tissues, 9

Humoral antibodies, 105

Humoral immunity, 62, 64
  B cell activation in, 100
  in invertebrates, 249–250
  major discoveries of, 64t
  outcome of responses in, 63t
  to parasites, 351
  theories of, 65–66

Hyaluronic acid, mucopolysaccharide, 279

Hyaluronidase, 279

Hybridization tests, 331

Hybridomas, 77, 431

antibody molecules produced by, 119–121

Hydatid cyst, 372

Hydrogen bonding, 5–6, 413

Hydrogen bonds, 95–96

Hydrogen-deuterium exchange technique, 95

Hydrogen peroxide
  in phagocytosis, 159
  in respiratory burst, 38, 39f

Hydrolytic enzymes, 8

Hydrophobic bonds, 413
  noncovalent, 107–108

Hydrophobic interactions, 5–6, 95

Hydroxyl radicals, 38

Hyperacute rejection, 214–215

Hypersensitivity, 198. *See also* Allergy;
  Delayed type hypersensitivity
  immediate, 184–190
    mediators of, 188–189
  preformed and newly formed mediators of, 188–189
  to tuberculin, 63
  type I, 184–190
  type II, 190–192
  type III, 192–194
  type IV, 194–197
  types and mechanisms of, 185t

Hypersensitivity reactions
  mechanisms mediating, 182–183
  to vaccine, 400–401

Hypervariable regions, 110

Hypobromite, 38

Hypochlorite, 38

Hypohalites, 38

Hypoiodite, 38

Hypoxanthine, 432f

ICAM-1, at inflamed site, 55

Icosahedral viruses, 319–320, 321f
  naked, 338

IcsA, 277

Idiotypic region, 111

IFA. *See* Immunofluorescence assays

Ig-superfamily domains, 110

IgA, 128
  in amphibians, 255
  in colostrum, 261–262
  functions of, 118–119

protease cleavage of, 279
secretory, in bacterial infection
  resistance, 313
transcytosis of, 120*f*
IgA antibody
  bacteriolytic, 162
  in immune response, 117
  pathogen-reactive, 3
  preventing parasite attachment to
    host cell, 161
IgE, 128, 185
  in immediate hypersensitivity
    reaction, 185–186
  in mast cell and basophil activation,
    187–188
IgE antibodies, 117
IgG
  in amphibians, 255
  B cell production of, 117
  in colostrum, 261–262
  DNP-specific antigen binding sites
    of, 94–95
  functions of, 118
IgG antibody, 7, 128
  antiviral, 161
  bacteriolytic, 162
  in fish, 254
  in hypersensitivity, 198
  in opsonization, 158
  in phagocytosis, 159
  in response to vaccination, 398
  in type II hypersensitivity, 190–192
IgG autoantibodies, 184
IgM
  in amphibians, 255, 256
  antibody secretion of, 116
  in fish, 252
  functions of, 118
IgM antibody
  bacteriolytic, 162
  in response to vaccination, 398
  in type II hypersensitivity, 190–192
IgM autoantibodies, 184
IgY antibody
  in amphibians, 255
  in fish, 253, 254
Immune adherence, 167–168
Immune complex
  in classical complement pathway,
    162, 164

cleared from erythrocytes, 168
clearing from circulation, 167
complement binding to, 165
diseases of, 192–194
in type III hypersensitivity, 193*f*
Immune effectors, 208–209
Immune evasion strategies, 7–8
Immune mediators, 4*f*
Immune response
  adaptive, 5–6
  affinity and antibody class changes
    during, 116–119
  in amphibians, 256
  in birds, 259
  escape of tumor cells from, 229–231
  genetics of, 77–78
  lymphoid organs and, 2*t*
  nonspecific, 80
  to parasites, 350–351
  in reptiles, 257
  to *Trypanosoma cruzi*, 356
  vaccine-induced, 242
Immune response genes, 99
Immune serum
  antibody specificity in, 97
  globulin of, 397
Immune system, 1–3
  adaptive, 5–6
  anatomy of, 137*f*
  anti-viral strategies of, 327–329
  antigen activation of, 145–154
  components of, 136–137
  constitutive, 3–5
  cross-reactivity of, 61
  development of, 138–145
  failure of, 8
  in graft rejection, 201–202
  major components of, 136–137
  neoplasia and, 223–242
  passive, 7
  primitive, 2
  in survival, 2–3
  tumors and, 223–224
  vaccination and, 6–7
Immunity
  in amphibians, 254–256
  to bacterial infections, 312–314
  in birds, 258–260
  cellular theory of, 62
  to feline leukemia virus, 238

in fish, 251–254
to hepatitis B virus, 240
hormonal substances induced by,
78–81
humoral theory of, 64
to intestinal protozoa, 351
in invertebrates, 247–251
to malaria, 358–359
in mammals, 260–262
in newborn mammals, 261–262
in reptiles, 256–257
to schistosomiasis, 366–368
side chain theory of, 64–65
to toxoplasmosis, 361
to virus-induced neoplasia,
231–238
Immunization, 61–62, 393
active, 394–396
agents in, 393–394
booster, 399
challenges for, 408–409
complications of, 400–401
against exotoxin-producing
microbes, 160
genetic, 407–408
host response to, 398–400
for occupational hazards, 400
passive, 394, 396–398
principles of, 394–398
risk/benefit evaluation of, 401
routine childhood, 400
against tumors, 224
vaccine development and
production for, 401–408
against viral infections, 331–333
Immunoblot assays, 330
Immunocompetence, 88
host response to immunization and,
399
Immunoelectrophoresis, 122–124,
414–416, 433
Immunofluorescence assays, 125–127,
330
direct, 126f
Immunofluorescent antibody assay,
419–420
Immunofluorescent staining, 388
Immunogen, 86
in active immunization, 404t
Immunogenicity, 89

Immunoglobulin, 74, 106. *See also*
Antibody
in adaptive immune system, 262–263
allotypes of, 112
in amphibians, 255
of B cell receptors, 113
in birds, 259
in camels, 261
characteristics of, 108t
Fab and Fc fragments of, 112–113
in fish, 252–253
functions of, 118–119
in glomerular capillary loops, 183
isotypes of, 109–110
in monotremes and marsupials, 260
in reptiles, 257
serum levels of, 118
structure of, 107–110
subclasses of, 110
Immunoglobulin fractionation
aggregates, 397
Immunoglobulin genes
arrangements of, 263
in fish, 253
segregation of, 78
Immunologic memory, 131
Immunological tests, 413–431, 431–433
Immunologically mediated disease,
181–184, 198
Immunology
comparative, 247–263
development of, 61–82
self-recognition in, 69–74
tumor, 224–229
Immunomagnetic separation assay,
428
Immunoprecipitation tests, 413–414
Immunoreagens, 423
Immunosuppression
bacterial disease and, 314
in clinical transplantation studies,
216–218
tumors in, 232
Immunosuppressive cells, induction
of, 8
Immunosuppressive chemotherapy,
387
Immunosuppressive drugs, 3
for acute allograft rejection, 215
for acute rejection, 204, 205

in graft rejection, 220
in tumor protection, 230–231
Immunosurveillance, 228–229
Immunotherapy
for allergies, 189–190
for immediate hypersensitivity
reaction, 189–190
Impetigo, 300
Incidence rate, 437
Inclusion bodies
of variola virus, 333
viral, 325
Inclusions, prokaryote, 291–293
Indirect binding assays, 121
Inducible defense system, 4f, 5–6
antibody molecules and antigen-
antibody reactions in, 105–128
antigen activation of, 145–154
antigens in, 85–102
cells of, 131–136
components of, 136–137
development of, 138–145
in host-parasite interaction, 61–82
to Marek's disease, 234–235
nature of, 62–64
theories explaining, 64–69
Infections
versus infestation, 17
initiation of, 266
Infectious agents, 444–445
as carriers of antigen-production
genes, 406–407
routs of entry of, 448
Infectious disease, 441–444
epidemiology of, 435–436
identification of cause of, 283
poverty and, 443–444
transmission mechanisms of,
450–454
Infective dose, 444
Infestation, 17
Inflammation, 251
Inflammatory mechanisms, 4
Inflammatory mediators, 51–54
carried by basophils, 34
sources of, 51t
Inflammatory response, 3–5, 10, 45–46
acute phase reactants induced by, 56
in bacterial resistance, 314

blood cells in, 54–55
cardinal signs of, 45, 57
local inflammatory events in, 46–55
mechanisms of, 56–57
molecules participating in, 45–46
purpose of, 57
systemic consequences of, 55–57
Inflammatory T cells
antigen-specific, 171–172
clonal expansion of, 169–170
in macrophage activation, 171–174
Influenza A virus, 336–337
pandemic, 337
Influenza pandemic, 337, 436
Influenza virus
external and internal antigens of,
395
hemagglutinin of, 407
vaccine target groups, 401t
Information dissemination, 441
Inhibition assay, 121
Insect vectors, 452
Insulin, 88
Integrins, 269
Intercellular adhesion molecule-1, 190
Interdigitating dendritic cells, 145–146
Interferon, 81
antiviral effect of, 327
in bacterial resistance, 314
in immune response, 5
natural killer cells and, 174
Interferon-α
for hepatitis B virus and hepatocellular carcinoma, 240
reducing viral protein synthesis, 232
Interferon-γ
antipathogen effect of, 275
Cytotoxic T cell production of, 153
in delayed hypersensitivity, 196
in macrophage activation, 41,
172–173, 351
in phagocytosis, 158–159
reducing viral protein synthesis, 232
Th1 cell production of, 135, 147
in toxoplasmosis immunity, 361
in tumor immunity, 241
Interleukin-1
in fever response, 55
inflammatory T cells and, 169–170

Interleukin-2
  in cell-mediated immunity, 170
  in delayed hypersensitivity, 196
  in graft rejection, 211
Interleukin-3, 139
Interleukin-4, 149
Interleukin-5, 149
Interleukin-7, 139
Interleukin-10, 149
Interleukin-12, 174
Interleukin-2 receptor, 147
  cytotoxic T lymphocyte expression
    of, 176–177
Interleukins, 81
  in hypersensitivity mediation, 190
  in invertebrates, 251
  T cell reactivity to, 254
  Th1 cell production of, 147
  in tumor immunity, 241
Intermediary metabolism, 286–287
Internalin A, 269
Internalin B, 269
Interventions, 457
Intestinal amoebae, 351–353
Intestinal coccidians, 354
Intestinal flagellates, 353–354
Invasin, 269–270
  in phagosome lysis, 277
Invertebrates
  defensive processes of, 247–249
  groups of, 247
  immunity in, 247–251
  phylogeny of, 248f
Ionic bonds, 95–96
IpaB protein, 270
  in phagosome lysis, 277
Iron acquisition, 277
Iron-binding proteins, 277
Iron-chelating agent, 277
Irrigation systems, 449–450
Isoantibodies, 87
Isoantigens, 87
Isoniazid, 304–305
Isonicontinic acid hydrazide, 304–305
Isospora belli, 354
Isotype-switching, 117
Itraconazole, 389

J chain, 118

J gene segments
  in birds, 259
  coding for B and T cells, 140
  random selection of, 142
Jenner, Edward, 61, 393

K88 antigen, E. coli expression of,
    268–269
Kallikrein, 51t
Kanamycin, 293
Ketoconazole, 389
Kidney
  allograft of, 203f
  in amphibians, 255
Kinin, 52f
  attracting phagocytes, 34
  in inflammatory response, 50f, 51
  neutrophil enzyme production of, 33
Kininase, 52f
Knock-out mice, 224
Koch, Robert, 62
Koch phenomenon, 62
Koch's postulates, 22–24
Kohler, Georges, 76–77
Kupffer cells, 33

Laboratory tests, fungal, 388–389
Lactic acid, 28
Lactic acid-producing bacteria, 30
Lactobacillus, 287
  intestinal, 21
  vaginal, 22
Lactoferrin
  in neutrophil granules, 33
  in oxygen-independent killing, 40
LAF. See Lymphocyte-activating factor
Lamprey complement system, 253
Landsteiner, Karl, 63, 89–91, 98
Langerhans' cells, 33
  in delayed hypersensitivity, 195–196
  in phagocytosis, 145–146
Large intestine, bacteria in, 29–30
Large pre-B-cell, 142
Lateral flow immunoassay, 428
  single step, 429f
Latex agglutination test, 388
Latex beads, 428–431
Lattice formation, 123f, 413
Lattice structure, 121

Lecithinase, 276, 279

Legionella
  micdadei, 303
  pneumoniae, 18
  pneumophila, 303
    transmission of, 454
Legionnaires' disease, 299, 303
  transmission of, 454
Lepidosaurs, 256
Leprosy, 24
Leptospirosis, 451
Leukemia-inducing viruses, 342–344
Leukocidin, 272–273
Leukocytes
  in Giemsa stained blood films, 31*f*
  polymorphonuclear, 33
  proliferation of, 80
  in pus, 54
Leukotrienes
  formation of, 49*f*
  in hypersensitivity mediation, 186, 190
  in inflammatory response, 47–50, 57
LFA-1 adhesion molecules, 147
Life expectancy
  global data on, 442–443
  increased, 283
Light chains, 107–108
  C region of, 112, 114–115
  DNA coding for, 114
  DNA recombination of, 116
  folding of, 110
  surrogate, 142
  V segments of, 114–115
  variable regions of, 110–111
Lincomycin, 293
Linnaeus, Carolus, 297
Lipid A adjuvant, 403
Lipids
  antigenic, 102
  immune response to, 85–86
  mediators of, 190
  oxidation of, 40
Lipolytic enzymes, 5
Lipopolysaccharide complex, 278
Lipopolysaccharides
  in bacteria cell envelopes, 289–290
  endotoxic, 160–161
  fish lymphocyte response to, 252

5-Lipoxygenase pathway, 190
Listeria
  binding to host cell, 270
  characteristics of, 316–317*t*
  monocytogenes
    cytolytic exotoxin release by, 276–277
    invasion of host cells, 269
    mechanism of immunity in, 170*f*
    in urinary tract infections, 309
Listeriolysin O, 276
Live-virus vaccines, 332
Liver flukes, 14*f*
Liver transplantation rejection, 218–219
LPS. *See* Lipopolysaccharides
Lumen, mucosa of, 28–29
Lung tissue, granulomatous reaction in, 197*f*
Lyme disease, 311, 446
Lymph nodes
  enlarged, 137
  in immune system, 136
  pig, 260–261
Lymphadenopathy-associated virus, 344
Lymphatic channels, 138
Lymphatic duct system, 138
Lymphatic filariasis, 364–365
Lymphatic vessels
  in birds, 258
  in inflammatory response, 46
Lymphoblasts, 134
Lymphocyte-activating factor, 80–81
Lymphocyte antigen-specific receptors, 135–136
Lymphocyte cross-match, 215–216
Lymphocyte trafficking. *See* Gut associated lymphoid tissue
Lymphocytes. *See also* B cells; T cells
  in adaptive immunity, 5–6
  in amphibians, 255
  antibody synthesis by, 67*f*
  in birds, 258–259
  classes of, 67–68
  electron micrographs of, 132–133*f*
  in fish, 252
  in Giemsa stained blood films, 31*f*
  graft-reactive, 218
  in immune response, 66, 131–136

large granular, 174–175
memory, 6–7, 131, 196
mixed cultures of, 213
   cytolytic lymphocytes generated
   in, 215f
morphology of, 131
in organ graft rejection, 63
progenitors for, 138–139
subsets of, 134t
tumor-infiltrating, 229–231
Lymphoid disorders, 324t
Lymphoid organs
in amphibians, 254–255
in birds, 258
embryologic development of, 138
in fish, 251–252
primary, 136
in reptiles, 257
secondary, 136–137
in vertebrate classes, 2t
Lymphoid tissues, embryologic
   development of, 138
Lymphokines, 80–81
in bacterial resistance, 314
Lymphoma, malignant, 342
Lymphoreticular system tumors, 229
Lymphotoxin, 177
Lysosomes
enzyme content of, 33t
fusion of
   with phagosomes, 41, 274
   prevention of, 168
at inflamed site, 54
in mononuclear phagocytes, 34
in oxygen-independent killing,
   40–41
secondary, 159
Lysozyme
in azurophilic granules, 33
in invertebrates, 249
in neutrophil granules, 33
in saliva, 29
in tears, 30

MAC. *See* Membrane attack complex
Macroconidia, 383
Macromolecular complex, 166
Macroparasites, 350
Macrophages, 145

activation of, 154, 168, 169, 171–174,
   351
angry, 158–159
blastoconidia in, 383
in delayed hypersensitivity, 194–195,
   196
enzyme content of lysosomes in, 33t
in immune response, 5, 137
   to Marek's disease, 234
at inflamed site, 55
in inflammatory response, 46, 56
maturation of, 32–33
in oxygen-independent killing, 41
recruitment of, 57
T cell activation of, 149f
T helper cells and, 149–150
in toxoplasmosis immunity, 361
tumoricidal activity of, 174
in various tissues, 33
yeast cells in, 382f
Macropinocytosis, 270, 276
MAGE, 241
Major histocompatibility antigens, 71
in allograft rejection, 210–211
in amphibian T cell responses, 256
genetic coding of, 99
in graft rejection, 206–207
in immune response, 6
polymorphic, 73–74
restriction of, 177
Major histocompatibility complex,
   69–71, 87
in adaptive immune system, 262–263
antigens encoded by, 205–208
Class I
   cytotoxic T lymphocytes and, 177
   genes of, 241
   in tumors, 223–224, 230f
Class II, 100, 101f, 145, 146f, 151f
   cytotoxic T lymphocytes and,
   176–177
   heterodimer, 206
   inflammatory T cells and, 169, 172
genes of, 205f
   in graft rejection, 206–208
   haplotype, 206–207
protein of, 82
   antigen attachment to, 70
   antigen fragments on, 92–93, 102

class I, structure of, 72*f*
in cytotoxic T lymphocyte
restriction, 177
restriction, 69
Malaria, 22
disease burden of, 441–442
host defense against, 358–359
immunity against, 161
life cycle of, 360*f*
mosquito vector of, 456*f*
parasites causing, 356–357
rainfall and, 450
susceptibility to, 358
vaccine against, 359–360
Mammals
immunity in, 260–262
lymphoid organs of, 2*t*
Mannose binding lectin, 53
Mannosidase, 34
Marek's disease, 231–232
herpesvirus, 232, 242
oncogenicity or virulence of and
genetic resistance, 235*f*
immune responses to, 234–235
pathogenesis of, 232, 233*f*
resistance to, 232–234
vaccine for, 235–236, 332
Marsupials, 260
MART-1, 241
Mast cells
activation of, 185–186
histamine and serotonin release
by, 46
hypersensitivity mediators released
by, 188–189
IgE-mediated activation of, 187–188
in immediate hypersensitivity
reaction, 186–187
Maternal antibodies, 7
Mazzotti reactions, 366
McDevitt, Hugh, 99
MDV. *See* Marek's disease virus
Measles
cases of before and after vaccine for,
394*t*
mortality from, 409
virus of, 337–338
Megakaryocytes, 31*f*
Melanin, 274

Membrane attack complex, 6
in classical complement pathway,
166
complement protein assembly into,
167*f*
Membrane-derived lipids, 189–190
Memory B cells, 117–118
Memory cells, 6–7, 131
Memory T cells, 196
Meningococcal meningitis, 450
transmission of, 454
Meningococcus polysaccharide
capsules, 406
Meront, 356–357
Merozoites, *Plasmodium malariae*, 356–
357
Mesosomes, 293
Messenger RNA
in prokaryotes, 292–293
viral, 325–326
Metabolism, bacterial, 286–287
Metamyelocytes, 30, 32*f*
Metazoa, 1–2, 445
Metchinikoff, Elie, 62, 63–64, 66, 249
MHC. *See* Major histocompatibility
antigens; Major histocompatibility
complex
MHC-antigen peptide complex, 73*f*
in graft rejection, 211
Microaerophilic bacteria, 287
Microbe-containing aerosols, 453–454
Microbes
disease-causing, 17–18
inhibited colonization of, 27
on and in multicellular organisms,
18–19
normally associated with humans,
19–22
oxygen-dependent killing of, 38–40
oxygen-independent killing of,
40–41
resident, 19
transient, 19
vitamin synthesizing, 22
Microcapsules, 270–271
Microcolonies, slime-covered, 271
Microconidia, 383
germination of, 381
Microfilaraemia, 364–365

Microfilariae, 365–366
Microglial cells, 33, 145
β-2 Microglobulin, 153
Microorganisms
    climate and development of, 450
    culture of, 24
    disease-causing, 18–19
    dissemination of, 444–445
    in mouth, 29
    rapid growth of, 284
    ubiquity and size of, 284–285
Microparasites, 350
Microplate assay format, 427
Microsporidians, 350, 361
Microsporum, 380
Migration, 449, 457
Milstein, Cesar, 76–77
Minor histocompatibility antigens, 71
Mites, 20
MNBDF, 94–95
Molecular genetics techniques, 77–78
Molecular technology, 242
Molecular weight, 89
Monoblasts, 30–32
    differentiation of, 32*f*
Monoclonal antibody, 75–77, 119–121
    competitive inhibition of, 95*f*
    ELISA detection of, 421
    in fluorescent assay, 420
    in microplate assays, 427
    production of, 431, 432*f*
    in viral diagnosis, 331
Monoclonal antibody secreting cells,
    431
Monoclonal antiserum, 433
Monocytes, 145
    in Giemsa stained blood films, 31*f*
    at inflamed site, 55
    maturation of, 32
Monokine, 80–81
Mononuclear phagocytes
    differentiation of, 32*f*
    lysosomes in, 34
Mononucleosis
    cross-reactions to, 97
    infectious, 342, 450
Monotremes, 260
Morbidity, 436–437
Morbillivirus genus, 324

Mortality rate, 436
Mosquitoes, 450
    as malaria vector, 456*f*
    spraying for, 455
Mouth
    bacterial infections of, 300–301
    in constitutive host resistance, 29
    normal microorganisms of, 20*f*, 21
Mucociliary escalator, 29
Mucoid-producing organisms, 304
Mucosa
    in constitutive host resistance,
    28–29
    of lung alveolar septa, 187*f*
    mast cells of, 186–187
    viral pathogens in, 324*t*
Mucous membranes, 27
Mucus, ciliated cells of, 29
Multicellular organisms, 18–19
Multiple sclerosis
    autoimmune pathogenesis of, 184
    pathogenesis of, 182*t*
Mumps
    cases of before and after vaccine for,
    394*t*
    virus in, 337
Muramyl dipeptide, 403
Mutation, 1
    natural selection and, 158
Mutual interdependence, 16
Mutualism, 16
Mutualistic microbes, 18
    pathogenic, 18–19
Myasthenia gravis
    antibodies in, 192
    autoimmune pathogenesis of, 182*t*
Mycobacteriosis, 304–305
Mycobacterium
    avium, 258
    avium complex, 304
    flavum, 291*f*
    fortuitum complex, 304
    leprae, 304–305
    phagocytosis of, 314
    tuberculosis, 304–305
        identification of, 62
Mycoplasma pneumoniae, 266
Mycoses
    agents causing, 380

opportunistic, 386–388
subcutaneous, 379, 381–382
superficial, 379, 380–381
systemic, 382–386
Mycotic disease
classification of, 379–388
diagnosis of, 388–389
therapy for, 389
Myeloblasts, 30, 32f
Myelocyte II cells, 30
Myeloma proteins, 76
Myelopathy, HTLV-1-associated, 344
Myeloperoxidase
in azurophilic granules, 33
deficiency of with candidiasis, 387
in respiratory burst, 38
Myosin, 37

N-acetyl-glucosaminidase, 34
N-nucleotide addition, 140, 142
NADPH-dependent oxidase enzyme
complex, 173
Naegleria fowleri, 18
NAP-lysine, 95
NAP-lysine-carrier complex, 95
Natural killer cells, 139, 174–175, 351
in amphibians, 255
antiviral effect of, 328
in immune response to Marek's
disease, 234, 236
precursors of, 175f
in tumor destruction, 230–231
tumors and, 224
Necator americanus, 362–363
Negative selection, 145
Neisseria gonorrhoeae, 310
adherence to host cells, 266–268
in healthy humans, 23
Nelfinavir, 329
Nematodes, 350
infestations of, 13
parasitic, 361–366
Neomycin, 293
Neoplasia
immune system and, 223–242
virus-induced, 231–238
Neuroaminidase, 336–337, 395
Neurological disorders, 324t
Neurotoxins, 306

Neurotrophic rabies virus, 16
Neutral proteases
in azurophilic granules, 33
in mononuclear phagocytes, 34
Neutralization, 417
outcome of, 63t
Neutralizing antibody, 127
in passive immunization, 394
Neutropenia, 387
Neutrophilic granules, 33
Neutrophils
chemotactic factor of, 190
enzyme content of granules in, 33t
fish, 251
Giemsa stained, 33
in immune response, 5
at inflamed site, 54–55
in inflammatory response, 46
polymorphonuclear, 31f, 33–34, 193
recruitment of, 57
Niacin, 22
Nicotinic acid dinucleotide, 287
Nitric oxide, 5
in immune response to Marek's
disease, 234
in macrophage activation, 351
in oxygen-independent killing, 41
Nitric oxide synthase, 275
Nitrocellulose membrane, 429f
Nocardia, 21
Nomenclature, 297
Northern blotting, 331
Nosocomial infections
enterobacterial, 307
prevention of, 315
Nuclear magnetic resonance
spectroscopy, 95
Nucleic acid genomes, viral, 320
Nucleic acid hybridization
procedures, 331
Nucleic acids
antigenic, 102
immune response to, 85–86
Nucleoside analogues, 329
Nucleoside inhibitors, 329
5'-Nucleotidase, 34
Nucleus, prokaryote, 291–292
Null cells, 174
Nutrient absorption, 29

Nutrition
   of bacteria, 286
   improved understanding of, 283

O polysaccharide, 270
Obligate intracellular organisms, 445
Old tuberculin, 62
Oligosaccharide synthesis, 87
onc genes, 236
Onchocerca volvulus, 364, 365–366
Onchocerciasis, 364, 365–366
Oncogenes, 225–227
Oncogenic RNA viruses, 225–227
Oncovirinae, 225*t*
Opportunistic diseases, 18
   in AIDS, 346
   fungal, 386–388
   pathogenicity and virulence of, 265
Opportunistic pathogens, 23
   in cystic fibrosis, 303–304
Opsonin, 35–36, 158
   in complement activation, 168
   in inflammatory response, 46
   in phagocytosis, 41
Opsonization, 35–36, 158
   of bacteria, 313
   of pathogens, 398
Opsonizing antibody, 118
   in passive immunization, 394
Organ graft rejection, 63
Organ transplants, 9
Orphan vaccine, 408
Orthomyxoviridae, 336
   properties of, 322*t*
Osteoarthritis, 184
Ouchterlony assay, 122, 123*f*
Outbreaks, 437–438
Oxidase
   activation of, 38
   in respiratory burst, 39*f*
Oxidation/reduction potential,
   287–288
Oxidative burst, 275
Oxidative metabolites, 274–275
Oxygen, bacterial, 287–288
Oxygen-dependent killing, 38–40

P adhesin, 268
P-nucleotide addition, 140, 142

P polysaccharide, 278
Pain, 5
Pancreas transplantation, 219
Pandemic, 436
Pantropic viruses, 325
Panzootic, 436
Papain, 112–113
Papilloma viruses, 338
Papillomatous tumors, viruses
   causing, 338
Papillomavirus, 225*t*, 227
Papovaviridae
   properties of, 322*t*
   tumors associated with, 225*t*
Paracortex, 137
Paramyxoviridae, 324, 337
   properties of, 322*t*
Parasites, 13, 445
   agglutination of, 162
   cell-mediated immunity against, 168
   disease production and, 24–25
   host immune systems and, 13–25
   immune response to, 350–351
   intracellular
      cell-mediated immunity against,
      169
      preventing attachment to host
      cells, 161
   life cycles of, 350
   mechanism of injury by, 15–16
   versus predators, 16–17
   variety of, 14*f*
Parasitic infections, 350
Parasitic protozoa, 349–373
   immunity to, 351
   types of, 351–361
Parasitic relationship, 16
Parasitic worms, 15, 18
   infestation of, 17
Parasitism, 13
   definition of, 349
   mechanisms resisting, 4*f*
Parasitosis, 16
Parvoviridae, 322*t*
Parvovirus, 320
Passive immunity, 4*f*, 7
Pasteur, Louis, 62
Pasteurization, 22
Pathogen-host interactions, 7–9

Pathogen-reactive antibodies, 3
Pathogenic bacteria
    common shapes and arrangements
    of, 286*f*
    identification of in disease, 62
Pathogenicity, 265–266, 281, 444
Pathogenicity islands, 280
Pathogens, 18–19, 440
    antibodies to, 6
    antiphagocytic components of, 36
    dispersal and transmission of,
    284–285
    dissemination of, 444–445
    encapsulated, 294–295
    evolution of, 7–8
    immune evasion strategies of, 7–8
    level of exposure to, 2–3
    mechanisms of, 10
    public and personal health and,
    9–10
    resistance of, 284
    selective pressure of, 2
    virulent, 17–18
Pauling, Linus, 68–69
Penicillin, 290–291
    antibodies against, 190–191
    for Lyme disease, 311
Penicillinase, 291
    gonococcal, 310
Pepsin, 113
Peptide immunotherapy, 190
Peptidoglycan, 290
Perforin, 153, 177
Periodic acid Schiff, 388
Periodontal infections, 301
Periodontitis, 301
Peritoneal macrophages, 33
Pernicious anemia, 182*t*
Peroxidase, 33
Peroxide ions, 38
Personal health measures, 9–10
Personal health practices, 3, 10
Pertussis, 301
    cases of before and after vaccine for,
    394*t*
    inactivated vaccine for, 404–405
Peyers patches, 136
Phagocytes
    binding of foreign objects to, 35–36

binding of opsonized bacterium to
    receptors of, 35*f*
    chemotactic factors and, 34
    in constitutive resistance, 27
    destruction of microorganisms by, 41
    ingestion by, 36–38
    mononuclear, 30–33
    morphology and development of,
    30–34
    oxygen-dependent killing by, 38–40
    oxygen-independent killing by,
    40–41
    pathogen survival within, 274–277
    polymorphonuclear, 30, 33–34
    professional, 269
        binding LPS by, 278
    survival within, 274–277
Phagocytosis, 5, 34–35, 158
    antibody-mediated, 158–159
    in bacterial infection resistance,
    313, 314
    in blastomycosis, 384
    host complement factors and, 8
    in invertebrates, 249
    Langerhans' cells, 145–146
    in multicellular animals, 88–89
    prevention of, 270–274
    yeast cell inhibition of, 382
Phagolysosome, 159, 274
    blastoconidia in, 383
    lowered pH of, 40
    pathogens surviving in, 275
Phagosome, 159
    acidification of, 40, 168
    escape from, 276–277
    fusion with lysosomes, 41, 274
    preventing maturation of, 275–276
Phagosome-lysosome fusion, 275–276
Pharyngitis, 304
Phospholipase A$_2$, 190
Phospholipase C, 276
    in hypersensitivity reaction, 188
Phospholipids, 49*f*
Phylogenetic tree, 296
Phylogeny, bacteria, 296–298
Physical barriers, 27–30
Phytohemagglutinin, 252
Picornaviridae, 335–336
    properties of, 322*t*

Pig lymph nodes, 260–261
Pili, 294–295
Pink eye, 300
Pityrosporum infection, 21
Placenta
    as barrier, 448
    in immunity, 261
Plague, 312
    prevention of, 455
    target groups for vaccine against, 401*t*
Plasma
    exudation of in inflammatory response, 46
    leakage of at inflammatory site, 46
Plasma cells, 135
    antibody-producing, 67*f*, 77
    antibody synthesis by, 66
    function and surface markers of, 134*t*
Plasmapheresis, 214–215
Plasmids, 292
Plasmin, 51–52
Plasminogen, 51–52
Plasmodia, 18
Plasmodium
    falciparum, 358
    falciparum malaria, 446
    life cycle of, 356, 357*f*, 360
    vivax, 358
Platelets
    clumping of, 31*f*
    in Giemsa stained blood films, 31*f*
    histamine and serotonin release by, 46
Platyhelminthes, 350
Pluripotential hematopoietic stem cells, 138–139
Pneumococcal pneumonia, 302–303
Pneumococcal polysaccharide vaccine, 401*t*
Pneumococcal vaccine, 396
Pneumococcus
    antibiotic resistant, 446
    polysaccharide capsules of, 406
Pneumocystis carinii
    in AIDS, 346
    macrophages in destruction of, 173–174
Pneumonia
    atypical, 303
    bacterial, 302–303
    hookworm and, 15
Point prevalence, 437
Poliovirus, 335
    cases of before and after vaccine for, 394*t*
    preventing attachment to host cells, 161
    vaccine against, 335–336
        route of administration of, 399
Poly-Ig receptor, 119
Polycationic proteins, 40
Polycations, 289
Polyclonal activators, 100
Polyclonal antibody, 76, 119
    ELISA detection of, 421
    in fluorescent assay, 420
Polyclonal antiserum, 94, 119, 433
Polymer adjuvants, 403–404
Polymerase chain reaction analysis
    in graft rejection, 216
    for viral diagnosis, 331
Polymorphism
    antigenic, 395–396
    cytokine promoter region, 212–213
Polymorphonuclear leukocytes. *See also* Granulocytes; Leukocytes
    differentiation of, 32*f*
    in inflammatory reaction, 56
Polymorphonuclear neutrophils, 33–34
    chemotaxic agents for, 193
    in Giemsa stained blood films, 31*f*
Polypeptide chains, 107–108, 128
    changes in, 108–109
    constant regions of, 112
    hinge region of, 112
    variable regions of, 110–111
Polypeptide chains, folding of, 110
Polyribosomes, 293
Polysaccharide capsules, 270, 406
Polysaccharide polymer, 293–294
Polysaccharide vaccines, 396
Polysaccharides
    in bacteria capsule, 293–294
    in bacteria cell envelope, 289–290
    in bacterial pneumonia, 303
    constituent monomers of, 101
    immune response induced by, 102

Polyspecific antiserum, 94
Population surveillance, 457
Pork tapeworm, 369–370
Portal of exit, 448
Positive selection, 145
Postcapillary venules, 47, 48f
Poverty, conditions of, 443–444
Poxviridae, 322t
Poxviruses, 320, 325
    intracytoplasmic inclusions of, 325
Pre-T cell β, 142
Preadaptation, 158
Precipitation, 413–414
    in gel matrix, 414–416
    outcome of, 63t
Precipitation assays, 121–123, 433
Precipitin-in-gel assays, 121–122, 123f
Predators, 16–17
Prednisone, 217
Pregnancy, immunity in, 399
Prevalence, 437
Prevention, 454–456, 457
Preventive measures, 9–10, 436
Priming antigen, 6–7
Pro-B cells, 114
Pro-T cells, 142
Progenitor cells, 138–139
Proinflammatory cytokines, 196
Prokaryotes
    cell envelope and Gram stain of,
    289–291
    cytoplasm, nucleus and inclusions
    of, 291–293
    versus eukaryotic cells, 288t
    shape and grouping among, 285–286
    structures of, 288–296
Prokaryotic kingdoms, 298
Promonocytes, 32f
Promyelocytes, 30
Properdin, 163
Properdin pathway, 164–166
Prophenoloxidase system, 249
Propionibacterium acnes, 20–21, 300
Prostaglandin D$_2$, 190
Prostaglandin E$_2$, 5
Prostaglandins
    in fever response, 56
    formation of, 49f
    in hypersensitivity mediation, 186

in inflammatory response, 46, 47–50,
57
Protease
    in azurophilic granules, 33
    in hypersensitivity reaction, 186, 190
    of P. aeruginosa, 279
Protease inhibitors, 329
Protectin, 168
Protein chains, 75, 76f
Protein-digesting organelles, 93
Protein immunogens, 102
Protein kinase C, 188
Protein tyrosine kinases, 187–188
Proteinase
    in aspergillosis pathogenesis, 387
    virulence and, 382
Proteins
    cell-mediated immune response to,
    85–86
    in serum, 106, 107f
    structural complexity of, 89
Proteolysis, 100
Proteolytic enzymes, 5
    fibronectin and, 36
Proteosome, 93, 153
Proteus
    preparations of, 97
    in urinary tract infections, 309
Protista, 298
Proto-oncogenes, 223
    point mutations of, 225
    transforming viruses and, 226–227
Protostomes, 247
    humoral immunity in, 250
Protozoa, 349–350
    in blood and body cavities, 14f
    genera of, 350
    parasitic, 18, 349–361
    preventing attachment to host cells,
    161
    unicellular, 13
Provirus, 342–343
Prozones, 121
Pseudomonas, 300
    aeruginosa, 300
        antiphagocytic exotoxins of,
        272–274
        binding to host cell receptors, 269
    capsule surrounding, 293f

cell envelope and extracellular polymer fibrils of, 292f
flagellum of, 295f
slime layer around, 294f
Pseudopods, 36–38
Psittacosis, 304
Public health, 9–10
bacterial disease and, 308–309
information dissemination on, 441
practices of, 3, 10
prevention and control programs of, 455–456
Pulmonary distress syndrome, 446
Purified protein derivative (PPD), 62
Pus, formation of, 54
Pyorrhea, 301
Pyoverdin, 277
Pyrazinamide, 304, 305
Pyrogen, 55

Q fever, 445
Quantitative precipitation methods, 75
Quarantine, 455
Quinine, antibodies against, 190–191

R factors, 280, 292
Rabies virus, 325, 334
neurotrophic, 16
vaccine for, 62, 397
hypersensitivity reaction to, 400–401
target groups for, 401t
Radial immunodiffusion, 415
Radiation therapy, 387
Radioimmunoassay, 125–127, 418–419, 421, 433
for fungal infections, 388
Raffel, Sidney, 66
RAG1 gene, 140
RAG2 gene, 140
Reactive nitrogen intermediates
formation of, 274
against intracellular pathogens, 275
Reactive oxygen intermediates, 5, 274–275
inactivation of, 8
Receptors, 1
Recombinant cloning technologies, 9
Recombinant DNA technology, 406

Recombination-activating genes, 140
Recombinational signal sequence, 140
Reduviid bug, 14–15f
Reemerging disease, 445–446, 457
geographical distribution of, 447t
Refugees, 449
Renal allograft, 203f
Reoviridae, 323t
Replicative form, 325–326
Reptiles
immunity in, 256–257
lymphoid organs of, 2t
subclasses of, 256
Reservoirs, 440, 455
Resistance, 312–314
Resistance transfer factor, 292
Respiratory burst, 159
events in, 38–40
Respiratory secretions, disrupted clearance of, 325
Respiratory syncytial virus, 454
Respiratory tract
in constitutive host resistance, 28f, 29
infections of
bacteria causing, 301–305
burden of, 441–442
mechanism of injury by, 15–16
pathogens causing, 299
precautions against, 9
viral pathogens in, 324t
Response gene activation, 1
Reticuloendothelial system, 66
Retransplantation, 218
Retroviruses, 320, 343–344
antiviral drugs for, 329
exogenous, 226–227
properties of, 323t
structure and genomic map of, 225–226
tumors associated with, 225t
Reverse transcriptase, 320
Rh blood group antigen, 191–192
Rhabdoviridae, 334
properties of, 322t
Rhabdoviruses, 320
Rhamnomannan, 382
Rheumatic fever, 302
streptococcal infection in, 99
Rheumatoid arthritis

autoimmune pathogenesis of, 182*t*

diagnosis of, 416

pathogenesis of, 184

Rheumatoid disease, secondary, 307

Rheumatoid factors, 184

Rhinoviruses, 335

RIAs. *See* Radioimmunoassays

Riboflavin, 22

Ribosomal RNA, 297–298

in prokaryotes, 292–293

Ribosomes, 292–293

Rickettsia, 445

detection of, 97

in typhus fever, 311

Rifampin, 304, 305

Ringworm, 381

RNA, 297–298

RNA-containing nucleoprotein, 336

RNA-containing virus, 334

RNA-dependent DNA polymerase, 343

RNA tumor viruses, 342–343

RNA viruses, 320

classification and properties of, 322–323*t*

enveloped, 337

leukemia-inducing, 343

nucleic acids of, 325

oncogenic, 225–227

Rocket immunoelectrophoresis, 415–416

Rous sarcoma virus, 225

Routes of entry, 448

Rubella

cases of before and after vaccine for, 394*t*

host response to vaccination against, 398

vaccine for, 397

Ruffling, 270

Ruminants

placenta of, 261

T cells in, 261

Sabine vaccine, 335

route of administration of, 399

Saccharomyces cerevisiae, 240

Saliva

bacteria of, 21

in host defense, 29

Salk polio vaccine, 335

complications of, 400

route of administration of, 399

Salmonella

avirulent strain of, 407

enteritidus, 308

paratyphi, 308

preparations of, 97

transmission of, 451

typhi, 308

in healthy humans, 23

typhymurium, 308

survival in phagosome, 276

Salmonellosis, 308

Sandwich assay, 121

Sandwich enzyme-linked immunosorbent assay, 422

Sandwich fluorescent test, 420

Sandwich radioimmunoassay, 419

Sanitation, improved, 283

Saprophytes, 16–17, 18, 379

Sarcinae, 285

Scarlet fever, 302

Schistosoma

eosinophils in defense against, 34

haematobium, 366

japonicum, 366

life cycle of, 453*f*

mansoni, 366–367

mattheei, 368

Schistosomes, 14*f*

Schistosomiasis, 366–368

transmission of, 451–452

Schizont, 356–357

SCID mice, 224

Sclerosing panencephalitis, subacute, 338

Sebum, lubricating skin, 28

Secretory component, 119

Sela, Michael, 99

Selection, 1

Self-antigens, 88

Self-reaction, 88

Self-recognition, 69–74, 177

Self-tolerance, 68, 86–88

breakdown of, 181–182

mechanisms of, 182

Septicemia, Gram-negative, 277–278

Sequence Specific Oligonucleotide

Probe typing, 216
Seroconversion, 398
Serologic cross-reactions, 97
    epitope similarity in, 98*f*
Serological assays
    antibody detection in, 119–127
    aspects of, 122*t*
    for fungal infections, 389
Serotonin, 46–47
Serum
    components of, 106
    electrophoresis of, 106, 107*f*
    enzymes of, 5
    globulins in, 397*t*
Serum factor, 66
Serum sickness, 193
Severe combined immune deficiency, 139
Severe combined immunodeficiency mice, 224
Sexual transmission, 450
Sexually transmitted disease, 441–442
Shigella
    binding to host cell, 270
    in diarrhea, 307
Sickle hemoglobin, 358
Side chain theory, 64–65
Siderophores, 277
Silver nitrate, 310
Simulium, 365
Sin Nombre virus, 446
SipB, 270
SipC, 270
SipD, 270
Skin
    allograft rejection of, 255
    bacterial infections of, 300
    in constitutive host resistance, 27–28
    failed transplantation of, 219
    graft rejection of, 71
        in reptiles, 257
    low pH of, 28
    normal microorganisms of, 20–21
    protection against dermatophytes, 380
    scrapings of for fungal infections, 388
    viral pathogens in lesions of, 324*t*
Slime layers, 293–294

Small intestine, alkaline pH of, 29
Small molecular weight molecules
    direct competitive ELISA detection of, 423–424
    indirect competitive ELISA detection of, 424–425
Smallpox
    immunity to, 61, 332, 393
    vaccine for, 393–394, 396
        contaminated, 333
    viruses causing, 333–334
Smooth muscle, histamine and serotonin effects on, 47
Sneezing, 29
Snell, George, 70–71
Social environment, 448–449, 457
Sodium cromolyn, 190
Somatic hypermutation, 117
Somatic mutation, 77–78
Sore throat, streptococcal, 302
Sowda, 366
Spirochaetes, 285
Spleen
    antigen filtering in, 136
    development of, 138
    in fish, 251–252
    in immune system, 136
Sporothricosis, 381–382
Sporothrix schenkii, 381–382
Sporozoans, 350
Staphylococcal food poisoning, 160
Staphylococcus, 285
    abscess formation with, 54
    aureus
        enterotoxins of, 100
        in impetigo, 300
        in toxic shock syndrome, 309–310
    cytotoxins of, 273
    enterotoxins of, 101*f*, 280
    epidermidis, 21
        in acne, 300
    in food poisoning, 305–306
    glycocalyx envelope of, 271, 272*f*
    of skin, 20
Stem cells
    committed, 32*f*
    cytokines and, 6
    differentiation of, 139*f*
    hematopoietic, 114

pluripotential hematopoietic, 138–139
producing mononuclear phagocytes, 30
producing polymorphonuclear leukocytes, 30
Sterilization methods, 455
Stomach, antimicrobial environment of, 29–30
Streptobacilli, 285
Streptococcal M protein, 270
Streptococcus, 54, 285
  in dental caries, 300
  enterotoxin of, 280
  Group A
    exotoxins of, 273
    fibrillae of, 271
  Group B, 271
    adherence to host cell, 269
  Group G, fimbrillae of, 267*f*
  intestinal, 21
  mutans, 21
  pneumoniae, 302–303
    capsules of, 294–295
  pyogenes, 302
    host defense against, 314
    in impetigo, 300
  virdians endocarditis, 301
Streptolysins, 273
Streptomycin, 293
Substance-A, slow-reacting, 49*f*
Subunit vaccines, 405–406
Sudden infant death syndrome, 306
Sulphonamides, 190–191
Superantigens, 99–100, 280
Superoxide, 38
  in respiratory burst, 39*f*
Superoxide anions, 274
  in phagocytosis, 159
Superoxide dismutase
  in aerobic organisms, 287
  pathogen production of, 274
  in phagocytosis, 159
Suppressor T cells, 68
Surface envelope proteins, 345
Surface markers, 134
Surveillance, 457
Survival, 2–3
Svedberg (S) units, 297–298

Swallowing, 29
Sweat, 28
Swine flu vaccine, 400
Swine flu variants, 337
Symbiosis, 24
Symbiotic relationships, 16
Syncytial agents, 445
Syncytial virus, 454
Syncytium formation, 325, 346
Syngeneic grafts, 202
Synthetic amino acid homopolymers, 89
Syphilis, 311
  toxins in, 310
Systematics, 296–297
Systemic disease, 445
  bacteria causing, 311–312
Systemic lupus erythematosus
  autoimmune pathogenesis of, 182*t*
  pathogenesis of, 183–184

T cell allorecognition pathways, 209–211
T cell growth factor, 80
  function of, 81
T cell leukemia/lymphoma, 342–344
T cell-mediated immune response, 8
  in amphibians, 256
  in birds, 259–260
  in reptiles, 257
T cell receptor/CD3 complex, 142
T cell receptors, 75, 135–136
  α/β, 136, 142–144
  in adaptive immune system, 262–263
  antibody molecules and, 141*f*
  antigen interaction with, 85
  in immune response, 81
  minigene segments of, 140*t*
  protein antigen recognition by, 92–93
  proteins chains of, 75, 76*f*
  specificity of for MHC protein, 93
T cells. *See also* Cytolytic T cells; Cytotoxic T cells; Inflammatory T cells; T helper cells
  activation of, 148*f*, 220, 398
    direct and indirect, 210*f*
    in graft rejection, 211–212
    indirect pathway in, 211*f*
  allospecific, 209

safety testing of, 402
for schistosomiasis, 368
for smallpox, 393–394
for specific groups, 401t
subunit, 405–406
types of, 404–408
Vaccinia virus, 61
recombinants of, 407
Vaccinology, 408–409
Vagina
bacterial infections of, 309
epithelium of, 30
lactic acid-producing bacteria in, 30
normal microorganisms of, 20f, 22
Vaginitis, candidal, 387
van der Waals forces, 95, 413
Vancomycin, 290
Variable segments, coding for B and T
cells, 140
Variable surface glycoprotein, 355–356
Varicella-zoster vaccine, 397
Variola virus, 333–334
Variolation, 61, 393
Vascular cell adhesion molecule-1, 190
Vascular permeability, 47–50
Vascularized grafts, hyperacute
rejection of, 202–203
Vasoactive amines
chemotactic for PMNs, 193
in inflammation, 46–47
synergistic action with
prostaglandins and leukotrienes, 47–
50
Vasoactive compounds, 34
Vasoactive molecules, 45–46
Vasodilation
at inflamed site, 48f
in inflammatory response, 45–46
vasoactive amines in, 47
VDJ rearrangement, 140, 144–145
Vector-borne protozoal disease,
449–450
Vector-borne transmission, 452–453
Vehicle-borne transmission, 450–451
Ventral cavity bodies, 255
Vertebrates, phylogeny of, 248f
Vertical flow-through immunoassay,
428–431
Vh genes, 253

Vibrio, 285
cholerae, 265
iron sequestering systems of, 277
toxins of, 308
transmission of, 451
parahaemolyticus, 308
Viral-induced neoplasia, 241
Viral infections, 346–347
acute, 333–337
cell susceptibility to, 326–327
diagnosis of, 329–331, 346
drugs for, 329
immunization against, 331–333
persistent, 341–346
that resolve or persist, 337–340
Viral neutralizing antibodies, 235
Viral nucleic acid strands, 320
Viral pathogens, 324–325
species-specific, 325
Viral proteins, 152f
Viridans streptococcus, 271
Virulence, 17–18, 265–266, 281, 444
encapsulation and, 270–271
Virulence factors, 158
in bacteria cell envelope, 289–290
Virus-induced neoplasia, 231–238
Virus neutralization assays, 330
Virus-neutralizing antibodies, 232
against HBsAg, 238–239
to poliovirus, 335
of smallpox vaccine, 333–334
Viruses, 319, 445
associated with naturally occurring
tumors, 225t
broken into proteins, 150–153
classification of, 320–325, 346
pathogenic, 324t
cytolytic T cells against, 168
cytopathic effects of, 325
enveloped, 320, 321f
host cell defense and immune
response to, 327–329
isolation of, 24, 331
latent, 326
morphology of, 319–320, 321f
nonenveloped, 320, 321f
oncogenic, 226–228
parasitic, 17
pathogenesis of, 325–327

in amphibians, 255
anti-self-reactive, 144–145
antigen-independent differentiation
of, 142–145
antigen presenting cells and, 146–147
antigen recognition by, 73f
antigen-specific receptors on,
135–136
antigens activating, 99–100
in birds, 258–259
chicken, 259–260
classes of, 169, 178
cytokine production by, 212
cytolytic, 168, 176–177
cytotoxic, generation and detection
of, 213–214
in delayed hypersensitivity, 194–196
development of, 138–139
in thymus, 144f
electron micrographs of, 132–133f
epitopes of, 145
in fish, 252, 254
functional subsets of, 135
γ/δ-positive, 136
graft-reactive, 204–205, 219–220
in immune response, 6, 10, 131, 135,
137
at inflamed site, 55
macrophage-induced sensitization
of, 171f
in pig, 261
ruminant, 261
superantigen and, 100, 280
viral infection of, 233f
T helper cells
activation of, 146–147
antiviral effect of, 328
differentiation of, 147–149
function and surface markers of, 134t
in cell-mediated immunity, 168
in immune response, 81–82
macrophages and, 149–150
recognizing Class II molecules, 151f
role of, 135
T-independent antigens, 89
Taenia
saginata, 369f, 370–373
solium, 369–370, 371–372
TAP1 protein, 153, 230

TAP2 protein, 153
in peptide transport, 230
Tapeworms, 350, 368–372, 373f
cysticercus of, 371f
mature, 373f
mature proglottids of, 370f
proglottids of, 373f
scolex of, 368, 369f, 373f
Taxonomic groups, bacterial, 296–298
TCGF. See T cell growth factor
TCR genes, fish, 254
TdT. See Terminal deoxynucleotidyl
transferase
Tears, 30
Template RNA, 297
Terminal deoxynucleotidyl transferase,
116, 140
Terminal electron acceptor, 287
Tetanus
cases of before and after vaccine for,
394t
immunization against, 160
toxoid, 405
vaccine for, 397
Tetracycline, 293
TGF-β. See Transforming growth
factor β
Th1 cells, 154
cytokines and, 147
function and surface markers of, 134t
helper, 212
production of, 147–149
role of, 135
Th2 cells, 154
B cell interaction with, 150
function and surface markers of,
134t
helper, 212
production of, 147–149
role of, 135
Thalassemia, 358
Theophylline, 190
Thiamine, 22
Thromboxane A₂, 49f
Thymidine, 432f
Thymocytes, 142
double-negative, 142
double-positive, 142
single-positive, 145

Thymus
  in amphibians, 255
  development of, 138
  in fish, 251
  in reptiles, 257
  T cell development in, 144*f*
Thymus-dependent immune system,
  229
Tickover, 168
TILs. *See* Tumor-infiltrating
  lymphocytes
Tinea capitis, 381
Tinea corporis, 381
Tinea pedis, 381
Tissue damage, 45–46, 56–57
Tissue fluids, antibody circulation in,
  105–106
Tissue matching, 215–216
Tissue necrosis, 203
Tissue transplantation, 201–202
Tissue tropism, 325
Tissue typing, 216
TNF. *See* Tumor necrosis factor
Tobacco mosaic virus, 320
Togaviridae, 322*t*
Togavirus, 337
Tongue, 29
Tourism, 457
Toxacara, 362
Toxic aldehydes, 40
Toxic shock syndrome, 280
  superantigens in, 100
  toxins in, 309–310
Toxin-antibody complexes, 160
Toxins
  antibody inactivation of, 159–161
  in food poisoning, 299
  neutralization of, 313–314, 398, 417
  pathogenicity and virulence of,
  277–280
Toxoid immunization, 160
Toxoids, 405
Toxoplasma gondii, 360–361
Toxoplasmosis, 360–361
Transcriptases, 320
Transferrin, 277
Transforming growth factor β
  in chronic rejection, 205
  in graft rejection, 212
  Th2 cell production of, 149

Transient normal flora, 19
Transmembrane domain, 113
Transmission, 436
  mechanisms of, 450–454
  mode of, 440
  route of, 455
Transplantation
  aspergillosis in, 387
  host response to, 201–220
  immunosuppressive strategies in,
  220
  rejection of, 201–202
  of specific tissues, 218–219
Traveler's diarrhea, 307
Trematodes, parasitic, 366–368
Trench mouth, 301
Treponema
  palladum, 310
  vincentii, 301
Trichinella, 18
  eosinophils in defense against, 34
  spiralis, 363, 364*f*
Trichinosis, 363
Trichomonas vaginalis, 309, 354
Trichophyton, 380
  mentagrophytes, 381
Tropical pulmonary eosinophilia, 365
Tropical spastic paraparesis, 344
Trypanosoma
  brucei, 354–356
    host specificity of, 17
  cruzi, 14–15*f*, 356
    transmission of, 453, 454*f*
Trypanosomes
  African, 354–356
  New World, 356
  VSG of, 355–356
Tuberculin skin test, 305
  hypersensitivity to, 63
  reaction to, 62
Tuberculosis
  bacteria in, 304–305
  burden of, 441–442
  transmission of, 450, 454
  vaccine for, 62
Tumor-associated antigens, 224
Tumor cells, 229–231
Tumor growth factor β, 213
Tumor-infiltrating lymphocytes, 231
  in tumor immunity, 241

Tumor necrosis factor
  in allograft rejection, 208–209
  in bacterial resistance, 314
  in invertebrates, 251
  overproduction of, 8
Tumor necrosis factor α
  in fever response, 55
  in hypersensitivity mediation, 190
  in macrophage activation, 173
  mast cell release of, 186
  suppression of, 275
  Th1 cell production of, 147
Tumor necrosis factor β, 173
Tumor necrosis factors, 81
Tumor-specific antigens, 224, 228, 229,
  241
Tumor suppressor genes, 223
Tumoricidal activity, 174
Tumors
  antigen processing and presentation
  in, 230*f*
  chemically-induced and spontaneous, 228
  DNA viruses and, 227–228
  immune system and, 223–224
  immunization against, 224, 229*f*
  immunological control of, 241–242
  immunology of, 224–229
  immunosurveillance of, 228–229
  in Marek's disease virus, 232–236,
  234*f*
  viral pathogens in, 324*t*
Tunicates, 250–251
Typhoid fever, 308
  carriers of, 23
  incidence of, 309
Typhus fever, 311
Tyrosine phosphorylation, 187–188

Ultraviolet radiation, 455
Urban crowding, 449
Urethritis, 309
Urinary tract
  infections of
    bacterial, 309
    fimbriae in, 268
    pathogens causing, 299
  normal microorganisms of, 20*f*, 22
Urine, flushing effect of, 30
Urodeles, 254–255

immune response in, 256
Urogenital tract
  in constitutive host resistanc
  infections of
    bacteria causing, 309–310
  protozoa of, 354

V genes, 78, 263
  segments of
    in birds, 259
    random selection of, 142
V region coding, 117
Vaccination, 455. *See also* Immunit
  Immunization; Vaccines
  diphtheria, 63–64
  discovery of, 62
  memory lymphocytes in, 6–7
  resistance to, 7
  route of administration of, 399
  timing of, 399
Vaccines
  adjuvants in, 101, 403–404
  AIDS, 346
  for anthrax, 312
  antigen preparations in, 332
  antiviral, 331–333
  for cancer, 242
  clinical studies of, 402–403
  against common pathogens, 9
  complications of, 400–401
  determinants of response to,
  399–400
  development of, 346–347
  early development of, 62
  effectiveness and safety of, 333
  for feline leukemia virus, 238
  against hepatitis B virus, 240–241
  host response to, 398–400
  inactivated, 404–405
  infectious disease incidence and,
  394*t*
  live, 404, 405
  for lymphatic filariasis, 365
  for malaria, 359–360
  against Marek's disease, 235–236
  measles, 338
  pneumococcal capsular polysaccharide, 396
  poliovirus, 335–336
  registration of, 403

preventing attachment to host cells, 161
properties of, 322–323*t*
replication of, 236*f*, 325
    rapid, 328
replication strategies of, 320–325
structure of, 319–320
vaccines for, 346–347
Visceral larval migrans, 362
Vitamin A deficiency, 399
Vitamin B$_{12}$, 22
Vitamin K, 22
Vitamins, microbe synthesis of, 22
VL-VH domain interaction, 110–111
von Behring, Emil, 63–64
VSG. *See* Variable surface glycoprotein

Wars, 449
Warts, viruses causing, 338
Water treatment, 308–309
Waterborne microorganisms, 451–452
    in intestinal disease, 305–306
Wax D, 305
Weil-Felix reaction, 97
West Nile virus, 446
Western blot assay, 91–92, 330

Wheal and flare reaction, 4–5, 184–185
White blood cells, 105
Whooping cough, 301
World Health Organization, global
    immunization program of, 393
Wound infections, 298–299
Wuchereria bancrofti, 364

Xenografts, 202
    in invertebrates, 250

Yeast cells
    in skin infection, 21
    surface polysaccharides of, 382
Yellow fever, 401*t*
Yersinia
    enterocolitica, 269–270
    pestis, 265, 312
        transmission of, 452
    pseudotuberculosis, 269–270
Yop proteins, 273–274

Zoonosis, 299, 436
Zoonotic disease, 449–450
Zoophilic dermatophytes, 380